D1263636

HANDBOOK OF
Cancer Control and Behavioral Science

HANDBOOK OF
Cancer Control and Behavioral Science

A Resource for Researchers, Practitioners, and Policymakers

EDITED BY
Suzanne M. Miller, Deborah J. Bowen, Robert T. Croyle, and Julia H. Rowland

American Psychological Association • Washington, DC

Published by
American Psychological Association
750 First Street, NE
Washington, DC 20002
www.apa.org

To order
APA Order Department
P.O. Box 92984
Washington, DC 20090-2984
Tel: (800) 374-2721; Direct: (202) 336-5510
Fax: (202) 336-5502; TDD/TTY: (202) 336-6123
Online: www.apa.org/books/
E-mail: order@apa.org

In the U.K., Europe, Africa, and the Middle East, copies may be ordered from
American Psychological Association
3 Henrietta Street
Covent Garden, London
WC2E 8LU England

Typeset in Goudy by Circle Graphics, Columbia, MD

Printer: McNaughton & Gunn, Inc., Ann Arbor, MI
Cover Designer: Mercury Publishing Services, Rockville, MD
Technical/Production Editor: Devon Bourexis

The opinions and statements published are the responsibility of the authors, and such opinions and statements do not necessarily represent the policies of the American Psychological Association.

Handbook of cancer control and behavioral science : a resource for researchers, practitioners, and policymakers / edited by Suzanne M. Miller . . . [et al.]. — 1st ed.
    p. ; cm.
  Includes bibliographical references and index.
  ISBN-13: 978-1-4338-0358-1
  ISBN-10: 1-4338-0358-5
  1. Cancer—Psychological aspects. 2. Cancer—Social aspects. 3. Medicine and psychology. I. Miller, Suzanne M. (Suzanne Melanie), 1951- II. American Psychological Association.
  [DNLM: 1. Neoplasms—prevention & control. 2. Neoplasms—psychology. 3. Behavioral Research. 4. Research Design. 5. Risk Factors. 6. Risk Reduction Behavior. QZ 200 H2345 2009]

  RC262.H273 2009
  616.99'4—dc22

2008005060

British Library Cataloguing-in-Publication Data

A CIP record is available from the British Library.

Printed in the United States of America
First Edition

To the patients and families whose lives have
been touched by cancer.

CONTENTS

Contributors .... *xiii*

Foreword .... *xvii*
David B. Abrams

Preface .... *xxi*

I. Introduction to Behavioral Science and Cancer 1

Chapter 1.   Overview, Current Status,
                 and Future Directions 5
                 Suzanne M. Miller, Deborah J. Bowen,
                 Robert T. Croyle, and Julia H. Rowland

Chapter 2.   Trends in Modifiable Risk Factors for Cancer
                 and the Potential for Cancer Prevention 23
                 Cynthia J. Stein and Graham A. Colditz

Chapter 3.   Creation of a Framework for
               Public Health Intervention Design 43
               Deborah J. Bowen, Carol Moinpour,
               Beti Thompson, M. Robyn Andersen,
               Hendrika Meischke, and Barb Cochrane

II. Methodology in Cancer Prevention and Control **57**

Chapter 4.   Designing and Evaluating Individual-Level
               Interventions for Cancer Prevention
               and Control 61
               Susan J. Curry, David W. Wetter,
               Louis C. Grothaus, Jennifer B. McClure,
               and Stephen H. Taplin

Chapter 5.   Design and Analysis of Group-Randomized
               Trials in Cancer Prevention and Control 85
               David M. Murray, Sherri L. Pals,
               and Jonathan L. Blitstein

Chapter 6.   Participation in Cancer Clinical Trials 103
               Electra D. Paskett, Mira L. Katz,
               Cecilia R. DeGraffinreid,
               and Cathy M. Tatum

Chapter 7.   Quality-of-Life Assessment in Cancer 115
               Carolyn C. Gotay

III. Primary Prevention: Reducing Cancer Incidence **129**

Chapter 8.   Understanding and Communicating
               About Cancer Risk 133
               Kevin D. McCaul, Renee E. Magnan,
               and Amanda Dillard

Chapter 9.   Prevention of Tobacco Use 151
               Robin Mermelstein and Sarah K. Wahl

Chapter 10.   Interventions for Smoking Cessation 167
               Lara K. Dhingra and Jamie S. Ostroff

Chapter 11.   Interventions to Modify Dietary Behaviors
               for Cancer Prevention and Control 189
               Marci Kramish Campbell, Jennifer Gierisch,
               and Lisa Sutherland

Chapter 12.   Interventions to Modify
               Skin Cancer–Related Behaviors 209
               David B. Buller

Chapter 13.   Behavioral Science Applications
               to Gynecologic Cancer Prevention............................. 225
               Lari Wenzel, Astrid Reina-Patton,
               and Israel De Alba

Chapter 14.   Interventions to Modify Physical Activity 237
               Bernardine M. Pinto, Carolyn Rabin,
               and Georita M. Frierson

IV. Secondary Prevention: Early Detection of Cancer **251**

Chapter 15.   Behavioral Research in Cancer Screening................... 255
               Sally W. Vernon, Jasmin A. Tiro,
               and Helen I. Meissner

Chapter 16.   Psychological Consequences of
               Cancer Screening.. 279
               Anne Miles, Jo Waller, and Jane Wardle

Chapter 17.   Psychological Issues in Genetic Testing...................... 303
               Catharine Wang and Suzanne M. Miller

V. Tertiary Prevention: Treating Clinical Cancer **323**

Chapter 18.   Practitioner–Patient Communication
               in Cancer Diagnosis and Treatment 327
               Walter F. Baile, Joann Aaron,
               and Patricia A. Parker

Chapter 19.   Behavioral Interventions for Side Effects
               Related to Cancer and Cancer Treatments 347
               Gary R. Morrow, Joseph A. Roscoe,
               Karen M. Mustian, Jane T. Hickok,
               Julie L. Ryan, and Sara Matteson

Chapter 20.   Psychosocial Response to Cancer Diagnosis
               and Treatment... 361
               Beth E. Meyerowitz and Sindy Oh

Chapter 21.   Reduction of Psychosexual Dysfunction
               in Cancer Patients 379
               Leslie R. Schover

Chapter 22.   Family Care During Cancer Care 391
               Barbara A. Given, Paula R. Sherwood,
               and Charles W. Given

VI. Quaternary Prevention: Cancer Survivorship **409**

Chapter 23.   The Experience of Survival for Patients:
               Psychosocial Adjustment 413
               Catherine M. Alfano and Julia H. Rowland

Chapter 24.   Physical Late Effects of Cancer:
               Implications for Care 431
               Jacqueline Casillas and Patricia Ganz

Chapter 25.   Psychosocial and Behavioral Issues
               in Cancer Survival in Pediatric Populations 449
               Anne E. Kazak, Melissa A. Alderfer,
               and Alyssa M. Rodriguez

Chapter 26.   Long-Term Effects of Cancer on Families
               of Adult Cancer Survivors 467
               Laurel L. Northouse, Suzanne Mellon,
               Janet Harden, and Ann Schafenacker

Chapter 27.   Health Promotion and Disease Prevention
               in Adult Cancer Survivors 487
               Wendy Demark-Wahnefried and Noreen M. Aziz

VII. Future Directions in Behavioral Science and Cancer **495**

Chapter 28.   Brain, Behavior, and Immunity in Cancer 499
               Michael Stefanek and Paige Green McDonald

Chapter 29.   Translation of Research Into Public
               Health Practice 517
               Carol R. White and Mark Dignan

Chapter 30.   Transdisciplinary Social and Behavioral
               Research for Cancer Prevention 531
               Colleen M. McBride

Chapter 31.   Interactive Health Communications
               for Cancer Prevention and Control 547
               Victor Strecher

Author Index 559

Subject Index 621

About the Editors... 651

CONTRIBUTORS

Joann Aaron, MA, The University of Texas M. D. Anderson Cancer Center, Houston

David B. Abrams, PhD, American Legacy Foundation, Washington, DC

Melissa A. Alderfer, PhD, The Children's Hospital of Philadelphia, Philadelphia, PA

Catherine M. Alfano, PhD, The Ohio State University, Columbus

M. Robyn Andersen, PhD, Fred Hutchinson Cancer Research Center, Seattle, WA

Noreen M. Aziz, MD, PhD, MPH, National Cancer Institute, Bethesda, MD

Walter F. Baile, MD, The University of Texas M. D. Anderson Cancer Center, Houston

Jonathan L. Blitstein, PhD, RTI International, Research Triangle Park, NC

Deborah J. Bowen, PhD, Fred Hutchinson Cancer Research Center, Seattle, WA

David B. Buller, PhD, Klein Buendel, Golden, CO

Marci Kramish Campbell, PhD, MPH, RD, University of North Carolina at Chapel Hill

Jacqueline Casillas, MD, University of California, Los Angeles

Barb Cochrane, PhD, Fred Hutchinson Cancer Research Center, Seattle, WA

Graham A. Colditz, MD, DrPH, Washington University School of Medicine, St. Louis, MO

Robert T. Croyle, PhD, National Cancer Institute, Bethesda, MD

Susan J. Curry, PhD, University of Illinois at Chicago

Israel De Alba, MD, MPH, University of California, Irvine

Cecilia R. DeGraffinreid, MHS, The Ohio State University, Columbus

Wendy Demark-Wahnefried, PhD, RD, LDN, University of Texas M. D. Anderson Cancer Center, Houston

Lara K. Dhingra, PhD, Beth Israel Medical Center, New York, NY

Mark Dignan, PhD, MPH, University of Kentucky, Lexington

Amanda Dillard, PhD, North Dakota State University, Fargo

Georita M. Frierson, PhD, Miriam Hospital and W. Alpert Medical School of Brown University, Providence, RI

Patricia Ganz, MD, University of California, Los Angeles

Jennifer Gierisch, MPH, University of North Carolina at Chapel Hill

Barbara A. Given, RN, PhD, FAAN, Michigan State University, East Lansing

Charles W. Given, PhD, Michigan State University, East Lansing

Carolyn C. Gotay, PhD, University of British Columbia, Vancouver, BC, Canada

Louis C. Grothaus, MA, Group Health Cooperative, Seattle, WA

Janet Harden, RN, MSN, Wayne State University, Detroit, MI

Jane T. Hickok, MD, University of Rochester, Rochester, NY

Mira L. Katz, PhD, The Ohio State University, Columbus

Anne E. Kazak, PhD, ABPP, The Children's Hospital of Philadelphia, Philadelphia, PA

Renee E. Magnan, PhD, North Dakota State University, Fargo

Sara Matteson, PsyD, University of Rochester, Rochester, NY

Colleen M. McBride, PhD, National Human Genome Research Institute, Bethesda, MD

Kevin D. McCaul, PhD, North Dakota State University, Fargo

Jennifer B. McClure, PhD, Group Health Cooperative, Seattle, WA

Paige Green McDonald, PhD, National Cancer Institute, Bethesda, MD

Hendrika Meischke, PhD, Fred Hutchinson Cancer Research Center, Seattle, WA

Helen I. Meissner, PhD, Office of Behavioral and Social Research, National Institutes of Health, Bethesda, MD

Suzanne Mellon, PhD, RN, University of Detroit, Detroit, MI

Robin Mermelstein, PhD, University of Illinois at Chicago

Beth E. Meyerowitz, PhD, University of Southern California, Los Angeles

Anne Miles, PhD, University College London, London, England

Suzanne M. Miller, PhD, Fox Chase Cancer Center, Philadelphia, PA

Carol Moinpour, PhD, Fred Hutchinson Cancer Research Center, Seattle, WA

Gary R. Morrow, PhD, MS, University of Rochester, Rochester, NY

David M. Murray, PhD, The Ohio State University, Columbus

Karen M. Mustian, PhD, University of Rochester, Rochester, NY

Laurel L. Northouse, PhD, RN, FAAN, University of Michigan, Ann Arbor

Sindy Oh, MA, University of Southern California, Los Angeles

Jamie S. Ostroff, PhD, Memorial Sloan-Kettering Cancer Center, New York, NY

Sherri L. Pals, PhD, U.S. Centers for Disease Control and Prevention, Atlanta, GA

Patricia A. Parker, PhD, The University of Texas M. D. Anderson Cancer Center, Houston

Electra D. Paskett, PhD, The Ohio State University, Columbus

Bernardine M. Pinto, PhD, Miriam Hospital and W. Alpert Medical School of Brown University, Providence, RI

Carolyn Rabin, PhD, Miriam Hospital and W. Alpert Medical School of Brown University, Providence, RI

Astrid Reina-Patton, PhD, Harbor-UCLA Medical Center, Torrance, CA

Alyssa M. Rodriguez, PhD, The Children's Hospital of Philadelphia, Philadelphia, PA

Joseph A. Roscoe, PhD, University of Rochester, Rochester, NY

Julia H. Rowland, PhD, National Cancer Institute, Bethesda, MD

Julie L. Ryan, PhD, University of Rochester, Rochester, NY

Ann Schafenacker, RN, MSN, University of Michigan, Ann Arbor

Leslie R. Schover, PhD, The University of Texas M. D. Anderson Cancer Center, Houston

Paula R. Sherwood, PhD, RN, CNRN, University of Pittsburgh, Pittsburgh, PA

Michael Stefanek, PhD, American Cancer Society, Atlanta, GA

Cynthia J. Stein, MD, MPH, Harvard University, Boston, MA

Victor Strecher, PhD, MPH, University of Michigan, Ann Arbor

Lisa Sutherland, PhD, University of North Carolina at Chapel Hill

Stephen H. Taplin, MD, MPH, National Cancer Institute, Bethesda, MD

Cathy M. Tatum, MA, The Ohio State University, Columbus

Beti Thompson, PhD, Fred Hutchinson Cancer Research Center, Seattle, WA

Jasmin A. Tiro, MPH, University of Texas Southwestern Medical Center, Dallas

Sally W. Vernon, PhD, University of Texas, Houston

Sarah K. Wahl, PhD, The University of Illinois at Chicago

Jo Waller, PhD, University College London, London, England

Catharine Wang, PhD, Fox Chase Cancer Center, Philadelphia, PA

Jane Wardle, PhD, University College London, London, England

Lari Wenzel, PhD, University of California, Irvine

David W. Wetter, PhD, University of Texas M. D. Anderson Cancer Center, Houston

Carol R. White, MPH, University of Kentucky, Lexington

FOREWORD

DAVID B. ABRAMS

Handbook of Cancer Control and Behavioral Science: A Resource for Researchers, Practitioners, and Policymakers is timely and unique in scope and focus. Its value and high quality owe much to the leadership and experience of the editors, the excellent choice of chapter authors, and its ambitious agenda to provide both depth and breadth of coverage. This handbook draws from new knowledge about cancer from the biological, behavioral, social, and population sciences to delineate how behavior interacts with both biology and the environment to either enhance health, longevity, and well-being, or cause disease, disability, and premature death. It also exemplifies the interdisciplinary and transdisciplinary "team science" approach pioneered by the National Cancer Institute to address complex diseases that defy single disciplinary solutions.

This handbook will be invaluable not only to those working in cancer but also to basic and translational researchers in other health care areas who address the role of biopsychosocial etiological factors to inform prevention, early detection, therapeutics, chronic disease management, and health policy. In 2008, the health care system in the United States is challenged by an aging population, unsustainable rises in health care costs, persistent tobacco use and health disparities, epidemic levels of obesity, and large segments of the population without health insurance coverage. Behavioral science as characterized in this handbook has an enormous role to play in the new models of medicine, health care delivery, and public health practice that are beginning to emerge to tackle these thorny public health issues.

This handbook fills a huge gap in knowledge synthesis about how behavioral and psychosocial methods and models can be employed to effectively and efficiently translate basic biomedical discoveries in cancer into cancer control practices and policies. It is a single source reference that surveys the enormous body of newly generated knowledge in this area (no small part of which derives from research supported by the National Cancer Institute, other National Institutes of Health organizations, as well as governmental and nongovernment funding agencies).

Individual and collective behavior and behavior change is the interconnecting link between biology, on the one hand, and society, on the other hand. The dramatic increase over a period of fewer than 50 years in the incidence and prevalence of several cancers (e.g., stomach, lung, uterine) and other chronic diseases (e.g., cardiovascular disease, Type 2 diabetes) provides a stark reminder of how powerful the interaction of multiple vulnerable genes and associated changes in behaviors and environmental exposures can be when they act in concert.

The emerging view for the 21st century, embraced in this handbook, is that the causes of chronic diseases such as cancer lie as much in socioecological models and the unintended consequences of human-made environments as in genetic and molecular biology models. This handbook points the way toward an integration of subsystems found both under and outside the skin, thereby extending systems biology to the behavioral, social, and population sciences.

This volume provides in-depth and rigorous coverage of the state of the science of large areas of behavioral and social science research in cancer. It reviews theory, models, methods, and empirical findings and documents the important progress that has been made in the field, as well as needed future research. Applications are covered across the entire cancer continuum, from primary prevention, early detection, and therapeutics, to posttreatment management of cancer patients and survivorship. The levels of analysis considered span a range from intraindividual mechanisms to individual and collective behavior patterns found in families, organizations, communities, and systems of health care delivery and health services research. This book is an evidence-based compendium, not only from bench to clinical bedside but beyond to the trenches of community-based dissemination, implementation, and policy research. Its panoramic treatment will strengthen basic science as well as the all-important science of dissemination and implementation. This volume will make a difference in people's lives by encouraging the widespread application of current knowledge to practices and policies designed to reduce the preventable burden of cancer on individuals, families, and populations.

New discoveries—such as the importance of epigenetics in understanding and more efficiently intervening at various critical periods within the human life span and across generations—are emerging almost daily at the microlevel of cellular and extracellular interactions; the mesolevel of psychoneuroimmunologic interactions among brain, hormone, endocrine, and immune systems; the macroenvironmental level of changes in lifestyle, diet, exercise, social stress and support, and tobacco use; and the macroeconomic and policy levels. As in many other fields, the past few decades have witnessed unprecedented growth in basic scientific knowledge as well as the use of that knowledge to improve interventions targeting the clinic, community, and policymakers. The more researchers learn about genes and gene expression, as well as about socioeconomics and population health, the more it is evident that knowledge about behavior and behavior change is critical to improving the health and well-being of individuals and populations. Understanding human behavior within its sociocultural and biological contexts is arguably the single most important frontier and grand challenge facing both those who work to reduce or eliminate the devastating preventable effects of cancer and those who confront other health-related challenges facing the world in the 21st century.

This handbook makes a powerful and convincing case for the pivotal role that the behavioral and social sciences can play at the basic science level, the clinical translational science level, and the population and policy levels in reducing the personal, societal, and economic burdens of cancer. It will engender a clear recognition that the behavioral and social sciences provide critical tools and approaches for understanding how to treat and reduce the incidence and prevalence of one of the leading preventable causes of premature death and disease burden in developed and developing nations.

PREFACE

The past 2 decades have been marked by the coming of age of behavioral science in cancer prevention and control. It is now widely accepted that the study of human behavior, in all its complexity, is central to the understanding of cancer risk and disease. Indeed, a vast literature attests to the fundamental role that behavioral and psychosocial factors play in cancer risk, the clinical management of cancer, and adjustment to cancer and its aftermath. Yet, the field lacks an integrative volume that systematically surveys and synthesizes the relevant literature. The *Handbook of Cancer Control and Behavioral Science: A Resource for Researchers, Practitioners, and Policymakers* is designed specifically to fill this gap.

Twenty years ago, this book could not have been written. It builds on the research literature in the intervening period—including studies that reach beyond the individual in the clinical setting and into the social, anthropological, and public health domains—while continuing to embrace the basic tenet that behavioral science is vital and integral to cancer control at the individual level. As we incubated the idea for this book, our conception of it evolved to include five primary goals based on insights from our own research as well as our joint perspectives on the field as a whole.

First, we wanted the book to span the field of cancer control but to do so within a unifying framework. Thus, we chose the cancer control continuum as the main organizational template. Second, we wanted the volume to be of value both to those new to the interface of behavioral science and cancer as well as to seasoned researchers and practitioners. To accommodate all groups of readers, the chapters were written to provide in-depth, state-of-the-science coverage but without the presumption of prior familiarity with the material. Third, consistent with the work's intended use as a handbook, we included an introductory section composed of conceptual and methodologic chapters to orient the reader to the constructs and tools that guide research in this area. Fourth, to systematically and integratively review the key clinical–research issues within each phase of the cancer control continuum, the bulk of the chapters summarize the evidence base in each domain, highlight the application of study findings to clinical and public health arenas, and provide directions for future research.

Finally, we wanted the volume to convey the need for progress along several fronts. Many of the chapters in the volume—especially those in the final part—address this objective by pointing out the current research priorities in several areas. These include (a) a greater focus on biobehavioral integration; (b) the design, evaluation, and dissemination of more tailored and targeted interventions; (c) the development of interventions that target risk and disease factors not only at the individual level but also at the broader ecological level; (d) a more systematic assessment and consideration of ethnic, social class, and cultural factors in cancer control; and (e) a more theory-driven research base.

We believe that if the promises of innovative biologic and technical advances in cancer prevention and control (e.g., new screening techniques, genetic testing, molecularly targeted therapies) are to be fully realized, the findings of behavioral research will need to be brought to bear to facilitate more informed decision making, enhance adjustment and quality of life, and motivate and sustain behavior change efforts among patients and their families, as well as the public at large. This volume provides the impetus, language, and infrastructure for the transdisciplinary communication among behavioral science researchers, health care providers, biological scientists, policymakers, advocacy groups, and other stakeholders that is essential for fostering the development and dissemination of behavioral interventions.

The book is intended to target a wide audience. The contributors have produced uniformly high-quality chapters that are not only scholarly but also practically useful, offering an overview of what behavioral science has thus far contributed to the achievement of cancer control goals, what it is poised to contribute, and specific strategies for furthering its impact on the field. As such, the volume provides behavioral scientists, as well as health and mental health professionals, with a reference work in the area of cancer control that has both breadth and depth. In particular, the volume will be a valuable source of guidance for scientists working at the interface of behavior and cancer in developing their research paradigms and agendas and for promoting a more evidence-based foundation for guiding the practice of health care providers, payers, and policy experts. The book is also intended to serve as a useful resource for clinicians working in cancer and related areas, including psychologists, psychiatrists, oncologists, nurses, social workers, health educators, and family therapists.

From our editorial perspective, we are championing cancer prevention and control at an especially opportune time. Multiple and diverse research funding mechanisms, publication outlets, and professional and policy groups are now available to behavioral and allied researchers in cancer control. This is an exciting time to be contributing to the literature and working with our colleagues in this uniquely transdisciplinary field. This book will help promote a synergy among cancer control researchers by serving as a cutting-edge yet accessible reference that reviews the burgeoning and multifaceted field of behavioral science and cancer control. Biobehavioral research in cancer has the potential to save lives, to make those lives more comfortable and satisfied, and to thereby reduce the human toll of this increasingly common and insidious disease. Our hope is that by benchmarking research progress to date, outlining research needs, and foreshadowing future research developments, this volume will play a pivotal role in enhancing and enlarging the application of behavioral science to cancer prevention and control. We are honored to be in a position to help contribute to the evolution of the interface between behavioral science and cancer.

We gratefully acknowledge the contributions of a number of people to this endeavor. First and foremost, we want to thank the individual chapter authors for their meticulously crafted and scientifically stellar chapters. We also recognize the contributions made by several individuals at the American Psychological Association who helped shepherd this book from conception to publication including Susan Reynolds (our acquisitions editor, who served as a valuable guide throughout this process), as well as Phuong Huynh, Ron Teeter, Devon Bourexis, and Tyler Aune. We also extend our gratitude to numerous friends and colleagues for their ideas and encouragement during the development of the book and for providing helpful input, including Andrea Barsevick, Keith Belizzi, Ronald Brown, Kenneth Chu, Michael Deifenbach, Joanne Dorgan, Brian Egleston, Ronit Elk, Andrew Godwin, Ellen Gritz, Paul Han, Jennifer Hay, Robert Hiatt, Shawna Hudson, Karen Hurley, Paul Jacobsen, Jeffrey Kendall, Jon Kerner, David Knowlton, Scott Leischow, Issac Lipkus, Grace Ma, Alfred Marcus, David Mohr, Melissa Napolitano, Wendy Nelson, Ellen Peterson, Bruce Rapkin, Elizabetta Razzaboni, William Redd, Pio Riccibitti, Barbara Rimer, Julia Hannum Rose, Eric Ross, Pagona Roussi, Kerry Sherman, James Spira, Bonnie Spring, Annette Stanton, Haley

Thompson, Carolyn Weaver, and Loni Zeltzer. We also gratefully acknowledge the input provided through the Fox Chase Cancer Center National Cancer Institute–funded Behavioral Core Facility by Joanne Buzaglo, Carolyn Fang, Linda Fleisher, Amy Lazev, Hua Min, Pamela Shapiro, Catharine Wang, and Kuang-Yi Wen.

Suzanne M. Miller also expresses her personal gratitude to her medical oncology colleagues and collaborators, especially Robert Beck, Paul Engstrom, and Michael Seiden, and also Cynthia Bergman, Angela Bradbury, Roger Cohen, Steven Cohen, Mary Daly, Crystal Denlinger, Veda Giri, Lori Goldstein, Richard Greenberg, Enrique Hernandez, Cory Langer, Neal Meropol, Mark Morgan, Monica Morrow, Alan Pollack, John Ridge, Jose and Irma Russo, Walter Scott, Michell Smith, Ramona Swaby, Rene Turchi, Michael Unger, Robert Uzzo, David Weinberg, Yu-Ning Wong, and Robert Young, among others, for their wisdom and commitment to highlighting, addressing, and incorporating psychosocial factors into their conceptions of clinical and community care.

We also thank Jennifer Lyle and Mary Anne Ryan at Fox Chase Cancer Center for their outstanding administrative support, and we are indebted to John Scarpato for his insightful and dedicated input on this volume. Finally, we extend our heartfelt appreciation to our families and friends who have sustained us during the arduous process of completing this work and whom we hope will benefit from the legacy of this field, directly as well as indirectly.

I

INTRODUCTION TO BEHAVIORAL SCIENCE AND CANCER

INTRODUCTION TO BEHAVIORAL
SCIENCE AND CANCER

Part I of this book lays the groundwork for the recognition that there are important behavioral causes of cancer, that those causes are in many cases modifiable through behavioral intervention, and that the interventions need to be designed on the basis of empirically supported theoretical models and theories. In chapter 1, Miller, Bowen, Croyle, and Rowland define the notion of cancer control, delineate the cancer control continuum, and provide an overview of the role of behavior in cancer control. They also present an integrative framework for a biobehavioral approach to cancer control and describe notable themes that emerge across the chapters of the volume. Chapter 2, by Stein and Colditz, documents that significant, and in some cases substantial, reductions in the incidence of specific cancers can be achieved through primary prevention at the population level. It also reviews temporal trends and demographic disparities in the population levels of major risk factors. Chapter 3, by Bowen, Moinpour, Thompson, Andersen, Meischke, and Cochrane, reviews theoretical models in cancer prevention and control and synthesizes them into a single theoretical framework for conceptualizing the design and evaluation of public health interventions to promote behavior change. It also illustrates how the framework can be tested and modified.

1

OVERVIEW, CURRENT STATUS, AND FUTURE DIRECTIONS

SUZANNE M. MILLER, DEBORAH J. BOWEN, ROBERT T. CROYLE, AND JULIA H. ROWLAND

Recent developments in biomedical cancer research have resulted in a rapid expansion of cancer prevention and control options (Curry, Byers, & Hewitt, 2003; Edwards et al., 2005). These advances have been accompanied by an explosion of psychosocial research in the areas of cancer risk, disease, and survivorship. The findings of this research have established a key role for behavioral and psychosocial variables in determining such outcomes as individuals' risk for cancer, their decision making about disease management and treatment options, and their behavioral choices and quality of life during and after treatment. The present volume is designed to synthesize what is known, what is suspected, and what is still unknown about the core biobehavioral and sociocultural aspects of cancer prevention and control. It provides a comprehensive and unifying overview of the main areas of research in this area, integrating basic and applied research in the behavioral and social sciences with biomedical advances.

BEHAVIORAL SCIENCE IN CANCER CONTROL RESEARCH

Cancer control has come to signify the programmatic role of the behavioral, social, and population sciences in reducing the burden of human cancer (Best,

Hiatt, Cameron, Rimer, & Abrams, 2003; Cullen, 1990; Greenwald & Cullen, 1984; Hiatt & Rimer, 1999). Although usage of *cancer control* varies, the operating definition employed by the National Cancer Institute (NCI; 2005, ¶ 3) is adopted in this volume: "the conduct of basic and applied research in the behavioral, social, and population sciences to create or enhance interventions that, independently or in combination with biomedical approaches, reduce cancer risk, incidence, morbidity, and mortality, and improve quality of life." These aims include the generation of "basic knowledge about how to monitor and change individual and collective behavior, and to ensure that such knowledge is translated into practice and policy rapidly, effectively, and efficiently" (NCI, 2005, ¶ 1).

This definition recognizes that *behavioral science* (used here as an umbrella term for the psychological and social sciences), in concert with the *population sciences* (e.g., epidemiology, surveillance, bioinformatics), is a scientific enterprise distinct from the biomedical sciences, reflecting its independent and complementary role in cancer control (Miller et al., 2004; Vernon, Meissner, & Miller, 2006). This approach highlights the fact that the behavioral and population sciences not only operate according to evidence-based scientific paradigms but also play a foundational role in understanding and addressing cancer risk and disease. An important element of this approach is the distinction between basic and applied behavioral and population science research. *Basic* research provides the conceptual, empirical, and methodological frameworks for identifying and developing relevant theoretical models, constructs, and measures, as well as for generating new empirical findings. The basic behavioral principles, methods, and findings delineated are then *applied* to the evaluation and dissemination of interventions designed to improve systems of care.

The Advisory Committee on Cancer Control of the National Cancer Institute of Canada (1994; NCI, 2005) developed a heuristic framework for conceptualizing how behavioral science contributes to cancer control. This framework identifies three major arms of cancer control research: (a) *fundamental research*, which provides the theoretical, methodological, and empirical basis for intervention development; (b) *surveillance research*, which provides data to inform the selection of cancer control intervention targets and the evaluation of their impact at the population level; and (c) *intervention research*, which includes the design of interventions to promote health-protective behaviors, support informed patient decision making, and mitigate the adverse psychosocial effects of cancer—this arm also includes the evaluation of the protocols developed, especially in terms of such factors as their efficacy, effectiveness, generalizability, and disseminability. The three arms of this framework interact reciprocally with each other, as well as with knowledge gained through application and program delivery, to contribute to the goal of reducing the burden of human cancer.

THE CANCER CONTROL CONTINUUM

The notion of the cancer control continuum is one of the most widely accepted paradigms for conceptualizing research in the behavioral sciences and cancer. It organizes the field in accordance with the temporal course of an individual's cancer experience, progressing from preventive actions to screening, diagnosis, and treatment and finally to health and disease management during the posttreatment, survivorship, and end-of-life periods (NCI, 2006a). Since its introduction in the 1970s, the cancer control continuum has been defined in somewhat different ways with respect to how it is segmented, that is, in terms of where along the continuum, and how finely, the lines delimiting successive phases are drawn (Canadian Strategy for Cancer Control, 2005; Holland, 2002; NCI, 2006a).

The definition of the *cancer control continuum* used in this volume, which is the basis for the book's organization, divides the continuum into four overarching phases: (a) *primary prevention* (i.e., reducing cancer incidence among cancer-free individuals), (b) *secondary prevention* (i.e., detecting cancer in its early, preclinical stages), (c) *tertiary prevention* (i.e., reducing morbidity and mortality through the diagnosis and treatment of clinical cancer), and (d) *quaternary prevention* (i.e., managing the disease and its effects following initial treatment: during remission, survivorship, recurrence, and palliative and terminal care). Using the cancer continuum as the organizing principle of the volume provides several advantages. First, the continuum has face validity and easy comprehensibility for a broad interdisciplinary audience, including not only behavioral and social scientists but also public health and policy researchers, social workers, nurses, genetic counselors, psychiatrists, oncologists, and primary care practitioners. Second, each phase of the continuum is characterized by psychosocial issues that cut across the specific cancer sites or organ systems involved.

As illustrated in Table 1.1, the main psychosocial issues for unaffected individuals at the primary prevention phase relate to the adoption of health-protective behaviors, for example, exercise, nutrition, smoking cessation, and so on. At the secondary prevention phase, the main psychosocial issues pertain to adhering to screening recommendations, making informed decisions about whether to undergo such technologies as genetic testing, coping with the results of screening and genetic tests, and dealing with the issues of communication of test results to family members. For cancer patients at the tertiary prevention phase, relevant psychosocial issues include the individual's adjusting to a cancer diagnosis, making informed decisions about treatment and management options, and coping with cancer and treatment-related symptomatology. Additional psychosocial issues in this phase include the effects of patients' cancer experiences on their caregivers and families. During the quaternary prevention phase, the psychosocial issues for patients include coping with

TABLE 1.1
The Cancer Control Continuum

Continuum phase	Medical goals of phase	Phase-specific behavioral and psychosocial issues
Primary prevention	Reducing cancer incidence among cancer-free individuals	Adopting health-protective lifestyle behaviors
Secondary prevention	Detecting cancer in its early, preclinical stages among those who are currently undiagnosed and particularly among those at high risk for the disease	Making informed decisions about whether to undergo screening and genetic testing Adhering to screening recommendations Understanding and coping with the results of screening and genetic testing Communicating genetic testing results to others
Tertiary prevention	Reducing morbidity and mortality through treatment of clinical cancer	Coping with the adverse psychosocial effects of a cancer diagnosis Making informed decisions about treatment options Coping with the adverse physical and psychosocial effects of cancer symptoms and treatment side effects Caregivers and family coping with the adverse psychosocial effects of the patient's cancer experience during diagnosis and treatment
Quaternary prevention	Monitoring for, and treating, late treatment side effects and other late-occurring morbidities, such as secondary cancers and cancer recurrence	Coping with the transition into the survivorship role Coping with the adverse psychosocial effects of late-occurring morbidities Making decisions about transitioning from curative to palliative care Coping with the psychosocial challenges of end-of-life issues, for example, confronting the prospect of death, and dealing with the physical, psychological, and existential concomitants of the dying experience Caregiver and family coping with the adverse psychosocial effects of the survivor's cancer experience

the transition into the survivorship role, coping with the adverse psychosocial effects of late-occurring morbidities, making decisions about transitioning from curative to palliative care, and coping with the psychosocial challenges of end-of-life issues, for example, confronting the prospect of death and dealing with the physical, psychological, and existential concomitants of the dying experience. Additional psychosocial issues raised during this period are the effects of the survivor's cancer experience on family and caregivers.

A further advantage of the cancer control continuum is that it helps to identify differences in psychological processes as a function of the particular cancer risk or disease challenge involved. For example, the issues that arise from behavior change efforts in the primary prevention phase for cancer-free individuals (who have not had personal experience with the disease) can differ in significant respects from the promotion of behavior change efforts among cancer survivors (who have had personal experience with the disease). Similarly, an individual's decisions about, and responses to, seemingly equivalent medical challenges can vary as a function of the phase of the cancer continuum at which they occur. For example, undergoing an unfamiliar follow-up procedure for an abnormal test result may have a very different meaning for a high-risk individual than for an affected individual experiencing a possible cancer recurrence.

THE ROLE OF BEHAVIOR IN CANCER CONTROL

Behavior both affects and is affected by cancer. Cancer control initiatives therefore target behavior as both a determinant and a consequence of cancer (Hiatt & Rimer, 1999). As a determinant, behavioral factors can play a critical role in cancer incidence, morbidity, mortality, and possibly, progression. The factors in question include lifestyle behaviors (e.g., smoking, diet), screening adherence (e.g., mammography), surveillance (monitoring for symptoms of recurrent or second cancers), and treatment adherence. The behavioral consequences of cancer are broad ranging, including the fear of cancer before it is diagnosed, as well as the psychosocial impact on patients, their families, and caregivers at the time of diagnosis, during cancer treatment, and throughout the posttreatment, survivorship, and end-of life periods.

In primary prevention, cancer control researchers are largely concerned with the role of behavior in contributing to risk exposure and therefore cancer incidence. Behavioral epidemiology (Sallis, Owen, & Fotheringham, 2000) has identified specific lifestyle behaviors that elevate an individual's risk for the development of cancer. These behaviors include tobacco use, physical inactivity, poor eating habits, excessive alcohol consumption, sun exposure, and unsafe sexual practices. Modifying these lifestyle behaviors is a central aim of cancer control efforts. Indeed, it is estimated that as much as 50% of cancer could be prevented through modification of these lifestyle behaviors (Colditz et al., 1996; see also chap. 2 and chaps. 8–14, this volume).

In secondary prevention, cancer control efforts address the importance of increasing the use of risk detection and early diagnostic technologies, which can lead to significant reductions in cancer morbidity and mortality.

Despite the availability of effective screening regimens for breast, cervical, and colorectal cancers, screening rates for breast and cervical cancers are less than optimal for major segments of the population, as are screening rates for colorectal cancer for the population at large (Swan, Breen, Coates, Rimer, & Lee, 2003). For individuals at elevated risk for hereditary cancer syndromes, additional options for risk detection and early diagnosis include genetic counseling and testing, and follow-up surveillance, risk reduction, and prevention regimens. The cancer control agenda is to promote awareness of these options and to support informed decision making about them. For example, research is under way to assess and address informed decision making concerning whether to undergo available prophylactic procedures (e.g., prophylactic surgery, chemoprevention), as well as how to mitigate the potential adverse psychosocial effects of the decision-making process and the consequences of the decisions that are made (see chaps. 15–17, this volume).

In tertiary prevention, research has shown that the effects of a cancer diagnosis before and during treatment can result in a range of adverse emotional and physical reactions for cancer patients, their caregivers, and their families. An important aim of cancer control efforts is to help patients respond adaptively to the challenges of diagnosis and treatment. An additional aim relates to the fact that patients vary in both the amount of information they prefer to be given about their diagnosis, treatment, and care and the degree of involvement that they prefer to have in decisions about their care. Cancer control efforts seek to understand these differences among patients, with a view to providing support for informed treatment decision making and responses (see chaps. 18–22, this volume).

In quaternary prevention, cancer survivors are at heightened risk not only for recurrence but also for secondary cancers, and they can therefore benefit from primary prevention efforts to promote the uptake of healthy lifestyle behaviors. Cancer control efforts therefore target the promotion of health-protective behaviors to reduce the risk of cancer recurrence, as well as screening and surveillance for both recurrences and secondary cancers, to reduce morbidity and mortality through early diagnosis and treatment. In addition, both the patient and his or her family often need to cope with the late-occurring psychological and physical effects of the disease and its treatment, including fatigue, pain, and suffering. In cases of advanced cancer, the patient and family must also cope with the difficult psychosocial issues that are involved in the transition from curative to palliative care, as well as those that arise during terminal care. Cancer control efforts seek to promote and support informed decision making concerning the transition to palliative care and also to contribute to the mitigation of the adverse psychosocial effects experienced by patient and family during both palliative and terminal care (see chaps. 23–27, this volume).

AN INTEGRATIVE FRAMEWORK FOR CANCER CONTROL AND BEHAVIORAL SCIENCE

The field of behavioral science and cancer as depicted in the chapters of this handbook can be viewed through the lens of an integrative framework that is based on several core concepts. One is the notion of *cancer control*, which represents the role of behavioral and allied sciences within the broader sweep of scientific efforts to reduce the burden of cancer. The second is the concept of *behavioral intervention*, the primary operational mechanism for achieving cancer control. The third is the *cancer control continuum*, a descriptive template for conceptualizing the areas that need to be addressed within the field of behavioral science and cancer. The fourth is *individual differences*, and more specifically, genetic and behavioral individual differences. The framework that we propose captures the interrelations among these concepts and does so in such a way as to provide an integrative approach to the field of behavioral science and cancer as presented in this handbook.

The proposed framework (see Figure 1.1) is organized into four pathways (see the columns in the figure), which correspond to the phases of the cancer control continuum. The pathways are designated as follows: (a) Predisease (i.e., primary prevention), (b) Early Disease (i.e., secondary prevention), (c) Clinical Disease (i.e., tertiary prevention), and (d) Survivorship/End of Life (i.e., quaternary prevention). The focus of cancer control efforts within each pathway is also indicated (e.g., see "Promoting health-protective behaviors" within the Predisease pathway).

Each pathway in Figure 1.1 begins with the individual's *molecular and behavioral signature*, which represents the interactive dynamic between the person's cancer-related genetic profile (e.g., susceptibility to developing certain cancers, responsiveness to certain therapies to alleviate pain) and his or her cancer-related behavioral profile (e.g., attitudes toward screening, values about treatment). Different elements of the behavioral component of the signature come into play at successive phases of the continuum; for example, lifestyle behaviors that are operative and of primary importance during Predisease may no longer be relevant during Early Disease. In addition, elements of the behavioral component of the signature may change over time as the individual traverses the successive phases of the continuum.

Each pathway then identifies the major foci (e.g., screening uptake, distress reduction) of the *behavioral interventions* that have been explored in that area. For ease of exposition, intervention content (e.g., how an intervention promotes screening) is not detailed within the framework, nor are the mechanisms by which these interventions are presumed to function. A bidirectional arrow connects the individual's molecular and behavioral signature with the behavioral interventions within each pathway. The arrow from the signature to the interventions signifies the potential influence of the

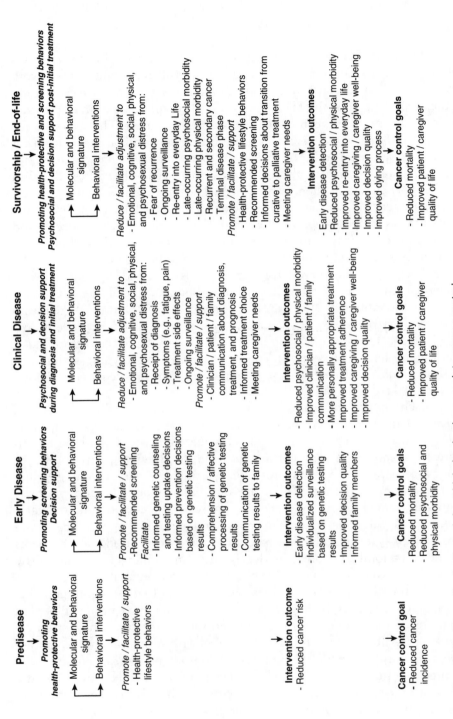

Figure 1.1. Integrative framework for a biobehavioral approach to cancer control.

signature in intervention design, as may occur in intervention tailoring and targeting on the basis of the psychosocial characteristics of the prospective intervention recipient. The arrow from the intervention to the signature reflects the potential of the intervention to modify the individual's behavior. For example, an intervention that is designed to promote lifestyle modification, by definition, changes the behavioral component of the signature through alteration of the individual's habit patterns.

Indicated next are the *intervention outcomes*, the target results of the interventions within each pathway. Finally, the framework specifies the ultimate goals of the interventions within each pathway, that is, the *cancer control goals*. The intervention outcomes (e.g., reduced cancer risk) are conceived of as intermediate milestones in the effort to achieve broader cancer control goals (e.g., reduced cancer incidence).

Within the first pathway (Predisease), the molecular component of the individual's signature includes the individual's hereditary or environmental susceptibility to cancer, as well as any genetic predisposition to engage in risk-elevating behaviors (e.g., genetic susceptibility to nicotine dependence). The behavioral elements of the signature include such factors as the individual's propensity for engaging in risk-taking behaviors (e.g., unhealthy diet, excessive sun exposure); his or her knowledge relating to cancer prevention (e.g., the risk-elevating effects of physical inactivity; genetic susceptibility to certain cancers); the individual's risk perceptions and expectancies about the efficacy of prevention regimens and his or her personal self-efficacy beliefs; his or her health-related values and goals (e.g., motivation to improve health); the individual's risk-related distress; and finally, his or her psychological and social resources to enact desired changes (e.g., coping skills, health literacy, social support network; Miller, Shoda, & Hurley, 1996).

Interventions in this context are primarily designed to promote and support the uptake and maintenance of health-protective lifestyle behaviors, including those related to smoking, diet, sun exposure, physical activity, and sexual practices. The individual's behavioral signature determines how effective a specific intervention is in motivating the uptake and maintenance of preventive regimens. The successful uptake of these regimens leads to reduced cancer risk, which in turn results in reduced cancer incidence, the goal of cancer control at this phase.

Within the second pathway (Early Disease), the molecular component of the individual's signature includes his or her status as having or not having a malignancy and, for an unaffected individual, his or her risk for developing a malignancy on the basis of hereditary susceptibility (e.g., being a carrier of a BRCA1 and BRCA2 genetic mutation) or environmentally induced susceptibility (e.g., because of smoking or infection with the human papillomavirus). The behavioral component of the individual's signature includes the factors listed earlier for the first pathway (i.e., knowledge, risk perceptions, expectancies, values and goals, affective states, and self-regulatory resources) as they relate to screening and genetic counseling and testing.

Interventions focus on promoting screening adherence for cancers for which there are current population-level screening recommendations, as well as supporting informed decision making about the uptake of genetic counseling and testing, and prevention and risk reduction options. Interventions are also designed to facilitate and support comprehension and affective processing of genetic testing results and the communication of such results to family members. The main target outcomes of these interventions are early disease detection, informed decision making about genetic testing and prevention regimens, and individualized surveillance through screening for above-average risk populations, which collectively contribute to reducing mortality and psychosocial and physical morbidity.

Within the third pathway (Clinical Disease), the molecular component incorporates such factors as the patient's genetically based responsiveness to available medical treatments as well as his or her genetically based susceptibility to treatment side effects. The behavioral component of the signature includes the elements of the patient's psychological profile that affect how he or she reacts to and deals with the psychosocial and symptom management challenges of this phase. Behavioral interventions are designed to reduce, and facilitate the patient's adjustment to, the distress caused by a cancer diagnosis, disease symptoms, treatment side effects, and/or surveillance regimens. Interventions are also available to facilitate and support communication with medical care providers and family about diagnosis, treatment and prognosis, and informed decision making about treatment choice in cases in which different medical options are available. Further, interventions have been designed to facilitate and support the development of caregiving skills and the efforts of caregivers to meet their own psychosocial needs as they provide caregiving.

The target outcomes of the interventions at this phase are to reduce psychosocial and physical morbidity; to improve communication among clinicians, patients, and family; to allow for more personally appropriate treatment and improve treatment adherence; and to enhance caregiving and caregiver well-being. These outcomes contribute to achieving the ultimate goals of diagnosis, which are to reduce mortality and improve patient and caregiver quality of life.

Within the final pathway (Survivorship/End-of-Life), the individual's molecular and behavioral signature includes those elements that were previously described with respect to the onset and management of clinical disease, but as they relate to issues of survivorship. Behavioral interventions are designed to reduce distress and provide support to the individual, but with a focus on issues of survivorship. Relevant target issues include decision making, fears of recurrence, the psychological impact of ongoing surveillance, reentry into everyday life, late-occurring psychosocial and physical morbidity, recurrent and secondary cancers, confronting terminal disease, transitioning from curative to palliative treatment, and family caregiving. The ultimate goals are improved patient and caregiver quality of life and, in end-of-life care, improved death and quality of bereavement. Survivorship is unique among the pathways within the framework because the issues and goals of the two initial pathways of the cancer control continuum are also relevant here, including the need to undertake preventive measures as in Predisease and screening measures as in Early Disease.

The proposed framework highlights the central role of behavioral interventions in cancer control and catalogs what they are designed to achieve. In addition, it delineates the importance of individual differences in cancer control, including those of genetic origin, by depicting the critical interplay between such differences and behavioral interventions. It also identifies the ultimate goals of cancer control, thereby elucidating the essential benchmarks for gauging the success of cancer control efforts. Finally, it clarifies the commonalities and differences in the behavioral interventions, target outcomes, and cancer control goals across the phases of the cancer control continuum.

EMERGING THEMES AND FUTURE DIRECTIONS

Across the chapters of this volume, a number of common themes emerge that have implications for future directions in research. We now provide an overview of these themes.

Efficacy and Effectiveness of Behavioral Interventions

At each phase of the cancer control continuum, behavioral interventions have been developed that have been demonstrated to significantly improve cancer outcomes. For example, in primary and secondary prevention, effective behavioral interventions have been developed to promote the uptake of cancer-related lifestyle behaviors and adherence to screening recommendations. However, questions remain about how to optimally tailor these interventions and target them to subgroups of individuals as well as how to maintain health behavior change and screening adherence over the long term. In tertiary prevention, behavioral interventions have shown success in improving adjustment to a cancer diagnosis, reducing cancer symptomatology and treatment side effects, and addressing the needs of the family and caregivers of cancer patients. Further research is needed to determine how best to help patients and their families make informed decisions about cancer treatment and management regimens as well as how to help high-risk individuals understand the pros and cons of increasingly available early detection, risk reduction, and prevention options. With respect to quaternary prevention, behavioral interventions have been developed that show promise in improving quality of life, especially in the short term. In addition, the effectiveness of behavioral interventions that promote lifestyle behavior modification among survivors has largely been supported, although the methodological rigor of some of the supporting studies is less than desirable. Further, the potential to extend life and reduce morbidity through the promotion of screening for cancer recurrence and secondary cancers remains an open question. Finally, clear conclusions cannot as yet be drawn regarding whether psychosocial interventions are effective in extending cancer survival.

As a field, behavioral science is in the process of organizing its evidence base with respect to issues of efficacy and effectiveness and identifying those areas in which the evidence is strong enough to begin the dissemination process and those in which additional and better designed studies are needed to support the implementation of particular interventions onto systems of care. This process is exemplified in the emergence of clinical practice guidelines for the psychosocial care of cancer patients (Hinds et al., 2003; Turner et al., 2005).

Tailoring and Targeting Interventions

Both the tailoring and targeting of interventions appear to provide major avenues for improving efficacy and effectiveness. Tailoring an intervention customizes or individualizes it to enhance its effectiveness for specific individuals, on the basis of the psychological profile of the intervention recipient. More formally, *tailoring* has been defined as "any combination of information or change strategies intended to reach one specific person on the basis of characteristics that are unique to that person, related to the outcome of interest, and . . . derived from an individual assessment" (Kreuter & Skinner, 2000, p. 1).

Targeting an intervention also involves customizing it to enhance its effectiveness, but instead of customizing it for an individual, it is customized for a target group, typically on the basis of demographic variables rather than individual-level variables. For example, if the target variable is ethnicity, the intervention would be modified to involve culturally sensitive messages for a particular group.

Some of the major challenges to be overcome in tailoring and targeting efforts include the selection of appropriate tailoring and targeting variables, how best to customize interventions with respect to these variables, and how to implement these interventions in a cost-effective manner (Rimer & Glassman, 1999). Print communications have been a major channel for tailoring and have shown great promise in cancer control research (Skinner, Campbell, Rimer, Curry, & Prochaska, 1999). Tailored print communications have been demonstrated to enhance intervention effectiveness in such areas as smoking cessation and genetic counseling (Dijkstra, De Vries, Roijackers, & van Breukelen, 1998; Lipkus, Lyna, & Rimer, 1999; Skinner et al., 2002). The research reported in this volume, particularly within primary and secondary prevention, suggests that targeting interventions to such group characteristics as ethnicity/race, gender, age, and risk status also holds great promise (Benowitz, 2002; Campell et al., 2002; Forbes, Jepson, & Martin-Hirsch, 1999; Lawrence, Graber, Mills, Meissner, & Warnecke, 2003; Worden et al., 1988).

Dissemination of Effective Cancer Control Interventions

Research into the dissemination of effective interventions has lagged behind research to develop and evaluate these interventions. The NCI has stressed the importance of identifying pathways and mechanisms for the dissemination of tested interventions, as indicated on their Web site (NCI, 2005). However, the process of dissemination has received limited attention in research on cancer control (Kerner, Rimer, & Emmons, 2005). Dissemination challenges that have yet to be successfully met are exemplified by the work on smoking cessation. This area of research has resulted in clinical practice guidelines; yet, the application of these guidelines by health care providers and insurers has been limited. More generally, most of the interventions reported in this handbook have yet to be put into place in clinical or public health practice.

One of the obstacles to progress in this area of research is the lack of agreement on terminology for dissemination research (Lee, Earle, & Weeks, 2000). Alternative terms include *diffusion, implementation*, and *knowledge transfer*. The lack of conceptual models and the lack of agreement on such issues as the importance of internal versus external validity (i.e., intervention efficacy vs. effectiveness) have also hampered this field (Glasgow, Klesges, Dzewaltowski, Bull, & Estabrooks, 2004). These issues are currently the focus of active debate and attention, which should result in improving the knowledge base in this area (Glasgow, Lichtenstein, & Marcus, 2003).

Use of Theories, Theoretical Models, and Mediation Hypotheses in Intervention Design

Behavioral research seeks to understand the factors that shape cancer-related health behavior to improve behavioral and psychosocial outcomes. The research reported in this handbook reflects a growing recognition that basic social and behavioral science is a critical foundation for intervention design and that using behavioral science–based theoretical models to inform behavior change strategies not only produces more effective interventions but also enhances understanding of the behavioral mechanisms that affect health outcomes. However, despite the increasing use of theory-driven intervention design, this approach has not been consistently applied in different areas of the cancer control continuum. For example, primary prevention interventions have largely been theory driven, particularly with respect to tobacco-use prevention (e.g., social inoculation theory, social learning theory), dietary behavior modification (e.g., socioecological model, health belief model, transtheoretical model), skin cancer–related behavior modification (e.g., health belief model, cognitive-social theory, extended parallel-processing communication model), and physical activity modification (e.g., environmental stress theories, restorative environment theory, behavior setting theory). Theory-based intervention design has also been used extensively in quaternary prevention. For example, cognitive–behavioral, cognitive-social, stress-coping, and family-stress theories have been used in the design of interventions to improve the psychosocial adjustment of adult survivors, and a traumatic stress model has been helpful in understanding and addressing the needs of parents of children with cancer. In addition, in the area of health promotion and disease prevention among adult cancer survivors, behavioral modification theory, cognitive-social theory, the transtheoretical model, and the theory of planned behavior have all served to inform intervention design.

In contrast, in secondary prevention theoretical models in intervention design have been applied to a more limited extent, with the exception of such models as the cognitive-social health information processing (C-SHIP) framework and the transactional model of stress and coping. In tertiary prevention, the concept of expectancy has been prominently used to provide a theoretical explanation for the efficacy of interventions to alleviate treatment-specific side effects. This construct is elaborated in the self-regulation and cognitive-social models (e.g., C-SHIP) as well as in locus of control theory, social learning theory, and schema theory. In this handbook, we argue for greater use of theory-driven intervention design across all of the phases of the cancer control continuum.

The evaluation of mediational hypotheses in intervention design is much more common than the evaluation of full-scale theoretical models. *Mediational hypotheses* draw from a knowledge base of scientific findings about the constructs that underlie maladaptive behaviors or psychosocial patterns, and they help to identify the active ingredients of interventions. For example, the research literature contains empirical findings concerning the impact of such constructs as coping, self-control, and self-regulation skills on behavior. These findings are used to generate hypotheses concerning how these skills facilitate or undermine behavior change efforts. In the case of adolescents' resistance to temptation to initiate smoking, the presence or absence of these skills serve as potential mediating mechanisms to explain why smoking prevention interventions that provide training in these skills are or are not effective. However, it is important to note that demonstrating the efficacy of an intervention does not necessarily imply that the hypothe-sized mediating mechanism of the intervention (e.g., change in coping skills) accounts for its efficacy.

Multilevel and Population–Level (Public Health–Level) Interventions

The cancer control area has seen a shift from a focus on prevention inter-ventions that target individuals to prevention interventions that target population segments, such as worksite or religious communities, as well as populations defined geographically or demographically. To date, most pre-vention programs have focused on individual risk factor considerations and individual-level change as important in both the short- and the long-term man-agement of behavior change. However, the focus on individual-level change and maintenance has not always been successful in achieving long-term improvements in behavior. The research reported in this handbook reflects an increasing trend toward the study of the environmental and societal contribu-tions to the adoption and maintenance of healthy lifestyles and behaviors. The emphasis on social, economic, and cultural environments is relatively new to cancer control and is reflected in the use of ecological models in this area, which focus on the environmental causes of health behavior and the identification of effective environmental interventions (Sallis & Owen, 2002).

Disparities in Cancer Control

Access to state-of-the-art care is essential for all genders, races, and eth-nic groups, regardless of abilities, disabilities, and sexual orientations, particu-larly for populations at risk for excess incidence of, or death from, cancer. However, considerable challenges exist in reaching vulnerable populations with information about cancer prevention, screening, and treatment, and there is a dearth of relevant knowledge and culturally sensitive interventions for improving access to care for underserved groups. In addition, significant progress remains to be made in assessing the applicability of existing cancer control research findings to minority populations, as noted in several chapters in this handbook. For example, ethnic minorities are markedly underrepre-sented in research on psychosocial responses to cancer diagnosis and treat-ment. Similarly, findings on survivorship are based largely on White samples, leaving the generalizability to survivors from other racial and ethnic back-grounds an open question. Further, racial and ethnic minority participation rates in clinical trials are significantly lower than those for the general popu-lation. Therefore, there is an urgent need to address underrepresentation of racial and ethnic minorities in cancer control research across all phases of the cancer control continuum.

REFERENCES

Advisory Committee on Cancer Control, National Cancer Institute of Canada. (1994). Bridging research to action: A framework and decision-making process for cancer control. *Journal of Canadian Medical Association, 151,* 1141–1146.

Benowitz, N. L. (2002). Smoking cessation trials targeted to racial and economic minority groups. *Journal of the American Medical Association, 288,* 497–499.

Best, A., Hiatt, R., Cameron, R., Rimer, B., & Abrams, D. B. (2003). The evolution of cancer control research: An international perspective from Canada and the United States. *Cancer Epidemiology, Biomarkers & Prevention, 12,* 705–712.

Campbell, M. K., Tessaro, I., DeVellis, B., Benedict, S., Kelsey, K., Belton, L., & Sanhueza, A. (2002). Effects of a tailored health promotion program for female blue-collar workers: Health Works for Women. *Preventive Medicine, 34,* 313–323.

Canadian Strategy for Cancer Control. (2005). *Establishing the strategic framework for the Canadian Strategy for Cancer Control.* Retrieved November 16, 2006, from http://209.217.127.72/cscc/work_reports1.html

Colditz, G. A., DeJong, W., Hunter, D. J., Trichopoulos, D., & Willett, W. C. (Eds.). (1996). Harvard report on cancer prevention. *Cancer Causes Control, 7*(Suppl.), 1–55.

Cullen, J. W. (1990). Phases in cancer control: Intervention research. In M. Hakama, V. Beral, J. W. Cullen, & D. M. Parkin (Eds.), *Evaluating effectiveness of primary prevention of cancer* (pp. 1–11). Lyon, France: International Agency for Research on Cancer.

Curry, S. J., Byers, T., & Hewitt, M. (2003). *Prevention and early detection.* Washington, DC: National Academies Press.

Dijkstra, A., De Vries, H., Roijackers, J., & van Breukelen, G. (1998). Tailoring information to enhance quitting in smokers with low motivation to quit: Three basic efficacy questions. *Health Psychology, 17,* 513–519.

Edwards, E. K., Brown, M. L., Wingo, P. A., Howe, H. L., Ward, E., Ries, L. A. G., et al. (2005). Annual report to the nation on the status of cancer, 1975–2002, featuring population-based trends in cancer treatment. *Journal of the National Cancer Institute, 97,* 1407–1427.

Forbes, C., Jepson, R., & Martin-Hirsch, P. (1999). Interventions targeted at women to encourage the uptake of cervical screening. *The Cochrane Database of Systematic Review, 3.* Available from http://www.cochrane.org

Glasgow, R. E., Klesges, L. M., Dzewaltowski, D. A., Bull, S. S., & Estabrooks, P. (2004). The future of health behavior change research: What is needed to improve translation of research into health promotion practice? *Annals of Behavioral Medicine, 27,* 3–12.

Glasgow, R. E., Lichtenstein, E., & Marcus, A. C. (2003). Why don't we see more translation of health promotion research to practice? *American Journal of Public Health, 93,* 1261–1267.

Greenwald, P., & Cullen, J. W. (1984). The scientific approach to cancer control. *CA: A Cancer Journal for Clinicians, 34*, 328–332.

Hiatt, R. A., & Rimer, B. (1999). A new strategy for cancer control research. *Cancer Epidemiology, Biomarkers & Prevention, 8*, 957–964.

Hinds, P. S., Gattuso, J. S., Barnwell, E., Cofer, M., Kellum, L., Mattox, S., et al. (2003). Translating psychosocial research findings into practice guidelines. *Journal of Nursing Administration, 33*, 397–403.

Holland, J. (2002). History of psycho-oncology: Overcoming attitudinal and conceptual barriers. *Psychosomatic Medicine, 64*, 206–221.

Kerner, J., Rimer, B., & Emmons, K. (2005). Dissemination research and research dissemination: How can we close the gap? *Health Psychology, 24*, 443–446.

Kreuter, M., & Skinner, C. S. (2000). Tailoring: What's in a name. *Health Education Research, 15*, 1–4.

Lawrence, D., Graber, J. E., Mills, S. L., Meissner, H. I., & Warnecke, R. (2003). Smoking cessation interventions in U.S. racial/ethnic minority populations: An assessment of the literature. *Preventive Medicine, 36*, 204–216.

Lee, S. J., Earle, C., & Weeks, J. C. (2000). Outcomes research in oncology: History, conceptual framework, and trends in the literature. *Journal of the National Cancer Institute, 92*, 195–204.

Lipkus, I. M., Lyna, P. R., & Rimer, B. K. (1999). Using tailored interventions to enhance smoking cessation among African-Americans at a community health center. *Nicotine and Tobacco Research, 1*, 77–85.

Miller, S. M., Bowen, J. B., Campbell, M. K., Diefenbach, M. A., Gritz, E. R., Jacobsen, P. B., et al. (2004). Current research promises and challenges in behavioral oncology: Report of the American Society of Preventive Oncology. *Cancer Epidemiology, Biomarkers & Prevention, 13*, 171–180.

Miller, S. M., Shoda, Y., & Hurley, K. (1996). Applying cognitive-social theory to health-protective behavior: Breast self-examination in cancer screening. *Psychological Bulletin, 119*, 70–94.

National Cancer Institute. (2005). *Division of Cancer Control and Population Sciences: 2005: Overview and highlights*. Retrieved August 1, 2006, from http://dccps.nci.nih.gov/bb/2005_bb.pdf#page=11

National Cancer Institute. (2006a). *Cancer Control and Population Sciences: Cancer control continuum*. Retrieved August 1, 2006, from http://cancercontrol.cancer.gov/od/continuum.html

National Cancer Institute. (2006b). *Cancer Control and Population Sciences: Research dissemination and diffusion*. Retrieved December 30, 2006, from http://cancercontrol.cancer.gov/d4d/

Rimer, B. K., & Glassman, B. (1999). Is there a use for tailored print communications in cancer risk communication? *Journal of the National Cancer Institute Monographs, 25*, 140–148.

Sallis, J. F., & Owen, N. (2002). Ecological models of health behavior. In K. Glanz, B. K. Rimer, & F. M. Marcus (Eds.), *Health behavior and health education, theory, research, and practice* (pp. 462–484). San Francisco: Jossey-Bass.

Sallis, J. F., Owen, N., & Fotheringham, M. J. (2000). Behavioral epidemiology: A systematic framework to classify phases of research on health promotion and disease prevention. *Annals of Behavioral Medicine, 22,* 294–298.

Skinner, C. S., Campbell, M. K., Rimer, B. K., Curry, S., & Prochaska, J. O. (1999). How effective is tailored print communication? *Annals of Behavioral Medicine, 21,* 290–298.

Skinner, C. S., Schildkraut, J. M., Berry, D., Calingaert, B., Marcom, P. K., Sugerman, J., et al. (2002). Precounseling education materials for BRCA testing: Does tailoring make a difference? *Genetic Testing, 6,* 93–105.

Swan, J., Breen, N., Coates, R. J., Rimer, B. K., & Lee, N. C. (2003). Progress in cancer screening practices in the United States: Results from the 2000 National Health Interview Survey. *Cancer, 97,* 1528–1540.

Turner, J., Zapart, S., Pedersen, K., Rankin, N., Luxford, K., & Fletcher, J. (2005). Clinical practice guidelines for the psychosocial care of adults with cancer. *Psycho-Oncology, 14,* 159–173.

Vernon, S. W., Meissner, H. I., & Miller, S. M. (2006). The role of behavioral science in cancer prevention research: Planning the next steps in the collaborative process. *Cancer Epidemiology, Biomarkers & Prevention, 15,* 413–415.

Worden, J. K., Flynn, B. S., Gellar, B. M., Chen, M., Shelton, L. G., Secker-Walker, R. H., et al. (1988). Development of a smoking prevention mass media program using diagnostic and formative research. *Preventive Medicine, 17,* 531–558.

2

TRENDS IN MODIFIABLE
RISK FACTORS FOR CANCER
AND THE POTENTIAL
FOR CANCER PREVENTION

CYNTHIA J. STEIN AND GRAHAM A. COLDITZ

More than 6 million people around the world die from cancer each year (Murray & Lopez, 1996). Overwhelming evidence suggests that lifestyle factors impact cancer risk and that positive, population-wide changes can significantly reduce the cancer burden (Curry, Byers, & Hewitt, 2003). Current epidemiologic evidence links behavioral factors to a variety of diseases, including the most common cancers diagnosed in the developed world: lung, colorectal, prostate, and breast cancers (Ezzati, Lopez, Rodgers, Vander Hoorn, & Murray, 2002). Because of the tremendous impact of modifiable factors on cancer risk, especially for the most common cancers, it has been estimated that 50% of cancer is preventable (Colditz, DeJong, Hunter, Trichopoulos, & Willett, 1996). However, to bring about dramatic reductions in cancer incidence, widespread lifestyle changes are necessary.

Evidence supports the success and benefit of population-wide prevention strategies. For example, reductions in lung cancer rates in the United States mirror changes in cigarette smoking patterns, with marked decreases seen first in young men, then older men, and finally in women (Wingo et al., 1999). Introduction of the Papaniculou test in the 1950s was followed by a dramatic decline in cervical cancer in those countries that made widespread screening available (Laara, Day, & Hakama, 1987). The decline in Australian melanoma mortality for those born after 1950 (Giles, Armstrong, Burton, Staples, & Thursfield, 1996) following strategies to limit sun exposure is another example of effective intervention at the population level.

Clearly, behavior change is possible and offers great potential for cancer prevention. This chapter summarizes (a) the major factors that can be modified to decrease cancer risk and (b) the recent trends in these risk factors across different segments of the population. Risk-reducing behaviors discussed include reducing tobacco use, increasing physical activity, maintaining a healthy weight, improving diet, limiting alcohol, avoiding excess sun exposure, using safer sex practices, and obtaining routine cancer screening tests.

Before discussing lifestyle issues, one important factor that must be noted is advancing age. Age is the dominant factor driving cancer risk; for all major malignancies, risk rises markedly with age. The importance of advancing age is exemplified by an estimate published by the American Cancer Society and National Cancer Institute, in which the aging U.S. population together with projected population growth will result in a doubling of the number of cancer cases diagnosed by the year 2050, assuming that incidence rates remain constant (Edwards et al., 2002). With this estimated growth in cancer from 1.3 million to 2.6 million cases per year, it is expected that both the number and the proportion of older persons with cancer will also rise dramatically. Diagnoses in individuals over age 75 are anticipated to increase from 30% to 42% of total cancer. Such projections further emphasize the importance of widespread interventions targeting individuals of all ages.

PREVENTION AND CESSATION OF TOBACCO USE

Use of tobacco is the major cause of premature death around the world, accounting for 4,907,000 deaths each year (Ezzati et al., 2002). In the United States, adult smokers lose an average of 13 years of life because of smoking, and approximately half of all smokers die of tobacco-related disease. Smoking is well known to cause over 90% of lung cancers in addition to a range of other malignancies. It causes about 30% of all the cancer in the developed world, including cancers of the lung, mouth, larynx, esophagus, pancreas, cervix, kidney, and bladder. Growing evidence also links smoking to increased risk for cancers of the colon, stomach, cervix, liver, and prostate, as well as to leukemia. In addition, smoking leads to many other health problems, including heart disease, stroke, lung infections, and pregnancy complications (Ezzati et al., 2002).

Avoiding initiation of tobacco use offers the greatest potential for disease prevention, and for those who use tobacco products, there are substantial health benefits that come with quitting. Extensive research has shown the effectiveness of a variety of cessation methods, and in the past 25 years,

50% of all living Americans who have ever smoked have successfully quit (U.S. Department of Health and Human Services [USDHHS], 1990). In a USDHHS 1990 report on smoking cessation, the U.S. Surgeon General concluded that quitting smoking has immediate and significant health benefits for men and women of all ages. Strategies to assist smoking cessation and decrease youth initiation from both a population and a clinical perspective are essential steps to reducing the burden of cancer (Curry et al., 2003).

Trends

Current smoking among U.S. adults has remained steady over the past decade. Once quite pronounced, gender disparity in smoking rates is now relatively small and has been stable since 1990. In 2002, 25.7% of men were current smokers compared with 20.8% of women (Centers for Disease Control and Prevention [CDC], 2003a; Holtzman, Powell-Griner, Bolen, & Rhodes, 2000).

During the 1990s, smoking decreased somewhat in smokers age 35 and older, but smoking rates among younger adults ages 18 to 25 rose to an alarming level (CDC, 2003a). Traditionally, almost 90% of adult smokers began smoking by age 18. In 2001, 28.5% of U.S. high school students were current smokers (defined as having smoked a cigarette in the past 30 days; CDC, 2003b). This marked the first time in 10 years that adolescent smoking fell below 30%. Unfortunately, young adults now appear to be at risk for smoking initiation beyond age 18. This escalation in smoking behaviors in the college-age population has emerged as a concern in the medical and public health communities (Rigotti, Lee, & Wechsler, 2000; Wechsler, Rigotti, Gledhill-Hoyt, & Lee, 1998). Tobacco industry strategies, such as promotions in bars and on college campuses, encourage smoking among this age group and seemed to intensify after the tobacco industry was specifically prohibited by the Master Settlement Agreement (see http://ag.ca.gov/tobacco/pdf/1msa.pdf) from marketing to youth under age 18.

Disparities

The National Health Interview Survey found that in 2000, approximately 24% of Whites and 23% of Blacks were current smokers (CDC, 2002). Alaskan Natives and American Indians had the highest rates of smoking (36%), whereas Asians and Hispanics had the lowest (14% and 19%, respectively; CDC, 2002).

Smoking rates are closely tied to measures of socioeconomic status (SES), including income and education level. Across both gender and race, people of lower income are more likely to smoke than people of higher income (CDC, 2002; USDHHS, 2001). In addition, adolescents who grow up in low-income households or who have parents with low levels of educational attainment are more likely to begin smoking (USDHHS, 1994; USDHHS, 2001).

As with active tobacco use, there are gender, racial/ethnic, and SES disparities in smoking cessation. For example, women are less likely than men to successfully quit smoking (USDHHS, 1990), and African Americans have a lower quit rate than Whites (USDHHS, 1998). Cessation rates are also associated with years of education: For individuals with 16 or more years of education, the quit rate is 57%, whereas for those with less than 12 years of education, the rate is only 35% (USDHHS, 1990).

Given the profound impact of smoking on cancer, disparities in smoking rates and in access to effective cessation methods will continue to translate directly into differences in the burden of smoking-related cancers.

Please see chapters 9 and 10 of this volume for more on prevention and cessation of tobacco use.

PHYSICAL ACTIVITY

Inactivity causes over 1,922,000 deaths each year around the world (Ezzati et al., 2002). People in the United States and in other developed nations are extremely inactive—over 60% of the U.S. adult population does not participate in regular physical activity, which includes 25% of adults who are almost entirely sedentary (USDHHS, 1999). Fortunately, the negative effects of a sedentary lifestyle are reversible: Evidence shows that increasing one's level of physical activity, even after years of inactivity, can reduce mortality risk (Paffenbarger et al., 1993).

Inactivity increases the risk for colon and breast cancers and likely endometrial cancer (International Agency for Research on Cancer [IARC], 2002), as well as diabetes, osteoporosis, stroke, and coronary heart disease. Overall, sedentary lifestyles have been linked to 5% of deaths from cancer (Colditz et al., 1996). Among both men and women, high levels of physical activity may decrease the risk for colon cancer by as much as 50% (Colditz, Cannuscio, & Frazier, 1997; IARC, 2002). Using a variety of measures of activity, studies have consistently shown a dose–response relationship between physical activity and colon cancer in different populations (IARC, 2002). Physical activity also appears to lower the risk for large adenomatous polyps, suggesting that it may influence the early stages of the adenoma–carcinoma sequence (Giovannucci, Colditz, Stampfer, & Willett, 1996). In addition, the relationship between physical activity and breast and colon cancers is seen across levels of obesity, suggesting that physical activity and obesity have independent effects on cancer incidence (IARC, 2002). In addition to these accepted causal relations, growing evidence suggests that physical activity may be protective against lung and prostate cancer (IARC, 2002; Marrett, Theis, & Ashbury, 2000).

The benefits of physical activity include the prevention of cancer and a large number of other chronic diseases. Increasing levels of physical activity reduces mortality risk (Hu et al., 2004), and as little as 30 minutes of moderate physical activity (e.g., brisk walking) per day significantly reduces disease risk (Hu et al., 1999, 2000; Manson et al., 1999).

Please see chapter 14 of this volume for a more in-depth discussion of physical activity.

Trends

One major determinant of activity level that has changed over time is the amount of activity required for work and daily living (Hill & Melanson, 1999). Advances in technology and the development of labor-saving devices have greatly reduced the need for physical activity for transportation, household tasks, and occupational requirements. Today, the overall prevalence of physical inactivity in the United States is remarkably high: In 1996, about 28% of Americans reported absolutely no participation in leisure-time physical activity (Holtzman et al., 2000). In addition, physical activity in schools has declined, and almost half of young Americans between the ages of 12 and 21 are not vigorously active on a routine basis (USDHHS, 1996).

Disparities

Disparities in physical activity are well documented in terms of gender, race/ethnicity, education, income, and place of residence (Bolen, Rhodes, Powell-Griner, Bland, & Holtzman, 2000; CDC, 1998; Holtzman et al., 2000). According to the 1996 Behavioral Risk Factor Surveillance System data, women have a higher prevalence of leisure-time inactivity than do men (Holtzman et al., 2000). Inactivity is also more prevalent among African Americans (38.2%) than any other ethnic groups (American Indians and Alaskan Natives, 37.2%; Hispanics, 34.2%; Asian or Pacific Islanders, 28.9%; Whites, 25.1%; Bolen et al., 2000). In addition, there appears to be a dose–response relationship between physical inactivity and both education and income: Lower education and income levels are independently associated with higher rates of inactivity. Individuals with more education tend to be less inactive (CDC, 1998). Finally, the prevalence of inactivity is higher in rural areas (with populations smaller than 2,500) than in large metropolitan areas (with populations exceeding one million; CDC, 1998). As with income and education, there appears to be a gradient in the prevalence of inactivity: The more rural the place of residence, the more likely an individual is to report being inactive.

WEIGHT CONTROL AND OBESITY PREVENTION

Obesity is increasing at epidemic rates both in the United States and worldwide and is estimated to account for 2,591,000 deaths each year (Ezzati et al., 2002). Currently, almost 65% of American adults are overweight (body mass index [BMI] ≥ 25), and over 30% are considered obese (BMI ≥ 30; Flegal, Carroll, Ogden, & Johnson, 2002). Evidence clearly shows that excess weight has severe health consequences. Overweight and obesity cause a variety of cancers: colon, postmenopausal breast, endometrial, renal, and esophageal (IARC, 2002). The population attributable risks linked to obesity range from 9% for postmenopausal breast cancer to 39% for endometrial cancer. A study by Calle, Rodriguez, Walker-Thurmond, and Thun (2003) suggested that obesity influences an even broader range of cancers, increasing the risk for death from cancers of the colon and rectum, prostate, breast, esophagus, liver, gallbladder, pancreas, kidney, stomach, uterus, and cervix, in addition to non-Hodgkin's lymphoma and multiple myeloma. Overall, Calle et al. estimated that obesity causes 14% of cancer deaths among men and 20% of cancer deaths among women. In addition to raising the risk for cancer, overweight and obesity also increase the risk for a multitude of other diseases and chronic conditions, such as stroke, cardiovascular disease, Type 2 diabetes, osteoarthritis, and pregnancy complications.

Please see chapter 14 of this volume for more on weight control and obesity.

Trends

In the United States, the prevalence of overweight and obesity has increased at a dramatic rate. Over the past 30 years, the prevalence of overweight among adults rose by 40% (i.e., from 46.0% to 64.5%) and that of obesity rose by 110% (i.e., from 14.5% to 30.5%; Flegal et al., 2002). Even more alarming, this trend is also being seen among children and adolescents. The number of overweight children has nearly doubled, and the number of overweight adolescents has almost tripled over the past 3 decades (CDC, National Center for Health Statistics, 2002). Currently, more than 10% of 2- to 5-year-olds and 15% of 6- to 12-year-olds are overweight (BMI ≥ 95th percentile for age and gender; Ogden, Flegal, Carroll, & Johnson, 2002).

Disparities

Overweight and obesity vary by gender. In the United States between 1999 and 2000, 67.2% of men and 61.9% of women were overweight (BMI ≥ 25), and 33.4% of women and 27.5% of men were obese (BMI ≥ 30; Flegal et al., 2002). The racial/ethnic composition of the increasing prevalence of adult obesity shows that among non-Hispanic Black women and among Mexican American women, the prevalence of obesity was approximately 20% higher than among non-Hispanic White women in 2000. Among men, the prevalence of obesity was comparable across ethnic groups, but overweight was more common among Mexican American men than among non-Hispanic White and non-Hispanic Black men (Flegal et al., 2002).

The influence of socioeconomic factors is also being studied. Lower SES of the individual and higher measures of community socioeconomic disadvantage are independently associated with an elevated risk for obesity (Robert & Reither, 2004). Data from the National Health and Nutrition Examination Surveys suggest that although significant disparities persist, the association between SES and obesity has weakened considerably over time (Q. Zhang & Wang, 2004).

DIETARY IMPROVEMENTS

The effects of multiple dietary factors on the risk of cancer have been studied extensively. In some cases the evidence is clear; in other cases, studies have failed to show an effect or have reached contradictory conclusions.

Fruits and Vegetables

The global burden of inadequate fruit and vegetable intake is estimated to be 2,726,000 deaths each year from a variety of diseases and conditions. Although evidence for cardiovascular benefits and reduced risk for diabetes is clear (World Cancer Research Fund & American Institute for Cancer Research, 1997), evidence for cancer risk reduction has become less convincing with the results of numerous prospective cohort studies (Feskanich et al., 2000; Smith-Warner et al., 2001).

Still, low intake of fruits and vegetables is probably related to increased risk for cancers of the pancreas, bladder, lung, colon, mouth, pharynx, larynx, esophagus, and stomach (Curry et al., 2003). For prostate cancer, the data on fruit and vegetable intake remain inconsistent, even though nearly 20 studies have examined this issue. Results of the majority of these studies suggest that overall fruit and vegetable intake has little, if any, effect on prostate cancer risk. However, individual fruits and vegetables may offer the potential for greater risk reduction, with tomatoes being the most promising (Giovannucci, 1999).

Folate

A number of studies have found that as folate intake increases, the risk for colorectal cancer (as well as polyps) decreases (Freudenheim et al., 1991;

Giovannucci et al., 1993). The Nurses' Health Study found that a high intake of folate from fruits and vegetables was sufficient to lower risk, but supplementation with a multivitamin that contained folate offered even greater risk reductions (Giovannucci et al., 1998). The underlying biological role of folate and its interaction with the methylenetetrahydrofolate reductase (aka MTHFR) gene add support to the causal relation between low folate and colon cancer. In addition to the reduction in colon cancer risk, growing evidence suggests that folate also reduces the adverse effect of alcohol intake on breast cancer (S. M. Zhang et al., 2003).

Dietary Fat

Variations in international cancer rates have often been attributed to differences in total fat intake, yet more detailed evaluations have shown no clear link between dietary fat and breast (Hunter et al., 1996), colon (Giovannucci et al., 1994), or prostate (Kolonel, 1996) cancers. Although dietary fat overall does not appear to impact cancer risk, some evidence suggests that certain types of fat, such as animal fat, may increase risk (Willett, Stampfer, Colditz, Rosner, & Speizer, 1990).

Fiber

Fiber has been shown to reduce the risk for heart disease and diabetes, but it does not appear to offer protection against cancer. Although fiber intake has long been believed to help prevent colon cancer, the data do not support this hypothesis (Fuchs et al., 1999; Giovannucci et al., 1994).

Red Meat

High intake of red meat—including beef, pork, veal, and lamb—is associated with an elevated risk for colorectal cancer (Chao et al., 2005; Willett et al., 1990). The mechanism of this increased risk is not well understood, but it may be related to high concentrations of animal fat or to carcinogens produced when the meat is cooked at high temperatures.

Calcium

Higher calcium intake has been linked to a reduced risk for colorectal adenomatous polyps (Baron et al., 1999) and colorectal cancer (Wu, Willett, Fuchs, Colditz, & Giovannucci, 2002). However, increased dietary calcium is also associated with an increased risk for prostate cancer (Chan et al., 1998; Rodriguez et al., 2003). Research indicates that a moderate level of intake protects against colorectal cancer without greatly increasing prostate cancer risk.

Whole Grains

The benefits of whole-grain foods in reducing cardiovascular disease and ischemic stroke are well established (World Cancer Research Fund & American Institute for Cancer Research, 1997). Although grain products in general have not been shown to affect cancer risk, whole-grain foods may provide some protection against stomach cancer (Jacobs, Slavin, & Marquart, 1995). Because most of the fiber, vitamins, and minerals are removed during the process of refining grain, whole-grain foods tend to be more nutrient-rich than refined foods and may offer more in terms of disease prevention (World Cancer Research Fund & American Institute for Cancer Research, 1997).

Vitamin A and Carotenoids

Isolated vitamin A and carotenoids are not likely to play a large role in cancer prevention. Some observational data support a probable inverse relation with lung cancer risk, but randomized trials of beta-carotene intake found either no effect or an increased risk for lung cancer (Hennekens et al., 1996; Omenn et al., 1996). It has also been suggested that beta-carotene impacts breast cancer risk; however, it seems that, at best, there is only a small decrease in breast cancer risk associated with a high intake of carotenoids (S. Zhang et al., 1999).

Selenium

Ecological studies have suggested that increased selenium intake is associated with decreased risk for colon and breast cancer (Clark, 1985). A randomized controlled trial of selenium for skin cancer prevention showed no effect of selenium on skin cancer incidence; however, it did show a reduction in incidence of lung, colon, and prostate cancers (Clark et al., 1996). Despite these promising results, the impact of selenium remains unclear. Fortification of the soil in Finland in the mid-1980s led to higher blood selenium levels in that region, but no decline in incidence or mortality has been noted for prostate or colon cancer (Willett, 1999).

Please see chapter 11 of this volume for more on the link between diet and cancer.

LIMITATION OF ALCOHOL USE

Globally, excessive alcohol intake is responsible for 1,804,000 deaths each year (Ezzati et al., 2002). Clear benefits of moderate alcohol intake have been shown in terms of reducing cardiac and diabetes risk, but alcohol remains a risk factor for cancer mortality (Thun et al., 1997). To balance the cardiovascular benefits with the risks of cancer and other negative consequences, it is recommended that those who drink alcohol should do so only in moderation. Intake should be limited to less than one drink per day for women and less than two drinks per day for men.

Trends and Disparities

Twenty percent of drinkers consume more than 85% of all the alcohol consumed in the United States (Greenfield & Rogers, 1999). Men tend to be the heaviest drinkers, accounting for about 75% of the country's total consumption. Young adults ages 18 to 29 are also disproportionately represented at the heaviest levels of consumption.

The National Health Interview Survey (National Center for Health Statistics, 1998) data indicate that at every age, the proportion of current drinkers is highest for non-Hispanic White men, followed by non-Hispanic Black men, and then Hispanic men (CDC, National Center for Health Statistics, 2000). Among women, the proportion of current drinkers is also highest among non-Hispanic White women at every age. Between the ages of 18 and 24, the proportion of Hispanic women who drink is higher than that of non-Hispanic Black women. This trend is reversed between the ages of 25 and 44. In women 45 and older, the percentage of current drinkers is similar among Hispanic and non-Hispanic Black women (~32%) but is still considerably lower than among non-Hispanic White women (51%). The national surveys on consumption patterns do not present data by SES.

SAFER SEX AND DECREASED VIRAL TRANSMISSION

Unsafe sex is responsible for 2,886,000 deaths each year (Ezzati et al., 2002), primarily because of the transmission of human immunodeficiency virus (HIV). However, unprotected sexual contact also results in the spread of multiple other sexually transmitted infections, including oncogenic viruses. Some of these viruses may also be spread through exposure to blood and blood products.

Human papillomavirus (HPV) causes cervical, vulvar, penile, and anal cancers; hepatitis B and C virus cause hepatocellular cancer; human lymphotropic virus–Type 1 is associated with adult T-cell leukemia; HIV-1 causes Kaposi's sarcoma and non-Hodgkin's lymphoma; and human herpes virus causes Kaposi's sarcoma and body cavity lymphoma.

Prevention strategies to contain the spread of these viruses should include behavioral and educational interventions to modify sexual behavior (U.S. Institute of Medicine, 1997) and structural and regulatory changes to promote safer sex and make condoms readily available. Biomedical interventions to develop and administer vaccines are also needed (Koutsky et al., 2002). For example, it is estimated that vaccination programs could reduce the global burden of liver cancer by 60% (Stuver, 1998). Additional strategies to prevent viral spread include needle exchange programs for intravenous drug users, regulation of tattooing and acupuncture, screening of blood donors, and the development of artificial blood products.

Please see chapter 13 of this volume for more on gynecological cancers.

Trends and Disparities

Current U.S. data on the prevalence of these different viruses is not adequate to predict trends in cancer incidence. In addition, the development of new technologies, such as vaccines against HPV, suggests that a new era in prevention of cervical cancer may be imminent. However, for success, such vaccines must be available and accessible to the entire population. Barriers for different segments of the population must be identified and overcome. Assuring such access remains a policy priority to maximize the potential benefit of this cancer prevention strategy.

SUN PROTECTION

The American Cancer Society estimates that more than 50,000 melanomas and more than 1 million non-melanomatous skin cancers are diagnosed each year in the United States. Exposure to solar radiation is the major modifiable cause of melanoma (English, Armstrong, Kricker, & Fleming, 1997) and other skin cancers. For most people, most lifetime sun exposure occurs during childhood and adolescence, and migrant studies clearly show that age at migration to high-risk countries has a strong impact on risk for this malignancy. For this reason, early intervention has the greatest potential for prevention.

Please see chapter 12 of this volume for more on melanoma and other skin cancers.

Trends and Disparities

The incidence of melanoma is rising more rapidly than that of any cancer in the United States. The increasing rates over the past 40 years reflect increasing sun exposure. Incidence rose through 1997 among both women and men, with the most rapid rise observed in older men.

The risk for melanoma and other less aggressive forms of skin cancer exists for all racial and ethnic groups, but skin cancers occur predominantly in the non-Hispanic White population. Constitutional characteristics, including hair color, nevus count, and family history, contribute to risk for melanoma. However, studies show that established risk factors alone do not identify a sufficient proportion of cases to focus prevention efforts on only a subset of the population (English & Armstrong, 1988). Because identifying high-risk individuals will miss the majority of cases, population-based efforts are likely to provide greater protection. Prevention efforts to limit sun exposure have been successfully implemented in numerous small studies. However, strategies to promote risk reduction through limiting sun exposure continue to be debated, and the potential to tailor messages to those with high-risk phenotypes remains an important question. Regardless of the resolution of this academic debate, there is tremendous potential to substantially reduce the burden of this common malignancy through effective prevention efforts.

SCREENING

Screening for cancer can provide protection in several ways. In the case of colorectal and cervical cancers, screening can detect premalignant changes that can be treated to prevent cancer from developing. This primary prevention has the potential to reduce the burden of cancer.

If cancer is already present, screening can act as a secondary prevention, facilitating early diagnosis and treatment, thereby decreasing morbidity and mortality. This type of prevention is an added benefit of colorectal and cervical screening, and it is the main goal of breast cancer and prostate cancer screening.

Please see chapters 15 and 16 of this volume for more on cancer screenings.

Trends and Disparities

Trends in cervical cancer screening have been impacted by the Breast and Cervical Cancer Prevention and Treatment Act (2000), which provided resources to states, through the CDC, to bring screening services to low-income women. National data suggest that low-income and Hispanic women are less likely to be current with screening recommendations (Swan, Breen, Coates, Rimer, & Lee 2003). Lack of access to care, defined as not having a usual source of care, was associated with significantly lower compliance with cervical screening. Evidence from the 1998 Health Interview Survey indicates that all U.S.-born women have comparable and high compliance with screening for cervical cancer. Foreign-born women, however, appear to be underscreened, accounting for the disparity among Hispanic women and suggesting a priority area for prevention as the United States continues to have a large immigrant population at risk for cancer (Goel et al., 2003).

CONCLUSION

Lifestyle changes offer tremendous potential to prevent cancer and many other chronic conditions. This potential is often underestimated, not only by the public but also by many health professionals. For behavioral change interventions to have the greatest impact possible, they must be multifaceted and have a broad reach. Approaches are needed to target individuals, communities, and systems, and to create an environment more conducive to healthy lifestyles. Social systems and regulatory efforts must complement individual behavior changes if these changes are to be sustained and the benefits of reduced disease burden realized (Atwood, Colditz, & Kawachi, 1997).

Outside of lifestyle factors, efforts must also continue to support the creation and enforcement of regulations controlling occupational and environmental hazards. Although such exposures account for a relatively small number of cancer cases compared with the lifestyle factors considered previously (Monson & Christiani, 1997), the burden of exposure to these harmful agents may be disproportionately high among low-income populations, accentuating their cancer risk. To be successful, we must largely reframe our approach to cancer prevention (Rockhill, Kawachi, & Colditz, 2000). The old paradigm of identifying risk factors and setting goals for reduction is only the beginning. Research and policy must now focus on bringing about population-wide lifestyle change, addressing the broad issues of disparities, and leaving no group or community behind.

REFERENCES

Atwood, K., Colditz, G., & Kawachi, I. (1997). Implementing prevention policies: Relevance of the Richmond model to health policy judgments. *American Journal of Public Health, 87,* 1603–1606.

Baron, J. A., Beach, M., Mandel, J. S., van Stolk, R. U., Haile, R. W., Sandler, R. S., et al. (1999). Calcium supplements for the prevention of colorectal adenomas: Calcium Polyp Prevention Study Group. *New England Journal of Medicine, 340,* 101–107.

Bolen, J. C., Rhodes, L., Powell-Griner, E. E., Bland, S. D., & Holtzman, D. (2000). State-specific prevalence of selected health behaviors, by race and ethnicity— Behavioral Risk Factor Surveillance System, 1997. *Morbidity and Mortality Weekly Report CDC Surveillance Summaries, 49,* 1–60.

Breast and Cervical Cancer Prevention and Treatment Act of 2000, Pub. L. No. 106–354, 114 Stat. 1381 (2000).

Calle, E. E., Rodriguez, C., Walker-Thurmond, K., & Thun, M. J. (2003). Overweight, obesity, and mortality from cancer in a prospectively studied cohort of U.S. adults. *New England Journal of Medicine, 348,* 1625–1638.

Centers for Disease Control and Prevention. (1998). Self-reported physical inactivity by degree of urbanization—United States, 1996. *Morbidity and Mortality Weekly Report, 47,* 1097–1100.

Centers for Disease Control and Prevention. (2002). Cigarette smoking among adults—United States, 2000. *Morbidity and Mortality Weekly Report, 51,* 642–645.

Centers for Disease Control and Prevention. (2003a, February 19). *Behavioral risk factor surveillance system.* Retrieved August 30, 2003, from http://apps.nccd.cdc.gov/brfss

Centers for Disease Control and Prevention. (2003b, May 29). *Youth risk behavior surveillance system.* Retrieved August 30, 2003, from http://apps.nccd.cdc.gov/yrbss

Centers for Disease Control and Prevention, National Center for Health Statistics. (2000, July 26). *Table 65. Alcohol consumption by persons 18 years of age and over, according to sex, race, Hispanic origin, and age: United States, 1997 and 1998.* Retrieved March 8, 2001, from http://www.cdc.gov/nchs/products/pubs/pubd/hus/hus.htm

Centers for Disease Control and Prevention, National Center for Health Statistics. (2002). *Prevalence of overweight among children and adolescents: United States, 1999–2000: Health e-stats.* Retrieved February 25, 2005, from http://www.cdc.gov/nchs/products/pubs/pubd/hestats/overwght99.htm

Chan, J. M., Giovannucci, E., Andersson, S. O., Yuen, J., Adami, H. O., & Wolk, A. (1998). Dairy products, calcium, phosphorous, vitamin D, and risk of prostate cancer (Sweden). *Cancer Causes Control, 9,* 559–566.

Chao, A., Thun, M. J., Connell, C. J., McCullough, M. L., Jacobs, E. J., Flanders, W. D., et al. (2005). Meat consumption and risk of colorectal cancer. *Journal of the American Medical Association, 293,* 172–182.

Clark, L. C. (1985). The epidemiology of selenium and cancer. *Federation Proceedings, 44,* 2584–2589.

Clark, L. C., Combs, G. F., Jr., Turnbull, B. W., Slate, E. H., Chalker, D. K., Chow, J., et al. (1996). Effects of selenium supplementation for cancer prevention in patients with carcinoma of the skin: A randomized controlled trial. Nutritional Prevention of Cancer Study Group. *Journal of the American Medical Association, 276,* 1957–1963.

Colditz, G. A., Cannuscio, C. C., & Frazier, A. L. (1997). Physical activity and reduced risk of colon cancer: Implications for prevention. *Cancer Causes Control, 8,* 649–667.

Colditz, G. A., DeJong, W., Hunter, D. J., Trichopoulos, D., & Willett, W. C. (Eds.). (1996). Harvard report on cancer prevention. *Cancer Causes Control, 7*(Suppl.), 1–55.

Curry, S., Byers, T., & Hewitt, M. (2003). *Fulfilling the potential of cancer prevention and early detection*. Washington, DC: National Academies Press.

Edwards, B. K., Howe, H. L., Ries, L. A., Thun, M. J., Rosenberg, H. M., Yancik, R., et al. (2002). Annual report to the nation on the status of cancer, 1973–1999, featuring implications of age and aging on U.S. cancer burden. *Cancer, 94*, 2766–2792.

English, D. R., & Armstrong, B. K. (1988, May 7). Identifying people at high risk of cutaneous malignant melanoma: Results from a case-control study in western Australia. *BMJ, 296*, 1285–1288.

English, D. R., Armstrong, B. K., Kricker, A., & Fleming, C. (1997). Sunlight and cancer. *Cancer Causes Control, 8*, 271–283.

Ezzati, M., Lopez, A. D., Rodgers, A., Vander Hoorn, S., & Murray, C. J. (2002, November 2). Selected major risk factors and global and regional burden of disease. *Lancet, 360*, 1347–1360.

Feskanich, D., Ziegler, R. G., Michaud, D. S., Giovannucci, E. L., Speizer, F. E., Willett, W. C., & Colditz, G. A. (2000). Prospective study of fruit and vegetable consumption and risk of lung cancer among men and women. *Journal of the National Cancer Institute, 92*, 1812–1823.

Flegal, K. M., Carroll, M. D., Ogden, C. L., & Johnson, C. L. (2002). Prevalence and trends in obesity among U.S. adults, 1999–2000. *Journal of the American Medical Association, 288*, 1723–1727.

Freudenheim, J. L., Graham, S., Marshall, J. R., Haughey, B. P., Cholewinski, S., & Wilkinson, G. (1991). Folate intake and carcinogenesis of the colon and rectum. *International Journal of Epidemiology, 20*, 368–374.

Fuchs, C. S., Giovannucci, E. L., Colditz, G. A., Hunter, D. J., Stampfer, M. J., Rosner, B., et al. (1999). Dietary fiber and the risk of colorectal cancer and adenoma in women. *New England Journal of Medicine, 340*, 169–176.

Giles, G. G., Armstrong, B. K., Burton, R. C., Staples, M. P., & Thursfield, V. J. (1996, May 4). Has mortality from melanoma stopped rising in Australia? Analysis of trends between 1931 and 1994. *BMJ, 312*, 1121–1125.

Giovannucci, E. (1999). Tomatoes, tomato-based products, lycopene, and cancer: Review of the epidemiologic literature. *Journal of the National Cancer Institute, 9*, 317–331.

Giovannucci, E., Colditz, G. A., Stampfer, M. J., & Willett, W. C. (1996). Physical activity, obesity, and risk of colorectal adenoma in women (United States). *Cancer Causes Control, 7*, 253–263.

Giovannucci, E., Rimm, E. B., Stampfer, M. J., Colditz, G. A., Ascherio, A., & Willett, W. C. (1994). Intake of fat, meat, and fiber in relation to risk of colon cancer in men. *Cancer Research, 54*, 2390–2397.

Giovannucci, E., Stampfer, M. J., Colditz, G. A., Hunter, D. J., Fuchs, C., Rosner, B. A., et al. (1998). Multivitamin use, folate, and colon cancer in women in the Nurses' Health Study. *Annals of Internal Medicine, 129*, 517–524.

Giovannucci, E., Stampfer, M. J., Colditz, G. A., Rimm, E. B., Trichopoulos, D., Rosner, B. A., et al. (1993). Folate, methionine, and alcohol intake and risk of colorectal adenoma. *Journal of the National Cancer Institute, 85,* 875–884.

Goel, M. S., Wee, C. C., McCarthy, E. P., Davis, R. B., Ngo-Metzger, Q., & Phillips, R. S. (2003). Racial and ethnic disparities in cancer screening: The importance of foreign birth as a barrier to care. *Journal of General Internal Medicine, 18,* 1028–1035.

Greenfield, T. K., & Rogers, J. D. (1999). Who drinks most of the alcohol in the U.S.? The policy implications. *Journal of Studies on Alcohol, 60,* 78–89.

Hennekens, C. H., Buring, J. E., Manson, J. E., Stampfer, M., Rosner, B., Cook, N. R., et al. (1996). Lack of effect of long-term supplementation with beta carotene on the incidence of malignant neoplasms and cardiovascular disease. *New England Journal of Medicine, 334,* 1145–1149.

Hill, J. O., & Melanson, E. L. (1999). Overview of the determinants of overweight and obesity: Current evidence and research issues. *Medicine and Science in Sports and Exercise, 31*(Suppl.), 515–521.

Holtzman, D., Powell-Griner, E., Bolen, J. C., & Rhodes, L. (2000). State- and sex-specific prevalence of selected characteristics—Behavioral risk factor surveillance system, 1996 and 1997. *Morbidity and Mortality Weekly Report CDC Surveillance Summaries, 49,* 1–39.

Hu, F. B., Sigal, R. J., Rich-Edwards, J. W., Colditz, G. A., Solomon, C. G., Willett, W. C., et al. (1999). Walking compared with vigorous physical activity and risk of Type 2 diabetes in women: A prospective study. *Journal of the American Medical Association, 282,* 1433–1439.

Hu, F. B., Stampfer, M. J., Colditz, G. A., Ascherio, A., Rexrode, K. M., Willett, W. C., & Manson, J. E. (2000). Physical activity and risk of stroke in women. *Journal of the American Medical Association, 283,* 2961–2967.

Hu, F. B., Willett, W. C., Li, T., Stampfer, M. J., Colditz, G. A., & Manson, J. E. (2004). Adiposity as compared with physical activity in predicting mortality among women. *New England Journal of Medicine, 351,* 2694–2703.

Hunter, D. J., Spiegelman, D., Adami, H. O., Beeson, L., van den Brandt, P. A., Folsom, A. R., et al. (1996). Cohort studies of fat intake and the risk of breast cancer—A pooled analysis. *New England Journal of Medicine, 334,* 356–361.

International Agency for Research on Cancer. (2002). *IARC handbook: Vol. 6. Weight control and physical activity.* Lyon, France: International Agency for Research on Cancer.

Jacobs, D. R., Jr., Slavin, J., & Marquart, L. (1995). Whole-grain intake and cancer: A review of the literature. *Nutrition and Cancer, 24,* 221–229.

Kolonel, L. N. (1996). Nutrition and prostate cancer. *Cancer Causes Control, 7,* 83–44.

Koutsky, L. A., Ault, K. A., Wheeler, C. M., Brown, D. R., Barr, E., Alvarez, F. B., et al. (2002). A controlled trial of a human papillomavirus type 16 vaccine. *New England Journal of Medicine, 347,* 1645–1651.

Laara, E., Day, N. E., & Hakama, M. (1987, May 30). Trends in mortality from cervical cancer in the Nordic countries: Association with organised screening programmes. *Lancet, 1*, 1247–1249.

Manson, J. E., Hu, F. B., Rich-Edwards, J. W., Colditz, G. A., Stampfer, M. J., Willett, W. C., et al. (1999). A prospective study of walking as compared with vigorous exercise in the prevention of coronary heart disease in women. *New England Journal of Medicine, 341*, 650–658.

Marrett, L. D., Theis, B., & Ashbury, F. D. (2000). Workshop report: Physical activity and cancer prevention. *Chronic Diseases in Canada, 21*, 143–149.

Monson, R. R., & Christiani, D. C. (1997). Summary of the evidence: Occupation and environment and cancer. *Cancer Causes Control, 8*, 529–531.

Murray, C., & Lopez, A. (1996). *The global burden of disease*. Geneva, Switzerland: World Health Organization.

National Center for Health Statistics. (1998). National Health Interview Survey. Available from http://www.cdc.gov/nchs/nhis.htm

Ogden, C. L., Flegal, K. M., Carroll, M. D., & Johnson, C. L. (2002). Prevalence and trends in overweight among US children and adolescents, 1999–2000. *Journal of the American Medical Association, 288*, 1728–1732.

Omenn, G. S., Goodman, G. E., Thornquist, M. D., Balmes, J., Cullen, M. R., Glass, A., et al. (1996). Effects of a combination of beta carotene and vitamin A on lung cancer and cardiovascular disease. *New England Journal of Medicine, 334*, 1150–1155.

Paffenbarger, R. S., Jr., Hyde, R. T., Wing, A. L., Lee, I. M., Jung, D. L., & Kampert, J. B. (1993). The association of changes in physical-activity level and other lifestyle characteristics with mortality among men. *New England Journal of Medicine, 328*, 538–545.

Rigotti, N. A., Lee, J. E., & Wechsler, H. (2000). U.S. college students' use of tobacco products: Results of a national survey. *Journal of the American Medical Association, 284*, 699–705.

Robert, S. A., & Reither, E. N. (2004). A multilevel analysis of race, community disadvantage, and body mass index among adults in the U.S. *Social Science & Medicine, 59*, 2421–2434.

Rockhill, B., Kawachi, I., & Colditz, G. A. (2000). Individual risk prediction and population-wide disease prevention. *Epidemiologic Reviews, 22*, 176–180.

Rodriguez, C., McCullough, M. L., Mondul, A. M., Jacobs, E. J., Fakhrabadi-Shokoohi, D., Giovannucci, E. L., et al. (2003). Calcium, dairy products, and risk of prostate cancer in a prospective cohort of United States men. *Cancer Epidemiology, Biomarkers & Prevention, 12*, 597–603.

Smith-Warner, S. A., Spiegelman, D., Yaun, S. S., Adami, H. O., Beeson, W. L., van den Brandt, P. A., et al. (2001). Intake of fruits and vegetables and risk of breast cancer: A pooled analysis of cohort studies. *Journal of the American Medical Association, 285*, 769–776.

Stuver, S. O. (1998). Towards global control of liver cancer? *Seminars in Cancer Biology, 8*, 299–306.

Swan, J., Breen, N., Coates, R. J., Rimer, B. K., & Lee, N. C. (2003). Progress in cancer screening practices in the United States: Results from the 2000 National Health Interview Survey. *Cancer, 97*, 1528–1540.

Thun, M. J., Peto, R., Lopez, A. D., Monaco, J. H., Henley, S. J., Heath, C. W., Jr., & Doll, R. (1997). Alcohol consumption and mortality among middle-aged and elderly U.S. adults. *New England Journal of Medicine, 337*, 1705–1714.

U.S. Department of Health and Human Services. (1990). *The health benefits of smoking cessation. A report of the Surgeon General.* Rockville, MD: Author.

U.S. Department of Health and Human Services. (1994). *Preventing tobacco use among young people: A report of the Surgeon General.* Atlanta, GA: U.S. Department of Health and Human Services, Public Health Service, Centers for Disease Control, Center for Chronic Disease Prevention and Health Promotion, Office on Smoking and Health.

U.S. Department of Health and Human Services. (1996). *Physical activity and health: A report of the Surgeon General.* Atlanta, GA: Author.

U.S. Department of Health and Human Services. (1998). *BRFSS tobacco use among US racial/ethnic minority groups.* Washington, DC: Author.

U.S. Department of Health and Human Services. (2001). *Women and smoking: A report of the Surgeon General.* Washington DC: Author.

U.S. Department of Health and Human Services, Centers for Disease Control and Prevention. (1999). *Promoting physical activity: A guide for community action.* Champaign, IL: Human Kinetics.

U.S. Institute of Medicine. (1997). *The hidden epidemic: Confronting sexually transmitted diseases.* Washington DC: National Academies Press.

Wechsler, H., Rigotti, N. A., Gledhill-Hoyt, J., & Lee, H. (1998). Increased levels of cigarette use among college students: A cause for national concern. *Journal of the American Medical Association, 280*, 1673–1678.

Willett, W. C. (1999). Goals for nutrition in the year 2000. *CA: A Cancer Journal for Clinicians, 49*, 331–352.

Willett, W. C., Stampfer, M. J., Colditz, G. A., Rosner, B. A., & Speizer, F. E. (1990). Relation of meat, fat, and fiber intake to the risk of colon cancer in a prospective study among women. *New England Journal of Medicine, 323*, 1664–1672.

Wingo, P. A., Ries, L. A., Giovino, G. A., Miller, D. S., Rosenberg, H. M., Shopland, D. R., et al. (1999). Annual report to the nation on the status of cancer, 1973–1996, with a special section on lung cancer and tobacco smoking. *Journal of the National Cancer Institute, 91*, 675–690.

World Cancer Research Fund & American Institute for Cancer Research. (1997). *Food, nutrition, and the prevention of cancer: A global perspective.* Washington, DC: American Institute for Cancer Research.

Wu, K., Willett, W. C., Fuchs, C. S., Colditz, G. A., & Giovannucci, E. L. (2002). Calcium intake and risk of colon cancer in women and men. *Journal of the National Cancer Institute, 94*, 437–446.

Zhang, Q., & Wang, Y. (2004). Trends in the association between obesity and socio-economic status in U.S. adults: 1971–2000. *Obesity Research, 12*, 1622–1632.

Zhang, S. M., Hunter, D. J., Hankinson, S. E., Giovannucci, E. L., Rosner, B. A., Colditz, G. A., et al. (1999). A prospective study of folate intake and the risk of breast cancer. *Journal of the American Medical Association, 281*, 1632–1637.

Zhang, S. M., Willett, W. C., Selhub, J., Hunter, D. J., Giovannucci, E. L., Holmes, M. D., et al. (2003). Plasma folate, vitamin B6, vitamin B12, homocysteine, and risk of breast cancer. *Journal of the National Cancer Institute, 95*, 373–380.

3

CREATION OF A FRAMEWORK FOR PUBLIC HEALTH INTERVENTION DESIGN

DEBORAH J. BOWEN, CAROL MOINPOUR, BETI THOMPSON,
M. ROBYN ANDERSEN, HENDRIKA MEISCHKE,
AND BARB COCHRANE

This chapter describes our application of Weiner's (1995) three-step process to develop an evidence-based theoretical framework for public health intervention design. Our first step was to read the literature on the use of health behavior and health behavior change theories and models in designing interventions. We focused on those theories and models that have been used to design published interventions and that have empirical support. Through this consideration, we identified a relatively small number of common variables that consistently predicted health behavior change and represented key research findings. Next, we ordered these variables into an initial framework, or classification system. We present this framework in this chapter. Our third step, actively applying this framework to intervention settings by measuring constructs in the intervention over time and using these measures to predict change in health behavior, will be conducted in future research programs. The organization of this chapter follows these three steps First, we discuss existing theories and their usefulness for intervention design. Then we combine these models into a single model, identifying commonalities among the models. Finally, we suggest future directions for research.

THE BASIS OF THE FRAMEWORK: EXISTING THEORIES

Individual-Level Theories

Investigators can choose multiple individual-level theories from which to choose when designing a framework for behavioral intervention. The idea behind the use of individual theories is that people make choices about health protection and health behaviors because of specific motivations, often thoughts or feelings. Understanding these thoughts and feelings and ultimately changing them in the appropriate directions will cause individuals' health behaviors to change as well.

Health belief models, like the original Health Belief Model are the most widely used in intervention design. The original formulation of the Health Belief Model in health promotion and disease prevention research addressed threat (i.e., perceived susceptibility and perceived severity) and outcome expectations (i.e., perceived benefits and perceived barriers). Other models were developed in response to the original Health Belief Model. One such example is the Protection Motivation Theory (R. W. Rogers & Mewborn, 1976), a cognitive theory (i.e., value expectancy theory) that posits that behavior is influenced by a person's subjective value of the outcome and by his or her subjective expectation that something he or she does will result in the desired outcome.

The Theory of Reasoned Action (Ajzen & Fishbein, 1980; Fishbein & Ajzen, 1975) explains individuals' health behavior as a function of their intentions, attitudes, and beliefs regarding health behavior, including nonhealth beliefs and beliefs about the social influences exerted by others. The Theory of Planned Behavior (Ajzen, 1991; Ajzen & Madden, 1986) builds on the Theory of Reasoned Action by adding to the model perceived behavioral control over the ability to perform the health behavior.

The Self-Regulation Model (Leventhal & Cameron, 1987; Leventhal, Diefenbach, & Leventhal, 1992) adds affect and the emotional response to the health problem as predictors in the equation. The Transactional Model of Stress and Coping, a cognitive behavior framework for addressing health promotion and disease prevention, describes a person's interaction with stressful environmental events through an appraisal of the stressor and its management, resulting in adaptation to the situation (Lazarus, 1991, 1993; Lazarus & Folkman, 1984).

The Transtheoretical Model of behavior change and the Precaution Adoption Model both hypothesize that people make changes in their health habits gradually, using different processes of change at different times and progressing through predictable stages of change (Prochaska & DiClemente, 1982, 1983; Weinstein, 1993). In addition, people in different stages of change perceive the pros and cons of changing their health behavior differently.

Miller, Shoda, and Hurley's (1996) Cognitive-Social Health Information Processing model goes beyond other models of behavior change in that it specifies characteristics of the individual, characteristics of the messages, and the basic elements of process among intermediate variables to explain and ultimately change behavior. Individuals who monitor their health and symptoms need more information, more attention, and more explanation than do those who simply want to move through an illness without observing and attending to its details and its associated symptoms and issues. A complex interplay of mechanisms is proposed to account for these differences, and this model has been used successfully in intervention design and evaluation to produce behavior change (Miller, Fang, Manne, Engstrom, & Daly, 1999; Miller et al., 1996).

Experimental psychology has contributed multiple theories of how individuals learn new behaviors to the design of health behavior interventions. The methods and strategies used in intervention research incorporate behavior modification and basic principles of conditioning (e.g., reinforcement; Abrams, Emmons, & Linnan, 1997; Pascale, Wing, Butler, Mullen, & Bononi, 1995; Redmon et al., 1999). According to social learning theory (Bandura, 1986, 1997), two basic belief systems drive behavior: *self-efficacy,* or the belief that the person has the resources to attain a proposed goal, and *outcome efficacy,* or the belief that the proposed goal is worth attaining. Indeed, values and goals represent a key, but understudied, component of decision making and behavior change in cancer risk and disease (Miller et al., 1996).

Community- or Group-Level Theories

Increasingly, there is recognition that a lifestyle behavior takes place in a complex web of formal and informal policies and actions that reflect a community's rules of conduct (Aarts, Paulussen, & Schaalma, 1997; Cohen, Scribner, & Farley, 2000; Thompson & Kinne, 1998). Community approaches to health behavior change have the potential to reach large numbers of people, to become widespread within a community, and to foster sustainability of behavior change as a particular behavior becomes normative in the community.

Ecological perspectives are specific about the influence of the environment: Behavior is greatly influenced by the social, cultural, and physical milieu within which individuals operate (McLeroy, Bibeau, Steckler, & Glanz, 1988; Stokols, 1992). Key concepts of theories within this perspective include (a) health is influenced by the social, physical, and interpersonal worlds; (b) environments are extremely complex, multidimensional, and difficult to measure; (c) environments can have many levels of aggregation from families to populations; and (d) there are reciprocal processes between the different levels of the environment. A specific example of an ecological model is the Diffusion of Innovations model. *Diffusion* is the process by which an innovation is communicated through certain channels over time among the members of a social system (E. M. Rogers, 1995). The *innovation* refers to an idea, practice, or object that is perceived as new by an individual or other unit of adoption.

The community organization approach (Minkler & Wallerstein, 1997; Rothman, 1979, 1996; Thompson & Kinne, 1998) includes four core constructs: (a) Community members must be engaged in problem solving (i.e., community participation); (b) all components of a community must be understood prior to any intervention (i.e., community analysis); (c) a process of intervention in which communities and their citizens gain control over their own problems should be used (i.e., empowerment); and (d) communities can be stimulated to take action toward solving their problems (i.e., mobilization). Community organization focuses on changing community structures, redistributing community resources, and instituting policies to ensure long-term change (Thompson et al., 1995).

Coalition building as a means to community change has received some attention (Carrell, Johnson, Stanley, Thompson, & Tosti, 1995; Salonen, Puska, Kottke, & Tuomilehto, 1981). A key assumption behind the coalition approach is that coalitions can have sufficient power to reach all community sectors and change community policies and norms. In the health field, coalitions are formed when diverse organizations within a community come together to address community health (National Cancer Institute, 1991; Pertschuk & Shopland, 1989). Community development theory has many similarities to a community organization approach. Historically, however, the main focus of community development is a community's economic development (Van Willigan, 1976). A secondary focus is in the area of education, seen as the key by which communities become stable and successful (i.e., the more educated a community, the more it will benefit; Chalmers & Bramadat, 1996; Kretzman & McKnight, 1993).

Social marketing is the design, implementation, and control of programs seeking to increase the acceptability of a social idea or practice in a target group. To maximize target group response, researchers use concepts of market segmentation, consumer research, idea configuration, communication, facilitation, incentives, and exchange theory (Walsh, Rudd, Moeykens, & Moloney, 1993). Successfully marketing ideas and behaviors in a social marketing campaign involves maximizing the four Ps—product, price, place, and promotion—by identifying the needs and wants of consumers. The roots of social marketing are found in the communication–persuasion matrix (McGuire, 1989). The underlying assumption of this theory is that people move through stages of exposure to postbehavioral consolidation in a conditional, sequential way. The persuasive context (e.g., source, messages) is assumed to allow for the questioning of the recipient's initial attitude, recommendation of the adoption of a new attitude, and provision of incentives (e.g., promises to reduce an unpleasant drive state such as fear) for attending to, understanding, yielding to, and retaining the new attitude (Petty & Cacioppo, 1996).

Finally, policy is a commonly used tool for implementing public health change. Public health policy (not to be confused with health care policy) focuses on attaining a broad vision of health. Policy advocates search for ways to reduce disparities in health attainment through changes at the structural level (Reutter & Williamson, 2000; Wallack, Dorfman, Jernigan, & Themba, 1993).

COMBINING THE EXISTING MODELS INTO A FRAMEWORK

Key Commonalities Among the Models

Common themes emerged from our reviews and discussions of the various theories and models and their contents. Many of the individual models were quite specific and well defined. We identified the key variables. This makes testing the usefulness of such models in predicting behavior change easier. Many larger level models (e.g., community and ecological models) presented principles and assumptions about factors related to behavior change but did not have detailed, testable hypotheses or specified variables with predeveloped measurement tools. The complexity of these approaches makes it difficult to explain how community-level events result in individual change. The evidence for models varied widely. Although the model or theory may have been used in the intervention design, it was not usually tested to evaluate the delivery and receipt of intervention strategies or the changes in key model variables and the behavioral outcomes. Several models (e.g., the Health Belief Model) provide key variables that should be targeted in interventions and that should change along with the main outcome variables. Others (e.g., community organization) simply provide principles of operation that should be used when delivering the intervention. A few models and theories (e.g., Transtheoretical, Self-Regulation, and Diffusion of Innovations models; some ecological approaches) have begun to describe the process of behavior change; however, in general, the steps or processes of changing health behavior over time are not clearly researched. Almost no framework or model truly integrates individual and societal perspectives, and very little research tests this combination of variables. This is perhaps the largest gap in the existing literature.

Synthesis Among the Models

Our next step was to summarize the common and divergent elements of the theories and models reviewed. This summary is presented in Figure 3.1. For each variable we have noted in Figure 3.1 where *any* attention has been paid

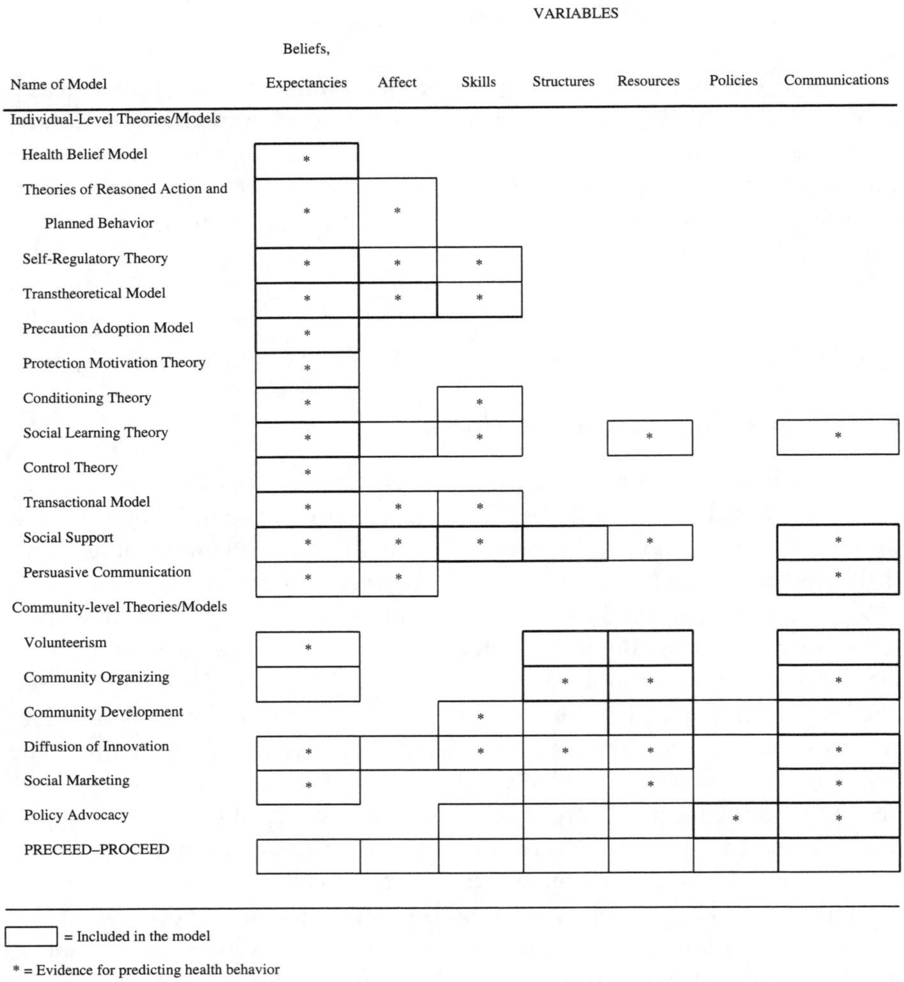

VARIABLES

Name of Model	Beliefs, Expectancies	Affect	Skills	Structures	Resources	Policies	Communications
Individual-Level Theories/Models							
Health Belief Model	*						
Theories of Reasoned Action and Planned Behavior	*	*					
Self-Regulatory Theory	*	*	*				
Transtheoretical Model	*	*	*				
Precaution Adoption Model	*						
Protection Motivation Theory	*						
Conditioning Theory	*		*				
Social Learning Theory	*		*		*		*
Control Theory	*						
Transactional Model	*	*	*				
Social Support	*	*	*		*		*
Persuasive Communication	*	*					*
Community-level Theories/Models							
Volunteerism	*						
Community Organizing				*	*		*
Community Development			*				
Diffusion of Innovation	*		*	*	*		*
Social Marketing	*				*		*
Policy Advocacy						*	*
PRECEED–PROCEED							

☐ = Included in the model

* = Evidence for predicting health behavior

Figure 3.1. Common variables across health behavior models and theories.

to measuring the construct (indicated by a box) and where some evidence exists in the literature to support the construct (indicated by an asterisk in the appropriate box). Beliefs are probably the most researched construct (most of the individual-level models include beliefs as a key construct), but these beliefs are often defined differently. For example, beliefs are named in the Health Belief Model and in the Precaution Adoption Model; however, similar constructs in the Self-Regulation Model are called *mental representations*. The two cornerstones of Social Learning Theory, self-efficacy and outcome efficacy, have been added to other models. Intentions to perform a behavior, identified through the theories of Reasoned Action and Planned Behavior, are very similar to a belief regarding one's future actions.

Both emotional and affective variables have been important in many models, including the Transtheoretical Model and the Transactional Model, and their relationship to each other and to health behavior outcomes needs to be better understood. Emotional or affective variables were proposed in four of the models we examined. Some models, such as the Transtheoretical Model, emphasize emotions as applied to specific issues, whereas the Transactional Model puts emphasis on general emotional reactions, such as anxiety or fear. The classic definition of *attitude*, central to much of social psychology, is a belief combined with a judgment of the importance of that belief, with that judgment being very similar to feeling or emotion.

Skills needed for behavior change include skills specific to the behavior as well as general skills to elicit social support, ask for help, and identify and use key coping strategies. Most of the models that explicitly identify skills as a component refer to them as *observable behaviors*. We define *cognitions* as skills and classify observations of these skills as collecting self-reported information. Cognitions are mutable under the same values and forces as are observable behaviors, thereby providing a method of changing beliefs.

We view constructs in the environmental-level theories as being organized around structures, resources, policies, and communications. *Structures* are the underlying systems within groups and organizations that facilitate or inhibit changes in health behavior. *Resources* are products within a system, community, or group that can be used to facilitate behavior change. Resources are necessary to ensure that the means for making changes are present in the environment and available to a substantial portion of the population. *Policies*, which correlate quite strongly with the social structures factor defined by Cohen et al. (2000), are rules and regulations at an organizational, community, or national level that make a behavior easier or more difficult to perform. Policies are both formal and informal. *Communications* are the processes whereby other aspects of the environment are made known to communities, organizations, and individuals. This term can refer to notifying a group regarding healthy behavior policies, appropriate structures for assistance in adopting a healthy behavior, or availability of resources. The importance of communication is recognized by the community organization approach, diffusion of innovations, social marketing, and policy advocacy views.

Figure 3.2 illustrates a framework that combines concepts from all the models and theories we identified and reviewed. There are two categories of critical variables identified within the framework: personal variables, which focus on individuals' ideas and thoughts, and environmental variables, which address the social setting within which people live. We assumed that some common influence among these variables existed, but identification of these kinds of correlations must wait for a full test of the framework.

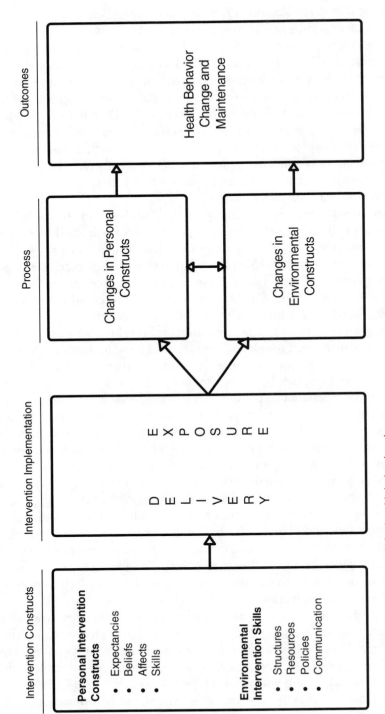

Figure 3.2. Potential framework for health behavior change.

Any intervention must be implemented to have an effect, and efforts have been made to define the process of implementation (Lichstein, Riedel, & Grieve, 1994). Here, we divided implementation into two parts, each measurable within the context of intervention research: (a) delivery (i.e., the intervention strategies must be delivered to the target population) and (b) exposure (i.e., the target population must be exposed to the strategies). Delivery can often be measured simply by counts of material sent, number of hours of contact time, interventionists' logbooks or other record keeping, or direct observations of content delivered. Delivery, however, is only a part of implementation. People must be exposed to the delivered intervention elements for them to produce an effect. Like delivery, exposure can be measured in multiple ways, such as by counting the number of people at events or actions resulting from the delivery of an intervention material or by simply asking target individuals whether they have seen or been part of intervention strategies. Then, of course, the intervention must be enacted or engaged by the target audience to have effect (Lichstein et al., 1994).

Finally, after intervention strategies have been delivered and exposure has occurred, we assume that key framework variables will change. Those changes will result in changes in the desired health behavior. The order in which these variables change, the importance of each variable in predicting outcome, and the relationships among intervention delivery and exposure and change in key framework variables are probably the least researched topics in this field. They are currently unknown for the framework we propose. This type of research, conducted using appropriate statistical techniques, should be a key part of every research project on health behavior interventions.

TAKING THE NEXT STEP

The next step in our systematic plan for developing a framework of health behavior change is to look for causal relationships among the variables in our current framework in an intervention setting. The variables identified from the literature have relationships between and among each other, and they need to be applied to a specific intervention and behavioral goal to be useful. Interventions occur at the individual level, the group or community level, or both, and the causal variables will likely interact to produce health behavior change (Emmons, 2000). In fact, the synergy of multiple components and levels of intervention is often assumed to produce successful change, although this is rarely tested.

This testing will allow us to identify and test specific hypotheses regarding the variables chosen for the initial framework. We will be able to confirm or disconfirm the usefulness of specific variables within constructs or, indeed, of entire constructs within the framework. This process will be laborious and will require application of the framework to multiple intervention settings. Several beliefs related to the specific health behavior would be measured both pre- and postintervention delivery. Each of those beliefs should change as a result of the intervention. Further, if we apply this framework we would hypothesize that the change in beliefs would predict change in health behavior. If change in only some of the beliefs predicts change in behavior, then the evidence for including those beliefs in the behavior-specific version of the framework is strengthened. If none of the beliefs predicts change in health behavior, then the evidence for including them as an important construct in the emerging framework is weakened. Finally, on the basis of previous research, we hypothesize that change in beliefs is related to change over time in specific resources that are intended to alter important beliefs, which then leads to a change in health behavior outcomes. Specific causal chains can and should be proposed a priori and tested as part of intervention evaluation and model building. A similar approach can be taken in assessing the influence of environmental factors. It will be important to understand, for instance, whether structures exist in communities to facilitate change. For example, if a number of studies indicate that specific health behavior change occurs even without an infrastructure to support such changes, the structural factor may not be a requirement for a comprehensive intervention.

Indeed, the process of changing health behavior is an understudied phenomenon in general. The analysis of interrelationships among the variables in this framework and their relative importance in any given behavior change setting is probably the most important aspect of our next step of applying the framework to intervention settings.

REFERENCES

Aarts, H., Paulussen, T., & Schaalma, H. (1997). Physical exercise habit: On the conceptualization and formation of habitual health behaviours. *Health Education Research, 12,* 363–374.

Abrams, D. B., Emmons, K. M., & Linnan, L. A. (1997). Health behavior and health education: The past, present, and future. In K. Glanz, F. M. Lewis, & B. K. Rimer (Eds.), *Health behavior and health education: Theory, research, and practice* (2nd ed., pp. 453–478). San Francisco: Jossey-Bass.

Ajzen, I. (1991). The theory of planned behavior. *Organizational Behavior and Human Decision Processes, 50,* 179–211.

Ajzen, I., & Fishbein, M. (1980). *Understanding attitudes and predicting social behavior.* Englewood Cliffs, NJ: Prentice Hall.

Ajzen, I., & Madden, T. J. (1986). Prediction of goal-directed behavior: Attitudes, intention, and perceived behavioral control. *Journal of Experimental and Social Psychology, 22,* 453–474.

Bandura, A. (1986). *Social foundations of thought and action: A social-cognitive theory.* Englewood Cliffs, NJ: Prentice Hall.

Bandura, A. (1997). *Self-efficacy: The exercise of control.* New York: Freeman.

Carrell, D. S., Johnson, C. L., Stanley, L. C., Thompson, J., & Tosti, S. (1995). *Changing public policy around tobacco control in the COMMIT communities. Community-based interventions for smokers: The COMMIT experience.* Bethesda, MD: U.S. Department of Health and Human Services.

Chalmers, K. I., & Bramadat, I. J. (1996). Community development: Theoretical and practical issues for community health nursing in Canada. *Journal of Advanced Nursing, 24,* 719–726.

Cohen, D. A., Scribner, R. A., & Farley, T. A. (2000). A structural model of health behavior: A pragmatic approach to explain and influence health behaviors at the population level. *Preventive Medicine, 30,* 146–154.

Emmons, K. M. (2000). Behavioral and social science contributions to the health of adults in the United States. In B. D. Smedley & L. S. Syme (Eds.), *Promoting health: Intervention strategies from social and behavioral research* (pp. 254–321). Washington, DC: National Academies Press.

Fishbein, M., & Ajzen, I. (1975). *Belief, attitude, intention, and behavior: An introduction to theory and research.* Reading, MA: Addison Wesley.

Kretzman, J., & McKnight, J. (1993). *Building communities from the inside out: A path toward finding and mobilizing a community's assets.* Evanston, IL: The Asset-Based Community Development Institute, Institute for Policy Research.

Lazarus, R. S. (1991). Progress on a cognitive–motivational–relational theory of emotion. *American Psychologist, 46,* 819–834.

Lazarus, R. S. (1993). Coping theory and research: Past, present, and future. *Psychosomatic Medicine, 55,* 234–247.

Lazarus, R. S., & Folkman, S. (1984). *Stress, appraisal, and coping.* New York: Springer Publishing Company.

Leventhal, H., & Cameron, L. (1987). Behavioral theories and the problem of compliance. *Patient Education and Counseling, 10,* 117–138.

Leventhal, H., Diefenbach, M. A., & Leventhal, E. A. (1992). Illness cognition: Using common sense to understand treatment adherence and affect cognition interactions. *Cognitive Therapy and Research, 16,* 143–163.

Lichstein, K. L., Riedel, B. W., & Grieve, R. (1994). Fair tests of clinical trials: A treatment implementation model. *Advances in Behavioral Research Therapy, 16,* 1–29.

McGuire, W. (1989). Theoretical foundations of campaigns. In R. E. Rice & C. K. Atkin (Eds.), *Public communication campaigns* (2nd ed., pp. 43–65). Newbury Park, CA: Sage.

McLeroy, K. R., Bibeau, D., Steckler, A., & Glanz, K. (1988). An ecological perspective on health promotion programs. *Health Education Quarterly, 15,* 351–377.

Miller, S. M., Fang, C. Y., Manne, S. L., Engstrom, P. E., & Daly, M. B. (1999). Decision making about prophylactic oophorectomy among at-risk women: Psychological influences and implications. *Gynecologic Oncology, 75,* 406–412.

Miller, S. M., Shoda, Y., & Hurley, K. (1996). Applying cognitive-social theory to health-protective behavior: Breast self-examination in cancer screening. *Psychological Bulletin, 119,* 70–94.

Minkler, M., & Wallerstein, N. (1997). Improving health through community organization and community building. In K. Glanz, F. M. Lewis, & B. K. Rimer (Eds.), *Health behavior and health education: Theory, research, and practice* (2nd ed., pp. 241–269). San Francisco: Jossey-Bass.

National Cancer Institute. (1991). *Assist program guidelines for tobacco-free communities.* Rockville, MD: Author.

Pascale, R. W., Wing, R. R., Butler, B. A., Mullen, M., & Bonomi, P. (1995). Effects of a behavioral weight loss program stressing calorie restriction versus calorie plus fat restriction in obese individuals with NIDDM or a family history of diabetes. *Diabetes Care, 18,* 1241–1248.

Pertschuk, M., & Shopland, D. R. (1989). *Major local smoking ordinances in the United States* (NIH Publication No. 90-479). Washington, DC: U.S. Department of Health and Human Services.

Petty, R. E., & Cacioppo, J. T. (1996). The message learning approach. In R. E. Petty & J. T. Cacioppo (Eds.), *Attitudes and persuasion: Classic and contemporary approaches* (pp. 59–94). Boulder, CO: Westview Press.

Prochaska, J. O., & DiClemente, C. C. (1982). Transtheoretical therapy: Toward a more integrative model of change. *Psychotherapy: Theory and Practice, 19,* 266–288.

Prochaska, J. O., & DiClemente, C. C. (1983). Stages and processes of self-change of smoking: Toward an integrative model of change. *Journal of Consulting and Clinical Psychology, 51,* 390–395.

Redmon, J. B., Raatz, S. K., Kwong, C. A., Swanson, J. E., Thomas, W., & Bantle, J. P. (1999). Pharmacologic induction of weight loss to treat Type 2 diabetes. *Diabetes Care, 22,* 896–903.

Reutter, L., & Williamson, D. L. (2000). Advocating healthy public policy: Implications for baccalaureate nursing education. *Journal of Nursing Education, 39,* 21–26.

Rogers, E. M. (1995). *Diffusion of innovations* (4th ed.). New York: Free Press.

Rogers, R. W., & Mewborn, C. R. (1976). Fear appeals and attitude change: Effects of a threat's noxiousness, probability of occurrence, and the efficacy of coping responses. *Journal of Personal and Social Psychology, 34,* 54–61.

Rothman, J. (1979). Three models of community organization practice. In F. M. Cox (Ed.), *Strategies of community organization: A book of readings* (3rd ed., pp. 86–102). Itasca, IL: F. E. Peacock.

Rothman, J. (1996). The interweaving of community intervention approaches. In M. Weil (Ed.), *Community practice: Conceptual models* (pp. 69–99). New York: Haworth Press.

Salonen, J. T., Puska, P., Kottke, T. E., & Tuomilehto, J. (1981). Changes in smoking, serum cholesterol, and blood pressure levels during a community-based cardiovascular disease prevention program—The North Karelia Project. *American Journal of Epidemiology, 114,* 81–94.

Stokols, D. (1992). Establishing and maintaining healthy environments. Toward a social ecology of health promotion. *American Psychologist, 47,* 6–22.

Thompson, B., & Kinne, S. (1998). Social change theory: Applications to community health. In N. F. Bracht (Ed.), *Health promotion at the community level* (2nd ed., pp. 29–46). Thousand Oaks, CA: Sage.

Thompson, B., Nettekoven, L., Ferster, D., Stanley, L. C., Thompson, J., & Corbett, K. K. (1995). *Mobilizing the COMMIT communities for smoking control community-based interventions for smokers: The COMMIT experience.* Bethesda, MD: U.S. Department of Health and Human Services.

Van Willigan, J. (1976). Applied anthropology and community development administration: A critical assessment. *Southern Anthropological Society Proceedings, 10,* 81–91.

Wallack, L., Dorfman, L., Jernigan, D., & Themba, M. (1993). *Media advocacy and public: Power for prevention.* Newbury Park, CA: Sage.

Walsh, D. C., Rudd, R. E., Moeykens, B. A., & Moloney, T. W. (1993). Social marketing for public health. *Health Affairs, 12,* 104–119.

Weiner, B. (1995). *Judgments of responsibility: A foundation for a theory of social conduct.* New York: Guilford Press.

Weinstein, N. D. (1993). Testing four competing theories of health-protective behavior. *Health Psychology, 12,* 324–333.

II

METHODOLOGY
IN CANCER PREVENTION
AND CONTROL

METHODOLOGY
IN CANCER PREVENTION
AND CONTROL

Part II reviews the major methodological topics in cancer control. Study design in intervention research has received increasing attention, given the recent emphasis on the evidence base for clinical and public health recommendations. In chapter 4, Curry, Wetter, Grothaus, McClure, and Taplin review the design of individual-level behavioral interventions for cancer control. They also discuss issues in the design of studies to evaluate such interventions, covering such topics as data collection, study participant recruitment and retention, data analysis and reporting, and the psychometric analysis of process and outcome measures. Chapter 5, by Murray, Pals, and Blitstein, reviews definitional, design, and statistical issues relating to group-randomized trials.

Finding effective ways to increase participation in clinical trials has been one of the main challenges in cancer control. A review of the issues and research findings in this area is the focus of chapter 6, by Paskett, Katz, DeGraffinreid, and Tatum. The chapter authors also offer recommendations for improving participation. Finally, quality-of-life assessment in cancer has burgeoned as an area of scientific focus in recent years. In chapter 7, Gotay discusses the major issues in the measurement of quality of life of cancer patients and also presents information on the intended use, content, and psychometric adequacy of quality-of-life instruments.

4

DESIGNING AND EVALUATING INDIVIDUAL-LEVEL INTERVENTIONS FOR CANCER PREVENTION AND CONTROL

SUSAN J. CURRY, DAVID W. WETTER, LOUIS C. GROTHAUS,
JENNIFER B. McCLURE, AND STEPHEN H. TAPLIN

Cancer prevention and control research is defined as "the conduct of basic and applied research in the behavioral, social, and population sciences that, independently or in combination with biomedical approaches, reduces cancer risk, incidence, morbidity, and mortality and improves quality of life" (Hiatt & Rimer, 1999, p. 957). Behavioral science is a cornerstone of cancer prevention and control efforts. One third of the annual cancer-related deaths are due to modifiable lifestyle factors such as tobacco use, alcohol consumption, poor nutrition, sun exposure, and behaviors resulting in cancer-related viral infections (e.g., hepatitis B, human papillomavirus, human immunodeficiency virus, human T-cell leukemia/lymphoma virus–1; American Cancer Society, 2000). Moreover, cancer survival rates could be increased through regular self-examination and screening behaviors (American Cancer Society, 2000). A recent Institute of Medicine Report estimates that 100,000 cancer cases and 60,000 cancer-related deaths could be prevented each year with modest increases in rates of behavioral risk factor reduction and increased participation in evidence-based screening (Curry, Byers, & Hewitt, 2003). More than 60% of the American Cancer Society's goals for reducing cancer incidence and mortality by the year 2015 could be met through behavioral changes such as smoking cessation, dietary modification, reduced drinking,

61

increased physical activity, and increased cancer screening (Byers et al., 1999).

Because behavior plays such an important role in reducing cancer risk, the modification of behavioral factors is the primary goal of most cancer prevention and control intervention studies. Greenwald and Cullen (1984) outlined five phases of cancer control research: hypothesis development, methods development, controlled intervention trials, defined population studies, and demonstration and implementation. Intervention research comprises two of these five phases (i.e., Phases III and IV) and so provides a bridge from basic biomedical research to national adoption and dissemination into health programs. This research must be well-designed, well-implemented, and well-evaluated if it is to advance knowledge of effective intervention strategies and techniques. This chapter discusses the application of behavioral science methods to intervention research in cancer prevention and control.

BEHAVIORAL INTERVENTIONS FOR CANCER PREVENTION AND CONTROL

Behavioral interventions for cancer prevention and control can be implemented at different levels. Winett, King, and Altman (1989) described a series of four levels: individual, interpersonal, organizational, and societal. Although the ultimate goal at each of these levels is to alter individual behavior, the intervention approaches differ for each level. Individual-level interventions target people either singly or in groups (e.g., one-on-one counseling or group therapy for dietary change). Interventions can also be delivered through interpersonal relations (e.g., physician advice to quit smoking), modifications of organizational structures (e.g., changes in health plan benefit policies or clinical practice infrastructure for promoting screening), or societal changes (e.g., tobacco control legislation, improved standards for school nutrition programs). Although each of these approaches is important in cancer prevention and control, this chapter focuses primarily on the design and evaluation of individual- and interpersonal-level interventions.

A well-designed behavioral intervention study has several key features. First, it is conceptually driven, meaning that the research questions and intervention components are developed on the basis of an explicit model of behavior change. Second, it uses a rigorous experimental or quasi-experimental design that allows the treatment to be compared with a control condition such as usual care. Third, the outcome measures are validated, replicable, and directly related to the cancer prevention objectives. Finally, the design allows for the assessment of process variables that can be used to evaluate the treatment's implementation and increase our understanding of the mechanisms that influence the target behavior(s).

CONCEPTUAL FRAMEWORKS

Sound behavioral research is conceptually driven. Depending on the nature of the behavior and intervention of interest, the conceptual framework may be based on one or more theoretical models. *Theory* has been defined as "a framework of interconnected concepts that gives meaning and explanation to relevant events and supports new insights and problem solving" (Lipsey, 1987). With respect to intervention studies for cancer prevention and control, one goal of theoretical models is to identify determinants of the target behavior, for example, biobehavioral models of health behavior (Baum & Posluszny, 1999), psychosocial models of compliance with mammography screening (McBride, Curry, Taplin, Anderman, & Grothaus, 1993), and anthropological models of dietary choices and modifications (Bennett, Smith, & Passin, 1943). Theoretical models also guide the measurement of key constructs, for example, scales to assess fat and fiber intake (Shannon, Kristal, Curry, & Beresford, 1997) or social normative influences on mammography screening (Montano & Taplin, 1991), and they define intervention components. Intervention components should logically flow from the theoretical determinants of the target behavior. For example, tobacco cessation interventions might include pharmacotherapy to address withdrawal due to nicotine dependence, dietary change interventions might teach skills related to food selection and preparation, and mammography screening interventions might target normative influences associated with participation in screening. Conceptual models help specify the variables that are expected to change as a result of the intervention and to determine the timing of data collection. Valid measures of intermediate or process outcomes allow researchers to assess whether changes in outcome are accompanied by changes in process. Equally important, they help researchers understand the lack of intervention effects. In addition, conceptual frameworks guide the selection of data-analytic strategies (e.g., decisions related to whether uniform results across all study participants or differing effects among different subpopulations are expected). Common conceptual frameworks can provide consistency in operational definitions of outcome measures, which facilitates cross-study comparisons and meta-analyses of study results.

COMMON INTERVENTION APPROACHES

In general, theoretical models of health behavior share two themes: Individuals must (a) be sufficiently motivated to attempt to change their behavior and (b) have, and perceive that they have, the requisite skills and supports to initiate and maintain changes in their behavior. Thus, behavioral interventions typically target individuals' motivation, self-efficacy, and skills to effect behavior change. Two of the most common intervention paradigms are motivational interviewing (Miller & Rollnick, 1991) and skills training (Marlatt & Gordon, 1985). Together, they offer a range of strategies targeting perceptions of personal risk, outcome expectations for change or the lack of change, self-efficacy, coping and problem-solving abilities, and enlisting social support. Motivational interviewing offers concrete strategies for working with individuals to enhance motivation for change and resolve ambivalence. This is accomplished by helping individuals articulate both their concerns about changing their behavior and their reasons for changing. According to Miller and Rollnick (1991), the active ingredients of motivational interviewing are providing feedback, enhancing personal responsibility, giving advice along with a menu of options, supporting self-efficacy, and providing a nonconfrontational and supportive context. Skills training is a commonly used cognitive behavior treatment approach. Unlike motivational interviewing, which is used to increase individuals' motivation or desire to change their behavior, skills training is used with individuals who are actively working to change. The core components of skills training include (a) training individuals to identify and cope with high-risk situations associated with the target behavior (e.g., urges to smoke or to overeat), (b) modifying cognitive expectancies and attributions associated with the target behavior, (c) teaching stress management skills, and (d) modifying general lifestyle activities (Elder, Ayala, & Harris, 1999).

INTERVENTION DESIGN

General Approach

The endpoint of nationwide prevention and health services programs of the continuum of cancer prevention and control speaks to an ultimate public health mandate. Achieving widespread adoption of proven interventions requires a practical and conceptually driven strategic process of intervention development. The RE-AIM framework conceptualizes the public health impact of interventions as a function of the five factors that form this acronym: reach (i.e., the proportion of the target population who receive an intervention), efficacy (i.e., the success rate of the intervention when delivered as intended), adoption (i.e., the proportion of intervention settings that will actually use the intervention), implementation (i.e., the extent to which the intervention is implemented as intended in real-world settings), and maintenance (i.e., the extent to which program effects [individual level] and the program itself [organizational level] are maintained over time; Glasgow, Vogt, & Boles, 1999).

Individual- and interpersonal-level cancer prevention and control interventions fall on a continuum from clinical to public health treatment models.

TABLE 4.1
Clinical and Public Health Treatment Models

Characteristic	Clinical perspective	Public health perspective
Problem definition	Individual, lifestyle	Community, environment
Target population	Self-referred or recruited	Populations or high-risk groups
Setting	Specialty, clinical	Natural environments
Provider	Trained professional	Lay, automated
Intervention	Intensive, multisession	Brief, low cost
Research design	Component analysis, comparative studies	Best shot or special intervention versus usual care
Outcome	Higher rates of change	Lower rates of change
Cost effectiveness	Lower	Higher

Note. Adapted from "Smoking Cessation: What Have We Learned Over the Past Decade?" by E. Lichtenstein and R. E. Glasgow, 1992, *Journal of Consulting and Clinical Psychology, 60,* p. 519. Copyright 1992 by the American Psychological Association.

Table 4.1 summarizes the characteristics of each end of this continuum as outlined by Lichtenstein and Glasgow (1992). Clinical interventions focus primarily on individual factors and lifestyle issues in behavior change. The target population includes individuals who are recruited or self-refer for interventions. Treatment is typically delivered by specially trained professionals in a medical or allied professional setting. Clinical interventions are often intensive and may involve multiple sessions. Treatment outcome studies are often comparative, so-called horse-race studies in which alternative treatments are compared with each other without no-treatment control groups. Clinical interventions often result in high rates of change among the self-selected participants; however, their effectiveness for producing population-based changes may be limited because of low penetration into the population.

At the public health end of the continuum, the target population includes all individuals or members of specific high-risk groups, regardless of their motivation to change their behavior. Interventions are delivered in natural settings, and the treatment providers are not necessarily specialists. Treatment outcome studies frequently compare a new intervention with usual care. Because public health interventions are often brief and low cost in an effort to reach the largest possible proportion of the target population, rates of change in these programs may be much lower than in more intensive clinical interventions.

Consideration of the RE-AIM model and the clinical–public health continuum makes it clear that there are myriad logistic, clinical, and methodological decisions to be made as part of intervention design. These decisions include (a) clarifying where the intervention fits on the public health to clinical intervention continuum, (b) defining the target population, (c) selecting where the intervention will be delivered and by whom, (d) deciding on the timing of intervention components, and (e) specifying the process and outcome targets for the intervention. These decisions can be guided by the integration of relevant scientific evidence from multiple disciplines such as epidemiology and surveillance, behavioral science, and medical research, as well as an understanding of the practical requirements for high-quality delivery of the intervention components.

In defining the target population and determining where on the clinical–public health continuum an intervention should fall, the relative importance of reach and efficacy in achieving the desired impacts of the intervention need to be considered. Behavioral scientists and their colleagues may choose to design interventions that are toward the public health end of the continuum (e.g., brief, low cost, delivered in community settings by nonspecialists) if modest changes in a large segment of the population could result in meaningful reductions in cancer incidence and mortality. Although much is to be gained in terms of reductions in cancer incidence and mortality from the development, evaluation, and dissemination of proven interventions to the general population, it is also important to develop interventions targeted to specific populations or tailored to individual participants. That is, to the extent that large changes are needed in highly selected groups of individuals, a more clinical intervention approach would be desirable. For example, there is increasing evidence that behavioral risk factors are disproportionately found in certain segments of the population, most notably among those with low income and lack of access to comprehensive medical services (American Cancer Society, 2000). Designing interventions that target these populations requires consideration of factors such as potential financial costs to individuals and/or institutional settings that have limited resources, the education level required to understand written materials, and the penetration of intervention modalities into the target population (e.g., telephones for outreach telephone counseling, home computers for Web-based interventions). From another perspective, advances in biomedical research may identify genetic predispositions that would lead researchers to target cancer prevention interventions to certain subgroups for which behavioral risk factors pose the greatest risk. For example, women with a family history of breast cancer that places them at higher risk may increase compliance with mammography screening through tailored interventions that personalize their risk profile (Curry, Taplin, Anderman, Barlow, & McBride, 1993).

Decisions about the organizational or community setting and personnel to deliver the intervention can have a profound effect on the ultimate impact of an intervention because they influence the likely adoption and implementation of an intervention with proven efficacy. The general goal is to select settings with a high potential to reach the target population and with missions and resources that would facilitate eventual adoption of the intervention. The efficacy of an intervention is best demonstrated when delivered by research staff; it is important to ensure that the protocols developed for research staff are compatible with the expertise and job responsibilities of individuals who would deliver the program in a nonresearch context.

The timing of delivery of intervention components is also important. One-shot interventions may be appropriate for relatively simple behaviors that occur in discrete time frames (i.e., do not have to be sustained over long periods of time). For example, interventions to enhance compliance with cancer screening tests may involve the simple mailing of reminder postcards or outreach reminder telephone calls (Tiffany, 1990). To the extent that the target behaviors are complex and the change process is one that must be sustained over an extended period of time (e.g., dietary change, physical activity, smoking cessation), it is important to relate the timing of intervention delivery to an understanding of the behavior change process. For example, smoking cessation interventions may have several intervention contacts delivered over a relatively short period of time during the initial cessation phase, followed by more infrequent, long-term contacts designed to enhance maintenance of nonsmoking.

Outcome targets range from actual health events (e.g., cancer incidence) to specifically defined behavioral targets (e.g., cessation of smoking, mammography, colonoscopy). Process targets are the intermediate (i.e., mediating) variables that the intervention is designed to change (e.g., beliefs and expectations, behavioral skills, amount of social support) to obtain the desired outcome. A clearly articulated conceptual model brings clarity to defining process and outcome targets and should be thought out early in the intervention development process.

Translating Conceptual Models for Intervention Development

One of the most intellectually stimulating aspects of intervention development is articulating the behavior change model that will guide the selection and design of specific intervention components. Several of the more commonly applied theoretical paradigms in health behavior research include value expectancy theories, social-cognitive theory, and the transtheoretical model (Glanz, Lewis, & Rimer, 1997). Most theory-driven interventions use conceptual frameworks that draw on multiple theories that are integrated into a single framework. For example, Gritz and Bastani (1993) described a framework for adherence that incorporates elements of several theoretical models, including the health belief model, the theory of reasoned action, and the transtheoretical model. Multidisciplinary team members inform the conceptual framework with theories from their respective disciplines. During this process, collaborations become more transdisciplinary as colleagues learn each other's frames of reference and terminologies.

At the simplest level, a conceptual framework provides a picture (literally and figuratively) of the key constructs believed to influence the target behavior. When illustrated, these frameworks are typically a series of boxes and arrows that show the relationships between the constructs and the target behavior(s). To the extent possible, the relationships outlined by the conceptual framework should be based on published findings from qualitative and quantitative research on factors associated with the target behavior. If such research is not available, or if the available research does not include data from the intended target population, then additional preliminary research is warranted. Focus group research is an important tool to evaluate the robustness of the conceptual framework in the target population. Providing even a primer on the conduct and interpretation of focus group research is beyond the scope of this chapter, but see Balch et al. (2004); Basch (1987); Karanja, Stevens, Hollis, and Kumanyika (2002); Morgan and Kreuger (1997); and Vuckovic, Harris, Valanis, and Stewart (2003).

TREATMENT–OUTCOME STUDY DESIGN

Effective cancer control efforts require well-designed, conceptually driven interventions that have been rigorously evaluated. This section briefly reviews some of the more common designs, data collection methods, measurement issues, and recruitment and retention issues. For a more detailed discussion of these issues, see Flay (1986) and Behar and Borkovec (2003).

Design Options

Perhaps the most important distinction among treatment–outcome study designs is between experimental designs and non- or quasi-experimental designs. Study groups in experimental designs are formed by random assignment of participant units, whereas groups in quasi-experimental designs are not formed by random assignment.

Randomized (Experimental) Trials

Randomized trials are generally considered to be the gold standard in evaluating cancer prevention and control interventions because they permit more powerful inferences about the causal effects of the treatment on outcome. An important distinction among randomized designs, although not always easy to determine, is between efficacy and effectiveness studies (Flay, 1986). Efficacy studies tend to be toward the clinical end of the clinical–public health continuum, whereas effectiveness studies tend to be toward the public health end (see Table 4.1, this volume). Efficacy studies are typically conducted in more research-oriented contexts (e.g., research clinics), whereas effectiveness studies are conducted in more naturalistic and ecologically valid settings (e.g., primary care, public health clinics, worksites).

Control groups in cancer prevention and randomized controlled trials frequently consist of usual care, although they might also consist of competing treatments, wait-list controls, or attention–placebo treatments. The use of a usual care control group is most appropriate when evaluating new treatments or when issues related to design efficiency are important. An intervention versus usual care design allows the investigator to determine whether the treatment under consideration could improve outcomes in a relatively efficient fashion in terms of cost, sample size, and complexity.

When the research question specifically addresses the efficacy of a particular treatment content or component relative to another content or component (e.g., motivational counseling vs. skills training), it can be argued that the control group(s) should adequately control for factors such as the length of contact, number of contacts, and treatment credibility. Including study groups that control for these variables allows researchers to make inferences directly related to treatment content.

Many cancer prevention and control interventions include multiple treatment components (e.g., physician or nurse advice to limit fat intake, nutritional counseling, self-help materials, tailored follow-up by mail) that may or may not be evaluated individually. Although both two-group and factorial designs can evaluate the overall impact of the multicomponent treatment, only the factorial design can tease apart the multicomponent treatment effect into its constituent components. In much the same way that a factorial design can be used to examine the individual components of a new multicomponent treatment, it can also be used in a dismantling strategy to partition the effects of a proven treatment. Understanding the effective and ineffective components of treatment is important because this information can be used to improve the allocation of resources and cost-effectiveness of cancer prevention and control interventions. As may be obvious, however, component studies can be considerably more costly in terms of money, sample size, and complexity.

Quasi-Experimental Designs

Treatment–outcome research may also compare treatments when participants have not been randomly assigned to study groups. Quasi-experimental designs can be used in numerous situations (e.g., when it is impractical or unethical to randomly assign participants) and are particularly useful in taking advantage of naturally occurring events. However, this type of design provides much weaker evidence for determining causality than does a randomized trial.

Pre–Post Observational Studies

Pre–post observational studies attempt to evaluate the effects of an intervention by conducting assessments both before and after treatment. Although this type of study provides information on the potential impact of the treatment, it does not allow any inferences regarding causality because there are numerous factors in addition to treatment that might account for pre–post changes (e.g., an increase in fruit consumption after introducing fruit in vending machines might also be attributable to a rise in the cost of dairy products). Nevertheless, pre–post observational studies are useful in generating hypotheses that can be tested in later experimental studies.

Data Collection

Data collection methods in behavioral intervention studies range from tissue samples (Audrain et al., 1997) to psychophysiological approaches (Coleman, Saelens, Wiedrich-Smith, Finn, & Epstein, 1997) to self-report measures (Velicer, Prochaska, Fava, Laforge, & Rossi, 1999). We address only self-report approaches because they reflect the most common approach in behavioral intervention studies.

Self-Report

Many of the constructs targeted by cancer prevention and control interventions (e.g., pros and cons of behavior change, self-efficacy, coping skills) are assessed using self-report measures. These measures are relatively inexpensive, easy to administer, and have contributed greatly to the understanding of cancer risk and preventive behavior. Self-report instruments can assess variables that occurred in the past (e.g., previous diet patterns), participant predictions about future variables (e.g., likelihood of smoking relapse in the next year), or current variables (e.g., present mood).

Retrospective self-report instruments can yield detailed information that covers long periods of time. However, there is evidence that numerous memory phenomena lead to biased and inaccurate recall (Stone et al., 1998). Prospective self-report measures eliminate some of the problems associated with retrospective recall, but they often involve recalling and synthesizing previous experience to arrive at predictions. Thus, prospective measures suffer from many of the same memory limitations as retrospective recall. Many biases and errors are reduced or eliminated by gathering data in near real time. Advances in technology have facilitated the use of near real-time assessments in naturally occurring settings using handheld computers, pagers, telephone hotlines, and so on. These *ecological momentary assessments* have been extraordinarily informative with respect to several cancer risk and protective behaviors such as coping (Stone et al., 1998) and relapse to smoking (Shiffman et al., 1997). Their potential for exploring participants' experiences and processes involved in preventing and controlling other aspects of cancer (e.g., current symptoms, mood, cognitions) remains largely untapped. Unfortunately, ecological momentary assessments can have several major disadvantages, including expense and participant burden. Moreover, even when conducting near real-time recording, the ability to access internal states may be limited (e.g., cognitions may be automatic and unconscious; Tiffany, 1990).

Assessment Intervals

The conceptual model underlying the effects of treatment should generally drive assessment intervals. Short-term assessments provide information on the initial effects of treatment, whereas long-term assessments yield information on the durability of treatment effects. The durability of treatment effects is particularly important for behavioral science research because many changes in behavior deteriorate after treatment completion (e.g., quitting smoking, losing weight). Even more frequent assessment intervals might be necessary if the research is concerned with treatment effects on putative mechanisms or intermediate outcomes. In sum, it is impossible to provide specific guidelines on appropriate assessment intervals (i.e., they differ on the basis of outcome, behaviors, study purpose, etc.). The study goals and conceptual framework underlying the research should form the basis of these decisions, but the appropriateness of both short-term and long-term follow-up should always be considered.

Measures

As with many other issues related to study design, the conceptual framework underlying treatment should guide the selection of process and outcome measures. Process measures reflect what is occurring during treatment and/or potential mechanisms underlying treatment effects, whereas outcome measures are consequences that result from treatment processes and reflect endpoints. In practice, distinctions between process and outcome measures can be difficult to make (i.e., biomarkers of carcinogenic activity may represent mechanisms underlying treatment effects or stand-alone endpoints). For example, in a study comparing tailored versus nontailored self-help interventions for smoking cessation, process measures might include whether the person read the self-help materials, the perceived relevance of the materials, and self-efficacy. Outcome measures are likely to be abstinence and, perhaps, quit attempts. However, it might be argued that tailored materials increase long-term abstinence rates not by increasing the abstinence rate for any one quit attempt but by increasing the number of quit attempts. In this case, quit attempts might be considered to be a process measure reflecting a treatment mechanism that leads to abstinence.

Psychometric Standards for Validity and Reliability

Measures should consistently do what they are intended to do. That is, they should assess the variable that they are hypothesized to assess (i.e., validity), and they should consistently assign the same number to the same observation (i.e., reliability).

Validity refers to the degree to which a measure assesses what it purports to assess. Validity is determined by examining the associations of the measure of interest with other measures that assess the same or similar constructs (e.g., a new measure of dietary intake should be highly correlated with other, independent observations of dietary intake) and by examining its hypothesized relations with other variables. Unfortunately, many cancer prevention and control research studies do not report the reliability and validity of the measures that were used. This is particularly problematic when measures have not been used in previous research or have not been evaluated in the target population. It is important to use measures with established reliability and validity, or if new measures are developed, to independently verify their reliability and validity in independent samples.

Reliability refers to how accurate a measure is in reflecting a participant's "true" score. Reliability can be computed in various ways. Two common methods in behavioral science research are test–retest reliability and internal consistency. *Test–retest reliability* refers to the concordance between scores when a measure is administered on separate occasions. For measurements collected in close temporal proximity or for variables that are posited to be relatively stable over time (e.g., personality traits, temperament), this can be an excellent method for determining reliability. Because most measures in behavioral science consist of multiple items and because the major source of measurement error is in the sampling of items (Nunnally, 1978), a key index of reliability is internal consistency (i.e., how well the items hang together). Reliability estimates from internal consistency are usually very close to estimates from alternate methods (e.g., test–retest, alternate forms; Nunnally, 1978). In behavioral science research, a reliability coefficient of .80 or greater is generally considered satisfactory, although lower reliabilities may be considered acceptable for measures with a limited number of items (e.g., fewer than five).

Validation of Self-Reported Outcomes

Because many cancer prevention and control interventions rely on self-reported outcomes (e.g., diet, screening, smoking) that are subject to misreporting either intentionally (e.g., smokers may misreport their smoking status) or involuntarily (e.g., individuals may be unable to accurately recall their food intake during a specified time period), those outcomes are often subject to verification. Common verification methods include unobtrusive measurement, collateral reports, and biochemical measures. The need for verification of self-reported outcomes depends on numerous factors such as the research purpose, social desirability of the behavior, and relationship between the participants and the investigators.

Study Population and Participants

Treatment–outcome research design involves a number of critical decisions related to adequate recruitment and retention of study participants. Key considerations include the size of the study samples, the unit being sampled, ways that participants are recruited into the study, and the requirements for participation.

Sample Size Considerations

Failure to have an adequate sample size (i.e., power) can result in a Type II error (i.e., deciding that the treatment does not improve outcome when in fact it does). Important factors that affect the requisite sample size include the level of statistical power desired, the estimated treatment effects, and the variability in outcome for the target population. Whenever possible, decisions on sample size should be based on power calculations using existing data. When data are not available, sample size should be based on having adequate power to detect clinically meaningful and reasonable effects on the basis of the literature that does exist. When determining sample size, the unit of analysis used in determining power should reflect the unit of randomization (e.g., when clinics are randomized to study arms, clinics should also be used as the unit of analysis in determining power).

Self-Selected Versus Nonvolunteer Samples

Random selection of a study sample from the target population maximizes the likelihood that the study sample will be representative of the population to whom conclusions are to be generalized. However, in treatment–outcome research, this often does not occur. Many cancer prevention and control studies use self-selected, volunteer samples that may not accurately reflect the characteristics of the target population. A biased sample can be problematic because it can affect outcomes, although it is not always easy to determine how a sample is biased or how the bias affects the results.

Response Burden

In any type of treatment–outcome research, minimizing the response burden placed on participants is important. However, the weight placed on this issue will vary on the basis of the purpose of each study. In a community-based effectiveness study, greater emphasis is placed on limiting the response burden. A burdensome assessment strategy could cause many potential participants to refrain from participating and thereby limit the generalizability of the findings, or it might reduce compliance with follow-up procedures and produce skewed results. In an efficacy study, however, the primary study aims might include identifying specific treatment mechanisms that necessitate more intensive assessment procedures. Without the increased response burden, it may be impossible to adequately measure these mechanisms.

Incentives

Incentives are frequently used in cancer prevention and control trials, particularly in efficacy trials. Incentives can be very valuable in that they can increase adherence to study procedures, increase participation rates, and minimize group differences in attrition or compliance that threaten a study's internal validity. However, by increasing adherence to study procedures, incentives may serve to increase treatment efficacy, and that efficacy may not translate to effectiveness trials or real-world applications of the treatment. Incentives also increase the cost of conducting the research. Therefore, the use of incentives needs to be carefully considered against the research question and the potential effects of the incentives.

DATA ANALYSIS

The most elegantly designed and carefully executed intervention study will contribute to improved methods for cancer prevention and control only to the extent that the study results are carefully analyzed and reported. This section discusses a number of critical issues in data analysis and reporting, including using analysis plans and appropriate bivariate and multivariate analytic strategies, testing for differential treatment effects among important population subgroups, using mediator analysis to test whether observed intervention effects are consistent with the overarching conceptual model, and handling missing outcome data.

General Analytic Considerations

It is imperative to have a plan for the outcome analyses before the analyses begin. One key element in such a plan is identifying the primary outcome measures for the study (Assmann, Pocock, Enos, & Kasten, 2000). In a typical trial, data on several outcome measures are collected and each measure is assessed at several follow-ups. As a result, it is not unusual for there to be 20 outcome measures that could be used to assess a treatment's effectiveness. This situation gives rise to what is called the *multiple comparison problem* (Breslow & Day, 1980, 1987; Meinert, 1986). For instance, if 20 outcomes were analyzed using the conventional .05 cutoff for statistical significance, a totally ineffective intervention would yield at least 1 outcome that displayed statistical significance 64% of the time (assuming the outcomes are uncorrelated).

Two approaches can be used to avoid the multiple comparison problem. The first is conceptual. Before looking at the data, investigators determine what will be the primary outcome or outcomes. These outcomes will be used to determine whether the intervention was effective. Primary outcomes should be chosen on the basis of clinical or practical importance and the likelihood of being affected by the intervention.

If investigators cannot or will not reduce the number of primary outcome measures to a small number (typically 1–3, but no more than 5), then the second approach applies statistical methods to adjust for multiple comparisons. The simplest and most commonly used is the Bonferroni method (Meinert, 1986), which replaces the usual $p = .05$ cutoff for significance with $p = .05$ divided by the number of outcomes being assessed. The drawback to this and similar approaches (e.g., *sequentially rejective Bonferroni* method; Hochberg, 1988) is a reduction in power. Another key aspect of the analysis plan involves the types of multivariate analyses to be done. In large randomized trials (i.e., hundreds of subjects per treatment group), the act of randomization ensures the comparability of the control and intervention groups. However, controlling for baseline covariates is often worthwhile because the standard error of the outcome variable tends to be reduced and power increased. Adjustments can be made for imbalances between treatment groups, which tend to occur in smaller trials or when losses to follow-up rates are high (Assmann et al., 2000).

The choice of variables to include should be based on which variables are imbalanced at baseline and on subject matter considerations. Baseline variables that prior knowledge of the subject matter suggests are correlated with the outcome should be included in the model to increase power. Another consideration is the rate of missing data for the covariate. Covariates with more than nominal rates of missing data may need to be excluded from the multivariate analyses because large numbers of observations will be dropped if numerous covariates have missing data. Such exclusions can distort estimates of the treatment effect by reducing the analysis to a nonrepresentative subset of the study population. Multiple imputation can also be used to avoid such problems (Little & Rubin, 1987).

Analysis of Discrete and Continuous Outcomes

For continuous or ordinal outcomes in a two-group design, the analysis can compare the means in the control and intervention groups using a t test. Regression analysis (i.e., least squares) can be used to determine whether the means are significantly different after adjusting for baseline covariates (Norman & Streiner, 1986).

For binary outcomes such as screened or not screened in a two-group design, chi-square tests can be used to compare the percent screened in the control and intervention groups. To compare the groups controlling for baseline characteristics, logistic regression can be used (Breslow & Day, 1980, 1987; Hosmer & Lemeshow, 2000; Kleinbaum, Kupper, & Morgenstern, 1982). Logistic regression results in an odds ratio that compares the odds of being screened in the intervention group with the odds of being screened in the control group.

When outcomes are assessed at multiple time points, each time point can be analyzed separately or data from multiple time points can be analyzed simultaneously to estimate the effect of the intervention. If the latter approach is used, there will be repeated measures of the outcome for each individual and those measures will be correlated. To handle these within-person correlations, mixed-model analyses (Ware, 1985) or generalized estimating equations (GEEs; Liang & Zeger, 1986) can be used with continuous outcomes, and GEEs can be used with binary outcomes. For example, in a screening study, one might want to compare screening rates using data from both the 12- and the 24-month follow-ups. Thus, each person would have two outcome values on screening status. GEEs could be used to do the equivalent of a logistic regression analysis to estimate a single odds ratio for the entire 24-month follow-up period.

Moderator and Mediator Analyses

Sometimes there is interest in determining whether an intervention was more effective in a subgroup of the study population. Although subgroup analyses can reflect a priori hypotheses, a common abuse of such analyses is when the intervention has no effect overall but the investigators divide the study population into subgroups (e.g., on the basis of age, health status, or amount smoked) and repeat the outcome analysis for each subgroup. This results in a number of independent analyses that increase the likelihood of finding a "significant" effect that is due to chance (Assmann et al., 2000). However, a principled way of doing a subgroup analysis is to, first, carefully determine whether there are subgroups for which there is a scientific basis for expecting a differential treatment response. For example, in a study assessing whether reminder calls increase the rate of screening mammograms, it might be hypothesized that the treatment effect varies depending on a woman's history of mammography. Such information could be used to target future interventions or clinical programs to the subgroups for which there would be the most impact. Second, to avoid the multiple comparison problem, the number of subgroup-defining variables should be kept small. Third, a formal test of an interaction between the intervention and the subgroup-defining variable should be done (Assmann et al., 2000). If this interaction test is significant, then the subgroup-defining variable is said to be an *effect moderator* (Kleinbaum et al., 1982). If and only if this interaction test is significant should analyses be done to test for intervention effects in each of the subgroups.

If there is a significant overall treatment effect, it is important to try to understand the mechanisms underlying that effect. For example, in a genetic counseling intervention, it is important to determine whether the intervention worked by increasing self-efficacy to perform protective behaviors or by reducing the negative emotions associated with testing. Such mechanisms can be explored by conducting mediator analyses (Baron & Kenny, 1986). To determine whether a variable mediates the treatment effect on outcome, treatment should influence the mediator, the mediator should influence outcome, and adjusting for the mediator should eliminate or substantially reduce the treatment effect on outcome (Baron & Kenny, 1986). Statistically, an analysis to identify a mediator variable is identical to an analysis to determine whether a variable is a confounder (Kleinbaum et al., 1982). However, a mediator variable should be measured after treatment begins (so that the treatment can affect it) but before assessment of the outcome. In addition, a mediator must appreciably reduce the treatment effect (i.e., the perfect mediator would drive the effect to zero), whereas a variable need only change the size of the effect to be considered a confounder. Although cause and effect cannot be established by demonstrating mediation, it suggests that the treatment influences the mediator variable, which in turn affects the outcome.

The Intention-to-Treat Principle and Missing Data

Intention to treat (Hollis & Campbell, 1999; Lewis & Machin, 1993; Roland & Torgerson, 1998) is an analytic approach for dealing with two problems that commonly arise in randomized trials: (a) noncompliance with the intervention and other deviations from study protocols and (b) missing outcome data. The first of two fundamental principles of intention-to-treat is to analyze as randomized, meaning that subjects are to be analyzed according to the treatment group they were randomized to regardless of their level of compliance with the intervention. The second principle is to collect and analyze follow-up outcome data on all study participants regardless of their level of participation in the study (Hollis & Campbell, 1999). Intention to treat is included in the CONSORT (i.e., the Consolidated Standards of Reporting Trials) statement (Begg et al., 1996), which authors must follow when reporting the results of clinic trials in prestigious medical journals and which has been adopted by behavioral medicine publications (Davidson et al., 2003). An important implication of this second principle is that even if someone refuses to continue participation in the intervention, every effort should be made to collect outcome data from that individual. However, even with careful implementation of a study protocol, there will be missing outcome data, particularly in randomized trials of behavioral interventions that involve nonvolunteers and/or minimal interventions devoid of face-to-face contact (e.g., unsolicited reminder calls to women who have been asked to schedule a screening mammogram; Taplin et al., 2000).

When reporting the results of clinical trials, it is important to provide data on the extent and causes of missing outcome data so the reader can better assess its impact on the validity of the findings. Key elements that should be reported by treatment group include the number of individuals providing outcome data at each time point, along with reasons for missing outcome data and dropout. The most commonly used approach to missing data, and the default method in statistical packages, is complete case analysis: Individuals with missing outcome data are simply dropped from the analysis. This approach can give valid results only when missing data rates are low (i.e., under 10%) and are similar across treatment groups. However, if participants who provide outcome data have consistently better or worse outcomes than those who do not, and if rates of attrition differ among study groups, the method can over- or underestimate treatment effectiveness.

A number of ad hoc methods to impute missing outcome data have been developed (Fairclough, 2002; Little & Rubin, 1987; Schafer & Olsen, 1998; Vach & Blettner, 1991), including worst-case imputation (e.g., assume all nonresponding participants in a smoking cessation trial are smoking), mean imputation (e.g., impute the group mean for missing outcomes), single regression imputation (e.g., predict missing outcomes on the basis of observed covariates), and last-value-carried-forward (e.g., impute last observed value for subsequent missing outcomes). We cannot recommend any of these methods because all treat the imputed values in the analysis as if they were real, not estimated, data, resulting in confidence intervals and p values which are too small. These methods also can underestimate treatment effects (e.g., worst-case imputation) and distort distributions (i.e., mean imputation).

Valid statistical methods for dealing with missing data include multiple imputation and maximum likelihood estimation (Fairclough, 2002; Little & Rubin, 1987; Rubin & Schenker, 1991; Schafer, 1997). Multiple imputation usually involves development of a regression-like model to predict missing outcome data (i.e., variables that predict "missingness" and/or are to be included in the analysis should be included in the imputation model). The model is used to impute missing values, resulting in a complete data set that can be analyzed using standard software. The imputation is done several times, resulting in a number of completed data sets, all different because the methods give different imputed values each time. Analyses are run on each completed data set, and then the results from each analysis are combined to get a single estimate and an appropriate standard error. Standard statistical software such as SAS and S-Plus can do multiple imputation. Maximum likelihood methods most commonly are done using mixed models (Fairclough, 2002; Verbeke & Molenberghs, 2000), which are also available in standard software packages (e.g., SAS's PROC MIXED; SAS Institute, 2008; see also Fairclough, 2002, and Verbeke & Molenberghs, 2000). No amount of statistical analysis or imputation can totally overcome the problems caused by missing outcome data. The best approach is to minimize missing data as much as possible.

CONCLUSION

Human behaviors are primary risk factors for cancer, accounting for at least one third of all cancer-related deaths. Even with exciting advances in molecular and genetic research, human behaviors will continue to be critical determinants of cancer risk (Curry et al., 2003). Therefore, the development, evaluation, implementation, and wide-scale adoption of effective interventions for behavioral risk factor modification is a crucial component of the cancer prevention and control arsenal. The core thesis of this chapter is that behavioral intervention research must be conceptually based and scientifically rigorous. The conceptual models underlying behavioral interventions must be evidence-based, and the link between theory and intervention development should be clearly articulated. Defining how conceptual models inform specific intervention components provides an important link from basic to applied behavioral research. To the extent that research paradigms are methodologically rigorous with valid and reliable assessments of key constructs and appropriate data analyses, the results from intervention studies can also inform basic behavioral research and theory development. Even though behavioral intervention research is conducted outside of controlled laboratory settings, adherence to basic scientific principles establishes the credibility of this research both within and outside the community of cancer prevention and control scientists.

REFERENCES

American Cancer Society. (2000). *Cancer facts & figures 2000.* Atlanta, GA: Author.

Assmann, S. F., Pocock, S. J., Enos, L. E., & Kasten, L. E. (2000, March 25). Subgroup analysis and other (mis)uses of baseline data in clinical trials. *Lancet, 355,* 1064–1069.

Audrain, J., Boyd, N. R., Roth, J., Main, D., Caporaso, N. F., & Lerman, C. (1997). Genetic susceptibility testing in smoking-cessation treatment: One-year outcomes of a randomized trial. *Addictive Behavior, 22,* 741–751.

Balch, G. I., Tworek, C., Barker, D. C., Sasso, B., Mermelstein, R., & Giovino, G. A. (2004). Opportunities for youth smoking cessation: Findings from a national focus group study. *Nicotine and Tobacco Research, 6,* 9–17.

Baron, R. M., & Kenny, D. A. (1986). The moderator–mediator variable distinction in social psychological research: Conceptual, strategic, and statistical considerations. *Journal of Personality and Social Psychology, 51,* 1173–1182.

Basch, C. E. (1987). Focus group interview: An underutilized research technique for improving theory and practice in health education. *Health Education Quarterly, 14,* 411–448.

Baum, A., & Posluszny, D. M. (1999). Health psychology: Mapping biobehavioral contributions to health and illness. *Annual Review of Psychology, 50,* 137–163.

Begg, C., Cho, M., Eastwood, S., Horton, R., Moher, D., Olkin, I., et al. (1996). Improving the quality of reporting of randomized controlled trials: The CONSORT statement. *Journal of the American Medical Association, 276,* 637–639.

Behar, E. S., & Borkovec, T. D. (2003). Psychotherapy outcome research. In J. A. Schinka & W. F. Velicer (Eds.), *Handbook of psychology: Research methods in psychology* (Vol. 2, pp. 213–240). New York: Wiley.

Bennett, J. W., Smith, H. L., & Passin, H. (1943). Food and culture in Southern Illinois—A preliminary report. *American Social Review, 7,* 645–660.

Breslow, N. E., & Day, N. E. (1980). *Statistical methods in cancer research: Vol. 1. The analysis of case-control studies.* Lyon, France: International Agency for Research on Cancer.

Breslow, N. E., & Day, N. E. (1987). *Statistical methods in cancer research: Vol. 2. The design and analysis of cohort studies.* Lyon, France: International Agency for Research on Cancer.

Byers, T., Mouchawar, J., Marks, J., Cady, B., Lins, N., Swanson, G. M., et al. (1999). The American Cancer Society challenge goals: How far can cancer rates decline in the U.S. by the year 2015? *Cancer, 86,* 715–727.

Coleman, K. J., Saelens, B. E., Wiedrich-Smith, M. D., Finn, J. D., & Epstein, L. H. (1997). Relationships between TriTrac-R3D vectors, heart rate, and self-report in obese children. *Medicine & Science in Sports and Exercise, 29,* 1535–1542.

Curry, S. J., Byers, T., & Hewitt, M. (Eds.). (2003). *Fulfilling the potential for cancer prevention and early detection.* Washington, DC: National Academies Press.

Curry, S. J., Taplin, S. H., Anderman, C., Barlow, W. E., & McBride, C. (1993). A randomized trial of the impact of risk assessment and feedback on participation in mammography screening. *Preventive Medicine, 22,* 350–360.

Davidson, K. W., Goldstein, M., Kaplan, R. M., Kaufmann, P. G., Knatterud, G. L., Orleans, C. T., et al. (2003). Evidence-based behavioral medicine: What is it and how do we achieve it? *Annals of Behavioral Medicine, 26,* 161–171.

Elder, J. P., Ayala, G. X., & Harris, S. (1999). Theories and intervention approaches to health-behavior change in primary care. *American Journal of Preventive Medicine, 17,* 275–284.

Fairclough, D. L. (2002). *Design and analysis of quality-of-life studies in clinical trials.* Boca Raton, FL: Chapman & Hall/CRC.

Flay, B. R. (1986). Efficacy and effectiveness trials (and other phases of research) in the development of health promotion programs. *Preventive Medicine, 15,* 451–474.

Glanz, K., Lewis, F. M., & Rimer, B. K. (Eds.). (1997). *Health behavior and health education: Theory, research, and practice* (2nd ed.). San Francisco: Jossey-Bass.

Glasgow, R. E., Vogt, T. M., & Boles, S. M. (1999). Evaluating the public health impact of health promotion interventions: The RE-AIM framework. *American Journal of Public Health, 89,* 1322–1327.

Greenwald, P., & Cullen, J. W. (1984). The scientific approach to cancer control. *CA: A Cancer Journal for Clinicians, 34,* 328–332.

Gritz, E. R., & Bastani, R. (1993). Cancer prevention—behavior changes: The short and the long of it. *Preventive Medicine, 22,* 676–688.

Hiatt, R. A., & Rimer, B. K. (1999). A new strategy for cancer control research. *Cancer Epidemiology, Biomarkers & Prevention, 8,* 957–964.

Hochberg, Y. (1988). A sharper Bonferroni procedure for multiple tests of significance. *Biometrika, 75,* 800–802.

Hollis, S., & Campbell, F. (1999, September 11). What is meant by intention-to-treat analysis? Survey of published randomised controlled trials. *BMJ, 319,* 670–674.

Hosmer, D. W., & Lemeshow, S. (2000). *Applied logistic regression* (2nd ed.). New York: Wiley.

Karanja, N., Stevens, V. J., Hollis, J. F., & Kumanyika, S. K. (2002). Steps to Soulful Living (Steps): A weight loss program for African American women. *Ethnicity and Disease, 12,* 363–371.

Kleinbaum, D. G., Kupper, L. L., & Morgenstern, H. (1982). *Epidemiologic research principles and quantitative methods.* London: Lifetime Learning Publications.

Lewis, J. A., & Machin, D. (1993). Intention to treat—Who should use ITT? *British Journal of Cancer, 68,* 647–650.

Liang, K. Y., & Zeger, S. L. (1986). Longitudinal analysis using generalized linear models. *Biometrika, 73,* 13–22.

Lichtenstein, E., & Glasgow, R. E. (1992). Smoking cessation: What have we learned over the past decade? *Journal of Consulting and Clinical Psychology, 60,* 518–527.

Lipsey, M. W. (1987, April). *Theory as method: Small theories of treatments.* Paper presented at the Health Services Research Conference: Strengthening Causal Interpretations of Non-Experimental Data, Tucson, AZ.

Little, R. J. A., & Rubin, D. B. (1987). *Statistical analysis with missing data.* New York: Wiley.

Marlatt, G. A., & Gordon, J. R. (1985). *Relapse prevention.* New York: Guilford Press.

McBride, C. M., Curry, S. J., Taplin, S., Anderman, C., & Grothaus, L. (1993). Exploring environmental barriers to participation in mammography screening in an HMO. *Cancer Epidemiology, Biomarkers & Prevention, 2*, 599–605.

Meinert, C. L. (1986). *Clinical trials design, conduct, and analysis*. New York: Oxford University Press.

Miller, W. R., & Rollnick, S. (1991). *Motivational interviewing: Preparing people to change addictive behaviors*. New York: Guilford Press.

Montano, D. E., & Taplin, S. H. (1991). A test of an expanded theory of reasoned action to predict mammography participation. *Social Science Medicine, 32*, 733–741.

Morgan, D. L., & Kreuger, R. A. (1997). *The focus group kit* (Vols. 1–6). Thousand Oaks, CA: Sage.

Norman, G. R., & Streiner, D. L. (1986). *PDQ statistics*. Toronto, Canada: B. C. Decker.

Nunnally, J. C. (1978). *Psychometric theory*. New York: McGraw-Hill.

Roland, M., & Torgerson, D. J. (1998, January 4). What are pragmatic trials? *BMJ, 316*, 285.

Rubin, D. B., & Schenker, N. (1991). Multiple imputation in health-care databases: An overview and some applications. *Statistics in Medicine, 10*, 585–598.

SAS Institute. (2008). *SAS/STAT® 9.2 user's guide*. Cary, NC: Author.

Schafer, J. L. (1997). *Analysis of incomplete multivariate data*. Boca Raton, FL: Chapman & Hall/CRC.

Schafer, J. L., & Olsen, M. K. (1998). Multiple imputation for multivariate missing-data problems: A data analyst's perspective. *Multivariate Behavioral Research, 33*, 545–571.

Shannon, J., Kristal, A. R., Curry, S. J., & Beresford, S. A. (1997). Application of a behavioral approach to measuring dietary change: The fat- and fiber-related diet behavior questionnaire. *Cancer Epidemiology, Biomarkers & Prevention, 6*, 355–361.

Shiffman, S., Hufford, M., Hickcox, M., Paty, J. A., Gnys, M., & Kassel, J. D. (1997). Remember that? A comparison of real-time versus retrospective recall of smoking lapses. *Journal of Consulting and Clinical Psychology, 65*, 292–300.

Stone, A. A., Schwartz, J. E., Neale, J. M., Shiffman, S., Marco, C. A., Hickcox, M., et al. (1998). A comparison of coping assessed by ecological momentary assessment and retrospective recall. *Journal of Personality and Social Psychology, 74*, 1670–1680.

Taplin, S. H., Barlow, W. E., Ludman, E., MacLehos, R., Meyer, D. M., Seger, D., et al. (2000). Testing reminder and motivational telephone calls to increase screening mammography: A randomized study. *Journal of the National Cancer Institute, 92*, 233–242.

Tiffany, S. T. (1990). A cognitive model of drug urges and drug-use behavior: Role of automatic and nonautomatic processes. *Psychological Review, 97*, 147–168.

Vach, W., & Blettner, M. (1991). Biased estimation of the odds ratio in case-control studies due to the use of ad hoc methods of correcting for missing values for confounding variables. *American Journal of Epidemiology, 134,* 895–907.

Velicer, W. F., Prochaska, J. O., Fava, J. L., Laforge, R. G., & Rossi, J. S. (1999). Interactive versus noninteractive interventions and dose–response relationships for stage-matched smoking cessation programs in a managed care setting. *Health Psychology, 18,* 21–28.

Verbeke, G., & Molenberghs, G. (2000). *Linear mixed models for longitudinal data.* New York: Springer-Verlag.

Vuckovic, N., Harris, E. L., Valanis, B., & Stewart, B. (2003). Consumer knowledge and opinions of genetic testing for breast cancer risk. *American Journal of Obstetrics and Gynecology, 189*(4, Suppl. 1), 48–53.

Ware, J. H. (1985). Linear models for the analysis of longitudinal studies. *The American Statistician, 39,* 95–101.

Winett, R. A., King, A. C., & Altman, D. G. (1989). *Health psychology and public health.* New York: Pergamon Press.

5

DESIGN AND ANALYSIS OF GROUP-RANDOMIZED TRIALS IN CANCER PREVENTION AND CONTROL

DAVID M. MURRAY, SHERRI L. PALS, AND JONATHAN L. BLITSTEIN

Group-randomized trials (GRT) are comparative studies in which investigators randomize identifiable groups to conditions and observe members of those groups to assess the effects of an intervention (Donner & Klar, 2000; Murray, 1998). In this context, an *identifiable group* refers to any group that is not constituted at random, so that there is some physical, geographic, social, or other connection among its members. Just as the randomized clinical trial (RCT) is the gold standard in public health and medicine when randomization of individuals to study conditions is possible, the GRT is the gold standard in public health and medicine when randomization of identifiable groups is required. Group randomization is required whenever the investigator wants to evaluate an intervention that operates at a group level, manipulates the social or physical environment, or cannot be delivered to individuals.

GRTs have become increasingly common in public health and medicine over the past 25 years. A review of GRTs published between 1990 and 1993 identified an average of 5.3 GRTs published each year in the *American Journal of Public Health* and *Preventive Medicine* (Simpson, Klar, & Donner, 1995). A more recent review covering articles published between 1998 and 2002 in the same journals identified an average of 12.0 GRTs published each year (Varnell, Murray, Janega, & Blitstein, 2004). For this chapter, we found 75 articles published in 25 peer-reviewed journals from 1998 through 2003 that reported the results of GRTs in the area of cancer prevention and control.

In this chapter, we identify the characteristics that distinguish GRTs from the more familiar RCT, review the implications of those characteristics in terms of design and analytic issues, and provide examples of GRTs in cancer prevention and control to illustrate those characteristics. We then review the GRTs related to cancer prevention and control that were published from 1998 to 2003, with particular attention to their design and analysis. Finally, we consider the implications for future GRTs in cancer prevention and control.

DISTINGUISHING CHARACTERISTICS

Several characteristics distinguish a GRT from the familiar RCT (Murray, 1998). First, the unit of assignment is an identifiable group rather than an individual. Such groups are not formed at random but rather through some physical, geographical, or social connection among their members. Second, different groups are allocated to each study condition. This creates a nested or hierarchical structure for the data, with different groups nested within each study condition. Third, the units of observation are members of those groups. This extends the nested structure to a second level, with different members nested in each group and different groups nested in each condition. Where the same members are measured repeatedly, there will be a third level of nesting, with repeat observations nested within members. Fourth, GRTs typically involve only a limited number of groups in each study condition. Although there are exceptions, it is uncommon to find a GRT with more than 25 assignment units allocated to each condition and quite common to observe GRTs with 12 or fewer groups allocated to each condition.

Together, these characteristics set the stage for the special issues of design and analysis that face investigators who conduct GRTs. These issues must be addressed as the trial is planned to ensure that it will provide a valid answer to the research questions of interest.

DESIGN ISSUES

There are four common threats to the internal validity of GRTs (Murray, 1998). The first is selection bias, which results from preexisting differences among the study conditions. Over many realizations, randomization has the opportunity to distribute all potential sources of confounding evenly between the two conditions, so that there should be no selection bias even in small GRTs. But because each GRT exists as just a single realization, and because GRTs often allocate only a limited number of often heterogeneous groups to each condition, randomization may not ensure that all sources of confounding are distributed evenly among the conditions. This makes confounding much more common in GRTs than in RCTs, particularly in smaller GRTs.

The second common threat is differential history, which refers to some external influence that can affect the primary endpoint and which operates differentially among the conditions. Most GRTs address topics important to the public health, such as dietary change, smoking cessation, or cancer screening. As such, these topics are of interest to many individuals and organizations quite apart from their interest to the investigators. When one or more of those individuals or organizations acts to change dietary intake, increase smoking cessation, or improve cancer screening, their actions may affect the primary outcome and create a plausible alternative explanation for the results of the trial.

The third common threat to internal validity is differential maturation, which reflects uneven secular trends among the groups in the trial that favor one condition over the other. Schools, worksites, communities, and other identifiable social groups may have an identifiable trajectory with respect to the outcome of interest. Some may be improving, whereas others may be declining. Absent steps to ensure that these trends will be balanced across the study conditions, they stand as a plausible alternative explanation for the results of the trial.

These first three threats to internal validity can either mask or mimic an intervention. They are best avoided by randomization of a sufficient number of groups to each study condition; careful matching or stratification can increase the effectiveness of the randomization, especially if the number of groups available is fewer than 20. Where confounding is detected after randomization, analytic techniques such as regression adjustment for confounding can be used to limit the effect of that confounding.

The fourth threat to internal validity is contamination, which occurs when components of the intervention find their way into the comparison condition, thereby biasing the estimate of the intervention effect toward the null hypothesis. Randomization will not protect against contamination, so monitoring exposure to activities that could affect the trial's endpoints in both the intervention and the comparison groups is especially important in GRTs because it will allow the investigators to detect contamination if it occurs.

ANALYTIC ISSUES

More than 25 years ago, Cornfield (1978) identified two issues (discussed in detail later in this section) that affect the analysis of GRTs that do not arise in RCTs. Both result from the physical, geographic, and social connections that exist among the members of any identifiable social group. Those connections create a component of variance attributable to the group in addition to the variance attributable to the members of those groups. That extra component of variance is indexed by the intraclass correlation coefficient (ICC), which is calculated as the proportion of variance attributable to the group (Kish, 1965). When the connections among the group members are weak, the ICC is small; when the connections among the group members are stronger, the ICC is larger. ICCs tend to be larger for measures of knowledge, attitudes, and beliefs; smaller for measures of behavior; and smaller still for physiological measures (Murray & Blitstein, 2003). ICCs also tend to be larger for small aggregates and smaller for large aggregates (Donner, 1982). It should not be surprising that spouses should have more in common in terms of attitudes or beliefs than in terms of physiological measures or that spouse pairs have more in common than unrelated residents of the same community.

Cornfield's (1978) first issue is that the variation in the condition-level statistic used to estimate the intervention effect must be assessed against the variation in the same statistic estimated at the group level; failure to do so will result in an inflated Type I error rate. Unfortunately, the variation of the group-level statistic is inflated in a GRT, both as a function of the ICC and as a function of the number of members per group (m). Donner, Birkett, and Buck (1981) defined the Variance Inflation Factor (VIF) to index the extra variation: $VIF = 1 + (m - 1)ICC$. As this formula indicates, VIF increases as m or ICC increases. It is important to note that any increase in the VIF will reduce power, other factors constant (Donner & Klar, 2000; Koepsell et al., 1991; Murray, 1998).

Cornfield's (1978) second issue is that there are often only a limited number of groups in each condition. This limits the degrees of freedom available for the test of the intervention effect; as those degrees of freedom decrease, power decreases, if other factors remain constant. In most RCTs, hundreds or thousands of participants are randomized to each condition and the degrees of freedom available for the test of the intervention effect are many. The typical GRT often has 12 or fewer groups (g) randomized to each of 2 conditions (c), so the degrees of freedom for a posttest-only analysis would be $c(g - 1) = 2(12 - 1) = 22$, with $g = 12$ and fewer with $g < 12$.

Together, these issues can make it difficult to detect important intervention effects in an otherwise well-designed and properly executed trial. This has led to some very creative, albeit misguided, strategies to try to avoid using methods that properly address the special issues inherent in a GRT.

Some have advocated testing to see whether the ICC is different from zero, and if it is not, to proceed with an analysis that ignored group and focused instead on the members (Hopkins, 1983). The problem is that the degrees of freedom for such tests are usually very limited so that they have low power. Further, the standard error for the group component of variance is not well estimated when the ICC is close to zero. So, the analyst using this strategy runs a real risk for falsely judging the ICC to be zero, ignoring it, and offering a test of the intervention effect that has an inflated Type I error rate. The prudent course is to retain all random effects associated with the design and sampling plan (Donner & Klar, 2000; Murray, 1998). After all, if the ICC really is close to zero, the extra variation will be limited unless the number of members per group is very large.

Some have noted that their groups contain subgroups and have based their analysis on the subgroups because there were more of them (Feldman, McKinlay, & Niknian, 1996). An example would be to analyze by classrooms instead of schools in a school-based GRT. This analysis rests on the strong assumption that the ICC at the subgroup level captures all of the ICC at the group level. Unfortunately, that assumption is usually not testable, and simulation studies have shown that if it is violated, the analyst risks an inflated Type I error rate (Varnell, Murray, & Baker, 2001).

Some prefer to ignore the group altogether. They argue that their study was not designed to be analyzed at the level of the unit of assignment, and so they should not be held to that standard. Others argue that their intervention was designed to change the behavior of individuals, and so their analysis should be based on individuals. Such arguments ignore the methodological realities of the GRT and are examples of exactly the kind of self-deception that Cornfield (1978) warned against 30 years ago. Ignoring the ICC will result in an inflated Type I error rate, and the investigator risks misleading their colleagues and policymakers alike.

Others attempt to address the problem of ICC by including group in the analysis, but as a blocking or stratification factor, modeled as a fixed effect (Siemer & Joormann, 2003). This is actually the worst of the misguided strategies, because it removes group variation from the error term but not from the variance of the condition means (Zucker, 1990). As a result, it carries the highest inflation in the Type I error rate of the strategies discussed in this section.

Others accept the extra variation reflected in the ICC but balk at using degrees of freedom calculated on the basis of the number of groups. The simulation results on this point are clear: The Type I error rate is protected only if the degrees of freedom are based on the number of groups (Murray, Hannan, & Baker, 1996).

How serious is this problem? Is it really necessary to attend to the problems of extra variation and limited degrees of freedom? Zucker (1990) showed that the Type I error rate can easily exceed 20% even with a modest ICC (e.g., .05) and a small number of members per group (e.g., 25); the inflation in the Type I error rate was more than 50% in larger studies or studies with larger ICCs (Zucker, 1990). Murray et al. (1996) reported similar findings. Simply put, ignoring Cornfield's (1978) warning will greatly increase the likelihood that investigators will falsely judge that their intervention was effective.

RECENT DEVELOPMENTS

The first comprehensive text on the design and analysis of GRTs did not appear until 1998, by Murray. It detailed the design considerations for the development of GRTs, described the major approaches to their analysis for both Gaussian and binary data, and presented methods for power analysis applicable to most GRTs. In the 5 years that followed, many articles discussed the methodological issues in GRTs generally or in design articles for new trials. The second textbook on the design and analysis of GRTs appeared in 2000, by Donner and Klar. That text provided a good history on GRTs and examined the role of informed consent and other ethical issues. It focused on extensions of classical methods, although it also included material on regression models for Gaussian, binary, count, and time-to-event data. Other textbooks on analysis methods germane to GRTs appeared during the same period (H. Brown & Prescott, 1999; Kreft & De Leeuw, 1998; McCulloch & Searle, 2001; Raudenbush & Bryk, 2002), as well as a large number of articles on new methods relevant to the design and analysis of GRTs. Murray, Varnell, and Blitstein (2004) summarized recent methodological developments for GRTs in public health and medicine.

A REVIEW OF RECENT GROUP-RANDOMIZED TRIALS PUBLISHED IN CANCER PREVENTION AND CONTROL

To evaluate the quality of the design and analytic methods in recent GRTs in cancer prevention and control, we conducted a review of recent GRTs published in the peer-reviewed literature between 1998 and 2002, inclusive. The methods used in this review were based on methods used in a recent review of GRTs published in the *American Journal of Public Health* and *Preventive Medicine* during the same period (Varnell et al., 2004). The Varnell et al. (2004) article considered all GRTs, regardless of content, and so was not restricted to studies on cancer prevention and control; it was also limited to just two journals. The current review examined a larger number of journals and was restricted to studies on cancer prevention and control.

Our review of peer-reviewed journals identified 75 such articles in 24 journals, ranging widely across medicine, public health, addiction research, and behavior. We identified the *American Journal of Public Health*, *Preventive Medicine*, and *Health Education & Behavior* as the three leading journals for the publication of GRTs in cancer prevention and control. We selected three other journals because of their high standing in the field of cancer prevention and control: *Journal of the National Cancer Institute*; *Cancer*; and *Cancer Epidemiology, Biomarkers & Prevention*. We then identified and reviewed all GRTs published in those journals from 1998 to 2002.

GRTs were defined as studies that randomized identifiable groups to study conditions but obtained observations from members of those groups; we use the term *group* to designate the unit of assignment and *condition* to designate the experimental condition to which the group is assigned. Articles reporting the results of studies in which groups were not randomly assigned to study conditions were excluded, as were studies involving only observations at the group, rather than individual, level because these studies do not involve group-level ICC.

Murray (1998) and Donner and Klar (2000) provided an extensive review of analytic methods appropriate for GRTs; Murray et al. (2004) provided a review of the most recent analytic developments. Table 5.1 (adapted from Varnell et al., 2004) presents the criteria used to judge whether the analytic approaches were appropriate. Methods considered appropriate for GRTs included but were not limited to mixed-model regression approaches including analysis of variance and analysis of covariance (ANOVA and ANCOVA) and random coefficients models, two-stage analyses (i.e., analysis on a summary statistic computed at the group level, including randomization-based tests), and generalized estimating equations (GEE). Because each of these methods may be applied incorrectly, we established additional criteria for rating analyses as appropriately applied; these depend on the design of the study, the assumptions underlying the analytic method, and the robustness of the method to violations of these assumptions. We considered mixed-model

TABLE 5.1

Analytic Methods Frequently Used in Group-Randomized Trials (GRTs) and the Conditions Under Which Their Use Is Appropriate

Method	Appropriate application in GRTs
Mixed-model methods	
ANOVA and ANCOVA	One or two time points
Random coefficients approach	More than two time points
Generalized estimating equations	
With correction for limited *df*	Fewer than 40 groups included in analysis
With no correction	40 or more groups included in analysis
Two-stage methods (analysis on group means or other summary statistic)	Applied at the level of the unit of assignment
Post hoc correction based on external estimates of ICC	Validity depends on validity of external estimates
Analysis at subgroup level, ignoring group-level ICC	Not appropriate for GRTs
Analysis at individual level, ignoring group-level ICC	Not appropriate for GRTs

Note. ANOVA = analysis of variance; ANCOVA = analysis of covariance; ICC = intraclass correlation coefficient. From "Design and Analysis of Group-Randomized Trials: A Review of Recent Practices," by S. P. Varnell, D. M. Murray, J. B. Janega, and J. L. Blitstein, 2004, *American Journal of Public Health, 94*, p. 395. Copyright 2004 by the American Public Health Association. Adapted with permission.

ANOVA and ANCOVA appropriate if variation at the condition level was assessed against variation at the group level, with degrees of freedom based on the number of groups and with one or two time points included in the analysis. If more than two time points are included in the analysis of a GRT, a random coefficients analysis preserves the nominal Type I error rate, whereas mixed-model ANOVA and ANCOVA may not (Murray, Hannan, Wolfinger, Baker, & Dwyer, 1998); thus, random coefficient analyses were considered appropriate for GRTs with more than two time points included in the analysis, whereas mixed-model ANOVA and ANCOVA were not. Two-stage approaches were considered appropriate if the second stage was conducted at the group level with degrees of freedom based on the number of groups. GEE was considered appropriate if the analysis included 40 groups or more or if special steps were taken to correct the downward bias in the empirical sandwich estimator when there are fewer than 40 groups in the study. This bias in the sandwich estimator is a problem whether in GRTs (Feng, Diehr, Peterson, & McLerran, 2001; Thornquist & Anderson, 1992) or in other designs involving correlated binary data (Emrich & Piedmonte, 1992; MacKinnon & White, 1985), and the problem only increases as the number of groups gets smaller (Murray et al., 1998). Several articles reporting less common methods referenced articles outlining these methods; we reviewed those articles for evidence that the analytic method described was suitable for the analysis of GRTs.

We reviewed a total of 51 GRT articles in the selected journals (e.g., see Allen, Stoddard, Mays, & Sorensen, 2001; Baranowski et al., 2002; Beresford et al., 2001; Biener et al., 1999; K. S. Brown et al., 2002; Buller et al., 1999; Cameron et al., 1999; Campbell et al., 2002; Cummings et al., 1998; Dietrich, Olson, Sox, Tosteson, & Grant-Petersson, 2000; D'Onofrio, Moskowitz, & Braverman, 2002; Duan, Fox, Derose, & Carson, 2000; Forster & Wolfson, 1998; Geller et al., 2001; Gritz et al., 1998; Hancock et al., 2001; Hennrikus et al., 2002; Hillman et al., 1998; Hunt et al., 2001; Kellam & Anthony, 1998; Lowe, Balanda, Stanton, & Gillespie, 1999; Manfredi, Crittenden, Cho, Engler, & Warnecke, 2000; Mayer et al., 1998; Noland et al., 1998; Resnicow et al., 2001; Reynolds et al., 2000; Segura et al., 2001; Sejr & Osler, 2002; Slater et al., 1998; Thomas et al., 2002; N. J. Thompson et al., 1999; Tilley et al., 1999; Walsh et al., 1999; Zhu et al., 2002), comprising 68% of the 75 GRT articles on cancer prevention and control published from 1998 to 2002. We also identified and reviewed 24 background articles cited in the selected articles (e.g., see Abrams et al., 1994; Allen, Sorensen, Stoddard, Peterson, & Colditz, 1999; Cameron et al., 1999; Campbell et al., 1998; Cullen et al., 2000; Demark-Wahnefried et al., 1998; Elder et al., 2000; Forster & Wolfson, 1998; Fox, Stein, Gonzalez, Farrenkopf, & Dellinger, 1998; Kramish Campbell et al., 1996; Reynolds et al., 1998; B. Thompson, Shannon, Beresford, Jacobson, & Ewings, 1995; B. Thompson, van Leynseele, & Beresford, 1997;

Tilley et al., 1997). Eighteen (35.3%) of the 51 articles were published in the *American Journal of Public Health*; 24 (47.1%) were published in *Preventive Medicine*; 4 (7.8%) in *Health Education & Behavior*; 3 (5.9%) in the *Journal of the National Cancer Institute*; and 1 each (2.0%) in *Cancer* and in *Cancer Epidemiology, Biomarkers & Prevention*.

Table 5.2 presents design characteristics from the 51 articles. Most GRTs published in the area of cancer prevention and control used a design with just two conditions (i.e., intervention vs. control); used a priori matching and/or stratification in their design; were conducted in schools or colleges, in worksites, or in communities or neighborhoods; included between 6 and 25 groups per condition; used a pretest–posttest design with repeat observations on the same individuals; and focused on tobacco use, dietary variables, or screening.

Sample Size Methods

Overall, only 7 (13.7%) of the 51 articles reported an ICC, group component of variance, or VIF, either in the reviewed article or in a background article. Authors of an additional 3 (5.9%) articles claimed either in the reviewed article or in a background article that variance had been inflated to account for the expected ICC, but they provided no evidence such as an ICC, variance component, or VIF. The remaining 41 (80.4%) articles either did not mention sample size calculations or did so without mention of any effort to account for the expected ICC.

Analytic Methods

We excluded one article published in *Preventive Medicine* from the analytic review because the authors did not provide enough detail to determine whether the analytic strategy was appropriate. Table 5.3 presents the numbers and percentages of the 50 remaining articles that reported only appropriate methods, reported some appropriate and some inappropriate methods, or reported only inappropriate methods.

Among the 50 articles, 33 (66.0%) reported only analyses that took ICC into account properly. The analytic methods used represented all of the methods described in Table 5.1 as appropriate under the proper conditions. GEEs were used less often than the other methods, which were used about equally often.

Ten (20.0%) articles reported some analyses that took ICC into account properly and some that did not. The most commonly used inappropriate analysis was an analysis at an individual level that ignored the unit of assignment altogether.

Seven (14.0%) articles reported only analyses that did not take ICC into account properly. Here too, the most commonly used inappropriate analysis was an analysis at the individual level that ignored the unit of assignment altogether.

TABLE 5.2

Characteristics of 51 Studies That Reported the Results
of Group-Randomized Trials, 1998–2002

Characteristic	N	%
Number of study conditions		
1	44	86.3
3	4	7.8
≥ 4	3	5.9
Matching or stratification in design		
Matching	23	45.1
Stratification	14	27.5
Matching and stratification	6	11.8
Randomization without matching or stratification	8	15.7
Type of group		
Schools or colleges	12	23.5
Worksites	16	31.4
Communities or neighborhoods	8	15.7
Health care practice	7	13.7
Housing projects or apartment buildings	3	5.9
Churches	3	5.9
Other	2	3.9
Number of groups per condition		
1	2	3.9
2–3	3	5.9
4–5	6	11.8
6–12	15	29.4
13–25	15	29.4
> 25	10	19.6
Number of members per group		
< 10	6	11.8
10–50	13	25.5
51–100	14	27.5
>100	18	35.3
Number of time points		
1	2	3.9
2	30	58.8
3	13	25.5
4–9	5	9.8
Number varies within study	1	2.0
Design		
Cohort	29	56.9
Cross-sectional	12	23.5
Combination of cohort and cross-sectional	10	19.6
Primary outcome variables		
Tobacco use	19	37.3
Dietary variables	12	23.5
Cancer screening	11	21.6
Sun protection	4	7.8
Dietary variables and tobacco use	3	5.9
Cancer mortality	1	2.0
Wood dust exposure	1	2.0

Note. From "Design and Analysis of Group-Randomized Trials: A Review of Recent Practices," by S. P.
Varnell, D. M. Murray, J. B. Janega, and J. L. Blitstein, 2004, *American Journal of Public Health, 94,*
p. 396. Copyright 2004 by the American Public Health Association. Adapted with permission.

TABLE 5.3
Distribution of Analytic Methods in 50 Articles That Reported the Results of Group-Randomized Trials, 1998–2002

Criteria	N	%
Articles reporting only appropriate methods	33	66.0
Mixed-model methods with baseline measurement as covariate	11	22.0
Mixed-model ANOVA and ANCOVA approach with one or two time points	10	20.0
GEEs with 40 or more groups	3	6.0
Two-stage analysis (analysis of group means or other summary statistics)	13	26.0
Articles reporting some appropriate and some inappropriate methods	10	20.0
Appropriate methods		
Mixed-model methods with baseline measurement as covariate	3	6.0
Mixed-model methods with one or two time points	3	6.0
GEEs with 40 or more groups	1	2.0
Two-stage analysis	2	4.0
Inappropriate methods		
Analysis at an individual level, ignoring group-level ICC	6	12.0
Analysis at a subgroup level, ignoring group-level ICC	0	0.0
GEE or other asymptotically robust method with fewer than 40 groups	1	2.0
Mixed-model ANOVA and ANCOVA approach with more than two time points	1	2.0
Other	5	10.0
Articles reporting only inappropriate methods	7	14.0
Analysis at an individual level, ignoring group-level ICC	5	10.0
Analysis at a subgroup level, ignoring group-level ICC	2	4.0
Analysis with group as a fixed effect	1	2.0
Mixed-model ANOVA and ANCOVA approach with more than two time points	0	0.0
GEEs with fewer than 40 groups	3	6.0

Note. ANOVA = analysis of variance; ANCOVA = analysis of covariance; GEE = generalized estimating equation; ICC = intraclass correlation coefficient. Percentages within subsections of this table may not add to the subsection total, because the categories were not mutually exclusive. From "Design and Analysis of Group-Randomized Trials: A Review of Recent Practices," by S. P. Varnell, D. M. Murray, J. B. Janega, and J. L. Blitstein, 2004, *American Journal of Public Health, 94,* p. 396. Copyright 2004 by the American Public Health Association. Adapted with permission.

Discussion

Our review indicated that fully 80.4% of the cancer prevention and control GRT articles published from 1998 to 2002 did not report enough information on sample size calculation to assure us that such calculations had been done appropriately. That does not necessarily mean that these studies were planned incorrectly, as the investigators might have used appropriate methods but chosen not to report them in their articles. Even so, 21.6% of the studies examined included fewer than six groups per condition, suggesting that appropriate sample size methods were not used in those studies.

Only 14.0% of the GRT articles published from 1998 to 2002 used consistently inappropriate analytic methods. Another 20.0% reported some inappropriate methods but also some appropriate methods. This suggests that between 14.0% and 34.0% of the analyses reported did not appropriately address the positive ICC and limited degrees of freedom often found in GRTs.

A natural question arises as to what to make of the studies that used inappropriate analytic methods. Are they misleading? Should their findings be discounted? It is quite likely that the Type I error rate in these analyses was higher than the ideal, nominal 5%, but it is impossible to say how much higher the true Type I error rate was. The only way to determine that, to any degree of certainty, would be to repeat those analyses using appropriate methods or to apply a post hoc correction to the analyses reported.

We are aware of only one article that performed such post hoc corrections to a collection of GRT articles. Rooney and Murray (1996) reviewed school-based adolescent smoking-prevention GRTs and found that 80.0% had not performed an appropriate analysis. Rooney and Murray reported two meta-analyses of these studies, with and without a post hoc correction for the likely ICC and limited degrees of freedom. They found that the correction made little difference because the many studies that had not performed appropriate analyses were usually much smaller than the more limited number of studies that had performed appropriate analyses. Because the meta-analyses were weighted by size, the weaker studies were discounted and the stronger studies were counted more heavily.

RECOMMENDATIONS TO IMPROVE THE QUALITY OF GROUP-RANDOMIZED TRIALS IN CANCER PREVENTION AND CONTROL

The most recent review of GRTs generally in public health and medicine (Varnell et al., 2004) covered the period from 1998 to 2002. That review reported that only 15.5% reported evidence of using appropriate methods for sample size estimation and that only 54.4% reported using only appropriate methods for data analysis. Our review found that a slightly lower proportion (13.7%) of the GRTs published in the area of cancer prevention and control during the same period reported evidence of using appropriate methods for sample size estimation but that an appreciably higher proportion (66.0%) reported using only appropriate methods for data analysis. From these results, it appears that the quality of the sample size and data analytic methods used in GRTs published in cancer prevention and control from 1998 to 2002 is at least as good and perhaps better than was observed across all of public health and medicine.

Even so, there remain important deficiencies in the methods used in GRTs in the area of cancer prevention and control. Fully 80.4% of these studies provided no information related to sample size estimation, and 34.0% reported at least some analytic methods that were inappropriate given the nature of the design and the state of the science.

What can be done to improve this situation? Certainly, reviews can continue to encourage investigators to attend to these issues. There are valid methods that are readily available and well documented for the design and analysis of GRTs. As noted earlier, there are now two textbook treatments of these issues (Donner & Klar, 2000; Murray, 1998), along with a number of other texts that provide supporting material (H. Brown & Prescott, 1999; Kreft & De Leeuw, 1998; McCulloch & Searle, 2001). Several more recent reviews have supplemented these sources (Feng et al., 2001; Feng & Thompson, 2002; Klar & Donner, 2001).

Investigators need not become methodologists or statisticians to improve the methods used in their studies. Indeed, they can benefit substantially by collaborating with methodologists or statisticians who know these issues well, just as they already benefit by collaborating with interventionists who understand their part of the health promotion and disease prevention research process.

In addition, reviewers both for agencies funding GRTs and for journals publishing these studies should ensure that studies are properly planned and that their reports provide evidence of that planning, both in terms of sample size estimation and in terms of data analysis. Editors can play a role as well, by assigning articles describing the results of a GRT to a statistician or other methodologist familiar with the special design and analytic issues facing these studies. That is now the policy of the *American Journal of Public Health*, and it would be helpful for other journals to adopt a similar policy.

REFERENCES

Abrams, D. B., Boutwell, W. B., Grizzle, J., Heimendinger, J., Sorensen, G., & Varnes, J. (1994). Cancer control at the workplace: The Working Well Trial. *Preventive Medicine, 23*, 15–27.

Allen, J. D., Sorensen, G., Stoddard, A. M., Peterson, K. E., & Colditz, G. (1999). The relationship between social network characteristics and breast cancer screening practices among employed women. *Annals of Behavioral Medicine, 21*, 193–200.

Allen, J. D., Stoddard, A. M., Mays, J., & Sorensen, G. (2001). Promoting breast and cervical cancer screening at the workplace: Results from the Woman to Woman Study. *American Journal of Public Health, 91*, 584–590.

Baranowski, T., Baranowski, J., Cullen, K. W., deMoor, C., Rittenberry, L., Hebert, D., & Jones, L. (2002). 5-a-day achievement badge for African-American Boy Scouts: Pilot outcome results. *Preventive Medicine, 34*, 353–363.

Beresford, S. A., Thompson, B., Feng, Z., Christianson, A., McLerran, D., & Patrick, D. L. (2001). Seattle 5 a day worksite program to increase fruit and vegetable consumption. *Preventive Medicine, 32*, 230–238.

Biener, L., Glanz, K., McLerran, D., Sorensen, G., Thompson, B., Basen-Engquist, K., et al. (1999). Impact of the Working Well Trial on the worksite smoking and nutrition environment. *Health Education & Behavior, 26,* 478–494.

Brown, H., & Prescott, R. (1999). *Applied mixed models in medicine.* Chichester, England: Wiley.

Brown, K. S., Cameron, R., Madill, C., Payne, M. E., Filsinger, S., Manske, S. R., Best, J. A. (2002). Outcome evaluation of a high school smoking reduction intervention based on extracurricular activities. *Preventive Medicine, 35,* 506–510.

Buller, D. B., Morrill, C., Taren, D., Aickin, M., Sennott-Miller, L., Buller, M. K., et al. (1999). Randomized trial testing the effect of peer education at increasing fruit and vegetable intake. *Journal of the National Cancer Institute, 91,* 1491–1500.

Cameron, R., Brown, K. S., Best, J. A., Pelkman, C. L., Madill, C., Manske, S. R., & Payne, M. E. (1999). Effectiveness of a social influences smoking prevention program as a function of provider type, training method, and school risk. *American Journal of Public Health, 89,* 1827–1831.

Campbell, M. K., Symons, M., Demark-Wahnefried, W., Polhamus, B., Bernhardt, J. M., McClelland, J. W., & Washington, C. (1998). Stages of change and psychosocial correlates of fruit and vegetable consumption among rural African-American church members. *American Journal of Health Promotion, 12,* 185–191.

Campbell, M. K., Tessaro, I., DeVellis, B., Benedict, S., Kelsey, K., Belton, L., & Sanhueza, A. (2002). Effects of a tailored health promotion program for female blue-collar workers: Health works for women. *Preventive Medicine, 34,* 313–323.

Cornfield, J. (1978). Randomization by group: A formal analysis. *American Journal of Epidemiology, 108,* 100–102.

Cullen, K. W., Baranowski, T., Baranowski, J., Warnecke, C., de Moor, C., Nwachokor, A., et al. (2000). "5 a day" achievement badge for urban Boy Scouts: Formative evaluation results. *Journal of Cancer Education, 13,* 162–168.

Cummings, K. M., Hyland, A., Saunders-Martin, T., Perla, J., Coppola, P. R., & Pechacek, T. F. (1998). Evaluation of an enforcement program to reduce tobacco sales to minors. *American Journal of Public Health, 88,* 932–936.

Demark-Wahnefried, W., McClelland, J., Campbell, M. K., Hoben, K., Lashley, J., Graves, C., et al. (1998). Awareness of cancer-related programs and services among rural African Americans. *Journal of the National Medical Association, 90,* 197–202.

Dietrich, A. J., Olson, A. L., Sox, C. H., Tosteson, T. D., & Grant-Petersson, J. (2000). Persistent increase in children's sun protection in a randomized controlled community trial. *Preventive Medicine, 31,* 569–574.

Donner, A. (1982). An empirical study of cluster randomization. *International Journal of Epidemiology, 11,* 283–286.

Donner, A., Birkett, N., & Buck, C. (1981). Randomization by cluster: Sample size requirements and analysis. *American Journal of Epidemiology, 114,* 906–914.

Donner, A., & Klar, N. (2000). *Design and analysis of cluster randomization trials in health research.* London: Arnold.

D'Onofrio, C. N., Moskowitz, J. M., & Braverman, M. T. (2002). Curtailing tobacco use among youth: Evaluation of Project 4-Health. *Health Education & Behavior, 29,* 656–682.

Duan, N., Fox, S. A., Derose, K. P., & Carson, S. (2000). Maintaining mammography adherence through telephone counseling in a church-based trial. *American Journal of Public Health, 90,* 1468–1471.

Elder, J. P., Campbell, N. R., Litrownik, A. J., Ayala, G. X., Slymen, D. J., Parra-Medina, D., & Lovato, C. Y. (2000). Predictors of cigarette and alcohol susceptibility and use among Hispanic migrant adolescents. *Preventive Medicine, 31*(2, Pt. 1), 115–123.

Emrich, L. J., & Piedmonte, M. R. (1992). On some small sample properties of generalized estimating equation estimates for multivariate dichotomous outcomes. *Journal of Statistical Computation and Simulation, 41,* 19–29.

Feldman, H. A., McKinlay, S. M., & Niknian, M. (1996). Batch sampling to improve power in a community trial: Experience from the Pawtucket Heart Health Program. *Evaluation Review, 20,* 244–274.

Feng, Z., Diehr, P., Peterson, A., & McLerran, D. (2001). Selected statistical issues in group randomized trials. *Annual Review of Public Health, 22,* 167–187.

Feng, Z., & Thompson, B. (2002). Some design issues in a community intervention trial. *Control Clinic Trials, 23,* 431–449.

Forster, J. L., & Wolfson, M. (1998). Youth access to tobacco: Policies and politics. *Annual Review of Public Health, 19,* 203–235.

Fox, S. A., Stein, J. A., Gonzalez, R. E., Farrenkopf, M., & Dellinger, A. (1998). A trial to increase mammography utilization among Los Angeles Hispanic women. *Journal of Health Care for the Poor Underserved, 9,* 309–321.

Geller, A. C., Glanz, K., Shigaki, D., Isnec, M. R., Sun, T., & Maddock, J. (2001). Impact of skin cancer prevention on outdoor aquatics staff: The Pool Cool program in Hawaii and Massachusetts. *Preventive Medicine, 33,* 155–161.

Gritz, E. R., Thompson, B., Emmons, K., Ockene, J. K., McLerran, D. F., & Nielsen, I. R. (1998). Gender differences among smokers and quitters in the Working Well Trial. *Preventive Medicine, 27,* 553–561.

Hancock, L., Sanson-Fisher, R., Perkins, J., Corkrey, R., Burton, R., & Reid, S. (2001). Effect of a community action intervention on cervical cancer screening rates in rural Australian towns: The Cart Project. *Preventive Medicine, 32,* 109–117.

Hennrikus, D. J., Jeffery, R. W., Lando, H. A., Murray, D. M., Brelje, K., Davidann, B., et al. (2002). The Success Project: The effect of program format and incentives on participation and cessation in worksite smoking cessation programs. *American Journal of Public Health, 92,* 274–279.

Hillman, A. L., Ripley, K., Goldfarb, N., Nuamah, I., Weiner, J., & Lusk, E. (1998). Physician financial incentives and feedback: Failure to increase cancer screening in Medicaid managed care. *American Journal of Public Health, 88,* 1699–1701.

Hopkins, K. D. (1983). A strategy for analyzing ANOVA designs having one or more random factors. *Educational and Psychological Measurement, 43,* 107–113.

Hunt, M. K., Lobb, R., Delichatsios, H. K., Stone, C., Emmons, K., & Gillman, M. W. (2001). Process evaluation of a clinical preventive nutrition intervention. *Preventive Medicine, 33*(2, Pt. 1), 82–90.

Kellam, S. G., & Anthony, J. C. (1998). Targeting early antecedents to prevent tobacco smoking: Findings from an epidemiologically based randomized field trial. *American Journal of Public Health, 88*, 1490–1495.

Kish, L. (1965). *Survey sampling.* New York: Wiley.

Klar, N., & Donner, A. (2001). Current and future challenges in the design and analysis of cluster randomization trials. *Statistics in Medicine, 20*, 3729–3740.

Koepsell, T. D., Martin, D. C., Diehr, P. H., Psaty, B. M., Wagner, E. H., Perrin, E. B., & Cheadle, A. (1991). Data analysis and sample size issues in evaluations of community-based health promotion and disease prevention programs: A mixed-model analysis of variance approach. *Journal of Clinical Epidemiology, 44*, 701–713.

Kramish Campbell, M., Polhamus, B., McClelland, J. W., Bennett, K., Kalsbeek, W., Coole, D., et al. (1996). Assessing fruit and vegetable consumption in a 5 a day study targeting rural Blacks: The issue of portion size. *Journal of the American Dietetic Association, 96*, 1040–1042.

Kreft, I., & De Leeuw, J. (1998). *Introducing multilevel modeling.* London: Sage.

Lowe, J. B., Balanda, K. P., Stanton, W. R., & Gillespie, A. (1999). Evaluation of a 3-year school-based intervention to increase adolescent sun protection. *Health Education & Behavior, 26*, 396–408.

MacKinnon, J. G., & White, H. (1985). Some heteroskedasticity-consistent covariance matrix estimators with improved finite sample properties. *Journal of Econometrics, 29*, 305–325.

Manfredi, C., Crittenden, K. S., Cho, Y. I., Engler, J., & Warnecke, R. (2000). The effect of a structured smoking cessation program, independent of exposure to existing interventions. *American Journal of Public Health, 90*, 751–756.

Mayer, J. A., Eckhardt, L., Stepanski, B. M., Sallis, J. F., Elder, J. P., Slymen, D. J., et al. (1998). Promoting skin cancer prevention counseling by pharmacists. *American Journal of Public Health, 88*, 1096–1099.

McCulloch, C. E., & Searle, S. R. (2001). *Generalized, linear, and mixed models.* New York: Wiley.

Murray, D. M. (1998). *Design and analysis of group-randomized trials.* New York: Oxford University Press.

Murray, D. M., & Blitstein, J. L. (2003). Methods to reduce the impact of intraclass correlation in group-randomized trials. *Evaluation Review, 27*, 79–103.

Murray, D. M., Hannan, P. J., & Baker, W. L. (1996). A Monte Carlo study of alternative responses to intraclass correlation in community trials: Is it ever possible to avoid Cornfield's penalties? *Evaluation Review, 20*, 313–337.

Murray, D. M., Hannan, P. J., Wolfinger, R. D., Baker, W. L., & Dwyer, J. H. (1998). Analysis of data from group-randomized trials with repeat observations on the same groups. *Statistics in Medicine, 17*, 1581–1600.

Murray, D. M., Varnell, S. P., & Blitstein, J. L. (2004). Design and analysis of group-randomized trials: A review of recent methodological developments. *American Journal of Public Health, 94*, 423–432.

Noland, M. P., Kryscio, R. J., Riggs, R. S., Linville, L. H., Ford, V. Y., & Tucker, T. C. (1998). The effectiveness of a tobacco prevention program with adolescents living in a tobacco-producing region. *American Journal of Public Health, 88*, 1862–1865.

Raudenbush, S. W., & Bryk, A. S. (2002). *Hierarchical linear models* (2nd ed.). Thousand Oaks, CA: Sage.

Resnicow, K., Jackson, A., Wang, T., De, A. K., McCarty, F., Dudley, W. N., & Baranowski, T. (2001). A motivational interviewing intervention to increase fruit and vegetable intake through Black churches: Results of the Eat for Life Trial. *American Journal of Public Health, 91*, 1686–1693.

Reynolds, K. D., Franklin, F. A., Binkley, D., Raczynski, J. M., Harrington, K. F., Kirk, K. A., & Person, S. (2000). Increasing the fruit and vegetable consumption of fourth-graders: Results from the High 5 Project. *Preventive Medicine, 30*, 309–319.

Reynolds, K. D., Raczynski, J. M., Binkley, D., Franklin, F. A., Duvall, R. C., Devane-Hart, K., et al. (1998). Design of "High 5": A school-based study to promote fruit and vegetable consumption for reduction of cancer risk. *Journal of Cancer Education, 13*, 169–177.

Rooney, B. L., & Murray, D. M. (1996). A meta-analysis of smoking prevention programs after adjustment for errors in the unit of analysis. *Health Education Quarterly, 23*, 48–64.

Segura, J. M., Castells, X., Casamitjana, M., Macia, F., Porta, M., & Katz, S. J. (2001). A randomized controlled trial comparing three invitation strategies in a breast cancer screening program. *Preventive Medicine, 33*, 325–332.

Sejr, H. S., & Osler, M. (2002). Do smoking and health education influence student nurses' knowledge, attitudes, and professional behavior? *Preventive Medicine, 34*, 260–265.

Siemer, M., & Joormann, J. (2003). Assumptions and consequences of treating providers in therapy studies as fixed versus random effects: Reply to Crits-Christoph, Tu, and Gallop (2003) and Serlin, Wampold, and Levin (2003). *Psychological Methods, 8*, 535–544.

Simpson, J. M., Klar, N., & Donner, A. (1995). Accounting for cluster randomization: A review of primary prevention trials, 1990 through 1993. *American Journal of Public Health, 85*, 1378–1383.

Slater, J. S., Ha, C. N., Malone, M. E., McGovern, P., Madigan, S. D., Finnegan, J. R., et al. (1998). A randomized community trial to increase mammography utilization among low-income women living in public housing. *Preventive Medicine, 27*, 862–870.

Thomas, D. B., Gao, D. L., Ray, R. M., Wang, W. W., Allison, C. J., Chen, F. L., et al. (2002). Randomized trial of breast self-examination in Shanghai: Final results. *Journal of the National Cancer Institute, 94*, 1445–1457.

Thompson, B., Shannon, J., Beresford, S. A., Jacobson, P. E., & Ewings, J. A. (1995). Implementation aspects of the Seattle "5 a day" intervention project: Strategies to help employees make dietary changes. *Topics in Clinical Nutrition, 11*, 58–75.

Thompson, B., van Leynseele, J., & Beresford, S. A. (1997). Recruiting worksites to participate in a health promotion research study. *American Journal of Health Promotion, 11*, 344–351.

Thompson, N. J., Boyko, E. J., Dominitz, J. A., Belcher, D. W., Chesebro, B. B., Stephens, L. M., & Chapko, M. K. (1999). A randomized controlled trial of a clinic-based support staff intervention to increase the rate of fecal occult blood test ordering. *Preventive Medicine, 30*, 244–251.

Thornquist, M. D., & Anderson, G. L. (1992). *Small sample properties of generalized estimating equations in group-randomized designs with Gaussian response.* Paper presented at the 120th Annual Meeting of the American Public Health Association, Washington, DC.

Tilley, B. C., Glanz, K., Kristal, A. R., Hirst, K., Li, S., Vernon, S. W., & Myers, R. (1999). Nutrition intervention for high-risk auto workers: Results of the Next Step Trial. *Preventive Medicine, 28*, 284–292.

Tilley, B. C., Vernon, S. W., Glanz, K., Myers, R., Sanders, K., Lu, M., et al. (1997). Worksite cancer screening and nutrition intervention for high-risk auto workers: Design and baseline findings of the Next Step Trial. *Preventive Medicine, 26*, 227–235.

Varnell, S. P., Murray, D. M., & Baker, W. L. (2001). An evaluation of analysis options for the one-group-per-condition design. Can any of the alternatives overcome the problems inherent in this design? *Evaluation Review, 25*, 440–453.

Varnell, S. P., Murray, D. M., Janega, J. B., & Blitstein, J. L. (2004). Design and analysis of group-randomized trials: A review of recent practices. *American Journal of Public Health, 94*, 393–399.

Walsh, M. M., Hilton, J. F., Masouredis, C. M., Gee, L., Chesney, M. A., & Ernster, V. L. (1999). Smokeless tobacco cessation intervention for college athletes: Results after 1 year. *American Journal of Public Health, 89*, 228–234.

Zhu, K., Hunter, S., Bernard, L. J., Payne-Wilks, K., Roland, C. L., Elam, L. C., et al. (2002). An intervention study on screening for breast cancer among single African-American women aged 65 and older. *Preventive Medicine, 34*, 536–545.

Zucker, D. M. (1990). An analysis of variance pitfall: The fixed effects analysis in a nested design. *Educational and Psychological Measurement, 50*, 731–738.

6
PARTICIPATION IN CANCER CLINICAL TRIALS

ELECTRA D. PASKETT, MIRA L. KATZ, CECILIA R. DEGRAFFINREID,
AND CATHY M. TATUM

Participation in cancer prevention, early detection, diagnostic, treatment, and survivor (i.e., nontreatment) clinical trials provides the opportunity to participate in state-of-the-art research and furthers scientific discovery. Thus, participation by all populations in clinical trials is critical for understanding the generalizability of trial findings. Despite the sound rationale for individuals to participate in the clinical trial process, overall participation rates are low for the adult general population. Between January 1991 and June 1994, only 2.5% of all cancer patients enrolled in a cooperative group clinical trial (Tejeda et al., 1996). A more recent review of a 1-year period (i.e., 1998–1999) indicated that this percentage has not changed (Sateren et al., 2002). This participation rate is even lower for minority and underserved populations. According to SEER (i.e., Surveillance Epidemiology and End Results) data, from 1991 to 1994 and from 1998 to 1999, approximately 14% to 19% of adults with cancer were non-White; of the total number of individuals participating in clinical trials, approximately 9% to 10% self-identified as Black and 4% to 6%, as Hispanic (Sateren et al., 2002; Tejeda et al., 1996). For cancer prevention trials, 1% to 5% of those approached participate (Schatzkin et al., 1996; Tangrea, 1997), and of those individuals that participate in a clinical trial, 3.7% (Fisher et al., 1998) to 18.5% (Rossouw & Hurd, 1999) are minorities. These participation rates are far from the national demographics of 25% non-White individuals in the 2000 Census (Grieco & Cassidy, 2001).

Improvement in cancer clinical trial participation rates would allow the statistical goals of the study to be achieved and the trial to be completed faster. It would also improve patient care because results could be published more quickly and new studies could be initiated in a timelier manner to answer current research questions (Demmy et al., 2004). In addition, improved participation rates would allow trials to be completed with fewer resources, thereby increasing the resources available for new clinical trials.

We have previously suggested effective recruitment strategies to increase participation of all individuals in the clinical trials process (Paskett, DeGraffinreid, Tatum, & Margitic, 1996). These strategies include adequately characterizing the target population, involving members of the target population in planning efforts, explaining the message to the target population, giving something back to the community, enhancing the study's credibility by using a community spokesperson, identifying and removing barriers to participation, improving staff sensitivity, and educating the target population about the importance of the trial.

RECRUITMENT FRAMEWORK

We developed the accrual to clinical trials (ACT) framework to understand and address difficulties in the recruitment of participants into cancer trials (see Figure 6.1; Paskett, Katz, DeGraffinreid, & Tatum, 2003). The ACT framework consists of targeting effective strategies to the participant or health care provider, system, community, and society levels. Because individuals are influenced by many factors, it is necessary to develop such a multilevel plan for the successful recruitment of potential participants.

The ACT framework was developed to reflect the fact that potential participants and their providers each have norms, beliefs, perceptions, and attitudes from (a) their own sphere (i.e., themselves and family), (b) the community they live in, and (c) society in general. The patient and provider must interact at a personal level and work within systems that influence that interaction, with both barriers and facilitators to participation. Thus, the patient–provider interaction may be influenced at several interacting but distinct levels: individual (i.e., patient and provider), system, community, and society. Work by Albrecht and colleagues (Albrecht, Franks, & Ruckdeschel, 2005; Albrecht, Penner, & Ruckdeschel, 2003) exemplifies the careful description and study of characteristics of the patient–provider relationship that could increase or decrease the effectiveness of that relationship.

Interventions can be implemented individually at each level or at multiple levels. Behavioral theories and models should be used to assist in design-

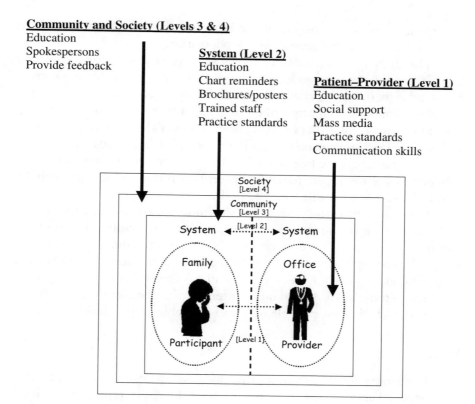

Community and Society (Levels 3 & 4)
Education
Spokespersons
Provide feedback

System (Level 2)
Education
Chart reminders
Brochures/posters
Trained staff
Practice standards

Patient–Provider (Level 1)
Education
Social support
Mass media
Practice standards
Communication skills

Society
[Level 4]

Community
[Level 3]

System ◄···[Level 2]···► System

Family

Office

Participant [Level 1] Provider

Figure 6.1. Intervention foci for the accrual to clinical trials (ACT) framework.

ing effective interventions. For minority populations especially, behavioral theories such as the minority health communication model (Alcalay, 1980) and models of community organization and community building (Minkler & Wallerstein, 2002) can be incorporated in the design and implementation of intervention strategies.

A CASE STUDY OF THE ACCRUAL
TO CLINICAL TRIALS FRAMEWORK:
RECRUITMENT OF AFRICAN AMERICAN CANCER SURVIVORS

The following example illustrates the value of using the ACT framework to achieve successful recruitment of potential participants into clinical trials. This example is from a multicenter trial that was conducted by a large cooperative group, Cancer and Leukemia Group B (CALGB No. 119901). The trial was designed to examine the quality of life of African American cancer survivors so that insights would be gained about the long-term effects of cancer and cancer treatments in this population.

This study aimed to enroll 500 cancer survivors from CALGB institutions and 500 community controls selected by random digit dialing. Inclusion criteria included participants (a) diagnosed with breast, colon, or prostate cancer or Hodgkin's lymphoma and treated on a CALGB treatment protocol or diagnosed with breast, colon, or prostate cancer, Hodgkin's lymphoma, or leukemia and not previously treated on a CALGB protocol; (b) diagnosed at least 3 years ago; (c) currently disease free; and (d) willing to complete a telephone survey conducted by research staff from the University of Illinois at Chicago, with the CALGB institution coordinating the study.

Before initiating the study at our institution, the levels included in the ACT framework (e.g., patient–provider, system, community, society) were identified. Determination of what would be necessary from patients or providers, the system (i.e., staff and institution), and community was assessed to ensure the successful completion of the study. A comprehensive list of potential barriers from each level that might interfere with completing the study was identified, as well as the possible resources available at each level.

Method

In addressing recruitment for this study, we first worked at the provider and system levels to prepare our institution for the research project. Then we approached the community and, finally, the individual patients. The interventions implemented at each level are explained in the following sections.

Provider Level

At the provider level, interventions consisted of presenting information about the importance of the trial and reassuring the providers that their patients would be treated respectfully by the research staff. An intervention was designed to gain cooperation and support. A short (10-minute) educational presentation was developed and presented at the relevant disease specific meetings, for example, breast cancer–specific meetings. This presentation included information about the purpose and the design of the study, physician and staff time commitment, and the importance and benefits of this trial to patients, health care providers, and science in general. The presentation served as a mechanism to educate providers (i.e., physicians and staff) about the study, to initiate a dialogue to address any concerns or issues related to the study, and to gain support prior to initiating recruitment activities. Starting at the provider level was essential because providers are the gatekeepers to the patient population, and thus their commitment was key to the success of the recruitment efforts.

Physicians and staff identified four important potential barriers to the recruitment of potential participants. First, they had concerns that their patients would not be willing to participate in phone interviews. Second, they did not think that their patients would be willing to talk with someone outside of their own institution. Third, they had poor experiences in the past trying to recruit African Americans into research studies. Finally, they did not think that patients would respond to receiving a letter as the first contact about a study. Each potential barrier was addressed by sharing examples based on previous trial recruitment experiences using effective strategies that targeted each of the concerns raised during the meetings. For example, we shared our experience that when an African American individual was eligible and approached in a respectful manner, he or she was as, or more, willing to participate in research projects than his or her Caucasian counterparts (Paskett et al., 1996).

System Level

At the system level, areas for interventions included access to parking, training of staff, and identification of eligible patients. Parking problems were thought to deter many individuals from meeting with us to explain the study and gain their consent. Therefore, the institution provided free valet parking for individuals coming to the medical center to discuss participation in the study.

To ensure successful recruitment of potential participants to this trial, interventions were also directed at the research staff. For this study, we presented the 10-minute educational presentation, previously described, to the comprehensive cancer center's clinical trials research staff. Although the clinical trials research staff would not be directly responsible for the recruitment activities involved in this study, awareness of the study, the eligibility criteria, and study requirements of the patients was essential for positive communication with potential participants. Discussion with the clinical trials research staff emphasized the importance of including women, minorities, and the underserved in clinical trials. The staff assisted in the identification of physicians in the system who would be the main source identifying patients who would be eligible to participate in this research trial.

After initiating these interventions, we needed to establish a mechanism to identify patients who were eligible and willing to participate in this study. Physicians or staff working in various specialties throughout the institution were asked to assist in the identification of potential participants. Once a physician provided us with a list of potential participants, a detailed review of the electronic and paper medical records was done to determine an individual's eligibility. After the record review, a list of individuals who were deemed eligible was forwarded to the physicians for their final approval to contact the identified patients. In addition, daily clinic schedules were reviewed, and individuals identified as potential participants were screened in the manner described earlier.

Community Level

At the community level, interventions include establishing good relationships and supporting communities. Interventions designed to establish commitment of time and support are needed to establish and cultivate good relationships with the surrounding communities, especially among minority and underserved populations. At our institution, we work closely with the Diversity Enhancement Program (DEP). The mission of this program is to make the minority and underserved communities aware of the importance of clinical trials and to establish trust. This has been accomplished by conducting education sessions in community settings, sponsoring community events, and hosting a radio show as a platform to establish trust and educate different communities about the importance of clinical trial participation.

An African American medical oncologist hosts the monthly radio show and has built trust through his broadcasts; thus, participants felt at ease with him and knew they could trust him in regard to his assessment of the benefits of participating in clinical trials. This African American Cancer Survivor study was specifically discussed on the radio show, and clinical trials had been discussed, in general, on each monthly broadcast.

Word of mouth about the trustworthiness of the study staff throughout the community was also valuable in getting participants to agree to take part in this study. Last, potential participants who questioned the validity of the study and the trustworthiness of the staff contacted DEP staff members to get their input. Thus, we built trust in the community by establishing avenues for the participants to be provided with information, seek answers to their questions, and gain reassurance and support.

Participant Level

Interventions at the participant level of the ACT framework were addressed in this study by fostering positive attitudes through proper communications strategies and by displaying concern for each participant and his or her specific needs or barriers to participation. Some patients were sent a letter that we developed to introduce the study and explain its purpose. The letter was printed on the patients' physician's letterhead and was signed by the physician. The letter clearly stated that a member of the research staff would be calling the patient, and it provided the name of this staff member so that the patient would be assured that the call was legitimate. These steps conveyed a measure of approval to the patient about the importance of his or her participation in the study and support from his or her physician.

Soon after the letters were mailed to the patients, some patients phoned the designated research staff member identified in the letter to discuss the study. The staff member also phoned the other patients to verify the receipt of the letter and to provide the opportunity to discuss participation in the study if the patient was interested. The phone calls were made in a respectful manner, and the patients were never addressed by their first name but were always addressed as Sir, Ma'am, Mr., Mrs., or Ms. If the patient could not discuss the study at the time of the initial telephone call, the research staff arranged an agreeable time to call the patient back.

During the initial or the arranged call, the patient was provided with a general description (i.e., purpose and requirements) of the study. Each patient was allowed the time he or she needed to discuss any issues about the study and ask questions until he or she was completely satisfied with the answers. In addition, the staff member explained that the patient had the right not to participate in the study or to withdraw at any time. If an individual stated that he or she was willing to participate, a day, time, and location were scheduled for him or her to meet with project staff to provide informed consent.

Prior to the scheduled meeting to provide consent, the consent form was mailed to the patient so he or she could review the form; consult family, friends, and physicians; and formulate any questions he or she might have had regarding participation in the study prior to the meeting. The visits to obtain the signed consent from the patient were made on a day and at a time and location that were convenient for the patient. Locations for the visit included Ohio State University's (OSU) main campus, an OSU hospital site closer to the community where the patient lived, or his or her home, having flexible early and late hours to accommodate schedules. Patients were approached during their clinic visit for consent.

During the consent process, each section of the consent form (i.e., purpose, requirements, benefits, risks, confidentiality, right to withdraw, and contact information) was explained to the patients. All potential participants were given an opportunity to ask questions until they were satisfied that all their questions were answered. Once the patient stated that he or she understood the requirements of the research study and understood each section of the consent form, he or she was asked to sign the consent. Structuring the consent process in this manner provided a patient-centered atmosphere.

Results

The following information outlines the impact of using the ACT framework for recruitment to the Quality of Life of African American Cancer Survivors study. A total of 178 patients were identified as potentially eligible for this study, and introductory letters were mailed to 168 of the survivors; 10 of the survivors were approached during their clinic visits. All 10 consented to participate in the study. Telephone calls were made to the 168 patients who were mailed the introductory letter, and we were able to speak with 114 (68%) of them. Of these additional 114 patients, 74 (65%) agreed to participate, thus giving us a combined total of 84 participants. The reason given most often for refusing to participate was that the interview would take too much time. Overall, our participation rate was 67% among those individuals with whom we had an opportunity to discuss the study.

The integration of strategies aimed at the patient–provider, system, and community levels included in the ACT framework was essential for the successful recruitment of the participants into this study. By directing strategies at multiple levels, this high participation rate was obtained.

Discussion

Efforts have been made to increase the proportion of patients and healthy persons to cancer treatment and prevention studies, respectively. Strategies, however, usually have focused on implementing one or several types of interventions, for instance, educational pamphlets or flyers, extending office hours, mass mailings, or physician education (Brewster et al., 2002; Maurer et al., 2001; Moinpour et al., 2000; Stallings et al., 2000). Recruitment rates for these efforts range from 1% to 5% for prevention trials and from 2% to 20% for clinical treatment trials (Adams, Silverman, Musa, & Peele, 1997; Sateren et al., 2002; Tangrea, 1997; Tejeda et al., 1996). Additionally, a variable cost is associated with the different recruitment strategies (Patrick, Pruchno, & Rose, 1998).

An individual's decision to participate in a cancer clinical trial is multifaceted and is based on the meaning that he or she has assigned to the importance of the trial, which is derived in part from his or her own social networks. Because of this complexity, it is important to recognize the clear and powerful connection between individuals, health care providers, and their communities. These important relationships play a significant role in successful recruitment efforts.

Few studies have used multiple strategies directed at the levels identified in the ACT framework. The Women's Health Initiative (WHI) mainly used mass-mailing strategies and physician referrals for recruitment and achieved a yield of approximately 3% (Hays et al., 2003). To recruit minority participants, however, multiple strategies were used, such as modifying eligibility criteria, creating dedicated minority clinics, establishing a recruitment study committee, and developing tips for staff and tailored material. These efforts resulted in 18.5% of WHI participants being minority (Hays et al., 2003; Rossouw & Hurd, 1999). Similar multilevel strategies were used in the Selenium and Vitamin E Cancer Prevention Trial study (Klein et al., 2001), with 21% of participants being from minority populations (Cook et al., 2005).

Little has been published on the success of the use of multiple-level strategies to accrue to cancer treatment studies. The example provided in this chapter demonstrates that a 67% participation rate can be achieved in a clinical trial with careful planning and use of the ACT framework. The use of the model for recruiting minority patients is also demonstrated. Thus, with the individualization of the components of the model, it can be adaptable to any population group or geographic area for various types of studies, such as prevention, treatment, or survivorship studies. The essential element for the recruitment of individuals from all population groups to participate in clinical trials is to develop continuing effective strategies aimed at the multiple levels identified in the ACT framework and their interrelationships. Successful recruitment to cancer clinical trials will not be achieved by a single intervention or multiple interventions addressed for one research study. Recruitment of all populations will occur by the recognition that it is a long-term process that includes different interrelated interventions that may appear independent.

FUTURE DIRECTIONS

Research on improving recruitment to cancer clinical trials in the future should focus on the application of the ACT framework. This entails focusing effective interventions at different and multiple levels simultaneously and in sequence. In previous behavioral research, barriers identified at the patient, provider, system, community, and society levels have been addressed one at a time, using various strategies, such as medical chart reminders or educational brochures. These types of strategies that address only barriers have failed to significantly increase the participation rates in cancer clinical trials. The ACT framework was designed as part of the emerging science of recruitment to design and deliver effective interventions at multiple levels (i.e., patient–provider, system, community, and society). Specific strategies will vary depending on the type of trial (i.e., prevention vs. treatment), the target population, and the resources available. By addressing important issues to participation at all levels, participation rates in all populations should increase in cancer clinical trials.

REFERENCES

Adams, J., Silverman, M., Musa, D., & Peele, P. (1997). Recruiting older adults for clinical trials. *Controlled Clinical Trials, 18*, 14–26.

Albrecht, T. L., Franks, M. M., & Ruckdeschel, J. C. (2005). Communication and informed consent. *Current Opinion in Oncology, 17*, 336–339.

Albrecht, T. L., Penner, L. A., & Ruckdeschel, J. C. (2003). Understanding patient decisions about clinical trials and the associated communication process: A preliminary report. *Journal of Cancer Education, 18*, 210–214.

Alcalay, R. (1980). *Rationale and guidelines for developing a minority health communication model*. Unpublished manuscript.

Brewster, W. R., Anton-Culver, H., Ziogas, A., Largent, J., Howe, S., Hubbell, F. A., & Manetta, A. (2002). Recruitment strategies for cervical cancer prevention study. *Gynecologic Oncology, 85*, 250–254.

Cook, E. D., Moody-Thomas, S., Anderson, K. B., Campbell, R., Hamilton, S. J., Harrington, J. M., et al. (2005). Minority recruitment to the Selenium and Vitamin E Cancer Prevention Trial (SELECT). *Clinical Trials, 2*, 436–442.

Demmy, T. L., Yasko, J. M., Collyar, D. E., Katz, M. L., Krasnov, C. L., Borwhat, M. J., Battershell, A., et al. (2004). Managing accrual in cooperative group clinical trials. *Journal of Clinical Oncology, 22*, 2997–3002.

Fisher, B., Costantino, J. P., Wickerham, D. L., Redmond, C. K., Kavanah, M., Cronin, W. M., et al. (1998). Tamoxifen for prevention of breast cancer: Report of the National Surgical Adjuvant Breast Cancer and Bowel Project P-1 Study. *Journal of the National Cancer Institute, 90*, 1371–1388.

Grieco, E. M., & Cassidy, R. C. (2001). *Overview of race and Hispanic origin, 2000*. Retrieved January 29, 2008, from http://www.census.gov/prod/2001pubs/c2kbr01-1.pdf

Hays, J., Hunt, J. R., Hubbell, A., Anderson, G. L., Limacher, M., Allen, C., & Rossouw, J. E. (2003). The Women's Health Initiative recruitment methods and results. *Annals of Epidemiology, 13*(9, Suppl.), 18–77.

Klein, E. A., Thompson, I. M., Lippman, S. M., Goodman, P. J., Albanes, D., Taylor, P. R., & Coltman, C. (2001). SELECT: The next prostate cancer prevention trial. *Journal of Urology, 166*, 1311–1315.

Maurer, L. H., Davis, T., Hammond, S., Smith, E., West, P., & Doolittle, M. (2001). Clinical trials in a rural population: Professional education aspects. *Journal of Cancer Education, 16*, 89–92.

Minkler, M., & Wallerstein, N. B. (2002). Improving health through community organization and community building. In K. Glanz, B. K. Rimer, & F. M. Lewis (Eds.), *Health behavior and health education: Theory, research, and practice* (3rd ed., pp. 279–311). San Francisco: Jossey-Bass.

Moinpour, C. M., Atkinson, J. O., Thomas, S. M., Underwood, S. M., Harvey, C., Parzuchowski, J., et al. (2000). Minority recruitment in the prostate cancer prevention trial. *Annals of Epidemiology, 10*(8, Suppl. 1), 85–91.

Paskett, E. D., DeGraffinreid, C., Tatum, C. M., & Margitic, S. E. (1996). The recruitment of African-Americans to cancer prevention and control studies. *Preventive Medicine, 25*, 547–553.

Paskett, E. D., Katz, M. L., DeGraffinreid, C. R., & Tatum, C. M. (2003). Participation in cancer trials: Recruitment of underserved populations. *Clinical Advances in Hematology & Oncology, 1*, 607–613.

Patrick, J. H., Pruchno, R. A., & Rose, M. S. (1998). Recruiting research participants: A comparison of the costs and effectiveness of five recruitment strategies. *The Gerontologist, 38*, 295–302.

Rossouw, J. E., & Hurd, S. (1999). The Women's Health Initiative: Recruitment complete—Looking back and looking forward. *Journal of Women's Health 8*, 3–5.

Sateren, W. B., Trimble, E. L., Abrams, J., Brawley, O., Breen, N., Ford, L., et al. (2002). How sociodemographics, presence of oncology specialists, and hospital cancer programs affect accrual to cancer treatment trials. *Journal of Clinical Oncology, 20*, 2109–2117.

Schatzkin, A., Lanza, E., Freedman, L. S., Tangrea, J., Cooper, M. R., Marshall, J. R., et al. (1996). The Polyp Prevention Trial: I. Rationale, design, recruitment, and baseline participant characteristics. *Cancer Epidemiology, Biomarkers & Prevention, 5*, 375–383.

Stallings, F. L., Ford, M. E., Simpson, N. K., Fouad, M., Jernigan, J. C., Trauth, J. M., et al. (2000). Black participation in the Prostate, Lung, Colorectal, and Ovarian (PLCO) Cancer Screening Trial. *Controlled Clinical Trials, 21*(6, Suppl. 1), 379–389.

Tangrea, J. A. (1997). Patient participation and compliance in cancer chemoprevention trials: Issues and concerns. *Proceedings of the Society for Experimental Biology and Medicine, 216*, 260–265.

Tejeda, H. A., Green, S. B., Trimble, E. L., Ford, L., High, J. L., Ungerleider, R. S., et al. (1996). Representation of African-Americans, Hispanics, and Whites in National Cancer Institute cancer treatment trials. *Journal of the National Cancer Institute, 88*, 812–816.

7

QUALITY-OF-LIFE ASSESSMENT IN CANCER

CAROLYN C. GOTAY

Quality-of-life (QOL) assessment has become an increasingly important aspect of cancer research and cancer care. This observation is supported by the burgeoning numbers of publications in this area—9,576 articles in MEDLINE indexed for "quality of life" and "cancer" between 2002 and 2006; increased numbers of clinical trials that include QOL measures; and the incorporation of QOL assessment into new areas, such as population monitoring and individual patient care. This chapter provides an overview of the use of QOL assessments in cancer. It discusses reasons QOL is currently receiving attention in cancer, uses of QOL data, definitions of QOL, approaches to QOL measurement, and future directions and research implications for this field.

WHY IS QUALITY-OF-LIFE ASSESSMENT IMPORTANT IN CANCER, AND HOW HAVE QUALITY-OF-LIFE DATA BEEN USED?

QOL assessment is increasingly incorporated in cancer research for several reasons. First, although eliminating death from cancer is the ultimate goal of cancer research, no magic bullet is on the horizon to cure cancer. The current reality of cancer therapeutics has led to a recognition of the significance of improving the quality, not only the quantity, of cancer patients' lives. Second, more individuals are surviving cancer for increasing lengths of time, because of earlier diagnosis and more effective treatment, with the assessment of long-term QOL in survivors increasingly needed. Third, consumers and advocates have assumed vocal and powerful roles in health care, including taking a greater role in treatment decision making and influencing research funding. For many consumers, QOL is a primary concern. Fourth, the burgeoning costs of health care have led to more accountability in health care systems, including attention to indicators of the quality of care such as QOL and satisfaction. And finally, research advances over the past 15 years have fostered increasing acceptance and use of QOL research, with the advent of validated and practical QOL questionnaires, quality control procedures to reduce missing data and other methodological problems (Moinpour & Lovato, 1998), and attention to the interpretation of QOL scores to guide cancer care (Tremaine, 2002). All of these reasons—and no doubt others—have led to an increased application of QOL research in cancer across a continuum of arenas of application, spanning the *macro level*, the population level; the *meso level*, which refers to use in specified populations; and the *micro level*, which refers to use in the context of the patient and clinician (Gotay, 2004; Lipscomb, Donaldson, & Hiatt, 2004).

At the macro level, QOL data can be used to monitor QOL in the population, including patients and survivors. Although there are many population-based surveys of health behaviors and health status sponsored by the federal government (e.g., Behavioral Risk Factor Surveillance Survey, Health Interview Survey; see Gotay & Lipscomb, 2005), these surveys include few cancer patients. Some attempts have been made to supplement cancer registries, which include detailed disease-related information, with QOL assessment (Potosky et al., 1999).

At the meso level, where most QOL research to date can be classified, studies include descriptive and analytic investigations of the impact of cancer, patterns of care, and effects of interventions, particularly clinical trials of cancer therapy (Barofsky & Sugarbaker, 1990; Day et al., 1999; Fisher et al., 1998; Goodwin, Black, Bordeleau, & Ganz, 2003; Lipscomb, Gotay, & Snyder, 2005; Sugarbaker, Barofsky, Rosenberg, & Gianola, 1982).

At the micro level, QOL data have been used to guide the care of individual patients. Applications have included identifying individuals who are at risk for or have QOL problems, patient–clinician decision making, and developing more effective therapy or supportive care (Detmar, Muller, Schornagel, Wever, & Aaronson, 2002).

WHAT IS MEANT BY *QUALITY OF LIFE?*

QOL is a term used to denote outcomes as experienced by the patient. Definitions of *QOL* vary and may focus on subjective evaluations (e.g., satisfaction), perceived health status (e.g., performance of daily activities), or both evaluations and health status (Ferrans, 2005). Despite definitional differences, virtually all investigators agree that the perspective of the patient is critical in any measurement of QOL and that QOL encompasses multiple domains, or areas, of well-being including, at a minimum, physical, psychological, and social functioning. Most measures also include cancer and cancer therapy symptoms as key components of QOL. Additional domains may be particularly appropriate for certain groups of cancer patients, such as sexuality in prostate cancer, spiritual concerns during end of life, and concerns about fertility for young adult cancer survivors.

Distinctions between QOL and two other terms are worth noting. Some investigators use *health-related quality of life* (HRQOL) for populations in which health issues are a primary concern, such as cancer patients. Also, in the past few years, a new term, *patient-reported outcome* (PRO), has surfaced in the literature, and this term seems to be especially favored by regulatory bodies such as the U.S. Food and Drug Administration (2007). PROs refer to any patient-reported outcomes and need not be multidimensional. This chapter uses the term *QOL* because it is the broadest and most encompassing.

Few conceptual models to identify predictors of QOL have been reported. This absence of theory stems largely from the pragmatic way that cancer QOL assessment developed. Most current widely used questionnaires were designed to serve a practical purpose in cancer care: to provide endpoints for cancer clinical trials that could be measured quickly and efficiently in the context of clinical practice. Empiricism rather than theory has guided work in this field to date.

HOW CAN QUALITY OF LIFE BE ASSESSED?

Measuring QOL differs in a number of ways from assessing other outcomes that are more traditionally used in cancer, such as incidence, mortality, survival, and disease-free survival, all of which are based on objective measures. QOL by its very nature requires input by the patient. The most common approach to QOL assessment in cancer patients is the use of standardized, self-report questionnaires. There are also other less frequently used modes of assessment: proxy ratings, behavioral indicators, and utility ratings.

Self-Report Questionnaires

QOL questionnaires ask patients to use quantitative response options to answer standardized questions. They may be administered by an interviewer (i.e., in person or by telephone) or may be self-completed through a number of approaches, for instance, in a clinic, through mailed surveys, or by using a computer. Little systematic attention has been given to possible effects of different modes of administration, although some information suggests that data collected through different modes are comparable (Kornblith & Holland, 1996).

Considerable methodological development of QOL questionnaires has occurred in the past decade, with extensive information available about validity, reliability, and responsiveness of many of the questionnaires (Bowling, 1995; Erickson, 2005; Spilker, 1996). Information about some of the most frequently used questionnaires is summarized in sections that follow. All of these questionnaires share some common properties: They were designed to be used in medical care settings and, as such, provide a very brief assessment of multiple QOL dimensions; the items were originally developed empirically through the input of patients and/or clinicians who determined what was important to assess; and all use well-accepted approaches to assess psychometric characteristics, such as internal consistency, construct validity, and external validity (Nunnally & Bernstein, 1994). Several kinds of QOL questionnaires have been used in cancer populations: generic instruments, general cancer tools designed for cancer patients, and cancer site–specific or treatment-specific tools. Table 7.1 provides a summary of relevant features of several questionnaires commonly used in cancer studies.

Generic Instruments

These questionnaires are designed to be used across populations and are not focused on aspects of QOL specific to cancer. Generic questionnaires can be used in addition to cancer-specific measures. Because these measures are often used in other populations, they can provide useful comparative data. Table 7.1 lists three examples of generic QOL questionnaires: The Medical Outcomes Study Short Form—36 (SF–36; Stewart, Hays, & Ware, 1988; Ware & Sherbourne, 1992), the Sickness Impact Profile (Bergner, Bobbitt, Carter, & Gilson, 1981; Gilson et al., 1975), and the Nottingham Health Profile (Hunt & McEwen, 1980).

Because the SF–36 has been used much more frequently than any other such questionnaire, discussion here is limited to this form. Detailed information about the SF–36 can be found on its Web site (SF–36 Health Survey, n.d.). This 36-item questionnaire was developed to provide a brief, multidimensional indication of patient functioning that would reflect the effects of health care interventions. According to its Web site, the SF–36 has been used in nearly 4,000 publications, and it is currently available in validated translation for 54 countries. National norms are available for the United States and are in process for 10 other countries. Extensive psychometric evaluation has been conducted, most of which provides strong support for construct

TABLE 7.1

Examples of Questionnaires Used to Assess Quality of Life in Cancer Patients

Type of measure	Questionnaire	No. of items	Domains (no. of items)	Sample psychological item
Generic	Medical Outcomes Study Short Form—36 (SF–36)	36	Physical functioning (10), role—physical (4), bodily pain (2), general health (5), vitality (4), social functioning (2), role–emotional (3), mental health (5), health change (1)	During the past 4 weeks, have you been a happy person? (all of the time, most of the time, a good bit of the time, some of the time, a little of the time, or none of the time)
	Sickness Impact Profile (SIP)	136	Alertness (10), ambulation (10), body care and movement (23), communication (9), eating (9), emotional behavior (9), home management (10), mobility (10), recreation and pastimes (8), sleep and rest (7), social interaction (20), work (9)	I act nervous or restless (yes or no for today, assigned a weighted score)
	Nottingham Health Profile	38	Emotional reactions (9), energy (3), pain (8), physical mobility (8), sleep (5), social isolation (5)	Things are getting me down (yes or no for today, assigned a weighted score)
Cancer specific	Functional Assessment of Cancer Therapy—General (FACT–G)	27	Emotional well-being (6), functional well-being (7), physical well-being (7), social well-being (7)	During the past 7 days, I feel sad (0 = not at all, 1 = a little bit, 2 = somewhat, 3 = quite a bit, 4 = very much)
	EORTC Quality of Life Questionnaire—Cancer 30 Items (QLQ–C30)	30	Physical functioning (5), role functioning (2), emotional functioning (4), cognitive functioning (2), social functioning (2), global QOL (2), symptoms (13)	During the past week: Did you feel depressed? (1 = not at all, 2 = a little, 3 = quite a bit, 4 = very much)
	Cancer Rehabilitation Evaluation System (CARES)	93–132 (Long Form), 38–57 (Short Form)	Physical (26; 7 subscales), psychosocial (44; 9 subscales), medical interaction (11; 3 subscales), marital (18; 5 subscales), sexual (8; 2 subscales), other (32; 5 subscales)	During the past month, indicate how much the statement applies to you: I frequently feel anxious. (0 = not at all, 1 = a little, 2 = a fair amount, 3 = much, 4 = very much)
	Rotterdam Symptom Checklist (RSCL)	38	Activity (8), psychological distress (8), physical distress (19), disease-specific symptoms (3)	How you have been feeling during the past 3 days: Tension (not at all, a little, quite a bit, very much)

Note. EORTC = European Organisation for Research and Treatment of Cancer.

validity and sensitivity of the questionnaire to differences in populations and effects of interventions. The SF–36 has been used in many cancer studies, including those on prevention (Day et al., 1999), treatment (Davis et al., 2002), and survivorship (Sarna et al., 2002).

Generic Cancer Questionnaires

A number of questionnaires have been developed to assess QOL in cancer patients, with items specific to concerns expressed by cancer patients. Four examples are shown in Table 7.1: the Functional Assessment of Cancer Therapy—General (FACT–G; Cella et al., 1993), the European Organisation for Research and Treatment of Cancer Quality of Life Questionnaire—Cancer 30 Items (EORTC QLQ–C30; Aaronson et al., 1993), the Cancer Rehabilitation Evaluation System (CARES; Schag, Ganz, & Heinrich, 1991; Schag, Heinrich, & Ganz, 1983), and the Rotterdam Symptom Checklist (de Haes, van Knippenberg, & Neijt, 1990). Of these, the FACT–G and EORTC QLQ–C30 have emerged as the most frequently used in recent years and are discussed in detail in this chapter.

The current version (Version 4) of the FACT–G has been evaluated and applied widely in the United States, particularly in the past 5 years. According to its Web site (http://www.facit.org/about/welcome.aspx), the FACT–G has been translated or translation is in process for 45 languages. The FACT–G has been used in many studies, particularly in clinical trials of cancer therapy. Psychometric evaluation has provided support for the FACT–G's postulated factor structure and has also supported its construct validity, reliability, and responsiveness.

The EORTC QLQ–C30 was developed by the EORTC, a clinical trials group based primarily in Europe. The QLQ–C30 has been used widely in Europe and Canada, particularly as an outcome measure in clinical trials. According to its Web site (EORTC Quality of Life, n.d.), the questionnaire has been translated and validated for 49 languages. Psychometric evaluation has provided support for the EORTC QLQ–C30's postulated factor structure and has also supported its construct validity, reliability, and responsiveness.

Although both the FACT–G and the EORTC QLQ–C30 share a number of similarities, several head-to-head comparisons of these questionnaires (Kemmler et al., 1999; Sharp et al., 1999) suggest that they do not yield completely equivalent results. Differences in content and wording across the two questionnaires may account for these differences, and this needs to be carefully considered by investigators.

Cancer Site–Specific or Treatment-Specific Questionnaires

Although somewhat less common than general cancer questionnaires, a number of instruments are available to assess QOL in specific diagnoses, for instance, the Breast Cancer Questionnaire (Levine et al., 1988), the UCLA Prostate Cancer Index Prostate Cancer Treatment Outcome Questionnaire (Litwin et al., 1998), as well as some in pediatric populations, such as the Pediatric Quality of Life Inventory (Varni, Seid, & Kurtin, 2001). In general, these questionnaires have received less use and psychometric examination than the generic and general cancer scales. Although these scales are specific to and sensitive to issues that may be of particular concern in the specific groups for which they were developed, they do not enable comparison of findings in different cancer patient populations.

One approach that is receiving increased attention addresses this concern. Both the FACT–G and the EORTC QLQ–C30 have associated modules that include a limited number of items targeted to specific cancer diagnoses or therapies (Cella et al., 1995; Sprangers et al., 1998). The developers of these questionnaires advocate the use of the general cancer core questionnaire plus an appropriate module to provide both a sensitive assessment of disease-specific concerns and a broader QOL that can be compared with other cancer patient populations. The QLQ–C30 currently has 7 associated validated modules plus 15 others in development, and the FACT–G reports 19 cancer-specific modules, 12 symptom modules, 11 cancer-specific symptom indexes, and 4 treatment-specific modules.

Proxy Ratings

The Karnofsky score, a physician-rated score from 0 to 100 (in which 0 is *dead* and 100 represents *perfect functioning*; Karnofsky & Burchenal, 1949), is still widely used in oncology as an indicator of patient capacity and as an eligibility criterion for clinical trials. However, the use of proxy QOL ratings has been limited. The reason is that QOL is generally defined as a subjective evaluation, and research has demonstrated that the assessments of proxies such as physician and patient ratings are not the same (Sprangers & Aaronson, 1992). However, a recent meta-analysis (Sneeuw, Sprangers, & Aaronson, 2002) found that correspondence between proxy and patient ratings was better for concrete aspects of functioning (e.g., physical activity), and when ratings differed, patients tended to report higher QOL than observers.

Behavioral Assessment

Performance-based evaluations, such as participant observer ratings, naturalistic observation, analog observation, measures of activity, tests of performance, product-of-behavior measures, and psychophysiological measures, are common in psychological assessment and as indicators of mental health more generally (Gotay, 1996; Haynes, 1990). However, behavioral measures are uncommon in work on QOL in cancer.

One scale that does include both naturalistic observation and self-report is List, Ritter-Sterr, and Lansky's (1990) performance status scale for head and neck cancer patients. This instrument requires the interviewer to rate patient performance regarding normalcy of diet, eating in public, and understandability of speech. The eating behaviors ratings are based on patient self-reports regarding specific aspects of their diet and dining patterns, whereas the speech component is based on the interviewer's experience communicating with the patient during the interview.

Utility Assessment

With few exceptions, QOL assessment yields an unweighted score or set of scores; that is, patient responses are not modified on the basis of their preferences or values. The usefulness of QOL scores for economic evaluations that compare the resource implications of health care interventions is also limited by the lack of a consistent and interpretable unit of measurement (Patrick & Chiang, 2000). To address such concerns, some investigators have proposed the use of utilities in QOL assessment. The quality-adjusted life year (QALY) is one example of a utility approach. Each year of life can be given a score from 0 to 1, in which 0 equals death and 1 equals perfect health, and values between 0 and 1 represent degrees of disability. Gelber and Goldhirsch (1986) proposed a variant approach to the QALY: Time Without Symptoms and Toxicity. This approach is particularly relevant to the experience of cancer patients undergoing toxic cancer therapies. Such QALYs can be computed for any health condition to measure the respective effects of health care interventions on QALYs gained or lost.

There have been several approaches to calculating the weights associated with disability, including surveys of health professionals, the general public, and patients. Other approaches require raters (who may or may not be patients) to provide comparative evaluations of specific health states. In the standard gamble technique, individuals are asked to indicate the odds they would accept to achieve various outcomes: For example, if they had a 60% chance of experiencing perfect health with a new therapy and a 40% chance of death, would they accept the new treatment? Questions that ask for a time trade-off may also be posed; that is, raters evaluate outcomes that are experienced for certain periods of time, such as perfect health for 5 years followed by death, compared with a longer period of life with less perfect health.

The utility approach has received considerable criticism (see Bowling, 1995, for a concise review). Clearly, there are major concerns: This is not a direct measure of QOL, the appropriateness of values derived from any group of raters is open to criticism about generalizability and relevance in a specific situation, the standard gamble and related techniques are cognitively complex and may not reflect the way that individuals actually make decisions, and ratings for hypothetical situations may not be comparable to decision making in real circumstances. As a result of these concerns—as well as the challenges in incorporating this kind of assessment in the clinical research environment—use of the utility approach in cancer research has been limited, to date. Nonetheless, the potential strengths of incorporating patient values and generating a metric that can be used in health care policy and planning are considerable and deserve continued investigation.

WHAT ARE CHALLENGES IN QUALITY-OF-LIFE RESEARCH?

Considerable progress has been made in knowing how to measure QOL and use resultant data to improve the care and well-being of cancer patients. Nonetheless, this is still a young field, and many questions remain to be answered. Some of these include how to select an appropriate instrument to measure QOL, how to interpret findings, and how to develop theories of QOL. We discuss each of these areas and conclude with a recommendation for additional research.

How Does One Choose the Right Approach to Measure Quality of Life?

There is currently no gold standard for QOL assessment: No question-naire or other approach has been shown to be superior to all others. Table 7.1 provides a few examples of reasonable choices, and there are many more good questionnaires available.

Methodological developments hold promise for the future of QOL instrumentation. Techniques such as item response theory (IRT) have been long established in psychological testing but are only now being investigated for their use in QOL assessment (Hays, Morales, & Reise, 2000). Considerable work needs to be done to determine whether IRT is appropriate; in particular, it must be determined whether QOL domains satisfy IRT criteria for unidimensionality. Some research that supports the appropriateness of IRT for the physical functioning domain of QOL has recently been reported for headache patients (Ware et al., 2003). Further work in this area is under way and has been stimulated by a major initiative by the National Institutes of Health (n.d.). This area is one of the highest priorities for QOL research.

How Can Quality-of-Life Findings Be Interpreted?

To be useful in clinical practice and in interpreting the meaning of trial results, QOL scores and changes in scores need to have meaning in terms of implications for interventions. This issue has received considerable attention in the past few years (see Osoba, 2005; Tremaine, 2002). Two primary approaches to QOL score interpretation have been explored: distribution-based approaches (i.e., examining differences in effect sizes and score variability) and anchor-based approaches (i.e., tying a difference on QOL score to an external criterion such as patient perception of meaningful QOL change or change in clinical status). Several investigators have explored the relationship between distribution-based and anchor-based interpretations of the data and found converging results (Norman, Sridhar, Guyatt, & Walter, 2001). Differences of about half a standard deviation appear to meet these both statistical and perceptual criteria across various HRQOL questionnaires, and such figures are already being used as the basis for power calculations in some cooperative group trials.

Additional research is needed to confirm the robustness of a half deviation difference as a clinically significant finding. If the importance of this marker is upheld, this will be an important step in making QOL data easier to use and interpret. Ultimately, QOL data may be able to be interpreted and used in the same way as other clinical and laboratory data: in the context of all the other information about the patient, so that an out-of-range score on a QOL questionnaire, or a big change in scores from the last assessment, will trigger "triage," that is, follow up on this warning sign to determine whether treatment is required and, if so, provide referral to appropriate resources. The development and testing of effective interventions to address QOL needs is another important area of research.

Several methodological issues remain as complications when doing QOL research. One is the issue of nonrandom missing data. When patients die or become too ill to participate in follow-up, such dropouts are not at random, and these participants likely represent a subgroup that is different from the rest of the sample. Therefore, they must be accounted for in some way in the analytic methods. This is an active area of research and study.

SUMMARY

The sophistication of QOL assessment in cancer has improved enormously in a short period of time. QOL is being assessed in many aspects of cancer research and clinical practice, ranging the full spectrum from prevention to long-term survivorship. Investigators can choose among a number of validated questionnaires to measure QOL, depending on the objectives of a particular application. At the same time, numerous challenges remain, only a few of which have been discussed here. These include using modern measurement techniques and new technologies for QOL assessment, interpreting and acting on the results of QOL studies, and developing models to predict QOL. Although QOL may be the new kid on the block as far as cancer outcome assessments are concerned, psychological researchers, along with investigators from multiple disciplinary perspectives, have ensured that its assessment rests on firm methodological principles. It is only with increased use of QOL assessment in cancer research and practice that the full contributions of these data will be understood, recognized, and incorporated into cancer care.

REFERENCES

Aaronson, N. K., Ahmedzai, S., Bergman, B., Bullinger, M., Cull, A., Duez, N. J., et al. (1993). The European Organization for Research and Treatment of Cancer QLQ–C30: A quality-of-life instrument for use in international clinical trials in oncology. *Journal of the National Cancer Institute, 85*, 365–376.

Barofsky, I., & Sugarbaker, P. H. (1990). Cancer. In B. Spilker (Ed.), *Quality of life assessments in clinical trials* (pp. 419–439). New York: Raven Press.

Bergner, M., Bobbitt, R. A., Carter, W. B., & Gilson, B. S. (1981). The Sickness Impact Profile: Development and final revision of a health status measure. *Medical Care, 19*, 787–805.

Bowling, A. (1995). *Measuring disease*. Bristol, PA: Open University Press.

Cella, D. F., Bonomi, A. E., Lloyd, S. R., Tulsky, D. S., Kaplan, E., & Bonomi, P. (1995). Reliability and validity of the Functional Assessment of Cancer Therapy—Lung (FACT–L) quality of life instrument. *Lung Cancer, 12*, 199–220.

Cella, D. F., Tulsky, D. S., Gray, G., Sarafian, B., Linn, E., Bonomi, A., et al. (1993). The Functional Assessment of Cancer Therapy scale: Development and validation of the general measure. *Journal of Clinical Oncology, 11*, 570–579.

Davis, A. M., O'Sullivan, B., Bell, R. S., Turcotte, R., Catton, C. N., Wunder, J. S., et al. (2002). Function and health status outcomes in a randomized trial comparing preoperative and postoperative radiotherapy in extremity soft tissue sarcoma. *Journal of Clinical Oncology, 20*, 4472–4477.

Day, R., Ganz, P. A., Costantino, J. P., Cronin, W. M., Wickerham, D. L., & Fisher, B. (1999). Health-related quality of life and tamoxifen in breast cancer prevention: A report from the National Surgical Adjuvant Breast and Bowel Project P-1 Study. *Journal of Clinical Oncology, 17*, 2659–2669.

de Haes, J. C., van Knippenberg, F. C., & Neijt, J. P. (1990). Measuring psychological and physical distress in cancer patients: Structure and application of the Rotterdam Symptom Checklist. *British Journal of Cancer, 62*, 1034–1038.

Detmar, S. B., Muller, M. J., Schornagel, J. H., Wever, L. D., & Aaronson, N. K. (2002). Health-related quality-of-life assessments and patient–physician communication: A randomized controlled trial. *Journal of the American Medical Association, 288*, 3027–3034.

EORTC quality of life. (n.d.). Retrieved May 10, 2005, from http://www.eortc.be/home/qol

Erickson, P. (2005). Assessing health status and quality of life of cancer patients: The use of general instruments. In J. Lipscomb, C. C. Gotay, & C. Snyder

(Eds.), *Outcomes assessment in cancer* (pp. 31–60). Cambridge, England: Cambridge University Press.

Ferrans, C. E. (2005). Definitions and conceptual models of quality of life. In J. Lipscomb, C. C. Gotay, & C. Snyder (Eds.), *Outcomes assessment in cancer* (pp. 14–30). Cambridge, England: Cambridge University Press.

Fisher, B., Costantino, J. P., Wickerham, D. L., Redmond, C. K., Kavanah, M., Cronin, W. M., et al. (1998). Tamoxifen for prevention of breast cancer: Report of the National Surgical Adjuvant Breast and Bowel Project P-1 Study. *Journal of the National Cancer Institute, 90,* 1371–1388.

Gelber, R. D., & Goldhirsch, A. (1986). The concept of an overview of cancer clinical trials with special emphasis on early breast cancer. *Journal of Clinical Oncology, 4,* 1696–1703.

Gilson, B. S., Gilson, J. S., Bergner, M., Bobbit, R. A., Kressel, S., Pollard, W. E., & Vesselago, M. (1975). The Sickness Impact Profile: Development of an outcome measure of health care. *American Journal of Public Health, 65,* 1304–1310.

Goodwin, P. J., Black, J. T., Bordeleau, L. J., & Ganz, P. A. (2003). Health-related quality-of-life measurement in randomized clinical trials in breast cancer—Taking stock. *Journal of the National Cancer Institute, 95,* 263–281.

Gotay, C. C. (1996). Patient-reported assessments versus performance-based tests. In B. Spilker (Ed.), *Quality of life and pharmacoeconomics in clinical trials* (2nd ed., pp. 413–420). Philadelphia: Lippincott-Raven.

Gotay, C. C. (2004). Assessing quality of life in cancer across a spectrum of applications. *Journal of the National Cancer Institute Monographs, 33,* 126–133.

Gotay, C. C., & Lipscomb, J. (2005). Sources and mechanisms for collecting cancer-related outcomes data. In J. Lipscomb, C. C. Gotay, & C. Snyder (Eds.), *Outcomes assessment in cancer* (pp. 522–549). Cambridge, England: Cambridge University Press.

Haynes, S. (1990). Behavioral assessment of adults. In G. Goldstein & M. Hersen (Eds.), *Handbook of psychological assessment* (pp. 423–463). Elmford, NY: Pergamon Press.

Hays, R. D., Morales, L. S., & Reise, S. P. (2000). Item response theory and health outcomes measurement in the 21st century. *Medical Care, 38*(9, Suppl. 2), 28–42.

Hunt, S. M., & McEwen, J. (1980). The development of a subjective health indicator. *Sociology of Health & Illness, 2,* 231–246.

Karnofsky, D. A., & Burchenal, J. H. (1949). The clinical evaluation of chemotherapeutic agents in cancer. In C. M. MacLeod (Ed.), *Evaluation of chemotherapeutic agents* (pp. 191–205). New York: Columbia University Press.

Kemmler, G., Holzner, B., Kopp, M., Dunser, M., Margreiter, R., Greil, R., & Sperner-Unterweger, B. (1999). Comparison of two quality-of-life instruments for cancer patients: The Functional Assessment of Cancer Therapy—General and the

European Organization for Research and Treatment of Cancer Quality of Life Questionnaire—Cancer 30 Items. *Journal of Clinical Oncology, 17*, 2932–2940.

Kornblith, A. B., & Holland, J. C. (1996). Model for quality-of-life research from the Cancer and Leukemia Group B: The telephone interview, conceptual approach to measurement, and theoretical framework. *Journal of the National Cancer Institute Monographs, 20*, 55–62.

Levine, M. N., Guyatt, G. H., Gent, M., De Pauw, S., Goodyear, M. D., Hryniuk, W. M., et al. (1988). Quality of life in Stage II breast cancer: An instrument for clinical trials. *Journal of Clinical Oncology, 6*, 1798–1810.

Lipscomb, J., Donaldson, M. S., & Hiatt, R. A. (2004). Cancer outcomes research and the arenas of application. *Journal of the National Cancer Institute Monographs, 33*, 1–7.

Lipscomb, J., Gotay, C. C., & Snyder, C. (2005). *Outcomes assessment in cancer.* Cambridge, England: Cambridge University Press.

List, M. A., Ritter-Sterr, C., & Lansky, S. B. (1990). A performance status scale for head and neck cancer patients. *Cancer, 66*, 564–569.

Litwin, M. S., Hays, R. D., Fink, A., Ganz, P. A., Leake, B., & Brook, R. H. (1998). The UCLA Prostate Cancer Index: Development, reliability, and validity of a health-related quality of life measure. *Medical Care, 36*, 1002–1012.

Moinpour, C. M., & Lovato, L. C. (1998). Ensuring the quality of quality of life data: The Southwest Oncology Group experience. *Statistics in Medicine, 17*, 641–651.

National Institutes of Health. (n.d.). *Patient-reported outcomes measurement information system.* Retrieved September 11, 2007, from http://www.nihpromis.org

Norman, G. R., Sridhar, F. G., Guyatt, G. H., & Walter, S. D. (2001). Relation of distribution- and anchor-based approaches in interpretation of changes in health-related quality of life. *Medical Care, 39*, 1039–1047.

Nunnally, J., & Bernstein, I. (1994). *Psychometric theory* (3rd ed.). New York: McGraw-Hill.

Osoba, D. (2005). The clinical value and meaning of health-related quality-of-life outcomes in oncology. In J. Lipscomb, C. C. Gotay, & C. Snyder (Eds.), *Outcomes assessment in cancer* (pp. 386–405). Cambridge, England: Cambridge University Press.

Patrick, D. L., & Chiang, Y. P. (2000). Measurement of health outcomes in treatment effectiveness evaluations: Conceptual and methodological challenges. *Medical Care, 38*(9, Suppl. 2), 14–25.

Potosky, A. L., Harlan, L. C., Stanford, J. L., Gilliland, F. D., Hamilton, A. S., Albertsen, P. C., et al. (1999). Prostate cancer practice patterns and quality of life: The Prostate Cancer Outcomes Study. *Journal of the National Cancer Institute, 91*, 1719–1724.

Sarna, L., Padilla, G., Holmes, C., Tashkin, D., Brecht, M. L., & Evangelista, L. (2002). Quality of life of long-term survivors of non-small-cell lung cancer. *Journal of Clinical Oncology, 20*, 2920–2929.

Schag, C. A., Ganz, P. A., & Heinrich, R. L. (1991). Cancer Rehabilitation Evaluation System—Short Form (CARES–SF): A cancer specific rehabilitation and quality of life instrument. *Cancer, 68,* 1406–1413.

Schag, C. A., Heinrich, R. L., & Ganz, P. A. (1983). Cancer Inventory of Problem Situations: An instrument for assessing cancer patients' rehabilitation needs. *Journal of Psychosocial Oncology, 1,* 11–24.

SF–36 health survey. (n.d.). Retrieved May 10, 2005, from http://www.SF-36.org/

Sharp, L. K., Knight, S. J., Nadler, R., Albers, M., Moran, E., Kuzel, T., et al. (1999). Quality of life in low-income patients with metastatic prostate cancer: Divergent and convergent validity of three instruments. *Quality of Life Research, 8,* 461–470.

Sneeuw, K. C., Sprangers, M. A., & Aaronson, N. K. (2002). The role of health care providers and significant others in evaluating the quality of life of patients with chronic disease. *Journal of Clinical Epidemiology, 55,* 1130–1143.

Spilker, B. (Ed.). (1996). *Quality of life and pharmacoeconomics in clinical trials* (2nd ed.). Minnetonka, MN: Lippincott-Raven.

Sprangers, M. A., & Aaronson, N. K. (1992). The role of health care providers and significant others in evaluating the quality of life of patients with chronic disease: A review. *Journal of Clinical Epidemiology, 45,* 743–760.

Sprangers, M. A., Cull, A., Groenvold, M., Bjordal, K., Blazeby, J., & Aaronson, N. K. (1998). The European Organization for Research and Treatment of Cancer approach to developing questionnaire modules: An update and overview. EORTC Quality of Life Study Group. *Quality of Life Research, 7,* 291–300.

Stewart, A. L., Hays, R. D., & Ware, J. E., Jr. (1988). The MOS Short-Form General Health Survey: Reliability and validity in a patient population. *Medical Care, 26,* 724–735.

Sugarbaker, P. H., Barofsky, I., Rosenberg, S. A., & Gianola, F. J. (1982). Quality-of-life assessment of patients in extremity sarcoma clinical trials. *Surgery, 91,* 17–23.

Tremaine, W. (2002). *Symposium on the clinical significance of quality of life measures in cancer patients.* Paper presented at the Mayo Clinic Proceedings, Rochester, MN.

U.S. Food and Drug Administration. (2007). *Guidance for industry. Patient-reported outcome measures: Use in medical product development to support labeling claims.* Retrieved September 11, 2007, from http://www.fda.gov/cber/gdlns/prolbl.pdf

Varni, J. W., Seid, M., & Kurtin, P. S. (2001). PedsQL 4.0: Reliability and validity of the Pediatric Quality of Life Inventory Version 4.0 generic core scales in healthy and patient populations. *Medical Care, 39,* 800–812.

Ware, J. E., Jr., Kosinski, M., Bjorner, J. B., Bayliss, M. S., Batenhorst, A., Dahlöf, C. G., et al. (2003). Applications of computerized adaptive testing (CAT) to the assessment of headache impact. *Quality of Life Research, 12,* 935–952.

Ware, J. E., Jr., & Sherbourne, C. D. (1992). The MOS 36-Item Short-Form health survey (SF–36): I. Conceptual framework and item selection. *Medical Care, 30,* 473–483.

III

PRIMARY PREVENTION: REDUCING CANCER INCIDENCE

PRIMARY PREVENTION: REDUCING CANCER INCIDENCE

Primary prevention of cancer, the subject of Part III, has been a key area of growth in cancer control over the past 2 decades. Chapter 8, by McCaul, Magnan, and Dillard, summarizes research findings on cancer risk perceptions, including those relating to the effects of strategies for promoting risk communication, risk understanding, and risk perception modification. Tobacco use is the major cause of cancer-related morbidity and mortality in the United States. In chapter 9, Mermelstein and Wahl review advances in the prevention of tobacco use, with a focus on interventions targeting children and adolescents. Chapter 10, by Dhingra and Ostroff, on smoking cessation, details the shift from conducting basic research on smoking behavior, to the design of interventions that help addicted smokers reduce their consumption, to the implementation of public policy and international law supporting cessation. In Chapter 11, on dietary change, Campbell, Gierisch, and Sutherland summarize the literature on interventions to improve dietary behaviors, many of which have been designed for specific settings, notably the workplace, religious organizations, and physician offices. In chapter 12, Buller describes successful intervention programs for reducing sun exposure in public health settings, particularly those designed to target specific populations such as children and working adults. Wenzel, Reina-Patton, and De Alba, in chapter 13, review the prevention of gynecological cancers, focusing primarily on cervical cancer prevention in community settings. Chapter 14, by Pinto, Rabin, and Frierson, reports findings across a number of settings and population groups on interventions to enhance physical activity and highlights the need for more research into the factors that mediate the adoption, as well as the maintenance, of desired activity levels.

8

UNDERSTANDING AND COMMUNICATING ABOUT CANCER RISK

KEVIN D. McCAUL, RENEE E. MAGNAN, AND AMANDA DILLARD

In 1999, the *Journal of the National Cancer Institute* published an entire volume titled *Cancer Risk Communication: What We Know and What We Need to Learn,* which included more than 30 articles and commentaries. That volume reflected the depth and breadth of the topic and set up a daunting task in developing a single, brief chapter describing how people understand their cancer risk and how one can better communicate such information. As such, we decided to use the present chapter to describe recent themes in this literature. First, we discuss what researchers mean by *risk* and how people appraise their cancer risk. Second, we address the connection of risk to behavior, with an emphasis on the strength of the link between risk perceptions and actions taken to protect one's health. Third, we deal with theory and research about how people respond to overt attempts to communicate new risk information. Fourth, we touch on presentation strategies intended to improve risk communication. The chapter concludes with a summary of how different theoretical approaches might improve the appreciation of risk, accompanied by a list of research needs.

UNDERSTANDING ONE'S RISK

People learning about cancer need to know how probable the threat is so they can decide whether to engage in available behaviors to mitigate the threat (Fischhoff, 1999). This notion of risk likelihood is at the heart of research into risk communication about cancer, and thus in this chapter we typically describe studies in which people learn about the likelihood that they might face cancer. However, it is important to recognize at the outset that understanding risk is a multifaceted task—it requires much more knowledge than researchers sometimes realize or acknowledge (Slovic, 1987). Perhaps because of the ubiquity of the health belief model (Strecher, Champion, & Rosenstock, 1997), researchers have focused on the single risk dimension of the likelihood that an event will occur. Even within this single domain, however, assessing risk is tricky. One could, for example, ask about absolute likelihood (i.e., a percentage estimate or simple magnitude judgments such as "high" or "low"), and these estimates could be measured for others and for oneself. Alternatively, one could ask about comparative likelihood (i.e., personal risk compared with others). Likelihood risk judgments are also more likely to predict self-protective outcomes if they are conditional on the basis of self-protective behavior. That is, rather than asking smokers, "What is the likelihood that you might develop lung cancer?" one is better served to ask, "What is the likelihood that you might develop lung cancer *if you continue to smoke?*" Failing to take precautionary behavior into account means that different people may interpret the risk question itself differently. Those planning on quitting smoking, for example, will compute their risk much differently than those without plans to quit (Ronis, 1992).

Recent evidence attests to the importance of these seemingly subtle differences in likelihood judgments. Compared with absolute measures, comparative measures correlate more strongly with actual risk factors such as one's odds of being diagnosed with cancer (Weinstein et al., 2004; Woloshin, Schwartz, Black, & Welch, 1999). Comparative measures also have different implications for worry associated with risk (Lipkus, Klein, Skinner, & Rimer, 2005; McCaul, Canevello, Mathwig, & Klein, 2003). However, researchers do not know whether different likelihood beliefs have different influences on motivation to engage in risk-reduction behaviors (Radcliffe & Klein, 2002). One possible explanation for the comparatively lower value of numerical risk communication is that people simply do not understand such information (Fischhoff & de Bruin, 1999; Lipkus, Biradavolu, Fenn, Keller, & Rimer, 2001; Yamagishi, 1997).

Although likelihood judgments have received the most research attention, other features of risk judgments are equally important, including the seriousness of the risk (Kohn & Rogers, 1991), severity (Lipkus et al., 2005), and actions to reduce risk (Sennott-Miller, 1994; Weinstein, 1999). Weinstein (2004) listed 16 variables that might fall under the rubric of "understanding one's risk," including beliefs about whether the health threat is chronic, painful, disabling, disfiguring, unfamiliar, progressive, fatal, acute, imminent, infectious, uncertain, localized, stigmatizing, visible, with a known cause, random, new, symptomatic, or delayed. Moreover, researchers already know that people are sensitive to some of these variables, including controllability, familiarity, and the risk's catastrophic potential (Slovic, Fischhoff, & Lichtenstein, 1987). In short, there is much to learn about risk perceptions.

Finally, Slovic, Finucane, Peters, and MacGregor (2004) pointed out that one can conceive of risk as analysis (e.g., a probability or seriousness judgment) or feeling. Thus, as a person saunters down a dark street, he or she could evaluate the chances of encountering danger or he or she might merely sense danger. Both cognitive and affective approaches to risk perception are important, but the latter focus has been underweighted in research to date (Loewenstein, Weber, Hsee, & Welch, 2001). Some of our own research suggests that worry about risk is at least as important as cognitions (e.g., perceived vulnerability in predicting self-protective behavior; Bergstrom & McCaul, 2004; McCaul & Mullens, 2003).

An important question to ask about how people understand their risk is whether their understanding is accurate. Like most research on risk perceptions, this question has been asked primarily in terms of the risk likelihood dimension. And the answer to the question depends heavily on characteristics of the particular disease, individual characteristics of the person reporting his or her risk, and the precise way that one asks about risk. We can illustrate each of these variables by referring to lung cancer. Using percentage scales, smokers as a group overestimate their risk for lung cancer; that is, they rate the chances that they will be diagnosed with lung cancer as higher than diagnosis rates for smokers (Weinstein, 1999). Using comparative scales, however, smokers show various optimistic biases. Smokers rate their own success at quitting as higher than that of the average smoker (Williams & Clarke, 1997). Even when they recognize that a particular level of smoking is very risky—a level that characterizes their own smoking—they define their own risk as average (Hahn & Renner, 1998). Although risk estimates vary depending on the characteristics just mentioned, some themes run through such estimates, and we put them forth as fair generalizations about risk accuracy. First, as a group, people often show an optimistic bias when asked to compare their risk with that of similar others. More members of a defined group, such as smokers, will see themselves as less at risk than one would expect, given a normal distribution in the population (McCoy et al., 1992; Weinstein, 1998a). In other circumstances, people overestimate their risk. Overestimates are more likely to occur for absolute likelihood measures than for comparative measures (McCaul & O'Donnell, 1998). In addition, persons with a family history of the disease are more likely to overestimate their risk (e.g., Montgomery, Erblich, DiLorenzo, & Bovbjerg, 2003). Specifically, people may hold a general belief that genes = destiny, explaining the overestimates by those with a family history. This general belief probably spills over into the genetic testing context. Thus, the public overestimates the accuracy and predictive power of such testing (Bottorff, Ratner, Johnson, Lovato, & Joab, 1998). Finally, researchers know very little about whether different ethnic groups report strong variations in their levels of risk or responses to risk communication, although some data suggest that testing for such variation will show important results (Donovan & Tucker, 2000; Lerman et al., 1995).

RISK AND BEHAVIOR

The importance of risk communication is predicated partly on a value judgment—the belief that people should be able to make health decisions on the basis of an adequate understanding of the costs and benefits of their choices (or, informed decision making; Edwards & Elwyn, 1999). Based on the possibility that stronger risk perceptions lead to greater self-protective motivation, the most straightforward prediction of failing to correctly understand one's risk is that people will neglect to take actions that could protect their health. It is also true that overestimating one's risk can be a serious problem. Overestimating risk, for example, might lead to excessive self-protective behaviors. Researchers have occasionally identified such an effect in the breast cancer screening literature, in which some women, characterized by strong risk perceptions, examine their breasts daily (Epstein et al., 1997). In addition, risk overestimates might lead to excessive worry, which can determine self-protective actions. Although it is not entirely clear what excessive worry is, researchers know that risk and worry are connected (Katapodi, Lee, Facione, & Dodd, 2004; McCaul & Mullens, 2003). Moreover, in the context of ovarian cancer, Fry, Rush, Busby-Earle, and Cull (2001) discovered that worry overrode beliefs when people made oophorectomy decisions (i.e., decisions about removing the ovaries to prevent ovarian cancer).

Raising the issue of informed decision making also introduces an important and unresolved ethical issue in risk communication: whether a communicator should focus on persuasion or on the objective provision of complete information to the recipient. A persuasion focus implies that the communicator knows best what a recipient should learn, feel, and do about his or her risk. An argument can be made that experts are sometimes in the best position to make such decisions (Loewenstein, 2005). However, others emphasize the importance of giving message recipients autonomy in decision making (Siminoff & Step, 2005), a strategy that would force communicators to lay out all decision alternatives along with their costs and benefits while avoiding a recommendation about any one course of action. We do not take a position on these alternatives here; we simply note that such ethical issues should be considered by researchers and health professionals engaged in risk communication.

Beliefs About Risk Are Associated With Health-Protective Behavior

Do risk judgments in the cancer area predict precautionary behaviors? The answer is probably yes, but the relationship is modest, and a definitive answer to this question based on solid research is lacking (Weinstein, 2003). McCaul, Branstetter, Schroeder, and Glasgow (1996), for example, reported a meta-analytic relationship (Pearson's r) of .16 between risk judgments and mammography screening, a relationship that has been confirmed in a more recent meta-analysis (Katapodi et al., 2004). Stronger cancer risk beliefs are also associated with uptake of colon cancer screening (Lipkus, Lyna, & Rimer, 2000), use of the Internet for a breast cancer risk intervention (Bowen et al., 2003), interest in desire to quit smoking and quit attempts (McCaul et al., 2004), interest in spiral computed tomography screening for lung cancer detection (Schnoll et al., 2003), and interest in genetic testing and prophylactic mastectomy to prevent breast cancer (Katapodi et al., 2004).

Changes in Risk Beliefs Cause Changes in Health-Protective Behavior

If the field is lacking data about risk–behavior associations, it is not surprising that researchers have even less confidence that changes in risk perception will cause changes in precautionary behavior. Some data do show that manipulations intended to change risk can increase health-protective behaviors. For example, Weinstein, Sandman, and Roberts (1991) found that a risk manipulation increased levels of home radon testing. Curry, Taplin, Anderman, Barlow, and McBride (1993) provided HMO enrollees with personalized information that they were at risk for breast cancer, producing higher mammography rates. McClure (2002) reviewed eight studies in which experimenters confronted people with biomarker data (e.g., carbon monoxide feedback for smokers), which should strengthen judgments of personal risk. McClure discovered that biomarker feedback increased self-protective behaviors, especially when the information conveyed was "particularly relevant to participants' health" (p. 204). Finally, McCaul et al. (2004) uncovered more than 80 studies of smoking cessation following hospitalization for a variety of illnesses, including cancer. A cancer diagnosis or treatment produced immediate cessation rates of around 50%—a rate far exceeding estimates that 3% to 8% of smokers will quit in any 12-month period (Baillie, Mattick, & Hall, 1995). One reasonable speculation is that a cancer diagnosis brings home one's personal vulnerability in a way that no other risk communication can accomplish, and it may be the new appreciation of one's risk that helps create a teachable moment for promoting smoking cessation (McBride & Ostroff, 2003).

Although some evidence shows that risk changes will result in behavior change, it is important to recognize that risk communication theoretically causes increases in motivation, which in turn may—or may not—cause successful behavior change. Behavioral changes are dependent on factors other than motivation alone, especially when the behavior is difficult to change (e.g., smoking). We predict that risk interventions are more likely to lead to behavior change when the barriers to change are few and/or when the behavior only needs to be performed a limited number of times (e.g., a mammography screening; see Aiken, West, Woodward, & Reno, 1994).

CHANGING RISK PERCEPTIONS

Risk communication may work best in stages. Weinstein's (1988) stage model suggests that people must first become aware of a threat, then recognize its importance for others, and finally, acknowledge the threat for themselves. As we have suggested, the best way to change risk perceptions is to focus on many features of the threat, including its likelihood, magnitude, and how it can be dealt with. Most research, however, has focused exclusively on communicating likelihood to influence personal vulnerability.

Increasing Risk Perceptions

Risk communication may be most interesting to researchers when health professionals communicate to others that their risk is greater than the message recipients had expected. However, people resist these communications (Leventhal, Kelley, & Leventhal, 1999; Weinstein & Klein, 1995). Difficulties in this type of risk communication may be at least partly explained by the motivation that people have to minimize threatening feedback. Some of the best illustrations of how people defend against negative risk information come from true experiments in which the experimenters manipulated feedback (Croyle, Sun, & Louie, 1993; Jemmott, Ditto, & Croyle, 1986), indicating that people change risk perception if it is threatening, self-relevant, and so on.[1] People seem to engage in rationalizations to reduce the threat to a "safe" level that then allows consideration of self-precautionary behavior while minimizing emotionality. This dual response to risk communication (McCaul, Thiesse-Duffy, & Wilson, 1992) fits easily with Cameron and Leventhal's (2003) parallel response model of self-regulation, suggesting that people often respond to threat both by actively coping with negative emotion and by simultaneously

---

[1]Some of the research studies discussed in this chapter relied on college-student samples rather than older adults, who are at higher risk for most cancers and who are more likely to have had experience with cancer (e.g., with family members being diagnosed). Although one must be cautious in generalizing from these studies, it is important to recognize that the experimenters using college student samples are more typically using designs based on true experiments and using manipulations in theoretically driven hypothesis testing. If anything generalizes from such studies, it should be the theoretical generalizations (Mook, 1983).

engaging in active problem solving (Cameron & Leventhal, 2003). In the cancer arena, minimization has been most often observed among smokers responding to threat communications about the risks of smoking (e.g., Freeman, Hennessy, & Marzullo, 2001). The defensiveness exhibited by some smokers in the laboratory gets played out when looking at the ineffectiveness of cigarette warning messages (Malouf, Schutte, Frohardt, Deming, & Mantelli, 1992; Strahan et al., 2002). The data concerning reactions to increasing risk information led Rothman and Kiviniemi (1999) to state, "People are not passive, unbiased processors of information about their health states. They welcome favorable information about their health but often engage in strategies that minimize or discount unfavorable health information" (p. 44; see also Ditto & Lopez, 1992).

Decreasing Risk Perceptions

Rothman and Kiviniemi (1999) may be only half right. Although failure to accept higher estimates of one's risk is probably due to defensiveness, an intriguing parallel finding has been discovered when people are given information that their cancer risk is lower than they expected. In an important early study on this topic, Lerman et al. (1995) provided individualized breast cancer risk counseling to first-degree relatives of women who had been diagnosed with breast cancer. Twenty-six percent of the relatives who received the individualized counseling reduced their percentage risk estimates after counseling, but not nearly to the level of feedback. Other studies (Hopwood et al., 1998; Lipkus et al., 2001) have also illustrated that women at high risk fail to adjust breast cancer risk values downward to match feedback, and McCaul et al. (2003) showed a similar phenomenon among low-risk college students. Researchers are still exploring possible explanations for why people resist positive information (Dillard, McCaul, Kelso, & Klein, 2006; Lipkus et al., 2001). Weinstein et al. (2004) speculated that when familiar illnesses such as colon cancer have low numerical risk (e.g., 8 in 1,000 over a 20-year period), people may have difficulty believing the numbers.

Overall, the data from two literatures show the same phenomenon: People are seemingly resistant to risk communication that differs from their original beliefs—regardless of whether the communication indicates that risk is higher or lower than they believed initially. Renner (2004) proposed a theoretical resolution to these disparate literatures, proposing that the sign of the risk feedback—positive versus negative—is less important than whether the risk communication is surprising and unexpected. Renner also suggested an asymmetry between negative and positive information: Negative information provokes greater processing, regardless of whether it is expected, but positive feedback will cause greater processing only when it is unexpected; otherwise, people will readily accept it.

PRESENTING RISK INFORMATION

Recent research has focused on creating *decision aids* (i.e., different presentation methods to help recipients better understand their risk). Many strategies have been created, including simply providing more information about the disease, providing risk information tailored to the recipient's circumstances, providing information about others' opinions, and guidance or coaching in decision-making steps (O'Connor et al., 1999). Presentation methods have included written materials, computer-based programs, videotapes, audio-guided workbooks, and decision boards (Agency for Healthcare Research and Quality, 2002). Chao et al. (2003), for example, showed that presenting risk-reduction information about chemotherapy in terms of the absolute survival benefit led to better understanding than alternative presentation methods. Woloshin, Schwartz, and Welch (2002) created charts that compare the risk for dying across different diseases, proposing that such comparisons will help people estimate risk magnitude because they provide context and may minimize unwarranted concern about relatively small risks. Overall, though, researchers have no firm idea at this time about what type of decision aid might be more effective and for whom.

The issue of tailoring risk communication to individual characteristics of the message recipient is especially important. Edwards et al. (2000) conducted a meta-analysis of more than 80 one-to-one risk communication interventions, at least half of which were related to cancer (e.g., smoking, screening). Across diverse outcomes, including knowledge, risk perceptions, emotion, and behavior, Edwards et al. concluded that risk communication strategies produce stronger positive effects when they present individualized estimates. Researchers know that targeting a message to the qualities of a particular individual has some advantages in encouraging attention and processing (Skinner, Campbell, Rimer, Curry, & Prochaska, 1999). Moreover, tailoring—by definition—personalizes the risk message, which may minimize the tendency of people to see risks as very different for themselves compared with others. As Sjoberg (2003) has shown, people believe that they can control their risks, and they also believe that others cannot control their risks or do not wish to do so. Thus, providing risk information about others or people in general is unlikely to affect personal judgments, whereas providing tailored information may. However, researchers know far too little about the effectiveness of tailoring, much less the particular features of tailoring that are important. And the strategy does not always work (Lipkus et al., 2004).

Two other strategies for presenting risk information not based on tailoring deserve mention because they have shown some effectiveness. First, when providing risk feedback to reduce overestimates about a particular disease, it helps to provide risk information about other diseases as well. From a decision-making view, support theory (Rottenstreich & Tversky, 1997) suggests that a risk judgment can be composed on the basis of the perceived strength of evidence or support for one hypothesis (e.g., What are the chances I might get colon cancer?) versus the evidence for alternative hypotheses (e.g., What are the odds I will die from some other cancer or other disease?). This phenomenon has been demonstrated for perceptions of smoking-related diseases (see Windschitl, 2002). As suggested earlier, a second effective strategy is to provide data about other people (i.e., social comparison information; Suls & Martin, 2001). In several examples, comparison information successfully changed the personal risk judgments recipients reported (Dillard et al., 2006; Ubel, Jepson, & Baron, 2001; Weinstein, 1983).

RISK COMMUNICATION: WHAT DO RESEARCHERS KNOW?

We believe that risk perceptions are important. However, we recognize that risk judgments, even when assessed in all their complexity, still represent a single class of judgments in the context of other perceptions and a larger environment (Leventhal et al., 1999). Leventhal et al. (1999), for example, describe a number of important beliefs in their illness representation model that may carry at least as much weight as risk perceptions. These beliefs include identification of aspects of the disease (e.g., When does colon cancer start to appear? What causes colon cancer?), beliefs about the self (e.g., Can I control whether I get colon cancer?), and beliefs about prevention, treatment, and recovery (e.g., I believe colon cancer is preventable). All of these beliefs theoretically can motivate (or inhibit) action.

In terms of the larger environment, researchers have known for some time that other predictors of behavior may play a larger role than risk perceptions. An extensive database in breast cancer screening, especially mammography, has demonstrated this fact. For example, the best predictor of screening is whether one has been asked (or told) by a physician to obtain a screening (Fox, Murata, & Stein, 1991; Lerman, Rimer, Trock, Balshem, & Engstrom, 1990). Besides physician recommendations, other variables (e.g., cost, transportation to screening) are also important in predicting self-protective behavior. The point is simply that risk is just one of a multitude of variables.

Despite the identification of risk as only one in a constellation of variables, it is important to note that nearly every theory purporting to explain why people engage in health-protective behavior refers to some aspect of risk (see Weinstein, 1993). One theoretical model may help to place risk judgments and risk communication into a more comprehensive model: the cognitive-social health information processing model (C-SHIP; Miller, Shoda, & Hurley, 1996), a framework that integrates relationships between different constructs from various models of health behavior. C-SHIP includes a set of mediating cognitive–affective units, such as an individual's expectancies, affect, and goals. Thus, risk communication cannot focus exclusively on a single variable such as risk likelihood but instead needs to take into account the way different people are likely to interpret that information.

This chapter has hinted at other research needs, and here we lay out some of those ideas more explicitly, stating possible topics in the form of testable hypotheses. People can characterize cancer risk along many dimensions, and different dimensions have stronger (or weaker) associations with self-protective behaviors. Researchers need both basic and applied research in assessing the multiple features of what cancer risk means to people. For example, earlier we suggested that feelings about risk may be at least as important as likelihood judgments; indeed, feelings (e.g., worry, dread, anticipated regret) could be more potent motivators of behavior change. However, researchers have not routinely measured different features of risk, much less contrasted their predictive power.

In terms of risk likelihood (i.e., personal vulnerability), comparative risk judgments are more important than absolute measures, at least when the latter measures use percentage scales. Indeed, social comparison is a fundamental process (Suls & Martin, 2001) that deserves more attention in studies of risk understanding and risk communication. Researchers know surprisingly little, for example, about whom people select for risk comparisons and how people deal with the knowledge that others like them (e.g., family members) are at risk for, or have, cancer.

Stronger risk perceptions predict self-protective actions. For several reasons, cross-sectional correlations are totally inappropriate for testing this hypothesis (Weinstein, 1998b), and such data may have contributed to the relatively low relationships that have been observed between risk and behavior. Researchers need to test prospective relationships, and they need to examine the interplay between risk and behavior at multiple intervals. The question of whether increased risk prompts action is immediately followed by the question of whether action then results in lowered risk estimates, which should happen as long as the behavior reduces actual risk (e.g., smoking cessation as opposed to cancer screening).

Increasing risk perceptions will foster self-protective actions; decreasing risk perceptions will do the opposite. Researchers need to examine changes in risk perceptions as they relate to changes in behavior, and they need to test manipulated risk and subsequent behavioral effects. There is surprisingly little experimental data using cancer as a topic and testing these straightforward predictions, but such data are important. Theoretically, for example, reducing exaggerated risk perceptions might simultaneously reduce motivation to engage in self-protective actions. Schwartz, Rimer, Daly, Sands, and Lerman (1999) observed just such a phenomenon among a subset of women who became less interested in mammograms after learning that they had been overestimating their risk (see Bowen, Christensen, Powers, Graves, & Anderson, 1998).

Risk perceptions are more important in initial actions meant to protect one's health (e.g., cancer screening), whereas repeated behavior (e.g., returning for screening) may be more dependent on one's initial experiences with the health action. This proposal has not been tested, as far as we are aware, but it relies first on the general notion that risk is but one variable in a larger constellation of factors that predict health-protective behaviors. More specifically, however, Rothman (2000) cogently argued that the factors that motivate behavior change, such as smoking cessation, may be very different from those that sustain behavior change. Behavioral maintenance is dependent on the outcomes that one actually experiences while engaging in the behavior, which may have little to do with the thoughts and feelings that motivated the behavior in the first place. These ideas suggest, for example, that colon cancer screening may result from heightened risk perceptions but repeating such screening may depend on whether the screening experience itself was acceptable.

Communicating new risk information elicits resistance, and new strategies will be needed to persuade people about their risk. Given that risk communication depends on successful persuasion about risk, more tests of possible strategies, which could include conceptually derived approaches (e.g., presenting narrative social comparison information) but also different decision aids (e.g., survival concerns, presenting multiple risks), are needed. More generally, it is clear that people often respond defensively to risk communications— It is threatening to learn that one is at risk for cancer of any kind. One way to reduce defensiveness is by first reinforcing positive aspects of the message recipient, a self-affirmation strategy (e.g., Aspinwall, 1998). Such strategies have never been tested in the cancer domain, as far as we know. Research investigating communication strategies that might circumvent defensiveness would be welcomed.

REFERENCES

Agency for Healthcare Research and Quality. (2002). *Impact of cancer-related decision aids* (AHRQ Publication No. 02-E004). Rockville, MD: Author.

Aiken, L. S., West, S. G., Woodward, C. K., & Reno, R. R. (1994). Health beliefs and compliance with mammography-screening recommendations in asymptomatic women. *Health Psychology, 13,* 122–129.

Aspinwall, L. G. (1998). Rethinking the role of positive affect in self-regulation. *Motivation and Emotion, 22,* 1–32.

Baillie, A. J., Mattick, R. P., & Hall, W. (1995). Quitting smoking: Estimation by meta-analysis of the rate of unaided smoking cessation. *Australian Journal of Public Health, 19,* 129–215.

Bergstrom, R. L., & McCaul, K. D. (2004). Perceived risk and worry: The effects of 9/11 on willingness to fly. *Journal of Applied Social Psychology, 34,* 1846–1856.

Bottorff, J. L., Ratner, P. A., Johnson, J. L., Lovato, C. Y., & Joab, S. A. (1998). Communicating cancer risk information: The challenges of uncertainty. *Patient Education and Counseling, 33,* 67–81.

Bowen, D. J., Christensen, C. L., Powers, D., Graves, D. R., & Anderson, C. A. M. (1998). Effects of counseling and ethnic identity on perceived risk and cancer worry in African American women. *Journal of Clinical Psychology in Medical Settings, 5,* 365–379.

Bowen, D. J., Ludwig, A., Bush, N., Unruh, H. K., Meischke, H., Wooldridge, J. A., & Robbins, R. (2003). Early experience with a Web-based intervention to inform risk of breast cancer. *Journal of Health Psychology, 8,* 175–186.

Cameron, L. D., & Leventhal, H. (2003). Self-regulation, health, and illness: An overview. In L. D. Cameron & H. Leventhal (Eds.), *The self-regulation of health and illness behaviour* (pp. 1–14). New York: Routledge.

Cancer risk communication: What we know and what we need to learn. (1999). *Journal of the National Cancer Institute* (Monograph No. 25).

Chao, C., Studts, J. L., Abell, T., Hadley, T., Roetzer, L., Dinee, S., et al. (2003). Adjuvant chemotherapy for breast cancer: How presentation of recurrence risk influences decision-making. *Journal of Clinical Oncology, 21,* 4299–4305.

Croyle, R. T., Sun, Y.-C., & Louie, D. H. (1993). Psychological minimization of cholesterol test results: Moderators of appraisal in college students and community residents. *Health Psychology, 12,* 503–507.

Curry, S. J., Taplin, S. H., Anderman, C., Barlow, W. E., & McBride, C. (1993). Randomized trial of the impact of risk assessment and feedback on participation in mammography screening. *Preventive Medicine, 22,* 350–360.

Dillard, A. J., McCaul, K. D., Kelso, P. D., & Klein, W. M. P. (2006). Resisting good news: Reactions to breast cancer risk communication. *Health Communication, 19,* 115–123.

Ditto, P., & Lopez, D. F. (1992). Motivated skepticism: Use of differential decision criteria for preferred and nonpreferred conclusions. *Journal of Personality and Social Psychology, 63,* 568–584.

Donovan, K. A., & Tucker, D. C. (2000). Knowledge about genetic risk for breast cancer and perceptions of genetic testing in a sociodemographically diverse sample. *Journal of Behavioral Medicine, 23,* 15–36.

Edwards, A., & Elwyn, G. (1999). How should effectiveness of risk communication to aid patients' decisions be judged? A review of the literature. *Medical Decision Making, 19,* 428–434.

Edwards, A., Hood, K., Matthews, E., Russell, D., Russell, I., Barker, J., et al. (2000). The effectiveness of one-to-one risk-communication interventions in health care: A systematic review. *Medical Decision Making, 20,* 290–297.

Epstein, S. A., Lin, T. H., Audrain, J., Stefanek, M., Rimer, B., & Lerman, C. (1997). Excessive breast self-examination among first-degree relatives of newly diagnosed breast cancer patients. *Psychosomatics, 38,* 253–261.

Fischhoff, B. (1999). Why (cancer) risk communication can be hard. *Journal of the National Cancer Institute Monographs, 25,* 7–13.

Fischhoff, B., & de Bruin, W. B. (1999). Fifty–fifty = 50%? *Journal of Behavioral Decision Making, 12,* 149–163.

Fox, S., Murata, P. J., & Stein, J. A. (1991). The impact of physician compliance on screening mammography for older women. *Archives of Internal Medicine, 161,* 50–56.

Freeman, M. A., Hennessy, E. V., & Marzullo, D. M. (2001). Defensive evaluation of antismoking messages among college-age smokers: The role of possible selves. *Health Psychology, 20,* 424–433.

Fry, A., Rush, R., Busby-Earle, C., & Cull, A. (2001). Deciding about prophylactic oophorectomy: What is important to women at increased risk of ovarian cancer? *Preventive Medicine, 33,* 578–585.

Hahn, A., & Renner, B. (1998). Perception of health risks: How smoker status affects defensive optimism. *Anxiety, Stress, and Coping, 11,* 93–112.

Hopwood, P., Keeling, F., Long, A., Pool, C., Evans, G., & Howell, A. (1998). Psychological support needs for women at high genetic risk of breast cancer: Some preliminary indicators. *Psycho-Oncology, 7,* 402–412.

Jemmott, J. B., Ditto, P. H., & Croyle, R. T. (1986). Judging health status: Effects of perceived prevalence and personal relevance. *Journal of Personality and Social Psychology, 50,* 899–905.

Katapodi, M. C., Lee, K. A., Facione, N. C., & Dodd, M. J. (2004). Predictor of perceived breast cancer risk and the relation between perceived risk and breast cancer screening: A meta-analytic review. *Preventive Medicine, 38,* 388–402.

Kohn, L. S., & Rogers, R. W. (1991). Dimensions of the severity of a health threat: The persuasive effects of visibility, time of onset, and rate of onset on young women's intentions to prevent osteoporosis. *Health Psychology, 10,* 323–329.

Lerman, C., Lustbader, E., Rimer, B., Daly, M., Miller, S. M., Sands, C, & Balshem, A. (1995). Effects of individualized breast cancer risk counseling: A randomized trial. *Journal of the National Cancer Institute, 87,* 286–292.

Lerman, C., Rimer, B., Trock, B., Balshem, A., & Engstrom, P. F. (1990). Factors associated with repeat adherence to breast cancer screening. *Preventive Medicine, 19,* 279–290.

Leventhal, H., Kelley, K., & Leventhal, E. A. (1999). Population risk, actual risk, perceived risk, and cancer control. *Journal of the National Cancer Institute Monographs, 25,* 81–85.

Lipkus, I. M., Biradavolu, M., Fenn, K., Keller, P., & Rimer, B. K. (2001). Informing women about their breast cancer risks: Truth and consequences. *Health Communication, 13,* 205–226.

Lipkus, I. M., Klein, W. M. P., Skinner, C. S., & Rimer, B. K. (2005). Breast cancer risk perceptions and breast cancer worry: What predicts what? *Journal of Risk Research, 8,* 439–452.

Lipkus, I. M., Lyna, P. R., & Rimer, B. K. (2000). Colorectal cancer risk perceptions and screening intentions in a minority population. *Journal of the National Medical Association, 92,* 492–500.

Lipkus, I. M., Skinner, C. S., Green, L. S. G., Dement, J., Samsa, G. P., & Ransohoff, D. (2004). Modifying attributions of colorectal cancer risk. *Cancer Epidemiology, Biomarkers & Prevention, 13*, 560–566.

Loewenstein, G. F. (2005). Hot–cold empathy gaps and medical decision making. *Health Psychology, 24*(Suppl. 4), 49–56.

Loewenstein, G. F., Weber, E. U., Hsee, C. K., & Welch, E. (2001). Risk as feelings. *Psychological Bulletin, 127*, 267–286.

Malouf, J., Schutte, N., Frohardt, M., Deming, W., & Mantelli, D. (1992). Preventing smoking: Evaluating the potential effectiveness of cigarette warnings. *The Journal of Psychology, 126*, 371–383.

McBride, C. M., & Ostroff, J. S. (2003). Teachable moments for promoting smoking cessation: The context of cancer care and survivorship. *Cancer Control, 10*, 325–333.

McCaul, K. D., Branstetter, A. D., Schroeder, D. M., & Glasgow, R. E. (1996). What is the relationship between breast cancer risk and mammography screening? A meta-analytic review. *Health Psychology, 15*, 1–8.

McCaul, K. D., Canevello, A. B., Mathwig, J. L., & Klein, W. M. P. (2003). Risk communication and worry about breast cancer. *Psychology, Health & Medicine, 8*, 379–389.

McCaul, K. D., Hockemeyer, J. R., Johnson, R. J., Zetocha, K., Quinlan, K., & Glasgow, R. E. (2004). *Motivation to quit using cigarettes: A review.* Unpublished manuscript, North Dakota State University, Fargo.

McCaul, K. D., & Mullens, A. B. (2003). Affect, thought, and self-protective health behavior: The case of worry and cancer screening. In J. Suls & K. Wallston (Eds.), *Social psychological foundations of health and illness* (pp. 137–168). Malden, MA: Blackwell Publishers.

McCaul, K. D., & O'Donnell, S. (1998). Naïve beliefs about breast cancer risk. *Women's Health, 4*, 93–101.

McCaul, K. D., Thiesse-Duffy, E., & Wilson, P. (1992). Coping with medical diagnosis: The effects of at-risk versus disease labels over time. *Journal of Applied Social Psychology, 52*, 1340–1355.

McClure, J. B. (2002). Are biomarkers useful treatment aids for promoting health behavior change? *American Journal of Preventive Medicine, 22*, 200–207.

McCoy, S. B., Gibbons, F. X., Reis, T. J., Gerrard, M., Luus, C. A. E., & Sufka, A. V. W. (1992). Perceptions of smoking risk as a function of smoking status. *Journal of Behavioral Medicine, 15*, 469–488.

Miller, S. M., Shoda, Y., & Hurley, K. (1996). Applying cognitive-social theory to health-protective behavior: Breast self-examination in cancer screening. *Psychological Bulletin, 119*, 70–94.

Montgomery, G. H., Erblich, J., DiLorenzo, T., & Bovbjerg, D. H. (2003). Family and friends with disease: Their impact on perceived risk. *Preventive Medicine, 37*, 242–249.

Mook, D. G. (1983). In defense of external invalidity. *American Psychologist, 38,* 379–387.

O'Connor, A. M. Fiset, V., DeGrasse, C., Graham, I. D., Evans, W., Stacey, D., et al. (1999). Decision aids for patients considering options affecting cancer outcomes: Evidence of efficacy and policy implications. *Journal of the National Cancer Institute Monographs, 25,* 67–80.

Radcliffe, N. M., & Klein, W. M. P. (2002). Dispositional, unrealistic, and comparative optimism: Differential relations with knowledge and processing of risk information and beliefs about personal risk. *Personality and Social Psychology Bulletin, 28,* 836–846.

Renner, B. (2004). Biased reasoning: Adaptive responses to health risk feedback. *Personality and Social Psychology Bulletin, 30,* 384–396.

Ronis, D. L. (1992). Conditional health threats: Health beliefs, decisions, and behaviors among adults. *Health Psychology, 11,* 127–134.

Rothman, A. J. (2000). Toward a theory-based analysis of behavioral maintenance. *Health Psychology, 19,* 64–69.

Rothman, A. J., & Kiviniemi, M. T. (1999). Treating people with information: An analysis and review of approaches to communicating health risk information. *Journal of the National Cancer Institute Monographs, 25,* 44–51.

Rottenstreich, Y. S., & Tversky, A. (1997). Unpacking, repacking, and anchoring: Advances in support theory. *Psychological Review, 104,* 406–415.

Schnoll, R. A., Bradley, P., Miller, S. M., Unger, M., Babb, J., & Cornfeld, M. (2003). Psychological issues related to the use of spiral CT for lung cancer early detection. *Lung Cancer, 39,* 315–325.

Schwartz, M., Rimer, B., Daly, M., Sands, C., & Lerman, C. (1999). A randomized trial of breast cancer risk counseling: The impact of self-reported mammography use. *American Journal of Public Health, 89,* 924–926.

Sennott-Miller, L. (1994). Using theory to plan appropriate interventions: Cancer prevention for older Hispanic and non-Hispanic White women. *Journal of Advanced Nursing, 20,* 809–814.

Siminoff, L., & Step, M. M. (2005). A communication model of shared decision making: Accounting for cancer treatment decisions. *Health Psychology, 24,* 99–105.

Sjoberg, L. (2003). Neglecting the risks: The irrationality of health behavior and the quest for *La Dolce Vita. European Psychologist, 8,* 266–278.

Skinner, C. S., Campbell, M. K., Rimer, B. K., Curry, S., & Prochaska, J. O. (1999). How effective is tailored print communication? *Annals of Behavioral Medicine, 21,* 290–298.

Slovic, P. (1987, April 17). Perception of risk. *Science, 236,* 280–285.

Slovic, P., Finucane, M., Peters, E., & MacGregor, D. G. (2004). Risk as analysis and risk as feelings: Some thoughts about affect, reason, risk, and rationality. *Risk Analysis, 24,* 311–322.

Slovic, P., Fischhoff, B., & Lichtenstein, S. (1987). Behavioral decision theory perspective on protective behavior. In N. D. Weinstein (Ed.), *Taking care: Understanding and encouraging self-protective behavior* (pp. 14–41). Cambridge, England: Cambridge University Press.

Strahan, E. J., White, K., Fong, G. T., Fabrigar, L. R., Zanna, M. P., & Cameron, R. (2002). Enhancing the effectiveness of tobacco package warning labels: A social psychological perspective. *Tobacco Control, 11*, 183–190

Strecher, V. J., Champion, V. L., & Rosenstock, I. M. (1997). The health belief model and health behavior. In D. S. Gochman (Ed.), *Handbook of health behavior research: I. Personal and social determinants* (pp. 71–91). New York: Plenum Press.

Suls, J., & Martin, R. (2001). Social comparison processes in the physical health domain. In A. Baum, T. Revenson, & J. Singer (Eds.), *Handbook of health psychology* (pp. 195–208). Hillsdale, NJ: Erlbaum.

Ubel, P. A., Jepson, C., & Baron, J. (2001). The inclusion of patient testimonials in decision aids: Effects on treatment choices. *Medical Decision Making, 21*, 60–68.

Weinstein, N. D. (1983). Reducing unrealistic optimism about illness susceptibility. *Health Psychology, 2*, 11–20.

Weinstein, N. D. (1988). The precaution adoption process. *Health Psychology, 7*, 355–386.

Weinstein, N. D. (1993). Testing four competing theories of health-protective behavior. *Health Psychology, 12*, 324–333.

Weinstein, N. D. (1998a). Accuracy of smokers' risk perceptions. *Annals of Behavioral Medicine, 20*, 135–140.

Weinstein, N. D. (1998b). Using correlation to study relationships between risk perceptions and preventive behavior. *Psychology and Health, 13*, 479–501.

Weinstein, N. D. (1999). What does it mean to understand a risk? Evaluating risk comprehension. *Journal of the National Cancer Institute Monographs, 25*, 15–20.

Weinstein, N. D. (2003). Risk perceptions and preventive health behaviors. In J. Suls & K. A. Wallston (Eds.), *Social psychological foundations of health and illness*. Malden, MA: Blackwell.

Weinstein, N. (2004). *Risk perceptions: Conceptualization, measurement, and analysis*. Paper presented at the preconference State of the Art in Risk Perception at the 25th Annual Meeting of the Society of Behavioral Medicine, Baltimore, MD.

Weinstein, N., Atwood, K., Pueleo, E., Fletcher, R., Collditz, G., & Emmons, K. M. (2004). Colon cancer: Risk perceptions and risk communication. *Journal of Health Communication, 9*, 53–66.

Weinstein, N. D., & Klein, W. M. (1995). Resistance of personal risk perceptions to debiasing interventions. *Health Psychology, 14*, 132–140.

Weinstein, N. D., Sandman, P. M., & Roberts, N. E. (1991). Perceived susceptibility and self-protective behavior: A field experiment to encourage home radon testing. *Health Psychology, 10*, 25–33.

Williams, T., & Clarke, V. A. (1997). Do cigarette smokers have unrealistic perceptions of their heart attack, cancer, and stroke risks? *Journal of Behavioral Medicine, 18,* 45–54.

Windschitl, P. D. (2002). Judging the accuracy of a likelihood judgment: The case of smoking risk. *Journal of Behavioral Decision Making, 15,* 19–35.

Woloshin, S., Schwartz, L. M., Black, W. C., & Welch, H. G. (1999). Women's perceptions of breast cancer risk: How you ask matters. *Medical Decision Making, 19,* 221–229.

Woloshin, S., Schwartz, L. M., & Welch, H. G. (2002). Risk charts: Putting cancer in context. *Journal of the National Cancer Institute, 94,* 799–804.

Yamagishi, K. (1997). When a 12.86% mortality is more dangerous than 24.14%: Implications for risk communication. *Applied Cognitive Psychology, 11,* 495–506.

9

PREVENTION OF TOBACCO USE

ROBIN MERMELSTEIN AND SARAH K. WAHL

Tobacco use remains the leading preventable cause of premature morbidity and mortality in the United States and other developed countries today (Fagerstrom, 2002; McGinnis & Foegbe, 1993; Twombly, 2003; U.S. Department of Health and Human Services [USDHHS], 1990, 2001). The vast majority of smokers in the United States begin their tobacco use during the adolescent years (USDHHS, 1994), and the majority of those who will eventually become regular smokers also do so by age 18 (USDHHS, 1994). For many years, cigarette experimentation was seen as a normative rite of adolescence, with little concern about the potential health consequences or risks of continued smoking. However, as data about the longitudinal patterns of cigarette use and the health effects of smoking during adolescence started to emerge, it became increasingly clear that (a) many adolescents do not "mature out of" smoking, becoming dependent on nicotine quite early in their smoking "careers" (Mermelstein, 2003), and (b) adolescents do indeed experience health problems from their smoking, such as impaired lung function and increased incidence of respiratory problems (USDHHS, 1994). Thus, both researchers and public health professionals have reaffirmed the critical need for effective prevention efforts.

This chapter provides an overview of the approaches used to prevent tobacco use, examining the strength of the evidence base for different

151

approaches and highlighting representative studies. We conclude with recommendations for future research. Our focus is primarily on cigarette smoking, considering the higher prevalence of use of cigarettes compared with smokeless tobacco and the broader evaluation of prevention efforts that measure mainly cigarette smoking outcomes. This focus is not meant to imply that smokeless tobacco use is not a serious problem, and indeed, smokeless use among male teens remains an entrenched problem in many subgroups and areas (National Cancer Institute [NCI], 1992). Prevention programs, intervention, and evaluation efforts are clearly needed in this area.

PREVALENCE OF SMOKING AMONG ADOLESCENTS

Although significant strides have been made in reducing the prevalence of smoking among adolescents, rates of cigarette smoking remain unacceptably high. Data from the Monitoring the Future study show that 47.1% of 12th graders in 2006 reported ever smoking, a notable decline from the mid-1970s, when the prevalence of lifetime use was slightly greater than 75% (Johnston, O'Malley, Bachman, & Schulenberg, 2006). Daily smoking rates among 12th graders hover around 12%, an indication that many youth move beyond experimental smoking to more established patterns of tobacco use. These prevalence rates are likely to be underestimates of total population rates of smoking among this age group, because the Monitoring the Future study surveys adolescents who are still in school and there is a well-established association between school dropout and higher prevalence of smoking (USDHHS, 1994).

STAGES AND PREDICTORS OF ADOLESCENT SMOKING

Smoking initiation and uptake is often conceptualized as progression through a series of stages (Mayhew, Flay, & Mott, 2000; Pierce, Choi, Gilpin, Farkas, & Merritt, 1996; USDHHS, 1994). Most youth go beyond the contemplation state to trying, but far fewer move on to the subsequent stages of experimentation, regular use, and dependence. Although researchers know a great deal about predictors of initial trying, they know much less about predictors of progression beyond trying and experimentation to dependence (Turner, Mermelstein, & Flay, 2004). Predictors of initiation or ever smoking are multilayered and multifaceted and include demographic factors (e.g., age, family socioeconomic status), social contexts (e.g., peer, family), temperaments, emotional functioning, attitudes about smoking, and broad macroenvironmental factors as well (e.g., policies, access, costs; Turner et al., 2004; USDHHS, 1994). To date, no one theory has adequately integrated the multiple sources of influence on, and pathways to, adolescent smoking, although the theory of triadic influence provides a summary rubric for integrating the myriad of factors hypothesized to predict adolescent smoking (Flay & Petraitis, 1994). Early interventions for smoking prevention were often based on the assumption that finding a strong bivariate relationship between a given predictor variable and smoking would be sufficient to translate into a strong intervention. However, such approaches may be limited by their failure to consider whether critical mediating variables may be more directly related to risk or whether moderating factors may influence program outcomes. A critical link in moving from theory to intervention is a better understanding of the mediational and moderational processes involved in program effects. Fortunately, there has also been increasing attention paid in the literature to understanding these mechanisms of action as well.

OVERVIEW OF PREVENTION APPROACHES

Approaches to tobacco use prevention have broadened considerably over the past 3 decades, ranging from relatively intensive, individually oriented approaches to more macrolevel policy interventions. More recently, researchers have taken a more macrolevel view of changing population rates of tobacco use by attempting to influence policy change and the broader social culture of youth through tobacco countermarketing campaigns.

School-Based Prevention Programs

School-based prevention programs remain a mainstay of the tobacco control movement, despite their record of mixed success. There are several reviews of these programs (e.g., Bruvold, 1993; Flay, 2000; Tobler et al., 2000), and thus we do not attempt to review comprehensively their effects but rather to highlight some of the primary approaches and consistent findings. Social influence programs have been among the more theoretically grounded and rigorously evaluated approaches to tobacco use prevention. A primary premise behind these programs is that social pressures, from peers and the media, are key determinants of adolescent smoking. Thus, social influence–based programs emphasize teaching skills to resist these social pressures. Correcting misperceptions of the prevalence of smoking is also a key component of social influence programs. Three of the more rigorously evaluated and effective school-based prevention programs are Sussman and colleagues' (Dent et al., 1995; Sussman et al., 1993) Towards No Tobacco Use (TNT); Botvin, Schinke, Epstein, Diaz, and Botvin's (1995) Life Skills Training Program (LST); and Project ALERT (Ellickson & Bell, 1990; Ellickson, McCaffrey, Ghosh-Dastidar, & Longshore, 2003).

Implementation factors and context may also influence the outcomes of school-based prevention programs. These factors may include provider or facilitator characteristics, provider training, and school context, such as prevalence of the problem behavior in the school. Cameron et al. (1999) examined the effectiveness of a social influences prevention program considering the provider type (i.e., teacher vs. nurse), training type (i.e., 1.5-day workshop vs. self-preparation kit), and school type (i.e., high-risk vs. low-risk regarding smoking prevalence among senior students). Their results suggest that *low-risk schools*, defined as those with low levels of smoking, may not need or benefit from the social influences prevention program—given the context, strong local norms may not support or influence students to smoke. Alternatively, youth who do smoke in the context of such strong nonsmoking norms may need more intensive or tailored interventions than those that are universally developed and delivered to all youth in a school.

Cultural context, as reflected by both program development and school ethnic diversity, may also be an important moderator of the effectiveness of school-based prevention programs. The one-size-fits-all approach to tobacco prevention programs might not be as effective as programs that are more culturally matched to their audiences (Unger et al., 2002). However, very few studies have directly addressed the issue of the relative effectiveness of culturally tailored versus nontailored programs. Botvin et al. (1995) compared the effectiveness of a generic skills training program, a culturally focused intervention approach, and an information-only control group on alcohol and other drug use. Results from the 2-year follow-up suggested that the culturally tailored intervention had a greater impact on alcohol consumption compared with the generic skills intervention or with the information-only control condition. Although this study did not specifically address tobacco use, it suggests the potential importance of culturally tailored prevention programs (Unger et al., 2004).

Despite the relatively positive results from programs such as Project ALERT, TNT, and LST, conclusions about the effectiveness of school-based prevention programs need to be tempered by the consideration of findings from several well-designed studies that have yielded negative results (e.g., Flay et al., 1989; Peterson, Kealey, Mann, Marek, & Sarason, 2000). The failure of these interventions to influence smoking behavior should be considered in the context of comprehensive and relatively recent meta-analyses of prevention programs. Tobler et al. (2000) conducted a meta-analysis of 207 school-based drug prevention programs that were published or reported between 1978 and 1998. All 207 programs were classified into one of two categories for meta-analysis: (a) noninteractive (including knowledge only; affective only; decisions, values, and attitudes; knowledge plus affective; and Drug Abuse Resistance Education–type programs) or (b) interactive (including social influences, comprehensive life skills, and systemwide change programs). In addition, this meta-analysis included nine predictors of program effectiveness, including program sample size, type of leader, type of control group, amount of program attrition, population characteristics, type of drug targeted, school grade, intensity of program delivery, and level of substance use. Results of Tobler et al.'s meta-analysis indicated that interactive programs produced greater effect sizes than the noninteractive programs across the board for all drug abuse programs. It also indicated that interactive programs that focused only on tobacco were significantly more effective than interaction programs that dealt with tobacco plus other drugs, and it found that effectiveness of the interactive program declined as the program size increased, whereas noninteractive programs were not affected by program size. Within the interactive programs, effect sizes were largest for the systemwide change programs, followed by the comprehensive life skills, and then the social influence programs. Systemwide change programs included school-based programs with active family and/or community support components or those that provided a supportive school environment.

Although the Tobler et al. (2000) meta-analysis presents a relatively positive view of the outcomes of school-based programs, one must consider that their primary analyses used effect sizes from follow-up points that were within 1 to 12 months postintervention. Thus, the longer term effects, when decays are likely, were not evaluated. Rooney and Murray (1996) also conducted a meta-analysis of school-based prevention programs but with the methodological improvement of adjusting for the original unit of analysis, which was often neglected in many early prevention studies. Rooney and Murray also separated follow-up periods in their analyses, given the strong likelihood that effects vary by time of follow-up. Their results suggested that the overall effects of school-based programs were small but nevertheless potentially meaningful in the context of overall prevention efforts. Translating the average effect size into a more meaningful metric, Rooney and Murray estimated that the school-based programs might result in a 5% reduction in smoking.

In sum, the effects of school-based prevention programs alone are modest at best but nevertheless provide the backbone of tobacco use prevention efforts. Studies examining hypothesized mediators of significant intervention effects have also pointed to the importance of influencing perceived peer reactions and normative expectations in reducing tobacco use. Quality of implementation and contextual factors are also likely to influence the effectiveness of these programs. The limited results of school-based prevention programs are not surprising when one considers the multiple levels of influence on an adolescent's tobacco use—including family, the macrolevel social environment, media, and community norms—and the challenge for any single intervention channel to exert a large effect. Thus, researchers have acknowledged the need to supplement school-based prevention programs with additional intervention channels.

Family Prevention Programs

Parents are a major influence on an adolescent's tobacco use (Conrad, Flay, & Hill, 1992; USDHHS, 1994). Parental effects on adolescent smoking may be mediated by a combination of modeling of tobacco use itself, messages parents give to youth about smoking and its consequences, parental self-efficacy for providing antismoking norms and messages, and family rules about tobacco use (Kodl & Mermelstein, 2004). Given the significant role parents play in an adolescent's life, it is surprising that there have been relatively few controlled evaluations of family interventions that have been universally delivered and that could address the unique role of the family intervention apart from other components within a multicomponent prevention program.

One of the more notable tests of a family-based intervention is Bauman et al.'s (2001) Family Matters program. Family Matters was directed at families with adolescents ages 12 through 14, and it consisted of successive mailings of four booklets to families, along with telephone discussions with health educators after each mailing. The booklets were well grounded in a variety of social and behavioral theories covering motivation to participate, family characteristics known to influence tobacco use (including communication), social inoculation theory, and principles of social learning theory. The booklets included a variety of activities for parents and adolescents, and the phone calls from the health educators were geared toward reinforcing participation. At a 1-year follow-up, smoking onset was reduced by 25% for non-Hispanic Whites but not for other racial or ethnic groups. The lack of effect for these groups may be explained in part, as the authors suggest, by the inability of the project to match health educators to the ethnicity of the participant. Alternatively, other culturally relevant tailoring factors may need to be considered. A challenge for all family-directed interventions is to engage and maintain the participation of parents at a high enough level to make a difference in their patterns of interacting with their children. The Family Matters program was implemented without the pairing of a school-based prevention intervention or with other community efforts, all of which may, in combination, boost program effectiveness.

Community Approaches

Community context helps set social norms and attitudes toward tobacco use, both of which influence behavior. Community-level interventions tend to be multicomponent interventions that combine change strategies across a variety of settings and levels of intervention. Thus, community-level tobacco prevention interventions may include school-based programs, media campaigns that may target both adults and youth, and policy initiatives that may cover both clean indoor air acts and enforcement of laws prohibiting youth access to tobacco. For the most part, community interventions that have been research based have demonstrated good effects on reducing tobacco use prevalence, such as Biglan, Ary, Smoklowski, Duncan, and Black (2000), Pentz et al. (1989), and Johnson et al. (1990).

Media Approaches

Without a doubt, mass media influence youth culture, attitudes, and behaviors, including tobacco use. The entertainment media may be particularly important to youth attitudes and behaviors (Sargent et al., 2001). Media campaigns are useful as vehicles for reinforcing the messages and effects of other programs, for altering community norms, and for modeling important behavioral skills.

There are several excellent examples of effective mass media campaigns combined with school-based programs. Flynn et al. (1992, 1994) found that after a 4-year intervention of paid advertising, a mass media plus school intervention program resulted in a 41% reduction in weekly smoking rates compared with those in the school-only group and that these effects persisted through a 2-year follow-up. The effectiveness of their intervention may be attributed, in part, to their careful development of media messages targeted to adolescents (Worden et al., 1988).

Hafstad et al. (1997) reported the positive results of a relatively extensive media campaign conducted in Norway and aimed at adolescents ages 14 through 18. Three consecutive yearly media campaigns were conducted in an intervention county and were aimed at preventing the onset of smoking. The campaigns included TV spots, full-page newspaper advertisements, posters sent to schools and youth organizations, and movie theater advertisements. Two of the three campaigns were targeted to girls. The messages were designed to evoke affective reactions and to promote communication among peers. At the end of the 3 years, a significantly lower proportion of adolescents in the intervention county had started to smoke (10.2% of boys and 14.6% of girls) compared with those in the control county (14.5% of boys and 25.6% of girls). Among those who were already smokers at baseline, more girls in the intervention county, compared with the control, had stopped smoking at the 3-year follow-up. However, no significant differences among smokers at baseline were found for boys. The results of the Hafstad et al. study suggest that provocative appeals and multiple exposures, across a variety of media, may be effective at reducing the prevalence of smoking and that tailoring messages by gender may be important for reducing smoking among youth who have already started to smoke.

Beyond the controlled experimental evaluations of mass media campaigns highlighted by the Flynn et al. (1992, 1994) and Hafstad et al. (1997) studies, the tobacco control landscape changed considerably during the 1990s as select states started to implement large-scale antismoking media campaigns. Siegel and Biener (2000) evaluated the impact of Massachusetts's statewide antismoking campaign on adolescents' progression to established smoking and found that the effects of exposure to the television advertising varied by age of the adolescent. Among younger adolescents, ages 12 to 13 years at baseline, recalled exposure to the advertisements was associated with a lower likelihood of progressing to established smoking 4 years later. However, exposure to the television advertising had no effects on smoking progression among slightly older adolescents (ages 14–15 at baseline). Neither radio nor outdoor smoking advertisements had an effect on smoking. There are numerous difficulties in evaluating the effects of these statewide mass media campaigns, one of which is noted by Siegel and Biener. Recalled exposure, as opposed to objectively measured actual exposure, may be subject to a variety of influences, including the possibility that youth who are at lower risk for smoking escalation may be more likely to recall or attend to the ads in the first place. The differential impact of the intervention for the younger and mid-age adolescents may also highlight the potential importance of segmenting messages to different audiences.

In 1998, the state of Florida began the Truth antitobacco countermarketing campaign, funded by Florida's settlement with the tobacco industry and combined with school-based and community-level tobacco use prevention efforts. This campaign focused on describing the tobacco industry's attempts to market a dangerous product to teens, and it portrayed ads with youth confronting the tobacco industry. In addition, the campaign had as a goal to empower teens by encouraging them to join statewide antitobacco efforts. Niederdeppe, Farrelly, and Haviland (2004) compared the smoking rates among Florida teens ages 12 to 17 years with those of teens from states without established comprehensive tobacco control programs, using the Legacy Media Tracking Survey, a national random-digit-dialed telephone survey of teens. They found that Florida teens were less likely than teens in other states to be current smokers, to have ever tried smoking, or to indicate a strong susceptibility to future smoking.

Florida's Truth campaign was followed in 2000 by the American Legacy Foundation's national tobacco countermarketing campaign. The Legacy's Truth campaign targets youth who are 12 to 17 years old who are susceptible to or considering smoking. The campaign features edgy, rebellious, multiethnic teens. A fundamental strategy of this campaign is to market its message as a brand, similar to other brands for youth products, and to feature hard-hitting facts about tobacco and tobacco industry marketing. The Truth advertisements feature teens confronting the tobacco industry, as a rebellious rejection of tobacco and tobacco advertising. For example, one of the better-known advertisements is Body Bags, in which youth pile body bags outside of a tobacco company's headquarters and loudly send the message that the bags represent the 1,200 people killed daily by tobacco. Farrelly et al. (2002) used data from two national telephone surveys of youth, ages 12 to 17, to assess whether exposure to the Truth countermarketing advertisements was associated with changes in antitobacco attitudes and intentions to smoke. Farrelly et al. found that exposure to the campaign was consistently associated with an increase in antitobacco attitudes but only a marginally significant decrease in nonsmokers' intention to smoke at any time in the next year. They concluded that an aggressive national countermarketing campaign can influence youth's attitudes toward tobacco and the tobacco industry and that these attitude changes may potentially predict future changes in smoking behavior, following longer exposure (as was seen in the Florida campaign).

An interesting component of Farrelly et al.'s (2002) evaluation of national countermarketing campaigns was their comparison of the effects of the Truth campaign to those of the Philip Morris tobacco company's Think, Don't Smoke campaign, which began in 1998. The Philip Morris campaign features a Just Say No approach to tobacco use for youth and ignores the health effects of tobacco and the addictive properties. Farrelly et al. found that the Truth campaign had much stronger effects on antitobacco attitudes than did the Think, Don't Smoke campaign and, it is important to note, that the Think, Don't Smoke campaign was associated with an increase in the odds of intentions to smoke in the next year. Furthermore, the dose–response relationship between exposure to Think, Don't Smoke and intentions to smoke was also significant. Farrelly et al. echoed the suggestion of tobacco control activists that the goals of the Think, Don't Smoke campaign may be more in line with promoting positive feelings toward the tobacco industry and buying them respectability, rather than discouraging youth from smoking.

In sum, both statewide and national countermarketing campaigns can exert notable population-wide changes not only in attitudes toward tobacco use but, potentially, in reducing the prevalence of tobacco use as well. In reviewing these campaigns and their effects, Farrelly, Niederdeppe, and Yarsevich (2003) noted that mass media prevention campaigns may be most effective when combined with school-based or community-level activities, although the evidence base behind this assertion is rather limited to date. What is still not known, too, is whether these campaigns can produce long-term behavioral changes or whether they simply delay the onset of tobacco use.

Policy Approaches

Policy approaches, with their potential for having broad reach at relatively low cost, have received increasing attention as possible vehicles for reducing youth tobacco use. Policy approaches include laws that attempt to prevent sales of tobacco to minors; that punish youth for tobacco possession, use, or purchase; or that increase taxes on tobacco products. Wakefield and Giovino (2003) reviewed the status and effects of tobacco possession, use, and purchase laws in the United States. These laws can be directed at both youth and vendors of tobacco products. Only a few studies have empirically evaluated these laws, and overall, Wakefield and Giovino concluded that it is difficult to see strong effects from them. As the researchers pointed out, these laws have notable theoretical and practical limitations, including implementation (e.g., having a long delay between the offense and the consequence, the distant and impersonal relationship between the punisher and the recipient) and detecting and enforcing transgressions. When the laws are aggressively enforced and compliance is higher, however, effects are seen on reducing youth tobacco use (e.g., Chaloupka & Grossman, 1996; Forster et al., 1998). In general, though, teens often find that it is easy to circumvent these laws (Crawford, Balch, & Mermelstein, 2002). Wakefield and Giovino suggested, too, that these laws may actually divert attention from other more effective tobacco control strategies.

In contrast, raising taxes on tobacco products and thus increasing their prices has been shown to have strong and consistent effects on youth smoking (Chaloupka & Warner, 2000). Work by Chaloupka and Grossman (1996) and by NCI (2001) suggested that youth are more sensitive to price increases than are adults and that a 10% price increase in cigarettes would likely reduce the prevalence of youth smoking by 5%, a remarkable effect.

Summary

There is now a strong consensus that comprehensive, multichannel programming is both needed and effective in reducing youth smoking (Backinger, Fagan, Matthews, & Grana, 2003). A large evidence base for the effects of school-based prevention programs comprises many rigorously designed and evaluated, and theoretically driven, programs. However, the magnitude of the effects of school-based programs alone is small at best. The addition of components that target other levels or channels of influence, such as families, media, and community policies, improves the success of school-based programs, although as Flay (2000) noted, few studies have been designed to isolate the effects of each of these components separate from the school program or by themselves. As antitobacco messages become more a part of the everyday culture, it may become increasingly difficult to demonstrate unique effects of any one intervention component. Among the policy approaches, the strongest effects seem to accrue from price increases. One must consider, though, that the conclusions about the impact of price increases on youth smoking come from a number of econometric studies of cross-sectional data, and there are far fewer longitudinal studies. Finally, the effects of aggressive countermarketing campaigns are promising in their potential to change the social norms surrounding tobacco use, along with youth attitudes toward tobacco. Over time, with sustained presence, countermarketing campaigns may also influence youth tobacco use behavior as well, although the evidence base here is still in its infancy.

ANALYSIS, CONCLUSIONS, AND FUTURE RESEARCH DIRECTIONS

Recent research examining how individual, temperamental factors (e.g., novelty seeking) may interact with broader social contextual variables (e.g., exposure to tobacco advertising) to increase risk for smoking (e.g., Audrain-McGovern et al., 2003) is one example of how investigating interactive effects of risk factors may have implications for designing more effective interventions. Researchers know that risk for tobacco use is not evenly distributed among the population, yet the vast majority of interventions are delivered universally. Researchers also know relatively little about the benefits of targeting more intensive or tailored interventions to high-risk groups, such as youth with comorbid disorders (e.g., attention-deficit/hyperactivity disorder, other substance use, depression) or those with smoking-intensive social networks or home environments. In addition, despite the increasing call in the literature for sensitivity to cultural issues in the development and delivery of interventions, there continues to be a lack of solid research evidence about how mechanisms of interventions may differ by ethnic or gender subgroups or even whether the content of the interventions should change. Furthermore, age of initiation may vary by ethnic group (USDHHS, 1998), thus further confounding the issue of tailoring by subgroup.

Prevention of tobacco use may best be thought of along the full uptake continuum, not just initial use or one-time use. For the most part, evaluations of interventions focus on unidimensional outcomes, such as past month use or lifetime use. Rarely do the interventions or evaluations consider interruptions in the progression from initial use to dependence as part of their outcomes. Yet, given recent data suggesting an increase in the rate of transitioning from ever use to more regular use (Lanz, 2003), researchers need to develop and evaluate interventions that specifically target adolescents who have already started to experiment with tobacco use. One notable example is Ellickson et al.'s (2003) separate examination of Project ALERT's effects on ever, past month, and weekly smoking and their finding that the intervention reduced rates of initial trying and progression to regular smoking. Understanding how interventions may affect transitions or trajectories of smoking may be increasingly important in having a more comprehensive approach to reducing overall rates of youth smoking.

One must also consider how changes in the broader social context and sources of influence in adolescent life may affect risk for smoking. For example, the Internet is becoming an increasingly important venue for promoting tobacco use (Ribisl, 2003), especially to adolescents and young adults. However, prevention efforts have yet to take full advantage of this potentially powerful medium both for counteracting the prosmoking messages and for promoting antismoking messages (Ribisl, 2003).

There also has been a relative lack of emphasis on improving the overall health picture of adolescents, in terms of helping youth to develop healthy sources of "rebellion" or satisfaction. Interventions that include training in general coping skills, self-control, and affect regulation throughout the period of risk for adolescents may be considered as a general preventive approach as well. Researchers know little, though, about how some of these more general prevention interventions may affect tobacco use specifically.

Finally, as the next generation of prevention interventions begins, there is an increasing call for a transdisciplinary perspective on interventions. Thus, intervention developers should attend to what is known about tobacco use vulnerabilities from biological through societal perspectives and incorporate lessons learned from these multiple disciplines (Jamner et al., 2003).

REFERENCES

Audrain-McGovern, J., Tercyak, K. P., Shields, A. E., Bush, A., Espinel, C. F., & Lerman, C. (2003). Which adolescents are most receptive to tobacco industry marketing? Implications for counter-advertising campaigns. *Health Communications, 15,* 499–513.

Backinger, C., Fagan, P., Matthews, E., & Grana, R. (2003). Adolescent and young adult tobacco prevention and cessation: Current status and future directions. *Tobacco Control, 12*(Suppl. 4), 46–53.

Bauman, K. I., Foshee, V. A., Ennett, S. T., Pemberton, M., Kicks, K., King, T. S., & Koch, G. G. (2001). The influence of a family program on adolescent tobacco and alcohol use. *American Journal of Public Health, 91,* 604–610.

Biglan, A., Ary, D. V., Smoklowski, T. D., Duncan, T., & Black, C. (2000). A randomized controlled trial of a community intervention to prevent adolescent tobacco use. *Tobacco Control, 9,* 24–32.

Botvin, G. J., Schinke, S. P., Epstein, J. A., Diaz, T., & Botvin, E. M. (1995). Effectiveness of culturally focused and generic skills training approaches to alcohol and drug abuse prevention among minority adolescents: Two-year follow-up results. *Psychology of Addictive Behaviors, 9,* 183–194.

Bruvold, W. H. (1993). A meta-analysis of adolescent smoking prevention programs. *American Journal of Public Health, 83,* 872–880.

Cameron, R., Brown, K. S., Best, J. A., Pelkman, C. L., Madill, D. L., Manske, S. R., & Payne, M. E. (1999). Effectiveness of a social influences smoking prevention program as a function of provider type, training method, and school risk. *American Journal of Public Health, 89,* 1827–1831.

Chaloupka, F., & Grossman, M. (1996). *Price, tobacco control policies, and youth smoking* (National Bureau of Economic Research Working Paper No. W5740). Cambridge, MA: National Bureau of Economic Research.

Chaloupka, F., & Warner, K. (2000). The economics of smoking. In A. J. Culyer & J. P. Newhouse (Eds.), *Handbook of health economics* (Vol. 1B, pp. 1539–1627). Amsterdam: Elsevier.

Conrad, K. M., Flay, B. R., & Hill, D. (1992). Why children start smoking cigarettes: Predictors of onset. *British Journal of Addiction, 87,* 1711–1724.

Crawford, M. A., Balch, G., & Mermelstein, R. (2002). Responses to tobacco control policies among youths. *Tobacco Control, 11,* 14–19.

Dent, C. W., Sussman, S., Stacy, A. W., Craig, S., Burton, D., & Flay, B. (1995). Two-year behavior outcomes of Project Towards No Tobacco Use. *Journal of Consulting and Clinical Psychology, 63,* 676–677.

Ellickson, P. L., & Bell, R. M. (1990, March 16). Drug prevention in junior high: A multi-site longitudinal test. *Science, 247,* 1299–1305.

Ellickson, P. L., McCaffrey, D. F., Ghosh-Dastidar, B., & Longshore, D. L. (2003). New inroads in preventing adolescent drug use: Results from a large-scale trial of project ALERT in middle schools. *American Journal of Public Health, 93,* 1830–1836.

Fagerstrom, K. (2002). The epidemiology of smoking: Health consequences and benefits of cessation. *Drugs, 62*(Suppl. 2), 1–9.

Farrelly, M. C., Healton, C. G., Davis, K. C., Messeri, P., Hersey, J. C., & Haviland, M. L. (2002). Getting to the truth: Evaluating national tobacco countermarketing campaigns. *American Journal of Public Health, 92,* 901–907.

Farrelly, M. C., Niederdeppe, J., & Yarsevich, J. (2003). Youth tobacco prevention mass media campaigns: Past, present, and future directions. *Tobacco Control, 12*(Suppl. 1), 35–47.

Flay, B. R. (2000). Approaches to substance use prevention utilizing school curriculum plus environment change. *Addictive Behaviors, 25,* 861–885.

Flay, B. R., Koepke, D., Thomson, S. J., Santi, S., Best, J. A., & Brown, K. S. (1989). Six-year follow-up of the first Waterloo school smoking prevention trial. *American Journal of Public Health, 79,* 1371–1376.

Flay, B. R., & Petraitis, J. (1994). The theory of triadic influence: A new theory of health behavior with implications for preventive interventions. In G. L. Albrecht (Ed.), *Advances in medical sociology: Vol. 4. A reconsideration of models of health behavior change* (pp. 19–44). Greenwich, CT: JAI Press.

Flynn, B. S., Worden, J. K., Secker-Walker, R. H., Badger, G. J., Geller, B. M., & Costanza, M. C. (1992). Prevention of cigarette smoking through mass media intervention and school programs. *American Journal of Public Health, 82,* 827–834.

Flynn, B. S., Worden, J. K., Secker-Walker, M. B., Pirie, P. L., Badger, G. J., Carpenter, J. H., & Geller, B. M. (1994). Mass media and school interventions for cigarette smoking prevention: Effects 2 years after completion. *American Journal of Public Health, 84,* 1148–1150.

Forster, J. L., Murray, D. M., Wolfson, M., Blaine, T. M., Wagenaar, A. C., & Hennrikus, D. J. (1998). The effects of community policies to reduce youth access to tobacco. *American Journal of Public Health, 88,* 1193–1198.

Hafstad, A., Aaro, L. E., Engeland, A., Andersen, A., Langmark, F., & Stray-Pedersen, B. (1997). Provocative appeals in anti-smoking mass media campaigns targeting adolescents—The accumulated effect of multiple exposures. *Health Education Research, 12*, 227–236.

Jamner, L. D., Whalen, C. K., Loughlin, S. E., Mermelstein, R., Audrain-McGovern, J., Krishnan-Sarin, S., et al. (2003). Tobacco use across the formative years: A road map to developmental vulnerabilities. *Nicotine & Tobacco Research, 5*(Suppl. 1), 71–87.

Johnson, C. A., Pentz, M. A., Weber, M. D., Dwyer, J. H., Baer, N., MacKinnon, D. P., et al. (1990). Relative effectiveness of comprehensive community programming for drug abuse prevention with high-risk and low-risk adolescents. *Journal of Consulting and Clinical Psychology, 58*, 447–456.

Johnston, L. D., O'Malley, P. M., Bachman, J. G., & Schulenberg, J. E. (2006, December 21). *Decline in daily smoking by younger teens has ended.* Ann Arbor, MI: University of Michigan News and Information Services.

Kodl, M., & Mermelstein, R. (2004). Beyond modeling: Potential psychosocial mediators of the relationship between parental smoking and adolescent smoking. *Addictive Behaviors, 29*, 17–32.

Lanz, P. M. (2003). Smoking on the rise among young adults: Implications for research and policy. *Tobacco Control, 12*(Suppl. 1), 60–70.

Mayhew, K. P., Flay, B. R., & Mott, J. A. (2000). Stages in the development of adolescent smoking. *Drug and Alcohol Dependence, 59*(Suppl. 1), 61–81.

McGinnis, J. M., & Foegbe, W. H. (1993). Actual causes of death in the United States. *Journal of the American Medical Association, 270*, 2207–2212.

Mermelstein, R. (2003). Teen smoking cessation. *Tobacco Control, 12*(Suppl. 1), 25–34.

National Cancer Institute. (1992). *Smokeless tobacco or health: An international perspective* (Smoking and Tobacco Control Monograph No. 2). Bethesda, MD: Author.

National Cancer Institute. (2001). *Changing adolescent smoking prevalence: Where it is and why* (Smoking and Tobacco Control Monograph No. 14). Bethesda, MD: Author.

Niederdeppe, J., Farrelly, M. C., & Haviland, M. L. (2004). Confirming "truth": More evidence of a successful tobacco countermarketing campaign in Florida. *American Journal of Public Health, 94*, 255–257.

Pentz, M. A., MacKinnon, D. P., Dwyer, J. H., Wang, E. Y. I., Hansen, W. B., Flay, B. R., & Johnson, C. A. (1989). Longitudinal effects of the Midwestern Prevention Project on regular and experimental smoking in adolescents. *Preventive Medicine, 18*, 304–321.

Peterson, A. V., Kealey, K. A., Mann, S. L., Marek, P. M., & Sarason, I. G. (2000). Hutchinson Smoking Prevention Project: Long-term randomized trial in school-based tobacco use prevention-results on smoking. *Journal of the National Cancer Institute, 92*, 1979–1991.

Pierce, J. P., Choi, W. S., Gilpin, E. A., Farkas, A. J., & Merritt, R. K. (1996). Validation of susceptibility as a predictor of which adolescents take up smoking in the United States. *Health Psychology, 15*, 355–361.

Ribisl, K. (2003). The potential of the Internet as a medium to encourage and discourage youth tobacco use. *Tobacco Control, 12*(Suppl. 1), 48–59.

Rooney, B. L., & Murray, D. M. (1996). A meta-analysis of smoking prevention programs after adjustment for errors in the unit of analysis. *Health Education Quarterly, 23,* 48–64.

Sargent, J. D., Beach, M. L., Dalton, M. A., Mott, L. A., Tickle, J. J., Ahrens, M. B., & Heatherton, T. F. (2001, December 15). Effect of seeing tobacco use in films on trying smoking among adolescents: Cross sectional study. *BMJ, 323,* 1394–1397.

Siegel, M., & Biener, L. (2000). The impact of an antismoking media campaign on progression to established smoking: Results of a longitudinal youth study. *American Journal of Public Health, 90,* 380–386.

Sussman, S., Dent, C. W., Stacy, A. W., Sun, P., Craig, S., Simon, T. R., et al. (1993). Project Towards No Tobacco Use one-year behavior outcomes. *American Journal of Public Health, 83,* 1245–1250.

Tobler, N. S., Roona, M. R., Ochshorn, P., Marshall, D. G., Streke, A. V., & Stackpole, K. M. (2000). School-based adolescent drug prevention programs: 1998 meta-analysis. *The Journal of Primary Prevention, 20,* 275–336.

Turner, L., Mermelstein, R., & Flay, B. (2004). Individual and contextual influences on adolescent smoking. *Annals of the New York Academy of Science, 1021,* 1–23.

Twombly, R. (2003). Tobacco use a leading global cancer risk, report says. *Journal of the National Cancer Institute, 95,* 11–12.

Unger, J. B., Chou, C., Palmer, P., Ritt-Olson, A., Gallaher, P., Cen, S., et al. (2004). Project FLAVOR: 1-year outcomes of a multicultural, school-based smoking prevention curriculum for adolescents. *American Journal of Public Health, 94,* 263–265.

Unger, J. B., Ritt-Olson, A., Teran, L., Huang, T., Hoffman, B. R., & Palmer, P. (2002). Cultural values and substance use in a multiethnic sample of California adolescents. *Addiction Research & Theory, 10,* 257–279.

U.S. Department of Health and Human Services. (1990). *The Surgeon General's 1990 report on the health benefits of smoking cessation executive summary—Introduction, overview, and conclusions.* Atlanta, GA: Author.

U.S. Department of Health and Human Services. (1994). *Preventing tobacco use among young people: A report of the Surgeon General.* Atlanta, GA: Author

U.S. Department of Health and Human Services. (1998). *Tobacco use among U.S. racial/ethnic minority groups—African Americans, American Indians and Alaska Natives, Asian Americans and Pacific Islanders, and Hispanics: A report of the Surgeon General.* Atlanta, GA: Author.

U.S. Department of Health and Human Services. (2001). *Women and smoking: A report of the Surgeon General.* Rockville, MD: Author.

Wakefield, M., & Giovino, G. (2003). Teen penalties for tobacco possession, use, and purchase: Evidence and issues. *Tobacco Control, 12*(Suppl. 1), 6–13.

Worden, J. K., Flynn, B. S., Gellar, B. M., Chen, M., Shelton, L. G., Secker-Walker, R. H., et al. (1988). Development of a smoking prevention mass media program using diagnostic and formative research. *Preventive Medicine, 17,* 531–558.

10

INTERVENTIONS FOR SMOKING CESSATION

LARA K. DHINGRA AND JAMIE S. OSTROFF

Smoking cessation has received the most research attention of any cancer-related behavioral outcome to date. Ample evidence has been found during the past decade on the effectiveness of approved pharmacologic and behavioral therapies for the treatment of tobacco dependence. However, there is still a need to enhance the dissemination of evidence-based treatments in real-world settings and to advance the training, preparedness, and accountability of health providers as they implement clinical practice guidelines for smoking cessation. Key challenges in this implementation include targeting intensive interventions to special high-risk populations and partnering with community-based medical and mental health care providers to improve readiness and capacity to deliver these interventions. This chapter provides a structure for the past 30 years of smoking cessation research, delineating areas in which progress has been achieved and areas that are still in need of research attention.

BACKGROUND

More than 40 years since the U.S. Surgeon General's report *Smoking and Health* was released in 1964 (U.S. Department of Health, Education, and

Welfare, 1964), major developments in smoking cessation research, theory, and practice have enhanced the field of tobacco treatment. The rigor and volume of smoking cessation research has escalated, with the number of published studies on tobacco treatment doubling in the past decade. Findings from clinical research have led to the systematic development of evidence-based guidelines for cessation and have prompted the investigation of new strategies to improve treatment implementation. Collaborative efforts at the public and private levels are under way to improve tobacco control, treatment use, and provider readiness to advance national quit rates for population change. National quit rates continue to increase, and for the first time in decades, more adults in the general population have quit than are currently smoking (Centers for Disease Control and Prevention, 2004).

Promising research is clarifying the pharmacologic, genetic, and behavioral determinants of smoking cessation and deciphering the complex nature of nicotine dependence. Findings from multidisciplinary studies will likely improve the understanding of smoking behavior change and maintenance and will advance potential interventions for smoking cessation and disease prevention. However, the scientific investigation of factors accounting for individual variation in smoking cessation is far from complete. Quit rates continue to differ widely across population subgroups and are lower among those with psychiatric comorbidity, alcohol and substance abuse disorders, poor socioeconomic status, and specific ethnic/racial backgrounds (Fiore et al., 2000; Husten, Jackson, & Lee, 2004). Additional research is needed regarding treatment efficacy for subgroups of smokers with the lowest cessation rates and greatest difficulty quitting, and targeted interventions for these groups may prove empirically justified. Furthermore, despite the release of evidence-based treatment guidelines for smoking cessation, behavioral and pharmacologic treatments are not routinely administered to many smokers (Fiore et al., 2000). Data suggest that most smokers quit without assistance and prefer not to enroll in formal treatment programs (Fiore et al., 1990). Unfortunately, the majority of ex-smokers relapse 1 year after quitting, with self-quitters relapsing at higher rates than treated smokers (Ockene et al., 2000). Strategies to improve the acceptability of smoking cessation treatments and minimize relapse rates are clearly needed. To this end, previous research has emphasized the critical importance of improving treatment access to reach those smokers motivated to quit and of boosting engagement in cost-effective tobacco interventions at the public health level. At the same time, because a one-size-fits-all approach to smoking cessation is not optimal and because many smokers are unmotivated to take action to quit, clinicians are challenged to maximize treatment efficacy by tailoring approaches to the individual needs and characteristics of the smoker within the context of his or her tobacco use. Despite advances in the treatment and understanding of nicotine dependence, there is much to be learned about smoking cessation in the decades to come.

In this chapter, we begin by reviewing current best practices for tobacco cessation treatment delivery. Then, we review research on provider readiness to deliver treatments for smoking cessation in real-world settings and strategies for increasing provider readiness and capacity. Given disparate rates of smoking prevalence and related morbidity among the general population, in the last section of this chapter we highlight research on cessation with specific subgroups. We summarize major findings within each section, followed by a discussion of existing gaps in the literature and topics for additional research. Because prevention and cessation among youth and adolescent populations are reviewed elsewhere in this volume, this review focuses on smoking cessation among adults. In addition, we direct our attention to cigarette smoking (for quality reviews on smokeless tobacco and other forms of tobacco, see Ebbert, Carr, & Dale, 2004; Ebbert, Rowland, et al., 2004; Hatsukami & Severson, 1999).

INTERVENTION APPROACHES FOR SMOKING CESSATION

A variety of approaches and models have guided the delivery of smoking interventions. Tobacco interventions have involved stepped-care strategies (Abrams et al., 2003; Orleans, 1993; Russell et al., 1993), treatment-matching strategies (Abrams, Clark, & King, 1999; Hall, Munoz, & Reus, 1994; Hall et al., 1996; Niaura, Goldstein, & Abrams, 1994; Spencer, Pagell, Hallion, & Adams, 2002), and tailored intervention strategies (Dijkstra, De Vries, Roijackers, & van Breukelen, 1998; Lipkus, Lyna, & Rimer, 1999). Stepped-care approaches represent a continuum of care ranging from minimal contact, self-help interventions to intensive counseling interventions by formal treatment programs (Abrams et al., 1996). Stepped-care approaches are cost-effective public health models developed to maximize the reach of efficacious tobacco treatments among the general population. Initial treatment involves minimally intensive interventions with more intensive treatments added in response to lapses, barriers, or specific patient characteristics (e.g., patient preference for more social support, presence of psychiatric comorbidity, high nicotine dependency; Abrams et al., 1996; Orleans, 1993). The goal of stepped-care methods is to expose treatment failures to successively more intense treatments in response to need (Fiore et al., 2000; Orleans, 1993). In treatment matching, smokers are assigned to specific interventions on the basis of their pretreatment characteristics and prognosis for cessation following assessment (Fiore et al., 2000). Treatment intensity and specific components may take into account differences in smoker readiness for cessation, motivation to quit, level of nicotine dependence, affective vulnerability, self-efficacy to quit, and social support (Abrams et al., 1996; Spencer et al., 2002). Similarly, tailored interventions use a variety of modalities (e.g., letters, phone counseling, interactive computer programs) to provide personalized feedback to the patient and are individualized to address dimensions such as stage of change, cultural influences, English literacy, and weight or health concerns (Dijkstra et al., 1998; Fiore et al., 2000; Lipkus et al., 1999). Although stepped-care approaches are widely accepted as effective, few empirical studies to date have evaluated their efficaciousness compared with brief interventions. A well-designed study by S. S. Smith et al. (2001) examined the efficacy of a stepped-care approach contrasting brief intervention treatment with two intensive treatments (i.e., cognitive behavior and skill training therapy, and motivational interviewing and supportive therapy). Intensive treatments for patients with high-risk profiles for relapse (e.g., greater nicotine dependency, past or current depression, greater tendency for negative affectivity) were no more efficacious than brief treatments, with results suggesting additional research on when to intensify treatment delivery is needed (S. S. Smith et al., 2001).

Other researchers have proposed the potential development of evidence-based guidelines for triaging patients to successive treatment steps (P. O. Smith, Sheffer, Payne, Applegate, & Crews, 2003; S. S. Smith et al., 2001). Such information would clarify the specific indicators or constructs to guide treatment intensity and identify when the critical opportunity for added intervention is too early or late. The development of assessment measures indicating the ideal time for progression along the continuum of care may be useful. Questions that should be addressed include (a) How do tailored strategies compare in efficacy with treatment-matching and stepped-care strategies? and (b) What is their advantage compared with nonindividualized or standard treatments? What patient characteristics should tailored strategies address, aside from factors such as ethnicity, age, gender, and health status, and what is the added benefit of using psychological profiles in terms of treatment acceptability and long-term abstinence? As knowledge about the differential impact of pretreatment patient characteristics on cessation advances, individualizing pharmacologic treatments may become routine (Lerman et al., 2004). Such topics will remain exciting areas of inquiry in the decades to come.

PROGRESS IN ENHANCING PROVIDER READINESS AND CAPACITY TO DELIVER SMOKING CESSATION INTERVENTIONS

Health care providers play a pivotal role in delivering state-of-the-art, brief, and intensive interventions for smoking cessation (Gorin & Heck, 2004). Progress in enhancing provider readiness and capacity to deliver clinical interventions for cessation has been promising. In 2000, the Public Health Service updated the clinical practice guidelines for the treatment of tobacco by health care providers. Evidence for the clinical practice guidelines was based on a systematic review of approximately 6,000 empirical studies, and the results established standards for tobacco treatment and recommendations for providers, systems, administrators, and insurers. Meta-analyses formulating the practice guideline highlighted that even brief interventions for smoking cessation could double national quit rates, with brief and effective interventions taking less than 3 minutes to deliver. Specifically, minimal interventions for smoking cessation (e.g., lasting less than 3 minutes) significantly increase tobacco abstinence rates, and higher intensity interventions (e.g., lasting more than 10 minutes) across multiple treatment sessions are nearly twice as effective as brief advice. Therefore, the clinical practice guidelines set forth standardized, evidence-based approaches for smoking cessation that are both clinically effective and cost-effective (Fiore et al., 2000).

Each year, an estimated 50% to 80% of tobacco users visit a health care provider (CDC, 1993; Fiore et al., 2000). Recognition of the cost efficacy of tobacco interventions and the promulgation of the clinical practice guidelines have supported the development of national objectives to enhance provider accountability for the delivery of tobacco interventions (Fiore, Croyle, et al., 2004; Pbert, 2003; Pbert, Vuckovic, Ockene, Hollis, & Riedlinger, 2003; U.S. Department of Health and Human Services, 2000). Scientific organizations have issued policy statements on tobacco intervention (American Psychiatric Association, 1994; Society for Research on Nicotine and Tobacco, n.d.). These targeted outcomes and policy statements encourage providers to have the knowledge, skills, and support systems necessary to assist patients in smoking cessation.

Training Health Care Providers in the Delivery of Interventions for Smoking Cessation

An emergent challenge for health providers and agencies is to delineate the combinations of community- and clinic-based services that are needed to achieve national population-based objectives for smoking cessation. Despite growing support from the public and the private sector and the promulgation of the clinical practice guidelines, surveys report that many health care providers feel unprepared to assist their patients in smoking cessation, and a majority of providers do not routinely advise or assist their patients in cessation attempts (Cantor, Baker, & Hughes, 1993; CDC, 1993; Fiore et al., 2000; Gilpin et al., 1992; Goldstein et al., 2003). Findings estimate smoking status is assessed in 50% to 66% of patient clinic visits (Anda, Remington, Sienko, & Davis, 1987; Frank, Winkleby, Altman, Rockhill, & Fortmann, 1991; Gilpin et al., 1992; Goldstein et al., 1997), and smoking cessation interventions are provided in 3% to 20% of smoker's visits (Goldstein et al., 1997; Thorndike, Rigotti, Stafford, & Singer, 1998). These patterns suggest there is compelling evidence for the incomplete uptake of clinical practice guidelines in many health care settings. Notably, most studies on provider adherence to delivering public health guidelines focus on practice patterns among primary care physicians, with only one known published study focusing on adherence by behavioral health professionals (Phillips & Brandon, 2004).

Graduate Education

The transfer of knowledge from the clinical practice guidelines to the delivery of therapeutic interventions for smoking cessation is central to advancing primary cancer prevention outcomes. There are multiple barriers to the implementation of smoking cessation interventions by health care providers. Recognizing and addressing different levels of provider training is one area for suggested action. Studies report only 21% of practicing physicians perceive that their formal medical education prepared them to assist patients in quitting smoking (Cantor et al., 1993), and several studies report medical schools and other professional programs in the United States are not adequately training graduates to develop skills in treating tobacco dependence (Cantor et al., 1993; Ferry, Grissino, & Runfola, 1999; Fiore, Epps, & Manley, 1994; Spangler, George, Foley, & Crandall, 2002). Nearly 33% of 126 medical schools spend 3 hours or less of instruction on tobacco cessation techniques over the 4-year curricula, and over 66% require no training in tobacco interventions (Ferry et al., 1999). Therefore, initiatives to augment and standardize medical training in evidence-based treatments for tobacco dependence appear necessary.

Pbert (2003) suggested three essential components of a comprehensive training approach for health care providers that will advance the delivery of tobacco interventions: (a) medical education, (b) professional education, and (c) community-based education. Of these methods, educational training methods using active learning techniques for cessation counseling are effective in improving provider confidence to deliver tobacco interventions and increasing quit rates (Ferry et al., 1999; Humair & Cornuz, 2003; Roche, Eccleston, & Sanson-Fisher, 1996; Spangler et al., 2002). For recent reviews of effective medical curricula educational techniques and training methods, see Geller et al. (2002), Ferry et al. (1999), and Spangler et al. (2002). In particular, training methods developed by Ockene and colleagues using simulated patient instructors (Ockene & Zapka, 1997; Yedidia et al., 2003) are innovative and effective approaches for establishing medical student proficiency in counseling and assessing competency in cognitive and behavioral endpoints (Eyler et al., 1997).

Postgraduate and Community-Based Education

Models for postgraduate clinical training in smoking interventions need to be advanced. Of the existing methods, didactic techniques (e.g., grand rounds) are practical dissemination methods to improve knowledge and familiarity, yet they are insufficient in affecting clinician behavior change (Pbert, 2003). More efficacious strategies to enhance provider adoption of clinical practice guidelines include more intensive skill-based workshops and academic detailing. A recent *Cochrane Review* suggests academic detailing (e.g., educational outreach visits designed to improve professional practice and patient outcomes) can significantly enhance the intervention skills of physicians (Thomson O'Brien et al., 2000). Successful interventions using this strategy have been published (DePue et al., 2002; Goldstein et al., 2003; Zapka, Goins, Pbert, & Ockene, 2004).

Additional Barriers to the Delivery of Smoking Cessation Interventions

In real-world settings, the effective dissemination of the clinical practice guidelines for smoking cessation and quality of care are associated with multiple organizational-, community-, and clinician-based factors affecting patient smoking outcomes (Cabana et al., 1999). General findings highlight that physician knowledge (e.g., lack of awareness or familiarity with the clinical practice guidelines), physician attitudes (e.g., lack of agreement with the clinical practice guidelines, lack of self-efficacy in counseling skills, lack of outcome expectancy, the inertia of previous practice), and other barriers (e.g., inconvenience of using clinical practice guidelines, patient-related barriers to guideline implementation, environmental barriers) may be targets of intervention (Cabana et al., 1999). From a practical perspective, the effective delivery of tobacco treatments may be compromised by short office visits or by competing demands for clinical attention. Unless smoking-related problems are at the forefront of the patient's health care needs, tobacco interventions may be absent during the health care visit. Zapka et al. (2004) and Pbert (2003) have conducted extensive work addressing the challenges of translating theoretically planned and tested programs into practice. According to their research, barriers to address in future research involve identifying effective strategies that are compatible with the culture of a community system. Further, Zapka et al. (2004) suggested examining the effectiveness of program implementation on process variables and patient outcomes, establishing consensus on the standards for the consistent delivery of interventions, alleviating barriers in office systems, and encouraging providers to participate in expected performance outcomes.

Alternative strategies for cessation that eliminate physician barriers, particularly time limitations, should be further investigated. Nonprovider-based interventions used as an adjunct to minimal counseling may enhance the dissemination of brief therapies for smoking cessation. For example, telephone quit lines (Ossip-Klein & McIntosh, 2003) have been shown to increase abstinence rates. In addition, three promising technological formats, hand-held computers (Curry, Ludman, & McClure, 2003), computer-based tailoring programs (Shiffman, Paty, Rohay, Di Marino, & Gitchell, 2001), and Internet-based interventions (Lenert, Munoz, Perez, & Bansod, 2004), also appear to be promising adjunct approaches to disseminating smoking cessation interventions. These advances in technology show the potential to reduce barriers to treatment dissemination, enhance delivery of evidence-based guidelines, and engage smokers in personalized interventions with tailored assistance at critical points during treatment and relapse.

Enhancing Future Treatment Delivery by Behavioral Health Providers

In contrast to emerging new innovations in pharmacological treatments for smoking cessation, there have been few recent advances in behavioral interventions for tobacco use. This is particularly troubling given evidence that nicotine replacement therapy alone or in combination with behavioral therapy may fail for a substantial percentage of smokers (Hughes, Shiffman, Callas, & Zhang, 2003). Scheduled reduced smoking (SRS) has been cited as one promising exception to this trend. Based on learning theory, SRS involves a progressive and systematic reduction in smoking rate by increasing the time between cigarettes (Cinciripini et al., 1995). By smoking on a reduction schedule, smokers develop more efficacious coping strategies in response to an increasing delay between cigarettes, relying less on smoking itself as a coping strategy (Cinciripini, Wetter, & McClure, 1997). We have applied SRS to our own research with heavily nicotine-dependent, newly diagnosed cancer patients and guided SRS treatment delivery using handheld computers. Preliminary results suggest patients perceive SRS using handheld computers as an acceptable means of treatment delivery and support, and we will evaluate the effectiveness of these methods on long-term abstinence.

Given that a recent survey of practicing psychologists found that few adhere to the clinical practice guidelines (Phillips & Brandon, 2004), the goal for behavioral health providers over the next few decades may be to improve the dissemination of smoking cessation therapies. We used the same search criteria used by Ferry et al. (1999) on training medical students in cessation treatments and found no published studies to date on enhancing smoking cessation education in behavioral health providers.

TARGETING SMOKING CESSATION INTERVENTIONS
TO POPULATION SUBGROUPS

Because quit rates continue to differ widely among population subgroups, the following sections in this chapter focus on potential individual differences in the mechanisms of smoking behavior and cessation.

Smoking Cessation Interventions for Racial/Ethnic Minorities

Tobacco produces a great burden on certain minority groups in the United States, with racial/ethnic status associated with differences in smoking prevalence, cessation, and adverse health effects. To date, smoking interventions for minority groups have focused primarily on African Americans but have largely ignored other racial/ethnic groups such as Asian Americans and American Indians (Lawrence, Graber, Mills, Meissner, & Warnecke, 2003). Although more African Americans tend to be light smokers (e.g., smoke fewer than three cigarettes per day) when compared with Caucasians, specific covariates of smoking behavior among African Americans may account for racial differences in cessation. These potential differences include (a) higher levels of nicotine dependence among African American smokers compared with Caucasian smokers (e.g., after controlling for the effects of cigarette consumption and environmental and demographic factors), (b) differences in smoking topography (e.g., African Americans may consume cigarettes more rapidly), (c) greater preference for mentholated cigarettes (e.g., potentially enhancing the rewarding aspects of smoking for African Americans), and (d) a stronger positive association between smoking and postcessation weight gain (e.g., increasing the perceived benefits of smoking; Payne & Diefenbach, 2003). According to recent research, African Americans may in fact be more receptive to formal cessation treatments and often report greater desire to quit than Caucasians, but specific barriers may impede African Americans from using tobacco treatments (Fiore, McCarthy, et al., 2004). It is possible that racial/ethnic status is a proxy for genetic and environmental factors that influence dependency and treatment response across all groups (Benowitz, 2002). Therefore, the deconstruction of racial/ethnic differences into common determinants shared by all individuals to some degree may provide meaningful information about cessation (Benowitz, 2002). Promising research by Benowitz (2002) suggests racial/ethnic status among African Americans, Caucasians, Chinese Americans, and Hispanics is associated with significant differences in nicotine intake per cigarette and metabolic differences in serum cotinine (i.e., a nicotine metabolite). Such metabolic differences may partly explain ethnic differences in cigarette consumption, smoking topography, and health-related effects (Benowitz, 2002). Findings from Benowitz (2002) suggest differences in nicotine metabolism may have implications for dosing with smoking cessation medications.

Despite the potential evidence to suggest that smokers of different racial/ethnic groups may differ in terms of level of nicotine dependence, readiness to quit, and treatment response, most clinical trials have not examined the relationship of racial/ethnic status with smoking cessation treatment efficacy (Piper, Fox, Welsch, Fiore, & Baker, 2001). Piper et al. (2001) highlighted that none of the 192 articles included in their meta-analyses of the clinical practice guidelines included results based on racial/ethnic status. The extent to which smoking cessation interventions developed for predominantly Caucasian samples can be extended to minority subgroups requires further examination.

Smoking Cessation and Alcohol Abuse and Dependence

The popular notion that smoking, alcohol, and substance abuse are positively associated is well-supported by empirical findings (Budney, Higgins, Hughes, & Bickel, 1993; Daeppen et al., 2000; Darke & Hall, 1995; Grant, Hasin, Chou, Stinson, & Dawson, 2004; Romberger & Grant, 2004). Genetic, physiologic, and psychological mechanisms have been proposed to characterize smoking and drinking interactions (Colby et al., 2004; Romberger & Grant, 2004). The biobehavioral relationship between alcohol use and smoking is complex, with results suggesting a cycle of continued addiction whereby alcohol and smoking perpetuate each other. Further research is needed to determine whether relationships between smoking and drinking are unidirectional or bidirectional in nature (Colby et al., 2004). There are mixed results about whether continued smoking following alcohol treatment and abstinence makes alcohol relapse more likely (Gulliver et al., 2000). Some studies suggest smoking may buffer newly sober individuals from alcohol relapse because smoking may be a strategy for coping with urges to drink (Gulliver et al., 2000). However, smoking may precipitate relapse for heavy drinkers later in recovery (Gulliver et al., 2000; Stuyt, 1997). Hence, the mitigating or harmful effects of smoking on alcohol recovery are associated with sobriety length and alcohol abuse severity (Gulliver et al., 2000; Sobell, Sobell, & Agrawal, 2002). In summary, concurrent and heavy alcohol dependence is associated with poorer smoking cessation outcomes (Sobell et al., 2002), but previous history of alcohol abuse does not appear to worsen smoking cessation efforts (Breslau, Peterson, Schultz, Andreski, & Chilcoat, 1996; Hughes & Callas, 2003). New evidence suggests that inclusion of smoking cessation interventions does not complicate, and in some cases may improve, the effectiveness of alcohol treatment (Bobo, McIlvain, Gilchrist, & Bowman, 1996; Burling, Burling, & Latini, 2001; Hurt et al., 1994; Romberger & Grant, 2004). Romberger and Grant (2004) presented a quality review of methodological issues related to the timing and proximity of tobacco and sobriety treatments, and they established the rationale for developing optimal strategies for concurrent treatment of both disorders. Despite increasing support for the delivery of smoking interventions in alcohol-dependent individuals, evidence-based guidelines for combined tobacco and alcohol treatment are not established. Many clinical trials for tobacco cessation and empirical studies have excluded individuals with comorbid alcohol and substance abuse disorders and have included those with severe alcohol dependence compared with few participants from community samples (Romberger & Grant, 2004; Sobell et al., 2002). Future research should examine prolonged nicotine replacement therapy (NRT) and other harm-reduction strategies in highly dependent smokers, given the high level of dependency observed among alcoholics and potential risk for relapse. Because of the high prevalence of depression among individuals with alcohol dependence and the hedonic or reinforcing properties of smoking in mood management, pharmacotherapy with bupropion may be effective, given its antidepressant effects. Implications for the concurrent treatment of alcohol and nicotine addiction are evolving areas of inquiry. The limited research on tobacco cessation and substance abuse has focused primarily on alcohol-dependent patients, with little published empirical data to date on other drugs of abuse (e.g., cocaine, heroin, cannabis; for recent work, see Sullivan & Covey, 2002; Ford, Vu, & Anthony, 2002; Unrod, Cook, Myers, & Brown, 2004).

Psychiatric Comorbidity and Smoking Cessation

Epidemiologic data highlight that individuals with psychiatric disorders have disproportionately high rates of tobacco use compared with individuals without psychiatric comorbidity. In particular, patients with mood, psychotic, substance abuse, and anxiety disorders report higher rates of current smoking (de Leon, Becona, Gurpegui, Gonzalez-Pinto, & Diaz, 2002; Grant et al., 2004; Lasser et al., 2000) and lower quit rates (Lasser et al., 2000) than do nonpsychiatric populations. Few studies have evaluated smoking cessation interventions for individuals with severe psychiatric disorders, as most patients with comorbidity have been excluded from clinical trials (Prochaska, Gill, & Hall, 2004). Spring, Pingitore, and McChargue (2003) recently evaluated smokers with schizophrenia, smokers with depression, and a nonpsychiatric reference group and observed no group differences in negative appraisals about smoking; however, both psychiatric groups weighted the rewarding aspects of smoking more heavily than the perceived negative consequences (Spring et al., 2003). Recent evidence suggests that patients with schizophrenia (de Leon et al., 2002) are more likely to have higher nicotine dependency than other populations of smokers. The clinical practice guidelines recommend that patients with psychiatric comorbidity be provided treatments validated with the general population. A comprehensive review by McChargue, Gulliver, and Hitsman (2002) concluded that abstinence-focused approaches may have little efficacy for patients with schizophrenia and that the benefits of reduction-focused approaches should be investigated, despite questions regarding the harm-reducing value of this strategy.

Ample research has evaluated the association between depression and smoking cessation among clinical samples and the general population (Brown et al., 2001; Glassman et al., 1988; Haas, Munoz, Humfleet, Reus, & Hall, 2004; Hitsman, Borrelli, McChargue, Spring, & Niaura, 2003). Several researchers have examined possible covariates of the relationship between depression and difficulty with cessation, including greater life stress, fewer coping skills, and lower quitting self-efficacy compared with nondepressed patients (Piper et al., 2001). Potential mechanisms to explain the complicating influence of depression on cessation have included the severe nature of nicotine withdrawal symptoms in depressed smokers, the impact of depressive symptoms on treatment response (Hitsman et al., 2003), and low self-efficacy among depressed smokers mediating abstinence (Cinciripini et al., 2003). Innovative studies using ecological momentary analysis show smoking behavior may be characterized by individual differences in negative affectivity (Shiffman, Paty, Gnys, Kassel, & Hickcox, 1996), with smokers who experience rapid spikes in negative affect rather than slow-changing shifts being more prone to relapse (Shiffman et al., 1996; Shiffman & Waters, 2004). Future research will elucidate the neurobiological, behavioral, and intrapersonal mechanisms moderating the effect of depression on smoking cessation (Piper et al., 2001).

Women and Smoking Cessation

Empirical studies suggest that women may experience more difficulty quitting smoking compared with men (Borrelli, Papandonatos, Spring, Hitsman, & Niaura, 2004; Cepeda-Benito, Reynoso, & Erath, 2004; Piper et al., 2001). A recent meta-analysis reported similar efficacy of NRT in both men and women at 3 and 6 months postcessation but observed long-term maintenance declined in women (from 3 to 12 months and 6 to 12 months; Cepeda-Benito et al., 2004). Of note, findings indicated women benefited more from NRT in conjunction with intensive versus minimal behavioral support, suggesting high-intensity support was more important for women than men (see Cepeda-Benito et al., 2004, for a systematic review of sex differences in nicotine replacement). Notably, the clinical practice guidelines observed no studies showed higher abstinence rates for women compared with men following formal cessation programs (Piper et al., 2001). Gender differences have also been evaluated across pharmacotherapies for cessation. S. S. Smith et al. (2003) evaluated data from a randomized clinical trial to determine the efficacy of bupropion sustained release and the nicotine patch in women and individuals with a history of depression. Bupropion was observed to be 3 times more effective than placebo for both groups at 1-year follow-up compared with no significant effects for NRT. Women both with and without depressive histories benefited from bupropion, and after controlling for gender effects, results suggested cessation success with bupropion may be somewhat more dependent on gender than depression.

Multiple theories have been proposed to explain sex-related variation in quitting and abstinence maintenance. General findings suggest women report lower quitting self-efficacy, lower commitment to quit, lower quit attempts, and higher relapse rates following cessation, compared with men (Borrelli et al., 2004; King, Borrelli, Black, Pinto, & Marcus, 1997). In addition, health care providers may be less likely to ask women about smoking status and to advise them to quit (Rogers, Johnson, Young, & Graney, 1997). Furthermore, the reinforcing properties of nicotine from cigarettes use may be associated with sex and gender differences (Perkins, 2001; Perkins, Donny, & Caggiula, 1999). The role of negative affect has been associated with tobacco use, and women report a higher prevalence of depression than men (King et al., 1997; Piper et al., 2001; Wetter et al., 1999). Gender differences in coping style and cognitive processing of negative affect may also account for variation in smoking rates (Piper et al., 2001). Collectively, the complexity of these factors suggests possible differences in the processes of reinforcement and dependence between men and women. Other potential barriers to consider in smoking cessation among women include the influence of hormones and menstrual cycles on cessation and negative affect (Perkins, 1996) and weight-related concerns (Bowen, McTiernan, Powers, & Feng, 2000). Women may benefit from tailored tobacco dependence treatments that address these specific areas. Because smoking is associated with elevated risks for certain health effects (e.g., greater risk for reproductive disorders, osteoporosis, and cervical cancer, particularly among minorities) and because smoking during pregnancy poses risks to both the woman and the developing fetus, clinicians can capitalize on motivation to quit by reinforcing the knowledge that cessation will reduce health risks to the woman and fetus and produce postpartum benefits for both the mother and the child. For a recent review on smoking cessation interventions with pregnant smokers, see Melvin and Gaffney (2004).

Smoking Cessation With Medically Ill Populations

The health risks of continued smoking in patients with various medical illnesses are well established. Perhaps less recognized and disseminated, however, is knowledge about the health benefits associated with smoking cessation following diagnosis of certain medical conditions. Among cancer patients, the health benefits of smoking cessation are considerable (Browman et al., 1993; Cox et al. 2002; Duffy et al., 2002; Gritz, Kristeller, & Burns, 1993; Stewart, King, Killen, & Ritter, 1995; Szarewski et al., 1996; Tucker et al., 1997; Videtic et al., 2003). Hospital-based smoking cessation trials suggest that medical admission is an effective time to deliver smoking cessation interventions (France, Glasgow, & Marcus, 2001; Munafo, Rigotti, Lancaster, Stead, & Murphy, 2001; Rigotti, Munafo, Murphy, & Stead, 2003). Research demonstrates higher cessation rates for patients in intervention compared with control conditions, with follow-up counseling (i.e., postdischarge) enhancing long-term abstinence rates (Rigotti et al., 2003). Cessation is positively associated with treatment dose and intensity, and intensive interventions show greater efficacy than minimal contact approaches (France et al., 2001). Furthermore, interventions delivered early in the hospital stay and closer to the time of medical diagnosis are positively associated with abstinence outcomes at 1 year (Rigotti et al., 2003). These results suggest a critical period, or teachable moment, for intervention that can enhance the potency of treatment delivery.

CONCLUSION

The past 4 decades have witnessed considerable progress in the development of interventions for smoking cessation. Future advances in the adoption of evidence-based guidelines and greater understanding of individual differences in the mechanisms of smoking cessation, long-term abstinence, and relapse will subsequently inform the innovation of efficacious new treatment strategies. Despite the availability of evidence-based treatment components for smoking cessation, dissemination of the evidence-based guidelines has fallen short. The future success and reach of smoking cessation programs relies heavily on the ability of mental health professionals to assist health care providers in increasing their capacity and readiness for the implementation of tobacco treatments. Increasing the availability of intensive smoking cessation programs community-wide and increasing special services to augment free-standing, hospital-based programs are other suggested areas for action. System enhancements also include supporting the routine assessment of tobacco by behavioral health professionals, establishing more intensive clinical programs to supplement brief clinical interventions, and developing strong models of service linkage between smoking cessation clinics and medically based cessation efforts. These advances, combined with advances in the cessation knowledge base and intervention by providers, will help to prevent significant smoking-related morbidity and mortality. Further examination of patterns or covariates of cessation in population subgroups, including ethnic minorities, patients with psychiatric comorbidity, women, and medically ill patients, to determine their response to smoking treatments are targeted areas for additional research. Therapies promoting smoking behavior change in these groups will refine understanding of the complex determinants of cessation and promote the development of optimal treatment approaches for the future.

REFERENCES

Abrams, D. B., Clark, M. M., & King, T. K. (1999). Increasing the impact of nicotine dependence treatment: Conceptual and practical considerations in a stepped-care plus treatment-matching approach. In J. A. Tucker, D. M. Donovan, & G. A.

Marlatt (Eds.), *Changing addictive behavior: Bridging clinical and public health strategies* (pp. 307–330). New York: Guilford Press.

Abrams, D. B., Niaura, R., Brown, R. A., Emmons, K. M., Goldstein, M. G., & Monti, P. M. (2003). *The tobacco dependence treatment handbook: A guide to best practices*. New York: Guilford Press.

Abrams, D. B., Orleans, C., Niaura, R., Goldstein, M. G., Prochaska, J., & Velicer, W. (1996). Integrating individual and public health perspectives for treatment of tobacco dependence under managed health care: A combined stepped-care and matching model. *Annals of Behavioral Medicine, 18*, 238–241.

American Psychiatric Association. (1994). *Nicotine dependence position statement* (APA Document Reference No. 940004). Retrieved September 8, 2004, from http://archive.psych.org/edu/other_res/lib_archives/archives/199404.pdf

Anda, R. F., Remington, P. L., Sienko, D. G., & Davis, R. M. (1987). Are physicians advising smokers to quit? The patient's perspective. *Journal of the American Medical Association, 257*, 1916–1919.

Benowitz, N. L. (2002). Smoking cessation trials targeted to racial and economic minority groups. *Journal of the American Medical Association, 288*, 497–499.

Bobo, J. K., McIlvain, H. E., Gilchrist, L. D., & Bowman, A. (1996). Nicotine dependence and intentions to quit smoking in three samples of male and female recovering alcoholics and problem drinkers. *Substance Use and Misuse, 31*, 17–33.

Borrelli, B., Papandonatos, G., Spring, B., Hitsman, B., & Niaura, R. (2004). Experimenter-defined quit dates for smoking cessation: Adherence improves outcomes for women but not for men. *Addiction, 99*, 378–385.

Bowen, D. J., McTiernan, A., Powers, D., & Feng, Z. (2000). Recruiting women into a smoking cessation program: Who might quit? *Women's Health, 31*, 41–58.

Breslau, N., Peterson, E., Schultz, L., Andreski, P., & Chilcoat, H. (1996). Are smokers with alcohol disorders less likely to quit? *American Journal of Public Health, 86*, 985–990.

Browman, G. P., Wong, G., Hodson, I., Sathya, J., Russell, R., McAlpine, L., et al. (1993). Influence of cigarette smoking on the efficacy of radiation therapy in head and neck cancer. *New England Journal of Medicine, 328*, 159–163.

Brown, R. A., Kahler, C. W., Niaura, R., Abrams, D. B., Sales, S. D., Ramsey, S. E., et al. (2001). Cognitive–behavioral treatment for depression in smoking cessation. *Journal of Consulting and Clinical Psychology, 69*, 471–480.

Budney, A. J., Higgins, S. T., Hughes, J. R., & Bickel, W. K. (1993). Nicotine and caffeine use in cocaine-dependent individuals. *Journal of Substance Abuse, 5*, 117–130.

Burling, T. A., Burling, A. S., & Latini, D. (2001). A controlled smoking cessation trial for substance-dependent inpatients. *Journal of Consulting and Clinical Psychology, 69*, 295–304.

Cabana, M. D., Rand, C. S., Powe, N. R., Wu, A. W., Wilson, M. H., Abboud, P. A., & Rubin, H. R. (1999). Why don't physicians follow clinical practice guidelines? A framework for improvement. *Journal of the American Medical Association, 282*, 1458–1465.

Cantor, J. C., Baker, L. C., & Hughes, R. G. (1993). Preparedness for practice: Young physicians' views of their professional education. *Journal of the American Medical Association, 270*, 1035–1040.

Centers for Disease Control and Prevention. (1993). Physician and other health-care professional counseling of smokers to quit—United States, 1991. *Morbidity and Mortality Weekly Report, 42*, 854–857.

Centers for Disease Control and Prevention. (2004). Smoking prevalence among U.S. adults. Retrieved January 4, 2004, from http://www.cdc.gov/od/oc/media/pressrel/r051110.htm

Cepeda-Benito, A., Reynoso, J. T., & Erath, S. (2004). Meta-analysis of the efficacy of nicotine replacement therapy for smoking cessation: Differences between men and women. *Journal of Consulting and Clinical Psychology, 72*, 712–722.

Cinciripini, P. M., Lapitsky, L., Seay, S., Wallfisch, A., Kitchens, K., & Van Vunakis, H. (1995). The effects of smoking schedules on cessation outcome: Can we improve on common methods of gradual and abrupt nicotine withdrawal? *Journal of Consulting and Clinical Psychology, 63*, 388–399.

Cinciripini, P. M., Wetter, D. W., Fouladi, R. T., Blalock, J. A., Carter, B. L., Cinciripini, L. G., & Baile, W. F. (2003). The effects of depressed mood on smoking cessation: Mediation by postcessation self-efficacy. *Journal of Consulting and Clinical Psychology, 71*, 292–301.

Cinciripini, P. M., Wetter, D. W., & McClure, J. B. (1997). Scheduled reduced smoking: Effects on smoking abstinence and potential mechanisms of action. *Addictive Behaviors, 22*, 759–767.

Colby, S. M., Rohsenow, D. J., Monti, P. M., Gwaltney, C. J., Gulliver, S. B., Abrams, D. B., et al. (2004). Effects of tobacco deprivation on alcohol cue reactivity and drinking among young adults. *Addictive Behaviors, 29*, 879–892.

Cox, L. S., Sloan, J. A., Patten, C. A., Bonner, J. A., Geyer, S. M., McGinnis, W. L., et al. (2002). Smoking behavior of 226 patients with diagnosis of Stage IIIA/IIIB non-small cell lung cancer. *Psycho-Oncology, 11*, 472–478.

Curry, S. J., Ludman, E. J., & McClure, J. (2003). Self-administered treatment for smoking cessation. *Journal of Clinical Psychology, 59*, 305–319.

Daeppen, J. B., Smith, T. L., Danko, G. P., Gordon, L., Landi, N. A., Nurnberger, J. I., Jr., et al. (2000). Clinical correlates of cigarette smoking and nicotine dependence in alcohol-dependent men and women: The collaborative study group on the genetics of alcoholism. *Alcohol and Alcoholism, 35*, 171–175.

Darke, S., & Hall, W. (1995). Levels and correlates of polydrug use among heroin users and regular amphetamine users. *Drug and Alcohol Dependence, 39*, 231–235.

de Leon, J., Becona, E., Gurpegui, M., Gonzalez-Pinto, A., & Diaz, F. J. (2002). The association between high nicotine dependence and severe mental illness may be consistent across countries. *Journal of Clinical Psychiatry, 63*, 812–816.

DePue, J. D., Goldstein, M. G., Schilling, A., Reiss, P., Papandonatos, G., Sciamanna, C., & Kazura, A. (2002). Dissemination of the AHCPR clinical practice guideline in community health centres. *Tobacco Control, 11*, 329–335.

Dijkstra, A., De Vries, H., Roijackers, J., & van Breukelen, G. (1998). Tailoring information to enhance quitting in smokers with low motivation to quit: Three basic efficacy questions. *Health Psychology, 17,* 513–519.

Duffy, S. A., Terrell, J. E., Valenstein, M., Ronis, D. L., Copeland, L. A., & Connors, M. (2002). Effect of smoking, alcohol, and depression on the quality of life of head and neck cancer patients. *General Hospital Psychiatry, 24,* 140–147.

Ebbert, J. O., Carr, A. B., & Dale, L. C. (2004). Smokeless tobacco: An emerging addiction. *Medical Clinics of North America, 88,* 1593–1605.

Ebbert, J. O., Rowland, L. C., Montori, V., Vickers, K. S., Erwin, P. C., Dale, L. C., & Stead, L. F. (2004). Interventions for smokeless tobacco use cessation. *Cochrane Database of Systematic Reviews, 3.* Available from http://www.cochrane.org

Eyler, A. E., Dicken, L. L., Fitzgerald, J. T., Oh, M. S., Wolf, F. M., & Zweifler, A. J. (1997). Teaching smoking-cessation counseling to medical students using simulated patients. *American Journal of Preventive Medicine, 13,* 153–158.

Ferry, L. H., Grissino, L. M., & Runfola, P. S. (1999). Tobacco dependence curricula in U.S. undergraduate medical education. *Journal of the American Medical Association, 282,* 825–829.

Fiore, M. C., Bailey, W. C., Cohen, S. J., Dorfman, S. F., Goldstein, M. G., Gritz, E. R., et al. (2000). *Treating tobacco use and dependence: Clinical practice guideline.* Rockville, MD: U.S. Department of Health and Human Services, Public Health Service.

Fiore, M. C., Croyle, R. T., Curry, S. J., Cutler, C. M., Davis, R. M., Gordon, C., et al. (2004). Preventing 3 million premature deaths and helping 5 million smokers quit: A national action plan for tobacco cessation. *American Journal of Public Health, 94,* 205–210.

Fiore, M. C., Epps, R. P., & Manley, M. W. (1994). A missed opportunity. Teaching medical students to help their patients successfully quit smoking. *Journal of the American Medical Association, 271,* 624–626.

Fiore, M. C., McCarthy, D. E., Jackson, T. C., Zehner, M. E., Jorenby, D. E., Mielke, M., et al. (2004). Integrating smoking cessation treatment into primary care: An effectiveness study. *Preventive Medicine, 38,* 412–420.

Fiore, M. C., Novotny, T. E., Pierce, J. P., Giovino, G. A., Hatziandreu, E. J., Newcomb, P. A., et al. (1990). Methods used to quit smoking in the United States: Do cessation programs help? *Journal of the American Medical Association, 263,* 2760–2765.

Ford, D. E., Vu, H. T., & Anthony, J. C. (2002). Marijuana use and cessation of tobacco smoking in adults from a community sample. *Drug and Alcohol Dependence, 67,* 243–248.

France, E. K., Glasgow, R. E., & Marcus, A. C. (2001). Smoking cessation interventions among hospitalized patients: What have we learned? *Preventive Medicine, 32,* 376–388.

Frank, E., Winkleby, M. A., Altman, D. G., Rockhill, B., & Fortmann, S. P. (1991). Predictors of physician's smoking cessation advice. *Journal of the American Medical Association, 266,* 3139–3144.

Geller, A. C., Prout, M. N., Miller, D. R., Siegel, B., Sun, T., Ockene, J., & Koh, H. K. (2002). Evaluation of a cancer prevention and detection curriculum for medical students. *Preventive Medicine, 35,* 78–86.

Gilpin, E., Pierce, J., Goodman, J., Giovino, G., Berry, C., & Burns, D. (1992). Trends in physicians' giving advice to stop smoking, United States 1974–87. *Tobacco Control, 1,* 185–196.

Glassman, A. H., Stetner, F., Walsh, B. T., Raizman, P. S., Fleiss, J. L., Cooper, T. B., & Covey, L. S. (1988). Heavy smokers, smoking cessation, and clonidine: Results of a double-blind, randomized trial. *Journal of the American Medical Association, 259,* 2863–2866.

Goldstein, M. G., Niaura, R., Willey, C., Kazura, A., Rakowski, W., DePue, J., & Park, E. (2003). An academic detailing intervention to disseminate physician-delivered smoking cessation counseling: Smoking cessation outcomes of the Physicians Counseling Smokers Project. *Preventive Medicine, 36,* 185–196.

Goldstein, M. G., Niaura, R., Willey-Lessne, C., DePue, J., Eaton, C., Rakowski, W., & Dubé, C. (1997). Physicians counseling smokers. A population-based survey of patients' perceptions of health care provider-delivered smoking cessation interventions. *Archives of Internal Medicine, 157,* 1313–1319.

Gorin, S. S., & Heck, J. E. (2004). Meta-analysis of the efficacy of tobacco counseling by health care providers. *Cancer Epidemiology, Biomarkers & Prevention, 13,* 2012–2022.

Grant, B. F., Hasin, D. S., Chou, S. P., Stinson, F. S., & Dawson, D. A. (2004). Nicotine dependence and psychiatric disorders in the United States: Results from the National Epidemiologic Survey on Alcohol and Related Conditions. *Archives of General Psychiatry, 61,* 1107–1115.

Gritz, E. R., Kristeller, J., & Burns, D. M. (1993). Treating nicotine addiction in high-risk groups and patients with medical co-morbidity. In C. T. Orleans & J. Slade (Eds.), *Nicotine addiction: Principles and management* (pp. 279–309). New York: Oxford University Press.

Gulliver, S. B., Kalman, D., Rohsenow, D. J., Colby, S. M., Eaton, C. A., & Monti, P. M. (2000). Smoking and drinking among alcoholics in treatment: Cross-sectional and longitudinal relationships. *Journal of Studies on Alcohol, 61,* 157–163.

Haas, A. L., Munoz, R. F., Humfleet, G. L., Reus, V. I., & Hall, S. M. (2004). Influences of mood, depression history, and treatment modality on outcomes in smoking cessation. *Journal of Consulting and Clinical Psychology, 72,* 563–570.

Hall, S. M., Munoz, R. F., & Reus, V. I. (1994). Cognitive–behavioral intervention increases abstinence rates for depressive-history smokers. *Journal of Consulting and Clinical Psychology, 62,* 141–146.

Hall, S. M., Munoz, R. F., Reus, V. I., Sees, K. L., Duncan, C., Humfleet, G. L., & Hartz, D. T. (1996). Mood management and nicotine gum in smoking treatment: A therapeutic contact and placebo-controlled study. *Journal of Consulting and Clinical Psychology, 64,* 1003–1009.

Hatsukami, D. K., & Severson, H. H. (1999). Oral spit tobacco: Addiction, prevention, and treatment. *Nicotine & Tobacco Research, 1*, 21–44.

Hitsman, B., Borrelli, B., McChargue, D. E., Spring, B., & Niaura, R. (2003). History of depression and smoking cessation outcome: A meta-analysis. *Journal of Consulting and Clinical Psychology, 71*, 657–663.

Hughes, J. R., & Callas, P. W. (2003). Past alcohol problems do not predict worse smoking cessation outcomes. *Drug and Alcohol Dependence, 71*, 269–273.

Hughes, J. R., Shiffman, S., Callas, P., & Zhang, J. (2003). A meta-analysis of the efficacy of over-the-counter nicotine replacement. *Tobacco Control, 12*, 21–27.

Humair, J. P., & Cornuz, J. (2003). A new curriculum using active learning methods and standardized patients to train residents in smoking cessation. *Journal of General Internal Medicine, 18*, 1023–1027.

Hurt, R. D., Eberman, K. M., Croghan, I. T., Offord, K. P., Davis, L. J., Jr., Morse, R. M., et al. (1994). Nicotine dependence treatment during inpatient treatment for other addictions: A prospective intervention trial. *Alcoholism, Clinical and Experimental Research, 18*, 867–872.

Husten, C., Jackson, K., & Lee, C. (2004). Cigarette smoking among adults—United States. *Morbidity and Mortality Weekly Report, 53*, 427–431.

King, T. K., Borrelli, B., Black, C., Pinto, B. M., & Marcus, B. H. (1997). Minority women and tobacco: Implications for smoking cessation interventions. *Annals of Behavioral Medicine, 19*, 301–313.

Lasser, K., Boyd, J. W., Woolhandler, S., Himmelstein, D. U., McCormick, D., & Bor, D. H. (2000). Smoking and mental illness: A population-based prevalence study. *Journal of the American Medical Association, 284*, 2606–2610.

Lawrence, D., Graber, J. E., Mills, S. L., Meissner, H. I., & Warnecke, R. (2003). Smoking cessation interventions in U.S. racial/ethnic minority populations: An assessment of the literature. *Preventive Medicine, 36*, 204–216.

Lenert, L., Munoz, R. F., Perez, J. E., & Bansod, A. (2004). Automated e-mail messaging as a tool for improving quit rates in an Internet smoking cessation intervention. *Journal of the American Medical Information Association, 11*, 235–240.

Lerman, C., Kaufmann, V., Rukstalis, M., Patterson, F., Perkins, K., Audrain-McGovern, J., & Benowitz, N. (2004). Individualizing nicotine replacement therapy for the treatment of tobacco dependence: A randomized trial. *Annals of Internal Medicine, 140*, 426–433.

Lipkus, I. M., Lyna, P. R., & Rimer, B. K. (1999). Using tailored interventions to enhance smoking cessation among African-Americans at a community health center. *Nicotine & Tobacco Research, 1*, 77–85.

McChargue, D. E., Gulliver, S. B., & Hitsman, B. (2002). Would smokers with schizophrenia benefit from a more flexible approach to smoking treatment? *Addiction, 97*, 785–793, 795–800.

Melvin, C., & Gaffney, C. (2004). Treating nicotine use and dependence of pregnant and parenting smokers: An update. *Nicotine & Tobacco Research, 6*(Suppl. 2), 107–124.

Munafo, M., Rigotti, N., Lancaster, T., Stead, L., & Murphy, M. (2001). Interventions for smoking cessation in hospitalised patients: A systematic review. *Thorax*, *56*, 656–663.

Niaura, R., Goldstein, M. G., & Abrams, D. B. (1994). Matching high- and low-dependence smokers to self-help treatment with or without nicotine replacement. *Preventive Medicine*, *23*, 70–77.

Ockene, J. K., Emmons, K. M., Mermelstein, R. J., Perkins, K. A., Bonollo, D. S., Voorhees, C. C., & Hollis, J. F. (2000). Relapse and maintenance issues for smoking cessation. *Health Psychology*, *19*(Suppl. 1), 17–31.

Ockene, J. K., & Zapka, J. G. (1997). Physician-based smoking intervention: A rededication to a five-step strategy to smoking research. *Addictive Behaviors*, *22*, 835–848.

Orleans, C. T. (1993). Treating nicotine dependence in medical settings: A stepped-care model. In C. T. Orleans & J. Slade (Ed.), *Nicotine addiction: Principles and management* (pp. 145–161). New York: Oxford University Press.

Ossip-Klein, D. J., & McIntosh, S. (2003). Quitlines in North America: Evidence base and applications. *The American Journal of the Medical Sciences*, *326*, 201–205.

Payne, T. J., & Diefenbach, L. (2003). Characteristics of African American smokers: A brief review. *The American Journal of the Medical Sciences*, *326*, 212–215.

Pbert, L. (2003). Healthcare provider training in tobacco treatment: Building competency. *The American Journal of the Medical Sciences*, *326*, 242–247.

Pbert, L., Vuckovic, N., Ockene, J. K., Hollis, J. F., & Riedlinger, K. (2003). Developing and testing new smoking measures for the health plan employer data and information set. *Medical Care*, *41*, 550–559.

Perkins, K. A. (1996). Sex differences in nicotine versus nonnicotine reinforcement as determinants of tobacco smoking. *Experimental and Clinical Psychopharmacology*, *4*, 166–177.

Perkins, K. A. (2001). Smoking cessation in women: Special considerations. *CNS Drugs*, *15*, 391–411.

Perkins, K. A., Donny, E., & Caggiula, A. R. (1999). Sex differences in nicotine effects and self-administration: Review of human and animal evidence. *Nicotine & Tobacco Research*, *1*, 301–315.

Phillips, K. M., & Brandon, T. H. (2004). Do psychologists adhere to the clinical practice guidelines for tobacco cessation? A survey of practitioners. *Professional Psychology: Research and Practice*, *35*, 281–285.

Piper, M. E., Fox, B. J., Welsch, S. K., Fiore, M. C., & Baker, T. B. (2001). Gender and racial/ethnic differences in tobacco-dependence treatment: A commentary and research recommendations. *Nicotine & Tobacco Research*, *3*, 291–297.

Prochaska, J. J., Gill, P., & Hall, S. M. (2004). Treatment of tobacco use in an inpatient psychiatric setting. *Psychiatric Services*, *55*, 1265–1270.

Rigotti, N. A., Munafo, M. R., Murphy, M. F., & Stead, L. F. (2003). Interventions for smoking cessation in hospitalised patients. *Cochrane Database of Systematic Reviews*, *1*. Available from http://www.cochrane.org

Roche, A. M., Eccleston, P., & Sanson-Fisher, R. (1996). Teaching smoking cessation skills to senior medical students: A block-randomized controlled trial of four different approaches. *Preventive Medicine, 25*, 251–258.

Rogers, L. Q., Johnson, K. C., Young, Z. M., & Graney, M. (1997). Demographic bias in physician smoking cessation counseling. *The American Journal of the Medical Sciences, 313*, 153–158.

Romberger, D. J., & Grant, K. (2004). Alcohol consumption and smoking status: The role of smoking cessation. *Biomedical Pharmacotherapy, 58*, 77–83.

Russell, M. A., Stapleton, J. A., Feyerabend, C., Wiseman, S. M., Gustavsson, G., Sawe, U., & Conner, P. (1993, May 15). Targeting heavy smokers in general practice: Randomised controlled trial of transdermal nicotine patches. *BMJ, 306*, 1308–1312.

Shiffman, S., Paty, J. A., Gnys, M., Kassel, J. A., & Hickcox, M. (1996). First lapses to smoking: Within-subjects analysis of real-time reports. *Journal of Consulting and Clinical Psychology, 64*, 366–379.

Shiffman, S., Paty, J. A., Rohay, J. M., Di Marino, M. E., & Gitchell, J. G. (2001). The efficacy of computer-tailored smoking cessation material as a supplement to nicotine patch therapy. *Drug and Alcohol Dependence, 64*, 35–46.

Shiffman, S., & Waters, A. J. (2004). Negative affect and smoking lapses: A prospective analysis. *Journal of Consulting and Clinical Psychology, 72*, 192–201.

Smith, P. O., Sheffer, C. E., Payne, T. J., Applegate, B. W., & Crews, K. M. (2003). Smoking cessation research in primary care treatment centers: The SCRIPT-MS project. *The American Journal of the Medical Sciences, 326*, 238–241.

Smith, S. S., Jorenby, D. E., Fiore, M. C., Anderson, J. E., Mielke, M. M., Beach, K. E., et al. (2001). Strike while the iron is hot: Can stepped-care treatments resurrect relapsing smokers? *Journal of Consulting and Clinical Psychology, 69*, 429–439.

Smith, S. S., Jorenby, D. E., Leischow, S. J., Nides, M. A., Rennard, S. I., Johnston, J. A., et al. (2003). Targeting smokers at increased risk for relapse: Treating women and those with a history of depression. *Nicotine & Tobacco Research, 5*, 99–109.

Sobell, L. C., Sobell, M. B., & Agrawal, S. (2002). Self-change and dual recoveries among individuals with alcohol and tobacco problems: Current knowledge and future directions. *Alcoholism, Clinical and Experimental Research, 26*, 1936–1938.

Society for Research on Nicotine and Tobacco. (n.d.). *SRNT statement of policy.* Retrieved November 5, 2004, from http://www.srnt.org/about/s_o_p.html

Spangler, J. G., George, G., Foley, K. L., & Crandall, S. J. (2002). Tobacco intervention training: Current efforts and gaps in US medical schools. *Journal of the American Medical Association, 288*, 1102–1109.

Spencer, L., Pagell, F., Hallion, M. E., & Adams, T. B. (2002). Applying the transtheoretical model to tobacco cessation and prevention: A review of literature. *American Journal of Health Promotion, 17*, 7–71.

Spring, B., Pingitore, R., & McChargue, D. E. (2003). Reward value of cigarette smoking for comparably heavy smoking schizophrenic, depressed, and nonpatient smokers. *American Journal of Psychiatry, 160*, 316–322.

Stewart, A. L., King, A. C., Killen, J. D., & Ritter, P. L. (1995). Does smoking cessation improve health-related quality-of-life? *Annals of Behavioral Medicine, 17,* 331–338.

Stuyt, E. B. (1997). Recovery rates after treatment for alcohol/drug dependence. Tobacco users vs. non-tobacco users. *American Journal of Addiction, 6,* 159–167.

Sullivan, M. A., & Covey, L. S. (2002). Current perspectives on smoking cessation among substance abusers. *Current Psychiatry Reports, 4,* 388–396.

Szarewski, A., Jarvis, M. J., Sasieni, P., Anderson, M., Edwards, R., Steele, S. J., et al. (1996). Effect of smoking cessation on cervical lesion size. *Lancet, 347,* 941–943.

Thomson O'Brien, M. A., Oxman, A. D., Davis, D. A., Haynes, R. B., Freemantle, N., & Harvey, E. L. (2000). Educational outreach visits: Effects on professional practice and health care outcomes. *Cochrane Database of Systematic Reviews, 2.* Available from http://www.cochrane.org

Thorndike, A. N., Rigotti, N. A., Stafford, R. S., & Singer, D. E. (1998). National patterns in the treatment of smokers by physicians. *Journal of the American Medical Association, 279,* 604–608.

Tucker, M. A., Murray, N., Shaw, E. G., Ettinger, D. S., Mabry, M., Huber, M. H., et al. (1997). Second primary cancers related to smoking and treatment of small-cell lung cancer: Lung cancer working cadre. *Journal of the National Cancer Institute, 89,* 1782–1788.

Unrod, M., Cook, T., Myers, M. G., & Brown, S. A. (2004). Smoking cessation efforts among substance abusers with and without psychiatric comorbidity. *Addictive Behaviors, 29,* 1009–1013.

U.S. Department of Health, Education, and Welfare. (1964). *Smoking and health: Report of the Advisory Committee to the Surgeon General of the Public Health Service* (PHS Publication No. 1103). Washington, DC: Author.

U.S. Department of Health and Human Services. (2000). *Healthy people 2010: Conference edition* (Vols. 1 and 2). Washington, DC: Author.

Videtic, G. M., Stitt, L. W., Dar, A. R., Kocha, W. I., Tomiak, A. T., Truong, P. T., et al. (2003). Continued cigarette smoking by patients receiving concurrent chemoradiotherapy for limited-stage small-cell lung cancer is associated with decreased survival. *Journal of Clinical Oncology, 21,* 1544–1549.

Wetter, D. W., Kenford, S. L., Smith, S. S., Fiore, M. C., Jorenby, D. E., & Baker, T. B. (1999). Gender differences in smoking cessation. *Journal of Consulting Clinical Psychology, 67,* 555–562.

Yedidia, M. J., Gillespie, C. C., Kachur, E., Schwartz, M. D., Ockene, J., Chepaitis, A. E., et al. (2003). Effect of communications training on medical student performance. *Journal of the American Medical Association, 290,* 1157–1165.

Zapka, J., Goins, K. V., Pbert, L., & Ockene, J. K. (2004). Translating efficacy research to effectiveness studies in practice: Lessons from research to promote smoking cessation in community health centers. *Health Promotion Practice, 5,* 245–255.

11

INTERVENTIONS TO MODIFY DIETARY BEHAVIORS FOR CANCER PREVENTION AND CONTROL

MARCI KRAMISH CAMPBELL, JENNIFER GIERISCH,
AND LISA SUTHERLAND

A large body of evidence indicates that what people eat can influence cancer risk (World Cancer Research Fund [WCRF], 2007). On the basis of this evidence, a number of dietary changes have been recommended to reduce cancer risk (Riboli & Norat, 2003; WCRF, 2007). A more detailed discussion of the relationship between diet and cancer is presented in chapter 2 in this volume. Improvements in the nutritional behaviors of all Americans have been recommended, but recent data suggest that changes are occurring slowly, if at all. For example, data from the Behavioral Risk Factor Surveillance System (2005; as cited in Centers for Disease Control and Prevention, 2007) revealed that only 32.6% of adults ate at least two servings of fruits daily, and only 27.2% ate at least three servings of vegetables daily. The corresponding Healthy People 2010 (U.S. Department of Health and Human Services, 2000) goals are 75% and 50%. Clearly, nutrition interventions are necessary to affect these trends.

WHY IS DIETARY CHANGE DIFFICULT?

Eating habits and patterns are notoriously complex and difficult to change. Dietary patterns and food preferences are established in early childhood, and research suggests that parent feeding practices and restrictions may influence later body weight and ability to modify dietary consumption (Birch & Fisher, 1998). Among adults, studies indicate that a variety of factors may influence dietary habits. Understanding the psychosocial determinants of dietary behavior is an important step in the process. However, many studies (Baranowski, 2006; Fuemmeler et al., 2006) have found that these determinants account for a relatively small proportion of the variance in behavior. Changing eating habits is especially complex because it involves continuing the overall behavior (i.e., eating) while making multiple daily decisions in a variety of sub-behavioral domains and settings. More basic theoretical research is needed to better understand how and why people change their eating habits and how best to promote these changes.

WHAT INTERVENTIONS WORK?

Ammerman, Lindquist, Lorn, and Hersey (2002) examined characteristics and findings across dietary intervention studies to attempt to identify common factors that may be most efficacious. It is not surprising that interventions focused on high-risk populations in more intensive clinical settings tended to have larger effects compared with population-based programs with average-risk individuals. Unfortunately, because of the broad diversity of study populations, methods, and intervention approaches and the requirements for inclusion in an evidence review, few conclusions could be drawn regarding efficacy of specific intervention strategies. Two approaches that did appear efficacious from this review were the use of small groups and individual goal setting. Despite evidence that cancer disproportionately affects certain populations, relatively few dietary intervention studies have been designed for specific ethnic populations (Agency for Healthcare Research and Quality, 2000). Issues of cultural, ethnic, and socioeconomic diversity are key for the design and evaluation of effective interventions to improve diet and reduce health disparities.

A growing body of evidence shows that human–environment interactions are essential components of dietary practices and that a social–ecological approach may be effective in dietary and other health promotion interventions. The Institute of Medicine, therefore, has recommended the use of a socioecological model, which provides a framework for intervening at multiple levels of influence, including the individual, interpersonal, institutional, community, and policy levels, and using multiple approaches for improving public health (Smedley & Syme, 2000). Health promotion programs that take into account the complexity of health problems, which are influenced by multiple levels, are more difficult to conceptualize and implement but might be more likely to result in lasting behavior change. In addition, interventions that draw from multiple theories and those that target multiple behaviors, such as nutrition and physical activity, have been a focus of recent research (Orleans, 2005). In the following sections, we present a summary of recent strategies and programs that have approached dietary intervention from the standpoint of various levels of the socioecological model.

Individual-Level Strategies

Individual-level approaches generally involve provision of personalized information and advice, delivered by an expert to a patient or individual community member. The paradigm of individual dietary behavior change is the clinic-based one-to-one counseling session between a trained nutrition or medical professional and a patient at high risk for a nutrition-related medical condition. As noted previously, such intensive individualized approaches, focused on high-risk individuals, are most likely to achieve significant effects (Ammerman et al., 2002).

Intensive Counseling and Education

A number of recent examples of individual-level interventions have been effective in promoting adherence to dietary patterns aimed at lowering cancer and chronic disease risk. These studies have generally used self-reported dietary information from food frequency questionnaires, food records, and/or 24-hour food recalls, and some studies also have included biomarkers of dietary intake such as serum carotenoid levels (Women's Health Initiative Study Group, 2004). Similarly, the Polyp Prevention Trial aimed to achieve significant dietary changes among participants who were deemed at increased risk for colorectal cancer because of previous polyp removal (Lanza et al., 2001).

Advantages of intensive individualized approaches include the ability to attain high rates of adherence over time and to achieve significant dietary changes. Such approaches are most warranted in clinical trials designed to assess the impact of dietary change on disease endpoints or in medical nutrition therapy with individuals who have or are at increased risk for diet-related diseases such as diabetes. The high cost and burden of mounting and implementing such intensive interventions, however, make it unlikely that such programs could ever be provided to the general population. Less intensive individual dietary change approaches with potential for broad population-wide dissemination, such as computer-tailored materials and telephone counseling, have therefore been the focus of a number of cancer prevention and control studies.

Tailored Nutrition Messages

The term *tailoring* is used to describe interventions that vary according to individual-level characteristics. Tailored communications are assessment based and should include personalized information that is relevant to the identified psychosocial constructs, as well as providing behavioral feedback (Kreuter, Farrell, & Olevitch, 1999). Computer-based tailoring, in which theory-based messages address the unique needs, interests, and concerns identified by the recipient, has been demonstrated in past research to improve dietary behaviors such as lowering fat and increasing fruit and vegetable (F&V) consumption (Brug, Oenema, & Campbell, 2003; Kroeze, Werkman, & Brug, 2006). These studies have been conducted in various settings, primarily health care (e.g., primary care practices, health maintenance organizations) and workplaces. Findings have generally shown that tailored print materials outperformed nontailored information in terms of process (e.g., attention, recall, readership, perceived relevance) and outcome (e.g., fat intake) measures. However, Kreuter, Oswald, Bull, and Clark (2000) found that group-targeted weight loss materials performed as well as individually tailored information when there was a good match between participant characteristics and the group-level targeting variables.

Currently, tailoring research includes a continued focus on the effectiveness of tailored printed communications, as well as assessing the impact of tailoring through new media such as the Internet, CD-ROM, and automated telephone systems. Studies also are investigating the importance of theories and constructs, methods, and mediating steps to better understand the link between exposure to tailored information and subsequent behavior change (S. M. Miller et al., 2004). These studies are important because they can lead to more parsimonious and effective interventions that can be disseminated broadly for cancer control. Studies generally suggest that one reason for the greater impact of tailored materials is greater perception of personal relevance, leading to greater attention to and use of the information (Brug et al., 2003; Heimendinger et al., 2005). In addition, findings indicate that providing more tailored materials over time produces more dietary change than does providing only one dose of tailored information (Brug et al., 2003). Several studies are under way to assess the relative impact of tailoring print materials to culturally specific characteristics among African Americans, such as ethnic identity, as compared with tailoring to psychosocial and behavioral constructs (Kreuter et al., 2004, 2005).

Several recent studies have evaluated computer-based interactive nutrition education among low-income women (Campbell, Carbone, et al., 2004; Jantz, Anderson, & Gould, 2002; Sutherland et al., in press) and in a Dutch population (Oenema, Brug, & Lechner, 2001). These studies consistently found program effects on psychosocial determinants (e.g., self-efficacy, knowledge, intentions to change). However, little effect was found for dietary change (Campbell, Carbone, et al., 2004; Campbell, Honess, Farrell, Carbone, & Brasure, 1999). Some studies have found that Web-based interventions led to dietary changes as well as weight loss (Baranowski et al., 2003; Tate, Jackvony, & Wing, 2003, 2006; Tate, Wing, & Winett, 2001). Typically, greater effects are found when interventions involve multiple sessions over time and when education is combined with tailored feedback (Tate et al., 2003, 2006). Other new and existing technologies have shown promise for delivering tailored interventions. One example is that of using automated telephone systems, which have been shown to promote adherence in disease self-management (e.g., diet and medication adherence for the control of conditions such as diabetes and hypercholesterolemia; Delichatsios et al., 2001; Friedman, 1998). One potential advantage of using the telephone as the delivery medium is its wide availability and familiarity as compared with the use of computers and high-speed Internet. This may be especially important among older, lower income, and minority populations.

Motivational Interviewing

A potential limitation of tailored interventions such as those previously described is that they are expert-based systems that use predetermined survey questions and feedback texts or scripts to provide feedback to participants. In such systems, assumptions are necessarily made about the best advice or information for a given person with a certain set of characteristics, and the participant has little opportunity to set the agenda or correct those assumptions. One alternative approach to behavior change interventions is motivational interviewing (MI), a counseling approach originally developed by W. R. Miller and Rollnick (2002) for dealing with addictive behaviors. MI first assesses each participant's readiness for and interest in engaging in change and then supports change at the level for which the participant is ready, encouraging open communication and future change if possible. It has been applied to brief interventions focused on chronic disease prevention and management, including programs to increase F&V intake, physical activity, cancer screening, and other lifestyle changes (W. R. Miller & Rollnick, 2002). MI integrates concepts from a variety of theories and counseling methods, including the transtheoretical model of Prochaska, DiClemente, and Norcross (1992), cognitive behavior therapy, and self-determination theory (Deci & Ryan, 1987; W. R. Miller & Rollnick, 2002). Growing evidence indicates that MI can help achieve dietary changes for cancer prevention and control (Resnicow et al., 2001).

Interpersonal and Social Network Interventions

Many studies point to the importance of social ties in influencing health behavior and suggest that intervention strategies that use social networks, family, friends, and churches can be an effective way to increase use of cancer prevention and control strategies. Building on existing social relationships with family members and others is one important strategy for promoting and sustaining dietary change. Intervention studies focused on childhood obesity prevention, for example, consistently suggest that at least one parent should be involved in any intervention (Golan, Weizman, Apter, & Fainaru, 1998). A systematic review of family involvement in weight-related interventions for adults and children found that interventions that included family members were more effective than those that focused only on the overweight individual (McLean, Griffin, Toney, & Hardeman, 2003).

Interventions that build on the social support functions of people's social networks may be especially important for minority women and for other individuals whose socioeconomic and/or cultural characteristics cause them to rely more heavily on others in their social environment (Tessaro, Eng, & Smith, 1994). Several studies have developed and evaluated dietary interventions based on social support models (Buller et al., 1999; Campbell, Demark-Wahnefried, et al., 1999; Haire-Joshu et al., 2003; Havas, Anliker, Damron, Feldman, & Langenberg, 2000; Tessaro et al., 2000).

Although social support may foster improved diet, the circumstances and mechanisms by which this influence may occur are not well understood (Kelsey et al., 1996; Thrasher, Campbell, Oates, Hudson, & Jackson, 2004). Resnicow et al. (2004) found that a possible mechanism of social influence is its effect on one's motivation to change. This study used social support to improve dietary behaviors. Examination of this study's secondary outcomes revealed an increase in both intrinsic and extrinsic motivation in the intervention group. On the basis of self-determination theory, increasing intrinsic motivation for change (e.g., feelings that one is responsible for, and able to improve, one's own health) would be a desirable outcome (Ryan & Deci, 2000). Another issue in social support that has not received much research attention is the potential adverse effect of binding ties that burden people and therefore might interfere with dietary change opportunity (Fiori, Antonucci, & Cortina, 2006). Such mechanistic areas need research attention.

Organizational Interventions and Settings

Dietary interventions for cancer and chronic disease prevention have been conducted in a variety of settings and contexts, including homes, schools, workplaces, religious organizations, health care provider offices, and public housing communities. Organizational settings provide a number of advantages for dietary change interventions, including access to participants, social and peer support, common communication and intervention delivery methods (e.g., paycheck stuffers, church bulletins), facilities such as cafeterias and gyms, management or leadership support (e.g., from pastors, teachers, or business owners), and potential for policy and environmental changes that may sustain the intervention over time. Most successful interventions within organizations have had multiple components (Reynolds et al., 2000). Such multicomponent programs are often expensive, and identifying the key elements that are essential for changing behavior may be difficult. These efficacy studies usually test interventions under researcher-controlled conditions to prove that change is possible. Careful process evaluation data can help to tease out the question of what worked, but subsequent effectiveness studies may also be necessary before programs can be disseminated under real-world conditions (Glasgow, Lichtenstein, & Marcus, 2003).

Schools

Because poor eating habits that originate in childhood usually track into adulthood, dietary interventions with children and youth are extremely important for cancer and chronic disease prevention (Nicklas, Arbeit, & Berenson, 1991). Advantages of school-based programs include access to the high proportion (95%) of children enrolled in school, access to school-based environmental resources such as cafeterias and gyms, the possibility of improving access to healthy options in these settings, opportunities for repeated contact with children over time for program implementation and data collection, and the mandate of most public school systems to offer health education as part of the curriculum. However, difficulties abound when working with schools. Many school systems restrict or closely regulate research access to schools, parental consent as well as child assent must be obtained, and there are many competing demands for time and priorities in the school day. In addition, school-based programs may modify children's dietary behaviors while they are in school but may have little or no impact on eating patterns outside of school. Obtaining parental and family participation and involvement can potentially multiply the effects of school-based interventions to change the home environment; however, it can be difficult to achieve such involvement (Reynolds, Baranowski, Bishop, Gregson, & Nicklas, 2001). Assessment of child diet is challenging as well, because dietary and psychosocial instruments may have lower validity when used with children (Baranowski, 2006; Baranowski et al., 1997).

A number of school-based dietary change studies have been successfully implemented among various populations of children, including elementary and middle-school age groups, and among a variety of ethnic groups (Caballero et al., 2003; Hoelscher et al., 2004; Lytle et al., 1996; Nader et al., 1999; Parcel et al., 2003; Perry et al., 1990; Reynolds et al., 2000, 2001). These studies have generally been rigorously conducted randomized trials that included a classroom curriculum component, school food service changes, and other out-of-school activities at home or in the community. Findings have generally shown positive changes in self-reported fat intake and nutrition knowledge among children. However, changes in objective measures such as body mass index or lipids have not been observed. A review by French and Stables (2003) examined studies that included interventions to change the school food environment and found that environment-only interventions targeting food choices at school have been effective for increasing F&V consumption among students. A more recent review of three additional studies found similar results (French, 2005).

Workplaces

Workplaces provide an important community setting for reaching adults with behavioral interventions. It is surprising that only a few randomized trials of dietary change through workplace interventions have been conducted, despite observation of consistent effects on intervention worksites (Beresford, Shannon, McLerran, & Thompson, 2000; Buller, Hunt, Sorensen, & Beresford, 2001; Patterson et al., 1997; Sorensen et al., 1999). Common themes derived from these workplace projects include the need for a multilevel strategy combining individual and environmental strategies, as well as the importance of social support from family and coworkers to promote dietary change (Buller et al., 2001).

Few worksite studies have specifically focused on lower income and minority workers, many of whom are employed in blue-collar occupations in small worksites that often lack resources such as cafeterias or fitness facilities. One intervention that specifically targeted blue-collar women for dietary change is Health Works for Women (Campbell et al., 2002). Using a combination of tailored print newsletters and a social support and natural helpers program delivered outside of work time, this program achieved significant improvement in F&V and fat intake. A subsequent study is examining whether the addition of more participatory strategies such as employee wellness committees and community advisory boards can enhance intervention effectiveness. Similar participatory approaches in another rural worksite resulted in significant increases in F&V consumption, self-efficacy for dietary change, as well as changes in social norms around dietary change (Fries, Ripley, Figueiredo, & Thompson, 1999).

Religious Organizations

Over the past 20 years, numerous health promotion and disease prevention research programs have been conducted through Black churches, with positive impact (Campbell, Demark-Wahnefried, et al., 1999; Campbell et al., 2007; Resnicow et al., 2001). The most successful interventions have formed partnerships with churches and have incorporated spiritual and cultural factors into interventions (Agency for Healthcare Research and Quality, 2000; Baskin, Resnicow, & Campbell, 2001). More recently, the National Cancer Institute (NCI) and American Cancer Society have adapted the essential elements of two community-based trials into a dissemination-ready program called Body and Soul. An effectiveness evaluation of Body and Soul, implemented primarily by church volunteers, showed significant improvement in F&V consumption, lower fat intake, and changes in psychosocial mediators

(Campbell et al., 2007; Fuemmeler et al., 2006; Resnicow et al., 2004). NCI is now offering Body and Soul to churches nationwide through a Web site (http://www.bodyandsoul.nih.gov) and the Cancer Information Service (1-800-4CANCER).

Recent research on faith-based dietary interventions has focused on several issues: expanding successful church-based programs to include multiple behaviors, dismantling multicomponent so-called kitchen-sink interventions to examine which components account for more effects, and reaching broader groups of religious organizations (Campbell, James, et al., 2004). Bowen et al. (2004) adapted dietary intervention strategies that had been tested in other settings (e.g., health maintenance organizations, workplaces) and designed a program called Eating for a Healthy Life that has been evaluated in a variety of religious organizations, including churches and synagogues. Faith-based dietary interventions have tremendous potential and will likely be the focus of future research. Several potential drawbacks exist, however, such as reaching only the population that attends religious organizations, which may be the population at lesser risk for a particular health problem. In addition, concerns about separation of church and state exist for both researchers and church leaders, especially when projects are federally funded (Campbell et al., 2007).

Environmental and Policy-Level Interventions

Environmental and policy interventions are important elements of a multilevel approach to dietary behavior change. Environmental nutrition interventions impact dietary behavior through access, availability, incentives, or information about foods at the point of purchase (Seymour, Yaroch, Serdula, Blanck, & Khan, 2004). Policy interventions promote change through the intentional enactment of legislation or rules that will impact the nutrition environment. In terms of environmental strategies, evidence suggests that changing availability and pricing of healthy foods in organizational and community settings such as those previously described can lead to dietary change (French & Stables, 2003). On the basis of experience from the antitobacco initiatives of the past 20 years, however, many experts believe that change will require broader and more controversial policy-level interventions such as restrictive food taxation (Nestle & Jacobson, 2000; Vanchieri, 1998).

Restrictive Food Taxation

Implementing restrictive taxes, or a "sin tax," on selected food items has been suggested as a viable mechanism to decrease individual consumption of low nutritional-value foods (Jacobson & Brownell, 2000; Nestle, 2003). Unlike tobacco taxes, which were implemented to decrease smoking, state budgetary shortfalls have been the primary impetus for implementing restrictive taxes on foods such as snack items and items high in sugar or fat. According to the State Tax Handbook (Commerce Clearing House, 2003) and the Center on Budget and Policy Priorities (Johnson, 2001), 13 states, including Maine, Ohio, Maryland, Oregon, and California, as well as the District of Columbia, have implemented and later repealed restrictive food taxes. In 1992, California voters repealed a sales tax on snack food and outlawed all future attempts to restrictively tax food. Reasons for tax failures have included difficulty with administration, the arbitrary nature of foods included, retailer and consumer confusion, limitation of consumer free choice, and disproportionate effect on households with low incomes. To date, no state has such taxes in place.

Controversy over what foods should be classified as "good" or "bad" for purposes of taxation has been at the center of the restrictive tax debate. For example, potato chips would likely be taxed because of high fat content, but Brie cheese would not. In 1991, the Maine legislature enacted a tax on "snack foods." The system taxed frozen baked apple pies but not fresh pies, and taxed blueberry muffins but not English muffins. In 2000, the law was repealed because of consumer confusion and disapproval, and retailer lack of compliance. The American Dietetic Association (2002) has declined to take a position on "good food, bad food" and instead advocates that all foods fit into a diet as long as moderation is exercised.

Although significant data support the financial benefit of these taxes, no scientific evidence exists to suggest that restrictive taxes impact food consumption. Jacobson and Brownell (2000) estimated that a 5% restrictive tax should result in a 2% decline in sales. However, U.S. food consumption data have not demonstrated that this is the case (Putnam, 2000). Although the jury is still out as to whether restrictive taxation will benefit consumer health, evidence indicates that manipulation of food and beverage pricing may hold promising results on the impact of improved dietary behavior.

Food Pricing

In the United States, as in other developed countries, household income is not associated with total food consumed but does influence the types of foods purchased. For example, as income increases, the proportion of income spent on at-home food decreases (Meade & Rosen, 1996). In addition, nations such as the United States that spend the most money on food receive the most dietary energy from foods high in added fats and sugars (Drewnoski, 2003).

Numerous studies have reported that price manipulation can achieve changes in dietary consumption patterns (French, 2003, 2005). For example, French, Jeffery, et al. (2001) and French and Stables (2003) found that favorable pricing and promotion strategies increased sales of low-fat packaged snacks from vending machines in worksites and high schools. Horgen and Brownell (2002) compared price changes and health messages in promoting healthy food selection and found effects from decreasing the price alone, with no additional effect from providing healthful messages. In addition to focusing on value and low cost of low-fat food items, however, taste, availability, and point-of-purchase labeling must also be addressed to promote healthier food choices (Shannon, Story, Fulkerson, & French, 2002).

Manipulating food prices (e.g., decreasing prices of fruits and vegetables and increasing the price of high-fat and high-sugar foods) has the potential to change dietary intake (Mhurchu, Blakely, Wall, Rodgers, & Jiang, 2007). However, it is important to point out that most studies to date have been limited to specific settings and target audiences. Further research should examine the population-wide impact of food pricing interventions, the impact on low socioeconomic groups, and the economic impact that price incentives may have on agriculture and commercial food companies (Drewnoski, 2003).

Regulating Food and Beverage Advertising

Television viewing by children has increased dramatically since the 1970s. During this same time, significant increases have been documented in snacking behavior (Francis, Lee, & Birch, 2003), physical inactivity (Eisenmann, Bartee, & Wang, 2002), and requests for nonnutritious foods (Clancy-Hepburn, Hickey, & Nevill, 1974). One study concluded that children who consumed fast food frequently also watched more television than other children (French, Jeffrey, et al., 2001). Increased television watching has also been associated with higher intakes of high-fat, sweet, and salty snacks (Coon, Goldberg, Rogers, & Tucker, 2001). Because television watching has been cited as a major factor contributing to decreased physical activity, increased snacking behavior, decreased F&V intake, increased energy intake, and overweight and obesity (Francis et al., 2003; Gortmaker et al., 1996), federal policies that would restrict or ban junk food advertisements during children's programming in the United States have been proposed.

Estimates of the percentage of U.S. households with television include 98.2% (Television Bureau of Advertising, 2007) and 99% (Herr, 2007), and most households have cable. It is estimated that U.S. adults and children are exposed to approximately 90 and 230 minutes of advertising per week, respectively (American Academy of Pediatrics, Committee on Public Education, 2001; French, Story, Neumark-Sztainer, Fulkerson, & Hannan, 2001). Studies report 45% to 91% of foods advertised during peak viewing hours for children are high in fat, sugar, and/or salt (Taras & Gage, 1995). Since 1972, the majority of foods advertised during Saturday morning children's television programming are high in sugar and fat (Gamble & Cotugna, 1999; Gussow, 1972). Commercials for convenience foods have tripled from 9% to 27%, and ads for snack foods have increased 30%. The findings are similar when advertising is examined during weekday peak children's programming hours (Taras & Gage, 1995). The major studies that have examined food advertising content have found that less than 5% of television commercials are for foods that promote a balanced diet, such as fruits, milk, vegetables, and cheese (Gamble & Cotugna, 1999).

Although limiting the advertising of specific food products in the United States is not likely in the foreseeable future, possible policy-level strategies could include increasing funding for public health campaigns and requiring television networks to set aside an allotment of minutes for healthy-food commercials. It may also be beneficial to restrict the advertising and marketing of unhealthful food items in controlled settings, such as schools and other environments oriented toward children. Schools could pass policies to incorporate mass media education, increase nutrition education, and mandate that physical education be a regular part of the curriculum. Such changes are examples of policy-level initiatives that could have a direct impact on individual behavior.

CONCLUSIONS AND NEXT STEPS

Healthy eating patterns and prevention of obesity will continue to be a major focus of future cancer and chronic disease prevention and control research. A strong body of evidence indicates that well-designed, theory-based dietary interventions can achieve behavior changes. Many questions remain, however, in terms of how to optimize such interventions for greatest efficacy and cost-effectiveness in different population groups with differing levels of disease risk. In addition, rather than looking for one magic-bullet intervention to be most efficacious, studies should examine possible combinations or interactive effects of low- to moderate-intensity interventions at various levels of change (e.g., through print, Internet, cell phones, and other interpersonal communications, as well as organizational and environmental changes) that can be delivered population-wide at reasonable cost. More research regarding optimal intervention types, doses, and timing (i.e., windows of opportunity) is needed to increase effectiveness with diverse populations.

Future research also should focus more attention on psychosocial factors and theoretical frameworks that may mediate the process of dietary change, to develop more efficient and effective interventions (Baranowski, Cullen, & Baranowski, 1999). Theory and methods development research also is urgently needed to better understand basic communication and processing of nutrition information and to improve measurement of nutrition-related behaviors and psychosocial mediators. Another important area for future research is the sustainability of dietary change. Although cancer risk most likely develops over many years, most studies have not followed participants for more than 1 or 2 years to assess long-term maintenance. Many aspects should be considered when developing interventions for dietary change that are sustainable over time. One primary issue is to involve the community in a participatory process from the outset, so that communities feel ownership of the project and a commitment to its sustainability (George, Daniel, & Green, 2007; George, Green, & Daniel, 1996). Research is needed to determine whether different behavioral theories are more useful for understanding long-term maintenance versus shorter term initiation of dietary change. Cost-effectiveness analyses and policy-based research also will be important for maintenance and dissemination of successful interventions, to convince stakeholders and legislators that investment in dietary change pays off over time in terms of reduced burden of illness and health care costs and improved quality of life.

REFERENCES

Agency for Healthcare Research and Quality. (2000). *Efficacy of interventions to modify dietary behavior related to cancer risk: Summary* (Evidence Report/Technology Assessment No. 25). Rockville, MD: Author.

American Academy of Pediatrics, Committee on Public Education. (2001). Children, adolescents, and television. *Pediatrics, 107,* 423–426.

American Dietetic Association. (2002). Position of the American Dietetic Association: Total diet approach to communicating food and nutrition information. *Journal of the American Dietetic Association, 102,* 100–108.

Ammerman, A., Lindquist, C. H., Lorn, K., & Hersey, J. (2002). The efficacy of behavioral interventions to modify dietary fat and fruit and vegetable intake: A review of the evidence. *Preventive Medicine, 35,* 25–41.

Baranowski, T. (2006). Advances in basic behavioral research will make the most important contributions to effective dietary change programs at this time. *Journal of the American Dietetic Association, 106,* 808–811.

Baranowski, T., Baranowski, J., Cullen, K. W., Marsh, T., Islam, N., Zakeri, I., et al. (2003). Squire's Quest! Dietary outcome evaluation of a multimedia game. *American Journal of Preventive Medicine, 24,* 52–61.

Baranowski, T., Cullen, K. W., & Baranowski, J. (1999). Psychosocial correlates of dietary intake: Advancing dietary intervention. *Annual Review of Nutrition, 19,* 17–40.

Baranowski, T., Smith, M., Baranowski, J., Wang, D. T., Doyle, C., Lin, L. S., et al. (1997). Low validity of a seven-item fruit and vegetable food frequency questionnaire among third-grade students. *Journal of the American Dietetic Association, 97,* 66–68.

Baskin, M. L., Resnicow, K., & Campbell, M. K. (2001). Conducting health interventions in Black churches: A model for building effective partnerships. *Ethnicity & Disease, 11,* 823–833.

Beresford, S. A., Shannon, J., McLerran, D., & Thompson, B. (2000). Seattle 5-a-Day Work-Site Project: Process evaluation. *Health Education & Behavior, 27,* 213–222.

Birch, L. L., & Fisher, J. O. (1998). Development of eating behaviors among children and adolescents. *Pediatrics, 101*(3, Pt. 2), 539–549.

Bowen, D. J., Beresford, S. A., Vu, T., Feng, Z., Tinker, L., Hart, A., Jr., et al. (2004). Baseline data and design for a randomized intervention study of dietary change in religious organizations. *Preventive Medicine, 39*, 602–611.

Brug, H., Oenema, A., & Campbell, M. K. (2003). The past, the present, and the future of computer-tailored nutrition education. *American Journal of Clinical Nutrition, 77*(Suppl. 4), 1028–1034.

Buller, D. B., Hunt, M. K., Sorensen, G., & Beresford, S. (2001). The 5 a Day Worksite Program. In *5 a Day for Better Health Program* (Monograph). Washington, DC: National Cancer Institute.

Buller, D. B., Morrill, C., Taren, D., Aickin, M., Sennott-Miller, L., Buller, M. K., et al. (1999). Randomized trial testing the effect of peer education at increasing fruit and vegetable intake. *Journal of the National Cancer Institute, 91*, 1491–1500.

Caballero, B., Clay, T., Davis, S. M., Ethelbah, B., Rock, B. H., Lohman, T., et al. (2003). Pathways: A school-based, randomized controlled trial for the prevention of obesity in American Indian schoolchildren. *American Journal of Clinical Nutrition, 78*, 1030–1038.

Campbell, M. K., Carbone, E., Honess-Morreale, L., Heisler-Mackinnon, J., Farrell, D., & Demissie, S. (2004). Randomized trial of a tailored nutrition education CD-ROM program for women receiving food assistance. *Journal of Nutrition Education and Behavior, 36*, 58–66.

Campbell, M. K., Demark-Wahnefried, W., Symons, M., Kalsbeek, W. D., Dodds, J., et al. (1999). Fruit and vegetable consumption and prevention of cancer: The Black Churches United for Better Health project. *American Journal of Public Health, 89*, 1390–1396.

Campbell, M. K., Honess, L., Farrell, D., Carbone, E., & Brasure, M. (1999). Effects of a tailored multimedia nutrition education program for low-income women receiving food assistance. *Health Education Research, 14*, 246–256.

Campbell, M. K., Hudson, M. A., Resnicow, K., Blakeney, N., Paxton, A., & Baskin, M. (2007). Church-based health promotion interventions: Evidence and lessons learned. *Annual Review of Public Health, 28*, 213–234.

Campbell, M. K., James, A., Hudson, M., Haughton, L., Jackson, E., Farrell, D., et al. (2004). Improving multiple behaviors for colorectal cancer prevention among rural African American church members. *Health Psychology, 23*, 492–502.

Campbell, M. K., Tessaro, I., DeVellis, B., Benedict, S., Kelsey, K., Belton, L., & Sanhueza, A. (2002). Effects of a tailored health promotion program for female blue-collar workers: Health Works for Women. *Preventive Medicine, 34*, 313–323.

Centers for Disease Control and Prevention. (2007). Fruit and vegetable consumption among adults [Electronic version]. *Mortality and Morbidity Weekly Report, 56*, 213–217.

Clancy-Hepburn, K., Hickey, A. A., & Nevill, G. (1974). Children's behavior responses to TV food advertisements. *Journal of Nutrition Education, 6*, 93–96.

Commerce Clearing House. (Eds.). (2003). *State tax handbook*. Chicago: Author.

Coon, K. A., Goldberg, J., Rogers, B. L., & Tucker, K. L. (2001). Relationship between use of television during meals and children's food consumption patterns. *Pediatrics, 107,* 1–9.

Deci, E. L., & Ryan, R. M. (1987). The support of autonomy and the control of behavior. *Journal of Personality and Social Psychology, 53,* 1024–1037.

Delichatsios, H. K., Friedman, R. H., Glanz, K., Tennstedt, S., Smigelski, C., Pinto, B. M., et al. (2001). Randomized trial of a "talking computer" to improve adults' eating habits. *American Journal of Health Promotion, 15,* 215–224.

Drewnoski, A. (2003). Fat and sugar: An economic analysis. *Journal of Nutrition, 133*(Suppl.), 838–840.

Eisenmann, J. C., Bartee, R. T., & Wang, M. Q. (2002). Physical activity, TV viewing, and weight in U.S. youth: 1999 Youth Risk Behavior Survey. *Obesity Research, 10,* 379–385.

Fiori, K. L., Antonucci, T. C., & Cortina, K. S. (2006). Social network typologies and mental health among older adults. *The Journals of Gerontology: Series B. Psychological Sciences and Social Sciences, 61,* 25–32.

Francis, L. A., Lee, Y., & Birch, L. L. (2003). Parental weight status and girls' television viewing, snacking, and body mass indexes. *Obesity Research, 11,* 143–151.

French, S. A. (2003). Pricing effects on food choices. *Journal of Nutrition, 133,* 841–843.

French, S. A. (2005). Public health strategies for dietary change: Schools and workplaces. *Journal of Nutrition, 135,* 910–912.

French, S. A., Jeffery, R. W., Story, M., Breitlow, K. K., Baxter, J. S., Hannan, P., & Snyder, M. P. (2001). Pricing and promotion effects on low-fat vending snack purchases: The CHIPS Study. *American Journal of Public Health, 91,* 112–117.

French, S. A., & Stables, G. (2003). Environmental interventions to promote vegetable and fruit consumption among youth in school settings. *Preventive Medicine, 37,* 593–610.

French, S. A., Story, M., Neumark-Sztainer, D., Fulkerson, J., & Hannan, P. (2001). Fast food restaurant use among adolescents: Associations with nutrient intake, food choices, and behavioral and psychosocial variables. *International Journal of Obesity, 25,* 1823–1833.

Friedman, R. H. (1998). Automated telephone conversations to assess health behavior and deliver behavioral interventions. *Journal of Medical Systems, 2,* 95–102.

Fries, E. A., Ripley, J. S., Figueiredo, M. I., & Thompson, B. (1999). Can community organization strategies be used to implement smoking and dietary changes in a rural manufacturing worksite? *Journal of Rural Health, 15,* 413–420.

Fuemmeler, B. F., Masse, L. C., Yaroch, A. L., Resnicow, K., Campbell, M. K., Carr, C. et al. (2006). Psychosocial mediation of fruit and vegetable consumption in the Body and Soul effectiveness trial. *Health Psychology, 25,* 474–483.

Gamble, M., & Cotugna, N. (1999). A quarter century of TV food advertising targeted at children. *American Journal of Health Behavior, 23,* 261–268.

George, M. A., Daniel, M., & Green, L. W. (2007). Appraising and funding partici-patory research in health promotion. *International Quarterly of Community Health Education, 26,* 171–187.

George, M. A., Green, L. W., & Daniel, M. (1996). Evolution and implications of participatory action research for public health. *Health Promotion and Education, 3,* 6–10.

Glasgow, R. E., Lichtenstein, E., & Marcus, A. C. (2003). Why don't we see more translation of health promotion research to practice? Rethinking the efficacy-to-effectiveness transition. *American Journal of Public Health, 93,* 1261–1267.

Golan, M., Weizman, A., Apter, A., & Fainaru, M. (1998). Parents as the exclusive agents of change in the treatment of childhood obesity. *American Journal of Clinical Nutrition, 67,* 1130–1135.

Gortmaker, S. L., Must, A., Sobol, A. M., Peterson, K., Colditz, G. A., & Dietz, W. H. (1996). Television viewing as a cause of increasing obesity among children in the United States, 1986–1990. *Archives of Pediatric Adolescent Medicine, 150,* 356–362.

Gussow, J. (1972). Counternutritional messages of TV ads aimed at children. *Journal of Nutrition Education, 4,* 48–52.

Haire-Joshu, D., Brownson, R. C., Nanney, M. S., Houston, C., Steger-May, K., Schechtman, K., & Auslander, W. (2003). Improving dietary behavior in African Americans: The Parents as Teachers High 5, Low Fat Program. *Preventive Medicine, 36,* 684–691.

Havas, S., Anliker, J., Damron, D., Feldman, R., & Langenberg, P. (2000). Uses of process evaluation in the Maryland WIC 5-a-day promotion program. *Health Education & Behavior, 27,* 254–263.

Heimendinger, J., O'Neill, C., Marcus, A. C., Wolfe, P., Julesburg, K., Morra, M., et al. (2005). Multiple tailored messages are effective in increasing fruit and vegetable consumption among callers to the Cancer Information Service. *Journal of Health Communication, 10*(Suppl. 1), 65–82.

Herr, N. (2007). *Television & health.* Retrieved February 5, 2008, from http://www.csun.edu/science/health/docs/tv&health.html

Hoelscher, D. M., Feldman, H. A., Johnson, C. C., Lytle, L. A., Osganian, S. K., Parcel, G. S., et al. (2004). School-based health education programs can be maintained over time: Results from the CATCH Institutionalization study. *Preventive Medicine, 38,* 594–606.

Horgen, K. B., & Brownell, K. D. (2002). Comparison of price change and health message interventions promoting health food choices. *Health Psychology, 21,* 505–512.

Jacobson, M. F., & Brownell, K. D. (2000). Small taxes on soft drinks and snack foods to promote health. *American Journal of Public Health, 90,* 854–857.

Jantz, C., Anderson, J., & Gould, S. M. (2002). Using computer-based assessments to evaluate interactive multimedia nutrition education among low-income pre-dominantly Hispanic participants. *Journal of Nutritional Education and Behavior, 34,* 252–260.

Johnson, N. (2001). *Which states tax the sale of food for home consumption in 2001?* Washington, DC: Center on Budget and Policy Priorities.

Kelsey, K. S., Kirkley, B. G., DeVellis, R. F., Earp, J. A., Ammerman, A. S., Keyserling, T. C., et al. (1996). Social support as a predictor of dietary change in a low-income population. *Health Education Research: Theory & Practice, 11,* 383–395.

Kreuter, M. W., Farrell, D., & Olevitch, L. (Eds.). (1999). *Tailored health messages: Customizing communication with computer technology.* Hillsdale, NJ: Erlbaum.

Kreuter, M. W., Oswald, D. L., Bull, F. C., & Clark, E. M. (2000). Are tailored health education materials always more effective than nontailored materials? *Health Education Research: Theory & Practice, 15,* 305–315.

Kreuter, M. W., Skinner, C. S., Steger-May, K., Holt, C. L., Bucholtz, D. C., Clark, E. M., & Haire-Joshu, D. (2004). Responses to behaviorally vs. culturally tailored cancer communication among African American women. *American Journal of Health Behavior, 28,* 195–207.

Kreuter, M. W., Sugg-Skinner, C., Holt, C. L., Clark, E. M., Haire-Joshu, D., Fu, Q., et al. (2005). Cultural tailoring for mammography and fruit and vegetable intake among low-income African-American women in urban public health centers. *Preventive Medicine, 41,* 53–62.

Kroeze, W., Werkman, A., & Brug, J. (2006). A systematic review of randomized trials on the effectiveness of computer-tailored education on physical activity and dietary behaviors. *Annals of Behavioral Medicine, 31,* 205–223.

Lanza, E., Schatzkin, A., Daston, C., Corle, D., Freedman, L., Ballard-Barbash, R., et al. (2001). Implementation of a 4-y, high-fiber, high-fruit-and-vegetable, low-fat dietary intervention: Results of dietary changes in the Polyp Prevention Trial. *American Journal of Clinical Nutrition, 74,* 387–401.

Lytle, L. A., Stone, E. J., Nichaman, M. Z., Perry, C. L., Montgomery, D. H., Nicklas, T. A., et al. (1996). Changes in nutrient intakes of elementary school children following a school-based intervention: Results from the CATCH Study. *Preventive Medicine, 25,* 465–477.

McLean, N., Griffin, S., Toney, K., & Hardeman, W. (2003). Family involvement in weight control, weight maintenance, and weight-loss interventions: A systematic review of randomised trials. *International Journal of Obesity and Related Metabolic Disorders, 27,* 987–1005.

Meade, B., & Rosen, S. (1996). Income and diet differences greatly affect food spending around the globe. *Critical Reviews in Food Science and Nutrition, 4,* 39–44.

Mhurchu, N. C., Blakely, T., Wall, J., Rodgers, A., & Jiang, Y. (2007). Strategies to promote healthier food purchases: A pilot supermarket intervention study. *Public Health Nutrition, 10,* 608–615.

Miller, S. M., Bowen, D. J., Campbell, M. K., Diefenbach, M. A., Gritz, E. R., Jacobsen, P. B., et al. (2004). Current research promises and challenges in behavioral oncology: Report from the American Society of Preventive Oncology Annual Meeting. *Cancer Epidemiology, Biomarkers & Prevention, 13,* 171–180.

Miller, W. R., & Rollnick, S. (2002). *Motivational interviewing: Preparing people for change* (2nd ed.). New York: Guilford Press.

Nader, P. R., Stone, E. J., Lytle, L. A., Perry, C. L., Osganian, S. K., Kelder, S., et al. (1999). Three-year maintenance of improved diet and physical activity: The CATCH cohort. Child and Adolescent Trial for Cardiovascular Health. *Archives of Pediatric and Adolescent Medicine, 153,* 695–704.

Nestle M. (2003, February 7). The ironic politics of obesity. *Science, 299,* 781.

Nestle, M., & Jacobson, M. F. (2000). Halting the obesity epidemic: A public health policy approach. *Public Health Reports, 115,* 12–24.

Nicklas, T. A., Arbeit, M. L., & Berenson, G. S. (1991). Dietary studies in children: Cardiovascular disease prevention. The Bogalusa Heart Study. *Comprehensive Therapy, 17,* 8–15.

Oenema, A., Brug, J., & Lechner, L. (2001). Web-based tailored nutrition education: Results of a randomized controlled trial. *Health Education Research, 16,* 647–660.

Orleans, C. T. (2005). The behavior change consortium: Expanding the boundaries and impact of health behavior change research. *Annals of Behavioral Medicine, 29*(Suppl.), 76–79.

Parcel, G. S., Perry, C. L., Kelder, S. H., Elder, J. P., Mitchell, P. D., Lytle, L. A., et al. (2003). School climate and the institutionalization of the CATCH program. *Health Education & Behavior, 30,* 489–502.

Patterson, R. E., Kristal, A. R., Glanz, K., McLerran, D. F., Hebert, J. R., Heimendinger, J., et al. (1997). Components of the Working Well trial intervention associated with adoption of healthful diets. *American Journal of Preventive Medicine, 13,* 271–276.

Perry, C. L., Stone, E. J., Parcel, G. S., Ellison, R. C., Nader, P. R., Webber, L. S., & Luepker, R. V. (1990). School-based cardiovascular health promotion: The Child and Adolescent Trial for Cardiovascular Health (CATCH). *Journal of School Health, 60,* 406–413.

Prochaska, J., DiClemente, C., & Norcross, J. (1992). In search of how people change: Applications to addictive behaviors. *American Psychologist, 47,* 1102–1114.

Putnam, J. (2000). Major trends in the U.S. food supply. *Critical Reviews in Food Science and Nutrition, 23,* 8–15.

Resnicow, K., Campbell, M. K., Carr, C., McCarty, F., Wang, T., Periasamy, S., et al. (2004). Body and soul: A dietary intervention conducted through African American churches. *American Journal of Preventive Medicine, 27,* 97–105.

Resnicow, K., Jackson, A., Wang, T., De, A. K., McCarty, F., Dudley, W. N., & Baranowski, T. (2001). A motivational interviewing intervention to increase fruit and vegetable intake through Black churches: Results of the Eat for Life trial. *American Journal of Public Health, 91,* 1686–1693.

Reynolds, K. D., Baranowski, T., Bishop, D., Gregson, J., & Nicklas, T. (2001). 5 A Day behavior change research in children and adolescents. In *5 a Day for Better Health Program* (Monograph). Washington, DC: National Cancer Institute.

Reynolds, K. D., Franklin, F. A., Binkley, D., Raczynski, J. M., Harrington, K. F., Kirk, K. A., & Person, S. (2000). Increasing the fruit and vegetable consumption of fourth graders: Results from the High 5 Project. *Preventive Medicine, 30*, 309–319.

Riboli, E., & Norat, T. (2003). Epidemiologic evidence of the protective effect of fruit and vegetables on cancer risk. *American Journal of Clinical Nutrition, 78*(Suppl. 3), 559–569.

Ryan, R. M., & Deci, E. L. (2000). Self-determination theory and the facilitation of intrinsic motivation, social development and well-being. *American Psychologist, 55*, 68–78.

Seymour, J. D., Yaroch, A. L., Serdula, M., Blanck, H. M., & Khan, L. K. (2004). Impact of nutritional environmental interventions on point-of-purchase behavior in adults: A review. *Preventive Medicine, 39*, 108–136.

Shannon, C., Story, M., Fulkerson, J. A., & French, S. A. (2002). Factors in the school cafeteria influencing food choices by high school students. *Journal of School Health, 72*, 229–234.

Smedley, B. D., & Syme, S. L. (2000). *Promoting health: Intervention strategies from social and behavioral research*. Washington, DC: National Academy Press.

Sorensen, G., Stoddard, A., Peterson, K., Cohen, N., Hunt, M. K., Stein, E., et al. (1999). Increasing fruit and vegetable consumption through worksites and families in the TreatWell 5-a-Day study. *American Journal of Public Health, 89*, 54–60.

Sutherland, L., Campbell, M. K., Haines, P., Wildemuth, B., Viles, C., & Symons, M. (in press). Creating healthy communities one byte at a time: An online tailored nutrition project. *Journal of the American Dietetic Association.*

Taras, H. L., & Gage, M. (1995). Advertised foods on children's television. *Archives of Pediatric and Adolescent Medicine, 149*, 649–652.

Tate, D. F., Jackvony, E. H., & Wing, R. R. (2003). Effects of Internet behavioral counseling on weight loss in adults at risk for Type 2 diabetes: A randomized trial. *Journal of the American Medical Association, 289*, 1833–1836.

Tate, D. F., Jackvony, E. H., & Wing, R. R. (2006). A randomized trial comparing human e-mail counseling, computer-automated tailored counseling, and no counseling in an Internet weight loss program. *Archives of Internal Medicine, 166*, 1620–1625.

Tate, D. F., Wing, R. R., & Winett, R. A. (2001). Using Internet technology to deliver a behavioral weight loss program. *Journal of the American Medical Association, 285*, 1172–1177.

Television Bureau of Advertising. (2007). *TV basics: Television households*. Retrieved February 5, 2008, from http://www.tvb.org/rcentral/mediatrendstrack/tvbasics/02_TVHouseholds.asp

Tessaro, I., Eng, E., & Smith, J. (1994). Breast cancer screening in older African-American women: Qualitative research findings. *American Journal of Health Promotion, 8*, 286–292.

Tessaro, I. A., Taylor, S., Belton, L., Campbell, M. K., Benedict, S., Kelsey, K., & DeVellis, B. (2000). Adapting a natural (lay) helpers model of change for worksite health promotion for women. *Health Education Research, 15*, 603–614.

Thrasher, J., Campbell, M. K., Oates, V., Hudson, M., & Jackson, E. (2004). Behavior-specific social support for healthy behaviors among African American church members: Applying optimal matching theory. *Health Education & Behavior, 31*, 193–205.

U.S. Department of Health and Human Services. (2000). *Healthy people 2010: Conference edition* (Vols. 1 and 2). Washington, DC: Author.

Vanchieri, C. (1998). Lessons from the tobacco wars edify nutrition war tactics. *Journal of the National Cancer Institute, 90*, 420–422.

Women's Health Initiative Study Group. (2004). Dietary adherence in the Women's Health Trial. *Journal of the American Dietetic Association, 104*, 654–658.

World Cancer Research Fund. (2007). *Food, nutrition, and the prevention of cancer: A global perspective.* Retrieved February 5, 2008, from http://www.wcrf-uk.org/research_science/expert_report.lasso

12

INTERVENTIONS TO MODIFY SKIN CANCER–RELATED BEHAVIORS

DAVID B. BULLER

Over the past 2 decades, strategies to prevent melanoma and non-melanoma skin cancers (NMSC) by increasing individuals' protection from excessive exposure to ultraviolet radiation (UVR) in sunlight have been the focus of study. Interest in this issue has been stimulated by the rising incidence of skin cancer in the United States, Australia, and Europe. In the United States, the American Cancer Society (2007) estimated that about 1 million cases of NMSC and 59,940 cases of melanoma would be diagnosed in 2007, with melanoma resulting in 8,110 deaths. Unfortunately, sun safety is not normative in many fair-skinned populations. The desire for suntans and ignorance of the dangers involved cause many to sunburn regularly, which greatly increases skin cancer risks (Saraiya, Hall, & Uhler, 2002).

In this chapter, research evaluating interventions intended to reduce UVR exposure (i.e., primary prevention) is reviewed. Some research has suggested that skin cancer prevention interventions are best aimed at children because they spend substantial time outdoors (Godar, Urbach, Gasparro, & van der Leun, 2003) and because severe sunburns at this age may increase risk for melanoma (Weinstock et al., 1989). However, sun safety remains important in adulthood. Estimates from the United States suggest that individuals receive three quarters of their lifetime exposure to UVR during adulthood, with exposure peaking in late middle age, especially for men (Godar et al., 2003). A variety of interventions aimed at children and their parents and caregivers have been investigated, with a large number being conducted in schools. For adults, interventions have been delivered and tested in community settings, such as by direct mail to homes, in medical practices, at worksites, at recreation venues, and at centers that care for children.

SUN PROTECTION INTERVENTIONS FOR CHILDREN

In two reviews of the sun protection programs for children I wrote with Ron Borland (D. B. Buller & Borland, 1998, 1999), we found that most of the evaluations had been performed in the United States and most focused on programs for preadolescents. The majority of these evaluations examined effects of the intervention on children's sun protection, and a few also reported the impact on parents' sun safety. The results of additional studies have been reported in the past 7 years, focusing on adolescents and adults.

Interventions for Infants and Preschool Children

Interventions for very young children tested in the past range from providing parents with simple guidelines for minimizing children's sun exposure issued through hospitals (Bolognia, Berwick, Fine, Simpson, & Jasmin, 1991), to sun safety curricula for children implemented in preschools (Gritz et al., 2007; Loescher, Emerson, Taylor, Christensen, & McKinney, 1995), to lectures on childhood sun safety for nursery school personnel (Boldeman, Ullen, Mansson-Brahme, & Holm, 1993). The hospital program reduced sun exposure of children reported by mothers, and direct instruction of children increased children's comprehension of sun safety information and preschool staff's sun protection of children. The nursery school program produced transmission of the sun safety information to other staff and parents.

Interventions for School-Age Children

A large proportion of sun safety interventions for school-age children have been implemented in schools, with the intention of teaching and motivating children to change their behavior. Although compulsory attendance laws make schools an attractive venue, shrinking resources, standards-based curricula, routine standardized testing, and other competing demands present barriers to such interventions. Currently, sun safety education is uncommon in elementary schools and is more frequent in secondary schools (D. B. Buller et al., 2002; D. B. Buller, Buller, & Reynolds, 2006). A few interventions have been used in other organizations that care for children, such as medical clinics, clubs, and outdoor recreation centers.

Short-Duration Interventions

Borland and I found it useful to distinguish programs of short duration, often presented at a single time or event and conveying a small amount of information, usually advice to protect oneself from the sun and how to do so (D. B. Buller & Borland 1998, 1999). In general, the short-duration programs improved children's knowledge related to sun protection but made little impact on their actual sun safety behaviors. Studies on interactive multimedia computer programs providing sun safety instruction suggest that they operate in a manner similar to short-duration programs delivered through more traditional means. The computer-based instruction mainly produced knowledge improvements (and possibly attitudes supporting sun safety) when compared with teacher-led lectures or no treatment (D. B. Buller et al., 1999; M. K. Buller et al., in press; Hewitt, Denman, Hayes, Pearson, & Wallbanks, 2001; Horning et al., 2000).

Multiunit Interventions

By contrast, multiunit programs presented over several days or weeks and containing large amounts of information—including instruction on the benefits and potential risks of the sun; methods for taking precautions; and strategies to improve the perceived benefits of sun protection, address common barriers, and set sun safety goals (D. B. Buller & Borland, 1998, 1999)—have by and large improved children's sun protection behavior, although mainly in primary school (D. B. Buller, Taylor, et al., 2006; English et al., 2005; Milne et al., 2001). Recently, this success has extended into early, but not late, secondary school (D. B. Buller, Taylor, et al., 2006; Geller et al., 2005). Changes achieved by multiunit school sun safety curricula may improve over successive years of instruction (D. B. Buller, Taylor, et al., 2006), but gains may plateau or retreat over several years as children age into adolescence (Lowe, Balanda, Gillespie, Del Mar, & Gentle, 1993). A curriculum may be more effective when coupled with environmental interventions such as recommending sunsafe policies to school (Giles-Corti et al., 2004). Tailoring of multiple prevention messages to children's perceived norms has also been successful (Norman et al., 2007).

Community-Based Interventions

Community interventions may also be effective. Sanson-Fisher (1995) reported that a mass media campaign for 11- to 16-year-old children in New South Wales, Australia, was successful in encouraging them to improve their sun protection and avoid sunburns. Community-wide sun safety programs also reduced sunburning by children under age 6 and increased use of sunscreen by children in Massachusetts (Miller, Geller, Wood, Lew, & Koh, 1999). These programs also improved parents' knowledge of the role of sun exposure in skin cancer formation, attitudes toward sun protection, and reports of children's sun protection in Scotland (Fleming, Newell, Turner, & MacKie, 1997). The outcomes of these studies are weakened by the lack of control groups in the evaluation design. However, in two randomized trials, community-wide sun safety programs delivered through schools, child care facilities, primary care practices, and at local beaches and pools enhanced the proportion of children in those communities protecting their skin compared with untreated control communities (Dietrich et al., 1998; Dietrich, Olson, Sox, Tosteson, & Grant-Petersson, 2000; Olson et al., 2007).

Directions for the Future in Research on Childhood Sun Protection Programs

The research conducted thus far on programs to improve childhood sun protection has documented that programs richer in content and instruction that occur over several sessions work best. Less attention has been paid to why this is the case or which components of these programs contribute most to their success. Certainly, theoretical models commonly used to explain how children learn suggest that learning new skills requires repeated presentation of the new behaviors with feedback as well as creating motivation and perceived ability to use the skills despite barriers to their implementation. Several authors have relied on principles of social-cognitive theory and other common theories used in health education, such as the health belief model, transtheoretical model, protection motivation theory, and participatory learning principles, to design comprehensive multiunit interventions for children (e.g., see D. B. Buller, Reynolds, et al., 2006; D. B. Buller, Taylor, et al., 2006; Gritz et al., 2007; Milne et al., 2001; Norman et al., 2007; Reynolds, Buller, Yaroch, Maloy, & Cutter, 2006). There is some suggestion that repeated presentation of sun safety advice is important (D. B. Buller, Taylor, et al., 2006), but how long these gains persist and whether it is the acquisition of skills, positive outcome expectations, ways of coping with potential barriers such as cultural beliefs that a suntan is attractive, or repeated reminders to take precautions that make these multiunit interventions successful is not known. It is essential to design instructional materials that satisfy state and local curricular mandates for them to be implemented by teachers.

SUN PROTECTION INTERVENTIONS FOR ADULTS

Evaluations of sun protection interventions for adults are showing promise, too. More recent work has tested interventions in workplace, recreation, and community settings. College-age populations were predominately used to test message formats to deliver sun safety content.

Interventions for College-Age Adults

College students' reactions to messages advocating skin cancer prevention have been tested in a few studies. These have been very short, single presentations of messages or lectures promoting sun safety rather than intensive interventions delivered over long periods of time. As with children, these short programs have primarily improved their knowledge of, and concern about, sun safety (Jones & Leary, 1994; Katz & Jernigan, 1991).

The research on college students provides insight into message strategies that may be persuasive about sun protection. For instance, undergraduate students were more concerned about the effects of the sun after reading appearance-based and unsupported warnings than a health-based admonition (Jones & Leary, 1994). Appearance-based information was even more convincing when accompanied by a photograph that showed skin damage from UVR (Mahler, Kulik, Gerrard, & Gibbons, 2007; Mahler, Kulik, Gibbons, Gerrard, & Harrell, 2003). An emotionally charged interview with people diagnosed with melanoma created intentions to take precautions among undergraduate students (Cody & Lee, 1990), as did messages with statistical and narrative evidence and a personal risk assessment (Greene & Brinn, 2003). College students' sun safety increased when receiving strong fear appeals that emphasized the effectiveness of sun protection behaviors (Stephenson & Witte, 1998), but threat-to-choice messages and vivid language in advice on sunscreen stimulated reactance that produced a boomerang effect (Quick & Stephenson, in press).

These studies were very limited in scope but were usually grounded in theoretical models about communication (e.g., extended parallel-processing model; Witte, 1992). The effectiveness of comprehensive sun safety programs might be improved by adopting these message strategies.

Interventions for Parents and Caregivers

A few programs that were designed to improve sun protection of children also showed that parents can be convinced to improve sun protection for their children (as well as increase their knowledge and create attitudes supporting sun safety). These programs have occurred in several venues, including in recreation centers (Glanz, Chang, Song, Silverio, & Muneoka, 1998; Glanz, Lew, Song, & Cook, 1999) and at swimming pools (Glanz, Geller, Shigaki, Maddock, & Isnec, 2002), through soccer leagues (Parrott et al., 1999) and ski and snowboard schools (Walkosz et al., 2007), by mail from schools and pediatric practices (D. B. Buller, Borland, & Burgoon, 1998; Reynolds et al., in press; Turrisi, Hillhouse, Robinson, Stapleton, & Adams, 2007b), and during pediatric well-child visits (Crane et al., 2006).

Other adult caregivers, such as child care personnel and school teachers and administrators, also respond favorably to sun safety interventions. A package of sun safety policy guidelines and educational materials, along with staff training for primary schools in New South Wales, elevated the adoption of comprehensive sun protection policies by schools but did not improve sun protection practices by the school staff when compared with sending the policy guidelines and educational materials alone (Schofield, Edwards, & Pearce, 1997). Information on etiology and prevention of melanoma sent to medical staff at child health centers in Sweden produced a desire for additional sun safety information by the staff. Almost all of the staff reported that they gave this information to parents; however, only one third of parents remembered actually receiving it from the staff (Boldeman et al., 1993).

Interventions for Working Adults

The occupational environment represents a relatively new venue for reaching adults with sun safety programs. Adults spend a large proportion of time at work, and worksites are among the most organized environments for diffusing prevention information through formal and informal communication channels. Recently, California passed legislation on claims for skin cancer by lifeguards on workers' compensation insurance, making this issue more important to employers there. Outdoor workers receive substantial amounts of sun exposure, often for many years, and many do not regularly protect themselves (Shoveller, Lovato, Peters, & Rivers, 2000; Stepanski & Mayer, 1998; Thieden, Philipsen, Heydenreich, & Wulf, 2004).

Sun safety interventions were evaluated with employee populations (Glanz, Buller, & Saraiya, 2007). Programs that educated staff at recreation centers on sun safety and provided education and environmental supports for children and parents increased the recreation center staff's sun protection knowledge and behaviors (Geller et al., 2001; Glanz et al., 1999; Glanz, Maddock, Lew, & Murakami-Akatsuka, 2001). Programs for lifeguards have improved the number of sun protection policies, increased sun protection behavior, and reduced sunburning by staff (Dobbinson, Borland, & Anderson, 1999; Winett et al., 1997). Also, sun safety interventions for postal workers in the United States (Mayer et al., 2007), utility workers in Israel (Azizi et al., 2000), and a general outdoor workers population in Australia (Girgis, Sanson-Fisher, & Watson, 1994) increased their sun protection. However, a sun safety education program for industry workers in Australia improved knowledge related only to sun protection (Hanrahan, 1995). My research team developed a sun safety program, Go Sun Smart, for employees in the North American ski industry. In a randomized trial, we witnessed a greater reduction in the number of employees at ski areas that deployed Go Sun Smart reporting that they had been sunburned during the winter season than at ski areas not assigned to use the program (D. B. Buller et al., 2005) and an increase in the number using sun protection at work during the following summer (Andersen et al., in press).

These workplace sun safety interventions were multifaceted, delivering several messages over several encounters with the audiences. Some were explicitly guided by theoretical models, such as social-cognitive theory (Glanz et al., 2001) and the diffusion of innovation model (D. B. Buller et al., 2005). Woolley, Lowe, Raasch, Glasby, and Buettner (2008) recently reported that a policy mandating sun protection by workers in Queensland reduced skin damage from UVR (i.e., solar keratoses, a precancerous skin lesion, and NMSC) compared to one that made sun protection voluntary, indicating that policy interventions may be potentially effective as well.

Interventions for Adults in Recreational and Community Settings

Reducing intermittent sun exposure during recreation and leisure is also a priority, for this exposure pattern has been associated with the formation of skin cancer (Kricker, Armstrong, English, & Heenan, 1995; MacKie & Aitchison, 1982; Rosso, Joris, & Zanetti, 1999; Weiss, Bertz, & Jung, 1991). Several recent interventions have successfully improved sun protection in this setting.

A multicomponent intervention that matched sun safety advice to beachgoers' readiness to change, using the transtheoretical model, improved their self-reported sun safety (Weinstock, Rossi, Redding, & Maddock, 2002). A photograph showing adults' damage to their skin from UVR, combined with appearance-based information, resulted in increased intentions to use sunscreen, more actual sun protection, and less reported sunbathing by beachgoers (Mahler et al., 2003). Requests for sunscreen and intentions to use sunscreen and reapply it were greater among beachgoers who received messages highlighting potential gains from sun protection as opposed to losses from sun exposure (Detweiler, Bedell, Salovey, Pronin, & Rothman, 1999). A program implemented at a zoo in the United States containing tip sheets for parents, children's activities, prompts, and discounted sun protection products increased sales of sunscreen and sun-protective hats when compared with a zoo that did not receive the intervention (Mayer et al., 2001). My multichannel sun protection program at ski areas improved sun safety by skiers and snowboarders who recalled seeing the messages (Walkosz et al., 2008). By contrast, one randomized study of people traveling on holiday found no effect of sun safety leaflets placed in the seatback pockets of airplanes flying from England to North America and Jamaica (Dey, Collins, Will, & Woodman, 1995).

In the United States, Australia, New Zealand, and Europe, UV indexes are being increasingly included in weather reports. This has shown some success in changing key behaviors (Branstrom, Ullen, & Brandberg, 2003). Other efforts to reach adults in community settings have had modest success (Robinson et al., 2004; Theobald, Marks, Hill, & Dorevitch, 1991).

Directions for the Future in Research
on Adult Sun Protection Programs

The research with adults showed that comprehensive, multifaceted sun safety programs can convince them to take precautions for themselves and their children. Once again, brief communication produced primarily changes in knowledge and beliefs about their risk for skin damage from overexposure to the sun. Some of the sun protection programs for adults have relied on theoretical models of behavior change, but researchers have also tested theoretically based communication strategies related to fear appeals, message framing, language intensity, logical style, and decision making. Several of these strategies could improve sun safety programs, but to date, they have not been explicitly integrated into many of the multifaceted sun protection programs.

The skin cancer prevention programs reported in the literature focused primarily on limiting exposure to ambient UVR in the outdoor environment. However, some individuals, predominately women, use indoor tanning facilities, and many users are adolescents (Demko, Borawski, Debanne, Cooper, & Stange, 2003; Lazovich et al., 2004). Efforts to control this risk behavior have involved public policy (Culley et al., 2001), not concerted educational efforts.

A limitation throughout this literature is an overreliance on self-reports of sun protection by adults and children (D. B. Buller & Borland, 1999; Creech & Mayer, 1997). More objective measures of sun exposure, such as mechanical measures of skin reflectance by a colorimeter (D. B. Buller, Taylor, et al., 2006; Eckhardt et al., 1996), counts of melanocytic nevi (i.e., moles), and ratings of the level of freckling performed by a trained observer examining photographs of the back, face, arms, and shoulders (English et al., 2005), have been used. These measures, though, have limitations; for instance, skin changes produced by UVR exposure can be too short lived to be detected by skin reflectance, and the time lag between sun exposure and melanocytic nevi formation may be too long to evaluate educational programs. Self-reports on sun protection behaviors by children have been validated using skin reflectance (D. B. Buller, Buller, Beach, & Ertl, 1996) and UVR detection devices (Yaroch, Reynolds, Buller, Maloy, & Geno, 2006), through correspondence with parental reports (Lower, Girgis, & Sanson-Fisher, 1998) and with cognitive interviewing techniques (Glanz et al., 2008). Reports by adults on sunburns and sun protection behavior have been validated (Brandberg, Sjoden, & Rosdahl, 1997; Oh et al., 2004). Although the self-report measures of sun protection may not accurately estimate the exact amount of sun protection a person practices, they appear to provide reasonable estimates of the relative amount of sun safety practiced by one person compared with another and therefore are useful in evaluating sun safety programs.

SUMMARY

Reducing excessive exposure to UVR in sunlight for light-skinned populations remains a priority. The Task Force on Community Preventive Services concluded that there was sufficient evidence from these studies to recommend educational and policy approaches in primary schools and in recreational or tourism settings but that there was insufficient evidence to recommend other forms of interventions to improve sun protection (Centers for Disease Control and Prevention, 2003). Several recent studies s uggest that these interventions can be successful in secondary schools and workplaces, as well as in multichannel community-wide efforts.

REFERENCES

American Cancer Society. (2007). *Facts and figures 2007*. Atlanta, GA: American Cancer Society.

Andersen, P. A., Buller, D. B., Voeks, J. H., Walkosz, B. J., Scott, M. D., Cutter, G. R., & Dignan, M. B. (in press). Testing the long term effects of the Go Sun Smart worksite health communication campaign: A group-randomized experimental study. *Journal of Communication*.

Azizi, E., Flint, P., Sadetzki, S., Solomon, A., Lerman, Y., Harari, G., et al. (2000). A graded work site intervention program to improve sun protection and skin cancer awareness in outdoor workers in Israel. *Cancer Causes and Control, 11*, 513–521.

Boldeman, C., Ullen, H., Mansson-Brahme, E., & Holm, L. E. (1993). Primary prevention of malignant melanoma in the Stockholm Cancer Prevention Programme. *European Journal of Cancer Prevention, 2*, 441–446.

Bolognia, J. L., Berwick, M., Fine, J. A., Simpson, P., & Jasmin, M. (1991). Sun protection in newborns: A comparison of educational methods. *American Journal of Diseases of Children, 145*, 1125–1129.

Brandberg, Y., Sjoden, P., & Rosdahl, I. (1997). Assessment of sun-related behaviour in individuals with dysplastic naevus syndrome: A comparison between diary recordings and questionnaire responses. *Melanoma Research, 7*, 347–351.

Branstrom, R., Ullen, H., & Brandberg, Y. (2003). A randomised population-based intervention to examine the effects of the ultraviolet index on tanning behaviour. *European Journal of Cancer, 39*, 968–974.

Buller, D. B., Andersen, P. A., Walkosz, B. J., Scott, M. D., Cutter, G. R., Dignan, M. B., et al. (2005). Randomized trial testing a worksite sun protection program in an outdoor recreation industry. *Health Education and Behavior, 32*, 514–535.

Buller, D. B., & Borland, R. (1998). Public education projects in skin cancer prevention: Child care, school, and college based. *Clinics in Dermatology, 16*, 447–459.

Buller, D. B., & Borland, R. (1999). Skin cancer prevention for children: A critical review. *Health Education and Behavior, 26*, 317–343.

Buller, D. B., Borland, R., & Burgoon, M. (1998). Impact of behavioral intention on effectiveness of message features: Evidence from the Family Sun Safety Project. *Human Communication Research, 24,* 433–453.

Buller, D. B., Buller, M. K., Beach, B., & Ertl, G. (1996). Sunny days, healthy ways: Evaluation of a skin cancer prevention curriculum for elementary school-aged children. *Journal of the American Academy of Dermatology, 35,* 911–922.

Buller, D. B., Buller, M. K., & Reynolds, K. D. (2006). A survey of sun protection policy and education in secondary schools. *Journal of the American Academy of Dermatology, 54,* 427–432.

Buller, D. B., Geller, A. C., Cantor, M., Buller, M. K., Rosseel, K., Hufford, D., et al. (2002). Sun protection policies and environmental features in US elementary schools. *Archives of Dermatology, 138,* 771–774.

Buller, D. B., Hall, J. R., Powers, P., Ellsworth, R., Beach, B., Frank, C., et al. (1999). Evaluation of the Sunny Days, Healthy Ways sun safety CD-ROM program. *Cancer Prevention and Control, 3,* 188–195.

Buller, D. B., Reynolds, K. D., Yaroch, A. L., Cutter, G. R., Hines, J. M., Geno, C. R., et al. (2006). Effects of the Sunny Days, Healthy Ways curriculum on students in grades 6–8. *American Journal of Preventive Medicine, 30,* 13–22.

Buller, D. B., Taylor, A. M., Buller, M. K., Powers, P. J., Maloy, J. A., & Beach, B. H. (2006). Evaluation of the Sunny Days, Healthy Ways sun safety curriculum for children in kindergarten through fifth grade. *Pediatric Dermatology, 23,* 321–329.

Buller, M. K., Kane, I. L., Martin, R. C., Giese, A. J., Cutter, G. R., Saba, L. M., & Buller, D. B. (in press). Randomized trial evaluating computer-based sun safety education for children in elementary school. *Journal of Cancer Education.*

Centers for Disease Control and Prevention. (2003). Preventing skin cancer: Findings of the Task Force on Community Preventive Services on reducing exposure to ultraviolet light and counseling to prevent skin cancer: Recommendations and rationale of the U.S. Preventive Services Task Force. *Morbidity and Mortality Weekly Report, 52,* 1–12.

Cody, R., & Lee, C. (1990). Behaviors, beliefs, and intentions in skin cancer prevention. *Journal of Behavioral Medicine, 13,* 373–389.

Crane, L. A., Deas, A., Mokrohisky, S. T., Ehrsam, G., Jones, R. H., Dellavalle, R., et al. (2006). A randomized intervention study of sun protection promotion in well-child care. *Preventive Medicine, 42,* 162–170.

Creech, L. L., & Mayer, J. A. (1997). Ultraviolet radiation exposure in children: A review of measurement strategies. *Annals of Behavioral Medicine, 19,* 399–407.

Culley, C. A., Mayer, J. A., Eckhardt, L., Busic, A. J., Eichenfield, L. F., Sallis, J. F., et al. (2001). Compliance with federal and state legislation by indoor tanning facilities in San Diego. *Journal of the American Academy of Dermatology, 44,* 53–60.

Demko, C. A., Borawski, E. A., Debanne, S. M., Cooper, K. D., & Stange, K. C. (2003). Use of indoor tanning facilities by White adolescents in the United States. *Archives of Pediatric and Adolescent Medicine, 157,* 854–860.

Detweiler, J. B., Bedell, B. T., Salovey, P., Pronin, E., & Rothman, A. J. (1999). Message framing and sunscreen use: Gain-framed messages motivate beachgoers. *Health Psychology, 18,* 189–196.

Dey, P, Collins, S., Will, S., & Woodman, C. B. J. (1995, October 21). Randomised controlled trial assessing effectiveness of health education leaflets in reducing incidence of sunburn. *BMJ, 311*, 1062–1063.

Dietrich, A. J., Olson, A. L., Sox, C. H., Stevens, M., Tosteson, T. D., Ahles, T., et al. (1998). A community-based randomized trial encouraging sun protection for children. *Pediatrics, 102*, E64.

Dietrich, A. J., Olson, A. L., Sox, C. H., Tosteson, T. D., & Grant-Petersson, J. (2000). Persistent increase in children's sun protection in a randomized controlled community trial. *Preventive Medicine, 31*, 569–574.

Dobbinson, S., Borland, R., & Anderson, M. (1999). Sponsorship and sun protection practices in lifesavers. *Health Promotion International, 14*, 167–176.

Eckhardt, L., Mayer, J. A., Creech, L., Johnston, M. R., Lui, K. J., Sallis, J. F., & Elder, J. P. (1996). Assessing children's ultraviolet radiation exposure: The potential usefulness of a colorimeter. *American Journal of Public Health, 86*, 1802–1804.

English, D. R., Milne, E., Jacoby, P., Giles-Corti, B., Cross, D., & Johnston, R. (2005). The effect of a school-based sun protection intervention on the development of melanocytic nevi in children: 6-year follow-up. *Cancer Epidemiology, Biomarkers & Prevention, 14*, 977–980.

Fleming, C., Newell, J., Turner, S., & MacKie, R. (1997). A study of the impact of Sun Awareness Week 1995. *British Journal of Dermatology, 136*, 719–724.

Geller, A. C., Glanz, K., Shigaki, D., Isnec, M. R., Sun, T., & Maddock, J. (2001). Impact of skin cancer prevention on outdoor aquatics staff: The Pool Cool program in Hawaii and Massachusetts. *Preventive Medicine, 33*, 155–161.

Geller, A. C., Shamban, J., O'Riordan, D. L., Slygh, C., Kinney, J. P., & Rosenberg, S. (2005). Raising sun protection and early detection awareness in Florida high schoolers. *Pediatric Dermatology, 22*, 112–118.

Giles-Corti, B., English, D. R., Costa, C., Milne, E., Cross, D., & Johnston, R. (2004). Creating SunSmart schools. *Health Education Research, 19*, 98–109.

Girgis, A., Sanson-Fisher, R. W., & Watson, A. (1994). A workplace intervention for increasing outdoor workers' use of solar protection. *American Journal of Public Health, 84*, 77–81.

Glanz, K., Buller, D. B., & Saraiya, M. (2007). Reducing ultraviolet radiation exposure among outdoor workers: State of the evidence and recommendations. *Environmental Health, 6*, 22.

Glanz, K., Chang, L., Song, V., Silverio, R., & Muneoka, L. (1998). Skin cancer prevention for children, parents, and caregivers: A field test of Hawaii's SunSmart program. *Journal of the American Academy of Dermatology, 38*, 413–417.

Glanz, K., Geller, A. C., Shigaki, D., Maddock, J. E., & Isnec, M. R. (2002). A randomized trial of skin cancer prevention in aquatics settings: The Pool Cool program. *Health Psychology, 21*, 579–587.

Glanz, K., Lew, R. A., Song, V., & Cook, V. A. (1999). Factors associated with skin cancer prevention practices in a multiethnic population. *Health Education and Behavior, 26*, 344–359.

Glanz, K., Maddock, J. E., Lew, R. A., & Murakami-Akatsuka, L. (2001). A randomized trial of the Hawaii SunSmart program's impact on outdoor recreation staff. *Journal of the American Academy of Dermatology, 44*, 973–978.

Glanz, K., Yaroch, A. L., Dancel, M., Saraiya, M., Crane, L. A., Buller, D. B., et al. (2008). Measures of sun exposure and sun protection practices. *Archives in Dermatology, 144*, 217–222.

Godar, D. E., Urbach, F., Gasparro, F. P., & van der Leun, J. C. (2003). UV doses of young adults. *Photochemistry and Photobiology, 77*, 453–457.

Greene, K., & Brinn, L. S. (2003). Messages influencing college women's tanning bed use: Statistical versus narrative evidence format and a self-assessment to increase perceived susceptibility. *Journal of Health Communication, 8*, 443–461.

Gritz, E. R., Tripp, M. K., James, A. S., Harrist, R. B., Mueller, N. H., Chamberlain, R. M., & Parcel, G. S. (2007). Effects of a preschool staff intervention on children's sun protection: Outcomes of Sun Protection Is Fun. *Health Education and Behavior, 34*, 562–577.

Hanrahan, P. F. (1995). The effect of an educational brochure on knowledge and early detection of melanoma. *Australian Journal of Public Health, 19*, 270–274.

Hewitt, M., Denman, S., Hayes, L., Pearson, J., & Wallbanks, C. (2001). Evaluation of "Sun-safe": A health education resource for primary schools. *Health Education Research, 16*, 623–633.

Horning, R. L., Lennon, P. A., Garrett, J. M., DeVellis, R. F., Weinberg, P. D., & Strecher, V. J. (2000). Interactive computer technology for skin cancer prevention targeting children. *American Journal of Preventive Medicine, 18*, 69–76.

Jones, J. L., & Leary, M. R. (1994). Effects of appearance-based admonitions against sun exposure on tanning intentions in young adults. *Health Psychology, 13*, 86–90.

Katz, R. C., & Jernigan, S. (1991). Brief report: An empirically derived educational program for detecting and preventing skin cancer. *Journal of Behavioral Medicine, 14*, 421–428.

Kricker, A., Armstrong, B. K., English, D. R., & Heenan, P. J. (1995). Does intermittent sun exposure cause basal cell carcinoma? A case-control study in Western Australia. *International Journal of Cancer, 60*, 489–494.

Lazovich, D., Forster, J., Sorensen, G., Emmons, K., Stryker, J., Demierre, M. F., et al. (2004). Characteristics associated with the use or intention to use indoor tanning among adolescents. *Archives of Pediatric and Adolescent Medicine, 158*, 918–924.

Loescher, L. J., Emerson, J., Taylor, A., Christensen, D. H., & McKinney, M. (1995). Educating preschoolers about sun safety. *American Journal of Public Health, 85*, 939–943.

Lowe, J. B., Balanda, K. P., Gillespie, A. M., Del Mar, C. B., & Gentle, A. F. (1993). Sun-related attitudes and beliefs among Queensland school children: The role of gender and age. *Australian Journal of Public Health, 17*, 202–208.

Lower, T., Girgis, A., & Sanson-Fisher, R. (1998). How valid is adolescents' self-report as a way of assessing sun protection practices. *Preventive Medicine, 27*, 385–390.

MacKie, R. M., & Aitchison, T. (1982). Severe sunburn and subsequent risk of primary cutaneous malignant melanoma in Scotland. *British Journal of Cancer, 46*, 955–960.

Mahler, H. I., Kulik, J. A., Gerrard, M., & Gibbons, F. X. (2007). Long-term effects of appearance-based interventions on sun protection behaviors. *Health Psychology, 26*, 350–360.

Mahler, H. I., Kulik, J. A., Gibbons, F. X., Gerrard, M., & Harrell, J. (2003). Effects of appearance-based interventions on sun protection intentions and self-reported behaviors. *Health Psychology, 22*, 199–209.

Mayer, J. A., Lewis, E. C., Eckhardt, L., Slymen, D., Belch, G., Elder, J., et al. (2001). Promoting sun safety among zoo visitors. *Preventive Medicine, 33*, 162–169.

Mayer, J. A., Slymen, D. J., Clapp, E. J., Pichon, L. C., Eckhardt, L., Eichenfield, L. F., et al. (2007). Promoting sun safety among U.S. postal service letter carriers: Impact of a 2-year intervention. *American Journal of Public Health, 97*, 559–565.

Miller, D. R., Geller, A., Wood, M. C., Lew, R. A., & Koh, H. (1999). The Falmouth Safe Skin Project: Evaluation of a community program to promote sun protection in youth. *Health Education and Behavior, 26*, 369–384.

Milne, E., English, D. R., Johnston, R., Cross, D., Borland, R., Giles-Corti, B., & Costa, C. (2001). Reduced sun exposure and tanning in children after 2 years of a school-based intervention (Australia). *Cancer Causes and Control, 12*, 387–393.

Norman, G. J., Adams, M. A., Calfas, K. J., Covin, J., Sallis, J. F., Rossi, J. S., et al. (2007). A randomized trial of a multicomponent intervention for adolescent sun protection behavior. *Archives of Pediatric and Adolescent Medicine, 161*, 146–152.

Oh, S. S., Mayer, J. A., Lewis, E. C., Slymen, D. J., Sallis, J. F., Elder, J. P., et al. (2004). Validating outdoor workers' self-report of sun protection. *Preventive Medicine, 39*, 798–803.

Olson, A. L., Gaffney, C., Starr, P., Gibson, J. J., Cole, B. F., & Dietrich, A. J. (2007). Sun safe in the middle school years: A community-wide intervention to change early-adolescent sun protection. *Pediatrics, 119*, e247–e256.

Parrott, R., Duggan, A., Cremo, J., Eckles, A., Jones, K., & Steiner, C. (1999). Communicating about youth's sun exposure risk to soccer coaches and parents. *Health Education and Behavior, 26*, 385–395.

Quick, B. L., & Stephenson, M. T. (in press). A test of psychological reactance on boomerang, vicarious, and related boomerang effects. *Human Communication Research.*

Reynolds, K. D., Buller, D. B., Yaroch, A. L., Maloy, J., & Cutter, G. R. (2006). Mediation of a middle school skin cancer prevention program. *Health Psychology, 25*, 616–625.

Reynolds, K. D., Buller, D. B., Yaroch, A., Maloy, J., Geno, C., & Cutter, G. R. (in press). Effects of program exposure and engagement with tailored prevention communication on sun protection by young adolescents. *Journal of Health Communication.*

Robinson, J. D., Silk, K. J., Parrott, R. L., Steiner, C., Morris, S. M., & Honeycutt, C. (2004). Health care providers' sun-protection promotion and at-risk clients' skin-cancer-prevention outcomes. *Preventive Medicine, 38,* 251–257.

Rosso, S., Joris, F., & Zanetti, R. (1999). Risk of basal and squamous cell carcinomas of the skin in Sion, Switzerland: A case-control study. *Tumori, 85,* 435–442.

Sanson-Fisher, R. W. (1995). *Me No Fry evaluation report.* Sydney, New South Wales, Australia: New South Wales Department of Health.

Saraiya, M., Hall, H. I., & Uhler, R. J. (2002). Sunburn prevalence among adults in the United States, 1999. *American Journal of Preventive Medicine, 23,* 91–97.

Schofield, M. J., Edwards, K., & Pearce, R. (1997). Effectiveness of two strategies for dissemination of sun protection policy in New South Wales primary and secondary schools. *Australian and New Zealand Journal of Public Health, 21,* 743–750.

Shoveller, J. A., Lovato, C. Y., Peters, L., & Rivers, J. K. (2000). Canadian National Survey on Sun Exposure and Protective Behaviors: Outdoor workers. *Canadian Journal of Public Health, 91,* 34–35.

Stepanski, B. M., & Mayer, J. A. (1998). Solar protection behaviors among outdoor workers. *American College of Occupational and Environmental Medicine, 40,* 43–48.

Stephenson, M. T., & Witte, K. (1998). Fear, threat, and perceptions of efficacy from frightening skin cancer messages. *Public Health Review, 26,* 147–174.

Theobald, T., Marks, R., Hill, D., & Dorevitch, A. (1991). "Goodbye Sunshine": Effects of a television program about melanoma on beliefs, behavior, and melanoma thickness. *Journal of the American Academy of Dermatology, 25,* 717–723.

Thieden, E., Philipsen, P. A., Heydenreich, J., & Wulf, H. C. (2004). UV radiation exposure related to age, sex, occupation, and sun behavior based on time-stamped personal dosimeter readings. *Archives of Dermatology, 140,* 197–203.

Turrisi, R., Hillhouse, J., Robinson, J., Stapleton, J., & Adams, M. (2006). Influence of parent and child characteristics on a parent-based intervention to reduce unsafe sun practices in children 9 to 12 years old. *Archives in Dermatology, 142,* 1009–1014.

Walkosz, B. J., Buller, D. B., Andersen, P. A., Scott, M. D., Dignan, M. B., Cutter, G. R., & Maloy, J. A. (2008). Increasing sun protection in winter outdoor recreation: A theory-based health communication program. *American Journal of Preventive Medicine, 34,* 502–509.

Walkosz, B. J., Voeks, J. H., Andersen, P. A., Scott, M. D., Buller, D. B., Cutter, G. R., & Dignan, M. B. (2007). Randomized trial on sun safety education at ski and snowboard schools in western North America. *Pediatric Dermatology, 24,* 222–229.

Weinstock, M. A., Colditz, G. A., Willett, W. C., Stampfer, M. J., Bronstein, B. R., Mihm, M. C., Jr., & Speizer, F. E. (1989). Nonfamilial cutaneous melanoma incidence in women associated with sun exposure before 20 years of age. *Pediatrics, 84,* 199–204.

Weinstock, M. A., Rossi, J. S., Redding, C. A., & Maddock, J. E. (2002). Randomized controlled community trial of the efficacy of a multicomponent stage-matched intervention to increase sun protection among beachgoers. *Preventive Medicine, 35,* 584–592.

Weiss, J., Bertz, J., & Jung, E. G. (1991). Malignant melanoma in southern Germany: Different predictive value of risk factors for melanoma subtypes. *Dermatologica, 183,* 109–113.

Winett, R. A., Cleaveland, B. L., Tate, D. F., Lombard, D. N., Lombard, T. N., Russ, C. R., & Galper, D. (1997). The effects of the Sun-safe program on patrons' and lifeguards' skin cancer risk-reduction behaviors at swimming pools. *Health Psychology, 2,* 85–95.

Witte, K. (1992). Putting the fear back into fear appeals: The extended parallel process model. *Communication Monographs, 59,* 329–349.

Woolley, T., Lowe, J., Raasch, B., Glasby, M., & Buettner, P. G. (2008). Workplace sun protection policies and employees' sun-related skin damage. *American Journal of Health Behavior, 32,* 201–208.

Yaroch, A. L., Reynolds, K. D., Buller, D. B., Maloy, J. A., & Geno, C. R. (2006). Validity of a sun safety diary using UV monitors in middle school children. *Health Education and Behavior, 33,* 340–351.

13

BEHAVIORAL SCIENCE APPLICATIONS TO GYNECOLOGIC CANCER PREVENTION

LARI WENZEL, ASTRID REINA-PATTON, AND ISRAEL DE ALBA

In 2007, an estimated 78,290 new diagnoses of invasive gynecological malignances were predicted in the United States, with 28,020 deaths expected (Jemal et al., 2007). Given the vast number of women at risk for developing gynecologic cancer, identification of risk factors, prevention strategies, and early detection approaches remain essential. In this chapter, we first review the epidemiology and specific risk factors of the most prevalent gynecologic malignancies (i.e., cervical, ovarian, and uterine). Then, we discuss behavioral science applications and conceptual models that specifically address prevention, detection, and screening among these malignancies. In so doing, we illustrate the complexities of research in gynecologic cancer prevention.

GYNECOLOGIC CANCERS: EPIDEMIOLOGY AND SPECIFIC RISK FACTORS

Cervical and endometrial cancer have been strongly associated with modifiable behavioral risk factors. Ovarian cancer risk factors are more difficult to identify. The sections that follow briefly describe known risk factors for the major gynecologic cancers.

Cervical Cancer

Despite a marked decrease in cervical cancer incidence and mortality rates in the past several decades (Schiffman, Brinton, Devessa, Fraumeni, & Joseph, 1996), an estimated 11,150 new cases of cervical carcinomas and 3,670 deaths were expected in the United States in 2007 (Jemal et al., 2007). With the majority of cases diagnosed at early stages, the relative 5-year survival rates for cervical cancer are as follows: 92% for localized disease, 56% for regional disease, and 15% for metastatic disease. Racial/ethnic health disparities exist in the case of cervical malignancies, with Latina women disproportionately sharing the disease burden (see chap. 3, this volume, for information on screening rates being selectively lower among immigrants; see also Bosch et al., 1994; Jemal et al., 2004; Mandelblatt, Andrews, Kerner, Zauber, & Burnett, 1991; Mitchell & McCormack, 1997; National Cancer Institute, 2001; Trapido et al., 1995).

Strong evidence indicates that the human papillomavirus (HPV) is causally related to cervical cancer (Bosch et al., 1995; Mandelblatt et al., 1991; National Institutes of Health Consensus Development Panel, 1996). Specifically, HPV Viral Types 16, 18, 45, and 56 have been identified as "high-risk," and Viral Types 31, 33, and 35 as "intermediate-risk," for cervical cancer development (Bosch et al., 1995; Liaw et al., 1995). Risk factors associated with increased risk for HPV infection in women include age at first sexual contact, number of lifetime sexual partners, number of partners' sexual partners (Bosch et al., 1996; Lorincz et al., 1992), and cigarette smoking (American Cancer Society, 2003; Giuliano et al., 2002; Hall, Bishop, & Marteau, 2003; Plummer et al., 2003; Schiffman, 1995; Winkelstein, 1977), all key behavioral issues.

A recent vaccination against the human papilloma virus has resulted in a recommendation from the Centers for Disease Control and Prevention that females between the ages of 11 and 26 years be vaccinated (Markowitz et al., 2007). The potential ability to reduce HPV-related disease has created important questions and concerns intersecting health promotion, social mores, and medical progress (Baden, Curfman, Morrissey, & Drazen, 2007). Behavioral science investigations are likely to provide significant contributions to the adoption of this vaccination in at-risk and underserved populations.

Ovarian Cancer

Ovarian cancer accounts for nearly 4% of all cancers among women and ranks second among the gynecologic cancers (American Cancer Society, 2003). In 2007, an estimated 22,430 new cases of ovarian cancer were noted, with 15,280 deaths expected (Jemal et al., 2007). The relative 5-year survival rates for localized, regional, and metastatic disease are 93%, 69%, and 30%, respectively (Jemal et al., 2004).

Ovarian cancer risk increases with age, peaking in approximately the late 70s. Women who have never had children are at greater risk for developing ovarian cancer, with pregnancy, tubal ligation, and oral contraception use appearing to function as protective factors (American Cancer Society, 2003). Further, use of fertility drugs and hormone replacement therapy appears to increase ovarian cancer risk, as does a family history of breast or ovarian cancer.

Endometrial Cancer

Endometrial carcinoma accounts for 6% of all cancers in women and is the most common gynecologic malignancy in the United States. Estimates for 2007 included 39,080 new cases and 7,400 deaths, with 5-year survival rates for localized, regional, and metastatic disease predicted at 96%, 67%, and 23%, respectively (Jemal et al., 2004).

Differences in epidemiology, tumor behavior, and relationship to hormonal stimulation suggest that there are two types of endometrial cancer. The first type is the most common, and its etiology is related to excess estrogen stimulation. Patients with this type of endometrial cancer tend to have risk factors such as obesity, nulliparity, endogenous or exogenous estrogen excess, diabetes mellitus, and hypertension (Smith et al., 2001). The second type of endometrial carcinoma appears unrelated to estrogen or endometrial hyperplasia and tends to present at more advanced stages. These patients are often multiparous and do not have an abnormal habitus or medical history.

Treatment of postmenopausal symptoms with unopposed estrogen has been associated with endometrial hyperplasia and endometrial cancer (Henderson, 1989). The risk is related to both estrogen dose and duration of treatment. Further, obesity and ovarian tumors are sources of endogenous unopposed estrogens and are also associated with increased risk for endometrial cancer (Siiteri, 1987), as are diets containing high amounts of fat (Potischman et al., 1993) and diabetes mellitus and hypertension (Soler et al., 1999).

BEHAVIORAL SCIENCE APPLICATIONS: PREVENTION, DETECTION, AND SCREENING

Behavioral science interventions have served as a springboard for improving cervical cancer screening rates. In contrast, behavioral aspects of endometrial cancer prevention focus primarily on weight management strategies. Screening adherence interventions for women at high risk for ovarian cancer may provide health benefits.

Cervical Cancer

As the only gynecologic malignancy with established and widely recognized detection and screening guidelines (i.e., the Papanicolaou, or Pap, smear), cervical cancer as a disease process is also the most amenable to direct intervention. A recent search of the literature in PubMed (http://www.ncbi.nlm.nih.gov/pubmed) yielded outcomes in excess of 540 results when the search terms *cervical cancer* and *prevention, detection, and screening* were used, in comparison with 142 and 52 results, respectively, when the terms *ovarian cancer* and *endometrial cancer* were used. Although cervical cancer clearly stands out as the most researched of the gynecologic cancers, the results of the intervention research conducted to date have been largely mixed (see Binstock, Geiger, Hackett, & Yao, 1997; Ornstein, Garr, Jenkins, Rust, & Arnon, 1991; Rimer et al., 1999). As a way to begin to understand the complexities involved in this area of the research, the following sections review the cervical cancer interventions aimed at screening and prevention or follow-up. Most of the literature has focused on secondary prevention of cervical cancer through increasing screening (e.g., Dignan et al., 1996; Margolis, Lurie, McGovern, Tyrrell, & Slater, 1998; Navarro et al., 1995, 1998). The field of primary prevention has only recently received research attention, and very little has been done in the area of prevention of endometrial or ovarian cancer.

In the past decade, a number of excellent review articles have attempted to summarize results for the numerous randomized controlled intervention trials conducted to increase cervical cancer screening (e.g., Marcus & Crane, 1998; Shepherd, Peersman, Weston, & Napuli, 2000; Snell & Buck, 1996; Somkin et al., 1997; Tseng, Cox, Plane, & Hla, 2001; Yarbroff, Mangan, & Mandelblatt, 2003). Interventions for cervical cancer screening and prevention run the gamut from being patient centered and physician focused to being community based and mass media driven. Such interventions have been developed to target the community at large (i.e., the community of women who are perceived to be underusing the Pap smear), as well as discrete samples of individuals in the workplace, inpatient settings, and outpatient clinics. Although different in scope, target population, and strategy, these numerous interventions fall into essentially three theoretical domains: behavioral, cognitive, and sociologic.

Behavioral cervical cancer screening interventions are those trials that "change stimuli associated with Papanicolaou smear use" (Yarbroff et al., 2003, p. 190). The hallmark strategy for behavioral interventions is the reminder, which has been delivered in a myriad of ways, from mail and telephone, to placement in patient charts. Cognitive interventions provide new cancer-related information and focus on educating women and clarifying existing misconceptions, and sociologic interventions target social norms or peers to increase Pap smear use.

CONCEPTUAL MODELS APPLIED
TO GYNECOLOGIC CANCER PREVENTION

Conceptual models provide a framework to develop a comprehensive theoretical strategy applied to cancer prevention, screening, or adherence. Two models, illustrated in the sections that follow, have been successfully applied to cervical cancer prevention and ovarian cancer screening adherence.

Cognitive-Social Health Information Processing Model

It is clear, particularly in the case of cervical cancer, that simply informing patients about the availability of cancer screening and management options does not automatically translate into improved health outcomes (Basen-Engquist et al., 2003; Miller et al., 1999; Miller, Mischel, O'Leary, & Mills, 1996). The recently developed cognitive-social health information processing (C-SHIP) model provides a conceptual framework for the organization of the relevant individual difference parameters that play a role in the process of coping with cancer threat and disease (Miller, Shoda, & Hurley, 1996), and it delineates the cognitive and affective processes involved in cancer-relevant information processing.

The units included in these processes include cancer-relevant encoding and self-construals, beliefs and expectancies, affects and emotions, goals and values, and self-regulatory competencies and skills. Miller, Shoda, and Hurley (1996) have focused on two dispositional attentional styles that influence adaptation by orienting and selectively filtering information. Through this work, they have demonstrated that in comparison with *blunters* (i.e., those who use distraction and minimization of threatening information), *monitors* (i.e., those who scan and amplify threatening cancer cues) manifest a cognitive–affective profile characterized by greater perceptions of threat, lower self-efficacy expectations, and greater cancer-related distress. They appear to fare better when provided with detailed information and enhanced self-efficacy expectations. Similarly, if cancer-relevant information is framed in a less negative, nonthreatening manner, distress is reduced. Blunters, however, do better when provided with more minimal information, framed to emphasize the costs of not adhering to recommended screening guidelines (Miller et al., 1999).

Specific to the gynecologic cancers, in a study of women at increased risk for ovarian cancer, monitoring was associated with heightened perceived risk for disease, intrusive thoughts, and distress (Schwartz, Lerman, Miller, Daly, & Masny, 1995). In the same study, perceived risk, an appraisal variable, mediated the effects of monitoring on psychological distress. Recent research has also shown that patients differentially benefit from how information is framed, depending on their dispositional style. In a study to enhance cervical dysplasia screening follow-up, recommendations were either loss framed (i.e., emphasizing cost), positively framed (i.e., emphasizing benefit), or neutrally framed (i.e., no emphasis). The results showed that monitors fared worse at the affective level when the message was presented in a loss frame, because the sense of risk was heightened. Blunters, however, fared better when the information was presented in a loss-framed manner (Miller et al., 1999). In short, the interaction of attentional style with message framing may motivate health practice actions.

Transactional Model of Stress and Coping

As suggested by Croyle and Lerman (1999), new theoretical models, measures of risk perception, stress associated with risk, and interventions may be needed to address issues of screening adherence that are unique to the mutation carrier group. For example, polygenic disorders challenge health psychologists to develop clinical research strategies that can integrate complementary conceptual approaches across disorders while addressing conceptual differences (see Wenzel & Glanz, 2004, for further discussion). However, the single-gene disorders (e.g., BRCA1 and BRCA2; hereditary nonpolyposis colorectal cancer mutations) also provide complexities as scientists attempt to discern where environment, genes, and behavior converge. The transactional model of stress and coping (Folkman & Chesney, 1995; Lazarus & Folkman, 1986) posits that an individual's response to a stressful event or situation (e.g., disclosure of positive test results) is dependent on three factors: (a) *primary appraisal*, which refers to an individual's perceptions of the level of risk and threat associated with the situation; (b) *secondary appraisal*, which refers to an individual's evaluation of his or her ability to exert control over the event and to manage emotional reactions; and (c) *coping efforts*, which refers to the strategies one uses to manage the event and/or one's feelings.

On the basis of this theoretical framework, a psychosocial telephone counseling (PTC) intervention was recently tested on women who had received news that they carried the BRCA1 and BRCA2 mutation. The model directed the process through which the intervention targeted three key areas impacted by the genetic testing result: emotional reactions, family concerns, and medical decision making. If effective, results of this structured intervention could, for example, be adopted in the clinical setting for implementation by genetic counselors or other health professionals. Further, subgroups of carriers most likely to benefit would help clinicians to target this intervention to their clients who are most in need.

Within this trial, it is noteworthy that of the 66 BRCA1 and BRCA2 mutation carriers who were randomized to receive the PTC intervention, 75.8% completed the PTC intervention and 24.2% did not. Cancer status, cancer-specific distress, and perceptions of appraisal support had significant independent associations with completion of the intervention. Compared with unaffected participants, those affected with breast and/or ovarian cancer were 76% less likely to complete the intervention. In addition, participants with higher levels of cancer-specific distress and those with greater perceptions of social support were most likely to complete the intervention (Halbert et al., 2004). The results of this study suggest that although most BRCA1 and BRCA2 mutation carriers are likely to complete an adjunctive psychoeducational program, personal history of cancer, cancer-specific distress, and perceptions of social support are likely to influence completion of the intervention.

AREAS OF FUTURE RESEARCH

Behavioral and psychosocial factors affect all aspects of gynecologic cancer prevention and control. This is perhaps most evident related to cervical cancer, in which behavioral prevention trials aimed specifically at HPV risk reduction can be planned, implemented, and tested on the basis of existing HIV/AIDS and general STD sexual risk reduction models. Prior behavioral research has also successfully aided at-risk populations in achieving screening. However, given the disproportionate burden among certain vulnerable populations, more work is needed to inform culturally sensitive public health campaigns, as well as culturally sensitive health messages specific to HPV infection for women and men. A novel community health approach to increasing awareness of HPV status among Latina women provided strong evidence that awareness of positive HPV status favorably impacts willingness to undergo screening and receipt of Pap smears among Latinas (DeAlba, Hubbell, & Manetta, 2006). Therefore, HPV testing may be an important tool to improve screening among women with persistent barriers to Pap smear use. It is important to note that in addition to the threat of cancer in general, cervical cancer in particular seriously jeopardizes women's capacity to reproduce. Among younger women, this incapacity has far-reaching implications that appear to extend to long-term quality-of-life disruption (Wenzel & Cella, 2005; Wenzel et al., 2005). Consequently, novel interventions should be directed at specific at-risk populations, such as minority youth, for whom disease rates are known to be prevalent and growing. To date, although both ovarian and endometrial cancers are not easily prevented or detected, promising avenues exist to explore pathways linking behavior, genetics, and environment. Behavioral scientists should be instrumental in shaping the future of this effort.

REFERENCES

American Cancer Society. (2003). *Cancer facts and figures, 2003*. Atlanta, GA: Author.

Baden, L. R., Curfman, G. D., Morrissey, S., & Drazen, J. (2007). Human papillomavirus vaccine—Opportunity and challenge. *The New England Journal of Medicine, 356*, 1990–1991.

Basen-Engquist, K., Paskett, E. D., Buzaglo, J., Miller, S. M., Schover, L., Wenzel, L. B., & Bodurka, D. C. (2003). Cervical cancer. *Cancer, 98*(Suppl. 9), 2009–2014.

Binstock, M. A., Geiger, A. M., Hackett, J. R., & Yao, J. F. (1997). Pap smear outreach: A randomized controlled trial in an HMO. *American Journal of Preventive Medicine, 13*, 425–426.

Bosch, F. X., Castellsague, X., Muñoz, N., de Sanjose, S., Ghaffari, A. M., Gonzalez, L. C., et al. (1996). Male sexual behavior and human papillomavirus DNA: Key risk factors for cervical cancer in Spain. *Journal of the National Cancer Institute, 88*, 1060–1067.

Bosch, F. X., Manos, M. M., Muñoz, N., Sherman, M., Jansen, A. M., Peto, J., et al. (1995). Prevalence of human papillomavirus in cervical cancer: A worldwide perspective. International Biological Study on Cervical Cancer (IBSCC) Study Group. *Journal of the National Cancer Institute, 87*, 796–802.

Bosch, F. X., Muñoz, N., de Sanjose, S., Guerrerro, E., Ghaffari, A. M., Kaldor, J., et al. (1994). Importance of human papillomavirus endemicity in the incidence of cervical cancer: An extension of the hypothesis on sexual behavior. *Cancer Epidemiology, Biomarkers & Prevention, 3*, 375–379.

Croyle, R. T., & Lerman, C. (1999). Risk communication in genetic testing for cancer susceptibility. *Journal of the National Cancer Institute Monographs, 25*, 59–66.

De Alba, I., Hubbell, F. A., & Manetta, A. (2006). Does awareness of HPV status improve willingness to have a Pap smear among Latinas? *Journal of General Internal Medicine, 21*(Suppl. 4), 40–41.

Dignan, M., Michielutte, R., Blinson, K., Wells, H. B., Case, L. D., Sharp, P., et al. (1996). Effectiveness of health education to increase screening for cervical cancer among Eastern-Band Cherokee Indian women in North Carolina. *Journal of the National Cancer Institute, 88*, 1670–1676.

Folkman, S., & Chesney, M. (1995). Coping with HIV infection. In M. Stein & A. Baum (Eds.), *Chronic diseases: Perspectives in behavioral medicine* (pp. 115–133). Hillsdale, NJ: Erlbaum.

Giuliano, A. R., Sedjo, R. L., Roe, D. J., Harris, R., Baldwin, S., Papenfuss, M. R., et al. (2002). Clearance of oncogenic human papillomavirus (HPV) infection: Effect of smoking (United States). *Cancer Causes and Control, 13*, 839–846.

Halbert, C. H., Wenzel, L., Lerman, C., Peshkin, B. N., Narod, S., Marcus, A., et al. (2004). Predictors of participation in psychosocial telephone counseling following genetic testing for BRCA1 and BRCA2 mutations. *Cancer Epidemiology, Biomarkers & Prevention, 13*, 875–881.

Hall, S., Bishop, A. J., & Marteau, T. M. (2003). Increasing readiness to stop smoking in women undergoing cervical screening: Evaluation of two leaflets. *Nicotine & Tobacco Research, 5*, 821–826.

Henderson, B. E. (1989). The cancer question: An overview of recent epidemiologic and retrospective data. *American Journal of Obstetrics and Gynecology, 161*(6, Pt. 2), 1859–1864.

Jemal, A., Siegel, R., Ward, E., Murray, T., Xu, J., & Thun, M. J. (2007). Cancer statistics, 2007. *CA: A Cancer Journal for Clinicians, 57*, 43–66.

Jemal, A., Tiwari, R. C., Murray, T., Ghafoor, A., Samuels, A., Ward, E., et al. (2004). Cancer statistics, 2004. *CA: A Cancer Journal for Clinicians, 54*, 8–29.

Lazarus, R. S., & Folkman, S. (1986). Cognitive theories of stress and the issue of circularity. In M. H. Appley & R. Trumbull (Eds.), *Dynamics of stress: Physiological, psychological, and social perspectives* (pp. 63–80). New York: Plenum Press.

Liaw, K. L., Hsing, A. W., Chen, C. J., Schiffman, M. H., Zhang, T. Y., Hsieh, C. Y., et al. (1995). Human papillomavirus and cervical neoplasia: A case-control study in Taiwan. *International Journal of Cancer, 62*, 565–571.

Lorincz, A. T., Reid, R., Jenson, A. B., Greenberg, M. D., Lancaster, W., & Kurman, R. J. (1992). Human papillomavirus infection of the cervix: Relative risk associations of 15 common anogenital types. *Obstetrics and Gynecology, 79*, 328–337.

Mandelblatt, J., Andrews, H., Kerner, J., Zauber, A., & Burnett, W. (1991). Determinants of late stage diagnosis of breast and cervical cancer: The impact of age, race, social class, and hospital type. *American Journal of Public Health, 81*, 646–649.

Marcus, A. C., & Crane, L. A. (1998). A review of cervical cancer screening intervention research: Implications for public health programs and future research. *Preventive Medicine, 27*, 13–31.

Margolis, K. L., Lurie, N., McGovern, P. G., Tyrrell, M., & Slater, J. S. (1998). Increasing breast and cervical cancer screening in low-income women. *Journal of General Internal Medicine, 13*, 515–521.

Markowitz, L. E., Dunne, E. F., Saraiya, M., Lawson, H. W., Chesson, H., Unger, E. R., et al. (2007). Quadrivalent human papillomavirus vaccine: Recommendations of the Advisory Committee on Immunization Practices (ACIP). *MMWR Recommendations and Reports, 56*, 1–24.

Miller, S. M., Buzaglo, J. S., Simms, S., Green, V., Bales, C., Mangan, C. E., et al. (1999). Monitoring styles in women at risk for cervical cancer: Implications for the framing of health-relevant messages. *Annals of Behavioral Medicine, 21*, 91–99.

Miller, S. M., Mischel, W., O'Leary, A., & Mills, M. (1996). From human papillomavirus (HPV) to cervical cancer: Psychosocial processes in infection, detection, and control. *Annals of Behavioral Medicine, 18*, 219–228.

Miller, S. M., Shoda, Y., & Hurley, K. (1996). Applying cognitive-social theory to health-protective behavior: Breast self-examination in cancer screening. *Psychological Bulletin, 119*, 70–94.

Mitchell, J. B., & McCormack, L. A. (1997). Time trends in late-stage diagnosis of cervical cancer: Differences by race/ethnicity and income. *Medical Care, 35*, 1220–1224.

National Cancer Institute. (2001). *Surveillance, epidemiology, and end results.* Retrieved January 31, 2001, from http://seer.cancer.gov

National Institutes of Health Consensus Development Panel. (1996). National Institutes of Health Consensus Development Conference Statement: Cervical cancer, April 1–3, 1996. *Journal of the National Cancer Institute Monographs, 21*, vii–xix.

Navarro, A. M., Senn, K. L., Kaplan, R. M., McNicholas, L., Campo, M. C., & Roppe, B. (1995). Por La Vida intervention model for cancer prevention in Latinas. *Journal of the National Cancer Institute Monographs, 18*, 137–145.

Navarro, A. M., Senn, K. L., McNicholas, L. J., Kaplan, R. M., Roppe, B., & Campo, M. C. (1998). Por La Vida model intervention enhances use of cancer screening tests among Latinas. *American Journal of Preventive Medicine, 15*, 32–41.

Ornstein, S. M., Garr, D. R., Jenkins, R. G., Rust, P. F., & Arnon, A. (1991). Computer-generated physician and patient reminders: Tools to improve population adherence to selected preventive services. *Journal of Family Practice, 32*, 82–90.

Plummer, M., Herrero, R., Franceschi, S., Meijer, C. J., Snijders, P., Bosch, F. X., et al. (2003). Smoking and cervical cancer: Pooled analysis of the IARC multi-centric case-control study. *Cancer Causes Control, 14*, 805–814.

Potischman, N., Swanson, C. A., Brinton, L. A., McAdams, M., Barrett, R. J., Berman, M. L., et al. (1993). Dietary associations in a case-control study of endometrial cancer. *Cancer Causes Control, 4*, 239–250.

Rimer, B. K., Conaway, M., Lyna, P., Glassman, B., Yarnall, K. S., Lipkus, I., & Barber, L. T. (1999). The impact of tailored interventions on a community health center population. *Patient Education and Counseling, 37*, 125–140.

Schiffman, M. H. (1995). New epidemiology of human papillomavirus infection and cervical neoplasia. *Journal of the National Cancer Institute, 87*, 1345–1347.

Schiffman, M. H., Brinton, L. A., Devessa, S. S., Fraumeni, J., & Joseph, F. (1996). Cervical cancer. In D. Schottenfeld, J. Fraumeni, & F. Joseph (Eds.), *Cancer epidemiology and prevention* (pp. 1090–1116). New York: Oxford University Press.

Schwartz, M., Lerman, C., Miller, S. M., Daly, M., & Masny, A. (1995). Coping disposition, perceived risk, and psychological distress among women at increased risk for ovarian cancer. *Health Psychology, 14*, 232–235.

Shepherd, J., Peersman, G., Weston, R., & Napuli, I. (2000). Cervical cancer and sexual lifestyle: A systematic review of health education interventions targeted at women. *Health Education Research, 15*, 681–694.

Siiteri, P. K. (1987). Adipose tissue as a source of hormones. *American Journal of Clinical Nutrition, 45*(Suppl. 1), 277–282.

Smith, R. A., von Eschenbach, A. C., Wender, R., Levin, B., Byers, T., Rothenberger, D., et al. (2001). American Cancer Society guidelines for the early detection of cancer: Update of early detection guidelines for prostate, colorectal, and endometrial cancers and update, 2001—Testing for early lung cancer detection. *CA: A Cancer Journal for Clinicians, 51*, 38–75, 77–80.

Snell, J. L., & Buck, E. L. (1996). Increasing cancer screening: A meta-analysis. *Preventive Medicine, 25*, 702–707.

Soler, M., Chatenoud, L., Negri, E., Parazzini, F., Franceschi, S., & la Vecchia, C. (1999). Hypertension and hormone-related neoplasms in women. *Hypertension, 34*, 320–325.

Somkin, C. P., Hiatt, R. A., Hurley, L. B., Gruskin, E., Ackerson, L., & Larson, P. (1997). The effect of patient and provider reminders on mammography and

Papanicolaou smear screening in a large health maintenance organization. *Archives of Internal Medicine, 157*, 1658–1664.

Trapido, E. J., Burciaga Valdez, R., Obeso, J. L., Strickman-Stein, N., Rotger, A., & Perez-Stable, E. J. (1995). Epidemiology of cancer among Hispanics in the United States. *Journal of the National Cancer Institute Monographs, 18*, 17–28.

Tseng, D. S., Cox, E., Plane, M. B., & Hla, K. M. (2001). Efficacy of patient letter reminders on cervical cancer screening: A meta-analysis. *Journal of General Internal Medicine, 16*, 563–568.

Wenzel, L., & Cella, D. (2005). Quality of life issues in gynecologic cancer. In W. J. Hoskins, C. A. Perez, R. C. Young, R. R. Barakat, M. Markman, & M. E. Randall (Eds.), *Principles and practices of gynecologic oncology* (4th ed., pp. 1333–1342). Philadelphia: Lippincott Williams & Wilkins.

Wenzel, L., Dogan-Ates, A., Habbal, R., Berkowitz, R., Goldstein, D., Bernstein, M., et al. (2005). Reproductive concerns and quality of life in female cancer survivors. *Journal of the National Cancer Institute Monographs, 34*, 94–98.

Wenzel, L., & Glanz, K. (2004). Behavioral aspects of genetic risk for disease: Cancer genetics as a prototype for complex issues in health psychology. In R. G. Frank, A. Baum, & J. L. Wallander (Ed.), *Handbook of clinical health psychology: Vol. 3. Models and perspectives in health psychology* (pp. 115–142). Washington, DC: American Psychological Association.

Winkelstein, W., Jr. (1977). Smoking and cancer of the uterine cervix: Hypothesis. *American Journal of Epidemiology, 106*, 257–259.

Yabroff, K. R., Mangan, P., & Mandelblatt, J. (2003). Effectiveness of interventions to Increase Papanicolaou smear use. *Journal of the American Board of Family Practice, 16*, 188–203.

14

INTERVENTIONS TO MODIFY PHYSICAL ACTIVITY

BERNARDINE M. PINTO, CAROLYN RABIN,
AND GEORITA M. FRIERSON

Given the overwhelming evidence for substantial benefits from physical activity[1], physical inactivity is still a national public health problem that has been addressed by the American Heart Association, American College of Sport Medicine, and Centers for Disease Control and Prevention (CDC). In chapter 2 of this volume, the link between physical activity and cancer incidence was briefly introduced. In this chapter, we examine in more depth recent developments in researchers' understanding of the benefits of physical activity both for primary prevention and for individuals with a previous diagnosis of cancer. There have been exciting developments in the promotion of physical activity among cancer survivors, primarily to improve functioning, promote quality of life, and reduce treatment sequelae (Courneya & Friedenreich, 1999; Galvao & Newton, 2005; Pinto & Maruyama, 1999). Recommendations have been made to increase the prevalence of physical activity, as seen in reports such as *Physical Activity and Health: A Report of the Surgeon General* (U.S. Department of Health and Human Services [USDHHS], 1996), *Physical*

---

[1]*Physical activity* has been defined as bodily movement that is the result of skeletal muscles contracting which noticeably increases energy expenditure (USDHHS, 1996).

237

Activity and Cardiovascular Health (National Institutes of Heath Consensus Development Panel on Physical Activity and Cardiovascular Health, 1996), and *Healthy People 2010* (USDHHS, 2000). However, it is estimated that only 25% of U.S. adults meet guidelines for moderate-intensity physical activity or vigorous-intensity physical activity (at least three times per week for at least 20 minutes each time) or both (CDC, 2001). In the next section, we highlight the efficacy or effectiveness of interventions in various settings, with a particular emphasis on interventions targeting certain hard-to-reach and minority groups characterized by sedentary lifestyles. Finally, we end this chapter with key points for new directions in physical activity research.

PHYSICAL ACTIVITY INTERVENTIONS: POPULATION BASED

Population-based interventions reach large segments of the population by, for example, taking advantage of the existing infrastructure in schools and work places or disseminating messages through various forms of media. The use of population-based strategies to promote physical activity is discussed in the sections that follow.

School

Schools provide an opportune setting in which to increase physical activity, as researchers can design interventions around the already existent physical education (PE) classes (Luepker et al., 1996; Marcoux et al., 1999; McMurray et al., 2002). For example, in the Child and Adolescent Trial for Cardiovascular Health, Luepker et al. (1996) provided PE teachers (in schools randomized to the intervention condition) with written materials, professional development sessions, and suggestions for activities that would increase the intensity of physical activity. These schools significantly increased the amount of time students spent in moderate-to-vigorous activity and vigorous-intensity activity as compared with control schools (Luepker et al., 1996). Other school-based interventions have also demonstrated success (Connor-Kuntz & Dummer, 1996; Flores, 1995; McMurray et al., 2002). There is some indication, however, that ease of implementation may be a critical variable in determining the success of these interventions; material that PE teachers find difficult to teach students (e.g., self-management skills) may not be fully implemented, compromising the intervention's success (Marcoux et al., 1999).

Worksite

Worksite interventions hold promise, as they have the ability to reach large sectors of the population. These interventions have been implemented in large companies (Peterson & Aldana, 1999), federal administration offices (Titze, Martin, Seiler, Stronegger, & Marti, 2001), and manufacturing plants (Emmons, Linnan, Shadel, Marcus, & Abrams, 1999). Worksite interventions vary in intensity from minimal programs (Peterson & Aldana, 1999) to intensive programs using a number of intervention strategies (e.g., Emmons et al., 1999; Titze et al., 2001) and are grounded in various theoretical orientations such as the transtheoretical model (Prochaska & DiClemente, 1983; see also Peterson & Aldana, 1999), social-cognitive theory (SCT; Bandura, 1977; see also Halam & Petosa, 1998), and environmental theory (Sallis, Bauman, & Pratt, 1998; see also Emmons et al., 1999; Titze et al., 2001).

The outcomes from worksite interventions are encouraging. The Working Healthy Project was one of the larger and more intensive worksite interventions conducted, involving 26 manufacturing sites (Emmons et al., 1999). This intervention targeted physical activity, smoking, and nutrition and used a combination of individual- and environmental-level strategies (e.g., self-assessments with feedback, allocation of space for exercise equipment; Emmons et al., 1999). Analyses revealed that workers receiving the intervention were significantly more likely than control participants to engage in regular exercise at posttest and to increase fruit, vegetable, and fiber consumption (Emmons et al., 1999). Other worksite interventions have produced similarly encouraging findings. For example, these interventions have increased the use of self-regulation strategies related to physical activity (Halam & Petosa, 1998) and have facilitated progression to a more advanced stage of change for physical activity adoption (Cole, Leonard, Hammond, & Fridinger, 1998; Emmons et al., 1999; Peterson & Aldana, 1999).

Media-Based Interventions

Media-based interventions also have the capability to reach large segments of the population. These interventions use television or radio advertisements, print materials, telephone contacts, or information technology (Marcus, Owen, Forsyth, Cavill, & Fridinger, 1998). The Internet has recently emerged as a tool for promoting health behavior change (Tate, Jackvony, & Wing, 2003). Marcus et al. (1998) reviewed 28 studies using media-based approaches to promote physical activity. They found that mass media campaigns may increase awareness of physical activity and its benefits but do not increase levels of physical activity. They also found, however, that the smaller scale studies using print media or telephone calls did produce increases in physical activity. The reviewers concluded that the greatest public health benefit may come from adapting the approaches used in smaller scale interventions (e.g., matching print materials to stage of readiness to adopt physical activity) to larger campaigns reaching a wider population.

Patient Populations

In addition to serving an important function in primary prevention, physical activity can be used to promote secondary prevention in certain patient populations. Physical activity has become a standard component of cardiac rehabilitation for patients with an acute cardiovascular event or cardiovascular disease (e.g., coronary artery disease, angina). Simons-Morton, Calfas, Oldenburg, and Burton (1998) reviewed 24 physical activity trials based in health care settings for patients with existing cardiovascular disease and concluded that interventions for this patient population effectively increased physical activity and improved cardiorespiratory fitness; further, this review indicated that gains are maintained for 12 months or longer. Physical activity is also recommended as an adjunctive treatment to diet for control of non-insulin dependent diabetes and is a useful adjunct to dietary management for weight loss (USDHHS, 1996). Improvements in symptoms and functioning following participation in exercise[2] programs have also been reported among patients with other chronic diseases such as osteoarthritis and rheumatoid arthritis (e.g., Ettinger et al., 1997; Holman, Mazonson, & Lorig, 1989). Among older adults, exercise adoption has the potential to improve balance and gait, reduce the number of falls, and counteract frailty and muscle weakness (Province et al., 1995; Tinetti et al., 1994). Finally, physical activity is also emerging as a strategy for secondary prevention in cancer populations (see the New Directions section and chap. 4, this volume).

COMMUNITY-BASED INTERVENTIONS

Findings supporting point-of-decision prompts and community-wide campaigns are strong and promising. Point-of-decision prompts include, for example, signs that contain messages that encourage the use of stairs to increase physical activity levels (Kahn et al., 2002; Russell & Hutchinson, 2000). Prompts are also designed to deter the use of elevators and escalators by describing them as being less accessible and attractive (Russell & Hutchinson, 2000). Kahn et al. (2002) reviewed six studies that used decision prompts in public areas such as malls, train stations, and a library. The review provided evidence that these messages are effective for obese and average-weight persons and should be tailored to specific groups (e.g., African Americans). Barriers (e.g., nonexistent artwork in stairwells, safety of stairwells, locked stairwells) and study limitations regarding decision prompts have been discussed by Kahn et al. (2002) and by Russell and Hutchinson (2000).

---

[2]*Exercise* is defined as planned, structured, and repetitive bodily movement done to improve or maintain one or more components of physical fitness (USDHHS, 1996).

Findings support the efficacy of community-wide campaigns (using multiple approaches, e.g., written materials and advertisements) in decreasing physical inactivity (Kahn et al., 2002). However, emerging literature suggests community-wide campaigns with adolescents are not as effective (Pate et al., 2003). The majority of studies reviewed by Kahn et al. (2002) involved interventions that included physical activity as part of multiple risk factor reduction programs. Cardiovascular disease risk factors such as smoking and diet have been targeted through nationally known cardiovascular disease interventions (e.g., Minnesota Heart Health Program, Pawtucket Heart Health Program). Concerns raised about these interventions are their huge undertaking (e.g., staffing, community involvement) and resources needed for implementation. As mentioned earlier, it has been recommended that these types of campaigns incorporate tailored messages for the targeted community.

Underserved Populations

The literature on physical activity interventions specific to diverse and underserved groups is growing. Development of efficacious interventions first requires appropriate and effective recruitment approaches, primarily tailoring recruitment methods for diverse groups. Several studies highlight that tailoring recruitment methods produced equal or greater accrual rates than did nontailored messages among African Americans (Coleman et al., 1997; Lee et al., 1997).

Poston et al. (2001) developed a culturally sensitive physical activity intervention for physically inactive and overweight Mexican American females. Unfortunately, this intervention was not successful, but the authors speculated that contamination (e.g., study conducted in a small community) and baseline activity levels affected their findings. Increases in female adolescent African Americans' and Latinas' physical activity levels (and improved weight management) have been achieved through aerobic dance activity and health education (Flores, 1995). Frenn et al. (2003) reported improvements in diet and physical activity levels among a multirace sample of adolescents attending low to middle income school systems.

Women with dependent children are another underserved community group with high levels of physical inactivity due to family constraints and dual roles (Cody & Lee, 1999). Cody and Lee (1999) conducted a 10-week physical activity intervention for mothers with dependent children. This intervention consisted of an exercise workbook and weekly, 60-minute low-to-moderate intensity physical activity sessions facilitated by an exercise instructor. Findings from this intervention demonstrated significant, positive effects for mothers on anthropometric measures (e.g., body mass index, resting heart rate) and maintenance effects for physical activity at 3 months. Ransdell, Dratt, Kennedy, O'Neill, and DeVoe (2001) conducted similar research from an SCT framework for mother-and-daughter pairs. The pairs participated in two sessions led by an instructor (engaging in physical and recreational activity and addressing ways to increase and maintain physically active lifestyles) each week for 12 weeks. This intervention did not affect the physical activity levels of the mother–daughter pairs. However, the participants reported improvements in their perceptions of sport competence, physical condition, and strength and muscularity. Subsequently, Ransdell et al. (2003) conducted another study for mother–daughter pairs participating in a 12-week either home-based or community-based intervention and found that the mother–daughter pairs in both interventions demonstrated greater participation in aerobic, muscular strength, and flexibility activities.

Physical inactivity has been documented as a significant problem for older people because of its association with physical decline, osteoporosis and fracture risk, and the onset of various medical conditions (Seeman & Chen, 2002; van der Bij, Laurant, & Wensing, 2002). In their review of 38 intervention studies among older people, van der Bij et al. (2002) concluded that home-based, group-based, and educational interventions are effective in promoting physical activity adoption. The effectiveness of these interventions in the adoption and maintenance of physical activity can be further enhanced by identifying reliable and sensitive measures of physical activity among older people; more closely examining how physical activity type, intensity, frequency, duration, and format affect subsequent physical activity participation; understanding the impact of life span events on the adoption and maintenance of physical activity; and identifying the determinants of physical activity among older subgroups (e.g., ethnic group members, those with low incomes or low levels of education, those with chronic illnesses; King, 2001; King, Rejeski, & Buchner, 1998).

NEW DIRECTIONS

As summarized in the preceding sections, physical activity intervention programs have had varying degrees of success. The Task Force on Community Preventive Services (Kahn et al., 2002) concluded that there are six types of interventions that have been shown to increase physical activity and cardiorespiratory fitness: point-of-decision prompts, community-wide education, school PE, community social support, individual health behavior, and enhanced access. In general, however, the U.S. population still remains largely sedentary, thus presenting a challenge to the progress made in physical activity intervention research.

Pragmatic Considerations in Physical Activity Research

An important issue to consider when designing interventions to reduce sedentary behavior in the United States is whether resources should be focused on initiating small changes in a large group of people (e.g., through point-of-decision prompts) or a larger change among a smaller group of people (e.g., through one-to-one exercise counseling). Although the latter may be associated with more health-related benefits for individuals receiving the intervention, increasing overall physical activity among large groups of people may ultimately accomplish more in terms of risk reduction for the population (McKinlay & Marceau, 2000). Thus, some argue that where chronic disease is concerned, resources should be distributed among upstream interventions (e.g., changes in health insurance reimbursement), which target the whole population; mid-stream interventions (e.g., physician education programs), which target large groups; and more intensive downstream interventions (e.g., physical activity interventions for patient populations), which target more circumscribed populations (McKinlay & Marceau, 2000). The type of intervention may influence whether the outcome is increased physical activity (e.g., as when point-of-decision prompts increase the use of stairs) or increased exercise (e.g., as when individuals increase their performance of planned physical exertion).

Strategies to Expand the Reach of Interventions

Some groups, such as ethnic minorities and older adults, have received much less attention in intervention development. The critical determinants of physical activity among these groups that will then allow the development of parsimonious but efficacious interventions need to be identified. Evidence suggests that interventions that go beyond face-to-face modalities (mediated interventions through print, telephone, Internet) may produce larger effect sizes while potentially expanding the reach of interventions. This has led to examining the role of interactive technology to enhance physical activity promotion. Interactive systems using mail or telephone to collect data to inform the intervention and telecommunication-based interactive interventions, such as those in which data are collected and feedback is delivered through telephones using computer-controlled speech and Web technology, are avenues that are open for further testing. There is also a growing interest in expert system interventions, which consist of feedback sections based on constructs that are believed to underlie behavior change. These systems can provide normative and ipsative feedback to the individual on the basis of decision rules developed by experts or by statistical analyses. Preliminary studies suggest that these interventions—for example, telecommunication-based interventions (e.g., Pinto et al., 2002) and Web-based interventions (Napolitano et al., 2003)—hold promise for physical activity promotion. These types of interventions may be attractive because they have the potential to provide participants individualized, tailored feedback when they need an intervention "dose." The reach of these interventions is, however, limited to the method of recruitment (i.e., reactive vs. proactive). Although expert systems can account for individual differences, use consistent decision rules, allow for new variables to be added, and are not expensive after the initial development, they do have their drawbacks, particularly in high development costs. Underserved groups' access to and use of interactive technology have not received much attention, although it is expected that the presence of public computers in libraries and schools will allow access by individuals who do not own personal computers.

Strategies to Increase the Efficacy of Interventions

Across target groups, much more needs to be done to identify and address the mediators of physical activity change that go beyond observational or cross-sectional designs (Lewis, Marcus, Pate, & Dunn, 2002). The study of mediators has hitherto focused on the adoption of physical activity, and less attention has been paid to the variables that mediate maintenance of behavior change. Unfortunately, mediator analyses suggest that researchers have yet to identify a large proportion of the variability in physical activity behavior (Baranowski, Anderson, & Carmack, 1998). Identifying the key mediators of physical activity interventions will contribute to increasing the efficacy of physical activity interventions.

In addition, the efficacy of interventions may be increased through creative strategies such as incentivizing physical activity. Various worksite interventions have used incentives in different ways to promote physical activity, including providing monetary incentives for engaging in a range of healthy behaviors including physical activity (Poole, Kumpfer, & Pett, 2001), offering monetary incentives to employees who participated in a health screening program (Pescatello et al., 2001), and offering a trophy (along with worksite-specific rewards or recognition) to the winners of an exercise competition between companies (i.e., to the company whose employees performed the greatest number of minutes of physical activity on average; Blake et al., 1996). Given the multicomponent nature of these interventions, it is difficult to determine the precise role of incentives in promoting physical activity; nonetheless, there is some indication that providing incentives may enhance physical activity participation (Poole et al., 2001).

Role of the Environment

Data on the efficacy of interventions have supported the call to go beyond a focus on individuals and to consider the larger environment and policies that support a sedentary lifestyle while making physical activity participation less attractive. These new approaches, based on ecological models, have begun investigating the effects of environmental variables (e.g., perceived presence of sidewalks, safe neighborhoods) on physical activity. Accordingly, measures have been developed to assess the impact of these environmental constructs on physical activity (e.g., Kirtland et al., 2003; Saelens, Sallis, Black, & Chen, 2003). Cross-sectional studies suggest environmental and policy variables are associated with physical activity behavior among youth and young adults (see a review by Sallis, Bauman, & Pratt, 1998). For example, access to parks and indoor gyms, sidewalks and pleasant scenery in the neighborhood, lack of unattended dogs in the environment, and having friends who exercise are all positively associated with physical activity (Brownson, Baker, Housemann, Brennan, & Bacak, 2001; King et al., 2000). Intervention studies have also been initiated primarily in the form of point-of-decision prompts such as signs prompting the use of stairs versus elevators or escalators (discussed in the Community-Based Interventions section). An example of a multicomponent physical activity intervention based on the structural ecological model examined the role of PE and physical activity promotion using environmental, policy, and social marketing interventions in schools (44% non-White students; Sallis et al., 2003). Over 2 years, the environmental and policy interventions increased physical activity at school among boys but not girls.

The potential to improve physical activity remains, but the barriers in implementing such multilevel interventions need to be identified (e.g., lack of, or inconsistent support for, policy change) and overcome (Sallis et al., 2003). At the local, state, and federal policy levels, several avenues could be explored to make physically active behaviors more attractive (e.g., making stairwells less intimidating, incentives to use bicycles vs. driving, increasing access to physical activity facilities). Legislative policies will also affect the sustainability of individual and group-level interventions by creating environments that encourage physical activity.

Need for an Interdisciplinary Focus

To disseminate and thereby expand the reach of effective interventions, the programs themselves need to be adapted to meet the needs of diverse groups and the costs and benefits of interventions have to be determined. An interdisciplinary focus is necessary for these efforts to succeed and to address the complex interaction of individual and contextual factors; for example, experts from marketing, economics, urban planning and policy, and scientists from other disciplines such as anthropology (Dunn & Blair, 2002) would need to be involved to address physical inactivity at the population level (i.e., upstream interventions). Concepts from these other arenas—for example, theories of environmental stress, neighborhood disorder, restorative environment theory, and behavior setting theory—can help identify environmental factors that may significantly influence physical activity (King, Stokols, Talen, Brassington, & Killingsworth, 2002). Observational studies can be conducted in those communities where factors that decrease physical activity (e.g., environmental stressors such as noise and heavy traffic) or foster activity (e.g., restorative environments such as open space, water, and accessible recreational facilities) have been modified compared with case-control communities where these types of environmental changes have not been made. Intervention studies will need to consider multiple environmental changes, perhaps selected for cost-effectiveness, so that the greatest increases in physical activity can be achieved at the lowest cost. Such macrolevel interventions will need to incorporate interventions at the individual level (i.e., downstream) to be maximally effective.

Besides an understanding of shared environmental factors, genetic factors have also begun to receive attention, with studies on gene–environment interactions and their effects on physical activity (Maia, Thomas, & Beunen, 2002) opening up yet another level of analysis. Hence, not only individual factors but also more distal contextual or environmental factors, by themselves and in interaction with individual biobehavioral and cognitive factors, may be required to move the field ahead (King, Bauman, & Abrams, 2002).

CONCLUSION

There is consensus that physical activity is beneficial to the health of Americans of all ages. Yet, a majority does not meet physical activity recommendations. Efforts have been invested in promoting physical activity on a large scale in various settings (such as schools and at worksites) in communities and among specific patient groups. The results have been promising, but there is more work to be done. Intervention development should continue to focus on underserved communities, including ethnic and racial minorities, older adults, and women with young children. In addition, given limitations on resources, choices must be made about whether to try to promote large changes in physical activity among a smaller group of individuals or smaller changes among a larger population. Ultimately, improving the efficacy of physical activity interventions may require that we identify additional mediators of physical activity adoption and maintenance, make the environment more hospitable to sustained physical activity, and identify and overcome barriers to physical activity at the policy level. This work will require interdisciplinary efforts to address the public health challenge of sedentary lifestyles.

REFERENCES

Bandura, A. (1977). Self-efficacy: Toward a unifying theory of behavioral change. *Psychology Review, 84*, 191–215.

Baranowski, T., Anderson, C., & Carmack, C. (1998). Mediating variable framework in physical activity interventions: How are we doing? How might we do better? *American Journal of Preventive Medicine, 15*, 266–297.

Blake, S. M., Caspersen, C. J., Finnegan, J., Crow, R. A., Mittlemark, M. B., & Ringhofer, K. R. (1996). The Shape Up Challenge: A community-based worksite exercise competition. *American Journal of Health Promotion, 11*, 23–34.

Brownson, R. C., Baker, E. A., Housemann, R. A., Brennan, L. K., & Bacak, S. J. (2001). Environmental and policy determinants of physical activity in the United States. *American Journal of Public Health, 91*, 1995–2003.

Centers for Disease Control and Prevention. (2001). Physical activity trends—United States, 1990–1998. *Mortality and Morbidity Weekly Reports, 50*, 166–169.

Cody, R., & Lee, C. (1999). Development and evaluation of a pilot program to promote exercise among mothers of preschool children. *International Journal of Behavioral Medicine, 6*, 13–29.

Cole, G., Leonard, B., Hammond, S., & Fridinger, F. (1998). Using "stages of behavioral change" constructs to measure the short-term effects of a worksite-based intervention to increase moderate physical activity. *Psychological Reports, 82*, 615–618.

Coleman, E. A., Tyll, L., LaCroix, A. Z., Allen, C., Leveille, S. G., Wallace, J. I., et al. (1997). Recruiting African American older adults for a community-based health promotion intervention: Which strategies are effective? *American Journal of Preventive Medicine, 13*(Suppl. 6), 51–56.

Connor-Kuntz, F. J., & Dummer, G. M. (1996). Teaching across the curriculum: Language-enriched physical education for preschool children. *Adapted Physical Activity Quarterly, 13*, 302–315.

Courneya, K. S., & Friedenreich, C. M. (1999). Physical exercise and quality of life following cancer diagnosis: A literature review. *Annals of Behavioral Medicine, 21*, 171–179.

Dunn, A. L., & Blair, S. N. (2002). Translating evidence-based physical activity interventions into practice: The 2010 challenge. *American Journal of Preventive Medicine, 22*(Suppl. 4), 8–9.

Emmons, K. M., Linnan, L. A., Shadel, W. G., Marcus, B., & Abrams, D. B. (1999). The Working Healthy Project: A worksite health-promotion trial targeting physical activity, diet, and smoking. *Journal of Occupational and Environmental Medicine, 41*, 5454–5555.

Ettinger, W. H., Jr., Burns, R., Messier, S. P., Applegate, W., Rejeski, W. J., Morgan, T., et al. (1997). A randomized trial comparing aerobic exercise and resistance exercise with a health education program in older adults with knee osteoarthritis: The Fitness Arthritis and Seniors Trial (FAST). *Journal of the American Medical Association, 277*, 25–31.

Flores, R. (1995). Dance for health: Improving fitness in African American and Hispanic adolescents. *Public Health Reports, 110*, 189–193.

Frenn, M., Bansal, N., Delgado, M., Greer, Y., Havice, M., Ho, M., et al. (2003). Addressing health disparities in middle school students' nutrition and exercise. *Journal of Community Health Nursing, 20*, 1–14.

Galvao, D. A., & Newton, R. U. (2005). Review of exercise intervention studies in cancer patients. *Journal of Clinical Oncology, 23*, 899–909.

Halam, J., & Petosa, R. (1998). A worksite intervention to enhance social cognitive theory constructs to promote exercise adherence. *American Journal of Health Promotion, 13,* 4–7.

Holman, H., Mazonson, P., & Lorig, K. (1989). Health education for self-management has significant early and sustained benefits in chronic arthritis. *Transactions of the Association of American Physicians, 102,* 204–208.

Kahn, E. B., Ramsey, L. T., Brownson, R. C., Heath, G. W., Howze, E. H., Powell, K. E., et al. (2002). The effectiveness of interventions to increase physical activity: A systematic review. *American Journal of Preventive Medicine, 22*(Suppl. 4), 73–107.

King, A. C. (2001). Interventions to promote physical activity by older adults. *The Journals of Gerontology: Series A. Biological Sciences and Social Sciences, 56,* 36–46.

King, A. C., Bauman, A., & Abrams, D. B. (2002). Forging transdisciplinary bridges to meet the physical activity challenge in the 21st century. *American Journal of Preventive Medicine, 23*(Suppl. 2), 104–106.

King, A. C., Castro, C., Wilcox, S., Eyler, A. A., Sallis, J. F., & Brownson, R. C. (2000). Personal and environmental factors associated with physical inactivity among different racial-ethnic groups of U.S. middle-aged and older-aged women. *Health Psychology, 19,* 354–364.

King, A. C., Rejeski, W. J., & Buchner, D. M. (1998). Physical activity interventions targeting older adults. *American Journal of Preventive Medicine, 15,* 316–333.

King, A. C., Stokols, D., Talen, E., Brassington, G. S., & Killingsworth, R. (2002). Theoretical approaches to the promotion of physical activity: Forging a transdisciplinary paradigm. *American Journal of Preventive Medicine, 23*(Suppl. 2), 15–25.

Kirtland, K. A., Porter, D. E., Addy, C. L., Neet, M. J., Williams, J. E., Sharpe, P. A., et al. (2003). Environmental measures of physical activity. *American Journal of Preventive Medicine, 24,* 323–331.

Lee, R. E., McGinnis, K. A., Sallis, J. F., Castro, C. M., Chen, A. H., & Hickman, S. A. (1997). Active vs. passive methods of recruiting ethnic minority women: A health promotion program. *Annals of Behavioral Medicine, 19,* 378–384.

Lewis, B. A., Marcus, B. H., Pate, R. R., & Dunn, A. L. (2002). Psychosocial mediators of physical activity behavior among adults and children. *American Journal of Preventive Medicine, 23*(Suppl. 2), 26–35.

Luepker, R. V., Perry, C. L., McKinlay, S. M., Nader, P. R., Parcel, G. S., Stone, E. J., et al. (1996). Outcomes of a field trial to improve children's dietary patterns and physical activity: The Child and Adolescent Trial for Cardiovascular Health (CATCH). *Journal of the American Medical Association, 275,* 768–776.

Maia, J. A., Thomas, M., & Beunen, G. (2002). Genetic factors in physical activity level: A twin study. *American Journal of Preventive Medicine, 23*(Supp. 2), 87–91.

Marcoux, M., Sallis, J. F., McKenzie, T. L., Marshall, S., Armstrong, C. A., & Goggin, K. J. (1999). Process evaluation of a physical activity self-management program for children: SPARK. *Psychology and Health, 14,* 659–677.

Marcus, B. H., Owen, N., Forsyth, L. H., Cavill, N. A., & Fridinger, F. (1998). Physical activity interventions using mass media, print media, and information technology. *American Journal of Preventive Medicine, 15,* 362–378.

McKinlay, J., & Marceau, L. (2000). U.S. public health and the 21st century: Diabetes mellitus. *Lancet, 356,* 757–761.

McMurray, R. G., Harrell, J. S., Bangdiwala, S. I., Bradley, C. B., Deng, S., & Levine, A. (2002). A school-based intervention can reduce body fat and blood pressure in young adolescents. *Journal of Adolescent Health, 31,* 125–132.

Napolitano, M. A., Fotheringham, M., Tate, D., Sciamanna, C., Leslie, E., Owen, N., et al. (2003). Evaluation of an Internet-based physical activity intervention: A preliminary investigation. *Annals of Behavioral Medicine, 25,* 92–99.

National Institutes of Health Consensus Development Panel on Physical Activity and Cardiovascular Health. (1996). Physical activity and cardiovascular health. *Journal of the American Medical Association, 276,* 241–246.

Pate, R. R., Saunders, R. P., Ward, D. S., Felton, G., Trost, S. G., & Dowda, M. (2003). Evaluation of a community-based intervention to promote activity in youth: Lessons from active winners. *American Journal of Health Promotion, 17,* 171–182.

Pescatello, L. S., Murphy, D., Vollono, J., Lynch, E., Bernene, J., & Constanzo, D. (2001). The cardiovascular health impact of an incentive worksite health promotion program. *American Journal of Health Promotion, 16,* 16–20.

Peterson, T. R., & Aldana, S. G. (1999). Improving exercise behavior: An application of the stages of change model in a worksite setting. *American Journal of Health Promotion, 13,* 229–232.

Pinto, B. M., Friedman, R., Marcus, B. H., Kelley, H., Tennstedt, S., & Gillman, M. (2002) Effects of a computer-based counseling system on physical activity. *American Journal of Preventive Medicine, 23,* 113–120.

Pinto, B. M., & Maruyama, N. C. (1999). Exercise in the rehabilitation of breast cancer survivors. *Psycho-Oncology, 8,* 191–206.

Poole, K., Kumpfer, K., & Pett, M. (2001). The impact of an incentive-based worksite health promotion program on modifiable health risk factors. *American Journal of Health Promotion, 16,* 21–26.

Poston, W. S. C., Haddock, K., Olevera, N. E., Suminski, R. R., Reeves, R. S., Dunn, J. K., et al. (2001). Evaluation of a culturally appropriate intervention to increase physical activity. *American Journal of Health Behavior, 25,* 396–406.

Prochaska, J. O., & DiClemente, C. C. (1983). Stages and processes of self-change of smoking: Toward an integrative model of change. *Journal of Consulting and Clinical Psychology, 51,* 390–395.

Province, M. A., Hadley, E. C., Hornbrook, M. C., Lipsitz, L. A., Miller, J. P., Mulrow, C. D., et al. (1995). The effects of exercise on falls in elderly patients: A pre-planned meta-analysis of the FICSIT Trials. Frailty and Injuries: Cooperative Studies of Intervention Techniques. *Journal of the American Medical Association, 273,* 1341–1347.

Ransdell, L. B., Dratt, J., Kennedy, C., O'Neill, S., & DeVoe, D. (2001). Daughters and mothers exercising together (DAMET): A 12-week pilot project designed to improve physical self-perception and increase recreational physical activity. *Women & Health, 33,* 101–116.

Ransdell, L. B., Taylor, A., Oakland, D., Schmidt, J., Moyer-Mileur, L., & Schultz, B. (2003). Daughters and mothers exercising together: Effects of home- and community-based programs. *Medicine and Science in Sports and Exercise, 35,* 286–296.

Russell, W. D., & Hutchinson, J. (2000). Comparison of health promotion and deterrent prompts in increasing use of stairs over escalators. *Perceptual and Motor Skills, 91,* 55–61.

Saelens, B. E., Sallis, J. F., Black, J. B., & Chen, D. (2003). Neighborhood-based differences in physical activity: An environment scale evaluation. *American Journal of Public Health, 93,* 1552–1558.

Sallis, J. F., Bauman, A., & Pratt, M. (1998). Environmental and policy interventions to promote physical activity. *American Journal of Preventive Medicine, 15,* 379–397.

Sallis, J. F., McKenzie, T. L., Conway, T. L., Elder, J. P., Prochaska, J. J., Brown, M., et al. (2003). Environmental interventions for eating and physical activity: A randomized controlled trial in middle schools. *American Journal of Preventive Medicine, 24,* 209–217.

Seeman T., & Chen X. (2002). Risk and protective factors for physical functioning in older adults with and without chronic conditions: MacArthur studies of successful aging. *The Journals of Gerontology: Series B. Psychological Sciences and Social Sciences, 57,* 135–144.

Simons-Morton, D. G., Calfas, K. J., Oldenburg, B., & Burton, N. W. (1998). Effects of interventions in health care settings on physical activity or cardiorespiratory fitness. *American Journal of Preventive Medicine, 15,* 413–430.

Tate, D. F., Jackvony, E. H., & Wing, R. R. (2003). Effects of Internet behavioral counseling on weight loss in adults at risk for Type 2 diabetes. *Journal of the American Medical Association, 289,* 1833–1836.

Tinetti, M. E., Baker, D. I., McAvay, G., Claus, E. B., Garrett, P., Gottschalk, M., et al. (1994). A multifactorial intervention to reduce the risk of falling among elderly people living in the community. *New England Journal of Medicine, 33,* 821–827.

Titze, S., Martin, B. W., Seiler, R., Stronegger, W., & Marti, B. (2001). Effects of a lifestyle physical activity intervention on stages of change and energy expenditure in sedentary employees. *Psychology of Sport and Exercise, 2,* 103–116.

U.S. Department of Health and Human Services. (1996). *Physical activity and health: A report of the Surgeon General.* Atlanta, GA: Author.

U.S. Department of Health and Human Services. (2000). *Healthy people 2010: Conference edition* (Vols. 1 and 2). Washington, DC: Author.

van der Bij, A. K., Laurant, M. G. H., & Wensing, W. (2002). Effectiveness of physical activity interventions for older adults. *American Journal of Preventive Medicine, 22,* 120–133.

IV

SECONDARY PREVENTION:
EARLY DETECTION
OF CANCER

SECONDARY PREVENTION: EARLY DETECTION OF CANCER

The secondary prevention of cancer, the subject of Part IV, is a well-researched area at the behavioral level. Chapter 15, by Vernon, Tiro, and Meissner, discusses the correlates and predictors of breast, cervical, and colorectal cancer screening adherence, as well as research on the efficacy of interventions to promote such behaviors. Miles, Waller, and Wardle, in chapter 16, review empirical findings on the psychosocial effects of breast, cervical, and colorectal cancer screening, including how these vary as a function of risk level and screening result. Chapter 17, by Wang and Miller, reviews research on the factors that influence the uptake of genetic testing for hereditary breast and ovarian cancer syndromes and discusses the psychological reactions to test results, including their effects on prevention-related decisions.

15

BEHAVIORAL RESEARCH
IN CANCER SCREENING

SALLY W. VERNON, JASMIN A. TIRO, AND HELEN I. MEISSNER

The primary purpose of this chapter is to review the evidence base for behavioral research in cancer screening and to identify directions for future research on the basis of this evidence. The overall goal of screening is to reduce morbidity and mortality from cancer. Thus, the focus in this chapter is on cancers for which the scientific evidence shows that the application of a screening test in a population reduces incidence or mortality. Those cancers include breast, cervical, and colorectal (Hartman, Hall, Nanda, Boggess, & Zolnoun, 2002; Humphrey, Helfand, & Chan, 2002; Pignone, Rich, Teutsch, Berg, & Lohr, 2002).

Screening entails the relatively quick and inexpensive use of tests or procedures to distinguish between people who are likely to have a disease and those who are not (Wilson & Jungner, 1968). Screening tests are not intended to be diagnostic but to distinguish those who may have the disease from those who probably do not. Some cancer screening tests, such as the Papanicolaou (Pap) test, can detect precursor lesions and thus have the

This work was supported in part by National Cancer Institute issued grants R01CA97263, to Sally W. Vernon, and R01CA76330, to Sally W. Vernon and Jasmin A. Tiro.

potential for primary prevention (i.e., they reduce the incidence of a disease), whereas others, such as mammography, are useful for secondary prevention (i.e., they detect disease at an early stage and reduce premature mortality). The decision to screen an at-risk population for cancer is based on well-established criteria first promoted by the World Health Organization (Wilson & Jungner, 1968), including the following: (a) The disease is an important public health problem in that it affects a substantial proportion of the population and causes significant morbidity or mortality, (b) there is a period in the natural history of the disease when it is detectable in asymptomatic persons, (c) treatment of occult disease offers advantages compared with treatment of symptomatic disease, (d) an affordable and cost-effective screening test is available, (e) characteristics of the test are acceptable to the target population (e.g., cost, invasiveness) and to health care professionals, (f) the test achieves an acceptable level of accuracy in the target population, and (g) the benefits outweigh the harms.

Evidence regarding test efficacy (i.e., application of the test in a population reduces incidence or mortality) is arguably the primary factor determining whether to promote a cancer screening test. Multiple organizations have established systematic review processes for evaluating evidence of efficacy (e.g., see U.S. Preventive Services Task Force: http://www.ahrq.gov/clinic/prevenix.htm; the *Cochrane Review:* http://www.cochrane.org). The reviews provide a basis for government, voluntary, and professional organizations to issue recommendations and guidelines for the use of cancer screening tests. As new scientific evidence becomes available and as new tests are developed, the guidelines are revised. Behavioral scientists interested in conducting research on cancer screening need to be aware of these changes so that their research will be based on sound scientific evidence that links a target screening behavior to a reduction in incidence or mortality (Meissner, Vernon, et al., 2004).

Of all cancer screening tests monitored by national surveys, the prevalence of recent (i.e., within the past 3 years) cervical cancer screening with the Pap test is the highest (Swan, Breen, Coates, Rimer, & Lee, 2003); prevalence has been over 70% every year since 1987. The prevalence of recent mammography (i.e., within the past 2 years) has increased steadily since 1987 among women over age 40 years and reached 70% in 2000. However, rates for consecutive, on-schedule mammograms (i.e., compliance with guidelines) are less than optimal. In a review of 37 studies, Clark, Rakowski, and Bonacore (2003) found that the weighted average prevalence estimate was only 46.1% (95% confidence interval: 39.4%, 52.8%). Despite evidence of efficacy, the uptake of colorectal cancer screening has been slow, but rates of endoscopy (i.e., sigmoidoscopy and colonoscopy) appear to be gradually increasing for both men and women since 2000 (Meissner, Breen, Klabunde, & Vernon, 2006).

CORRELATES, PREDICTORS, AND DETERMINANTS OF CANCER SCREENING BEHAVIORS

Many studies identify factors associated with cancer screening behaviors, but few have attempted to systematically review this literature. Two exceptions are Jepson et al. (2000), who conducted a systematic review of the determinants for mammography, the Pap test, and the fecal occult blood test (FOBT), and Hiatt, Klabunde, Breen, Swan, and Ballard-Barbash (2002), who summarized National Health Interview Survey data over a period of years. Three major categories of factors have been extensively studied in relation to cancer screening behaviors: sociodemographic, health care system, and psychosocial. Most of the research in cancer screening is based on cross-sectional study designs that can establish only associations or correlations.

The associations between cancer screening behaviors and sociodemographic and access factors, including race/ethnicity, socioeconomic status, immigration status, and insurance coverage, have been shown to be statistically independent; however, because the data are cross-sectional, it is not possible to unravel the causal sequence. Because minorities tend to have lower socioeconomic status, more frequently lack health insurance, and cite cost as an important barrier, it is important to understand whether and how race/ethnicity interacts with socioeconomic status and access to health care to affect screening behavior. Further, race/ethnicity and socioeconomic status may be markers for unmeasured social processes such as racial discrimination or attitudes toward health, such as fatalism, that mediate or moderate the relationship between access and screening (Hoffman-Goetz, Breen, & Meissner, 1998; Pearlman, Rakowski, Ehrich, & Clark, 1996; Weber & Reilly, 1997; Whitman et al., 1991). Evaluating mediators and moderators can help researchers understand the causal pathways linking factors to each other and to cancer screening behaviors, and can thereby refine and advance theories of behavior change (Rimer, 2002; Sallis, Owen, & Fotheringham, 2000).

As with the literature on sociodemographic and health care system characteristics, few studies of psychosocial factors have been based on prospective data (Jepson et al., 2000), making it difficult to infer causal relationships. Further, only a few studies have systematically tested conceptual models of hypothesized causal pathways between psychosocial variables and cancer screening behaviors (Aiken, West, Woodward, Reno, & Reynolds, 1994; Manne et al., 2003; Montano & Taplin, 1991). There is no consensus on the "best" model of theoretically important factors or even on the best set of psychosocial constructs that empirically predict screening behaviors (Curry & Emmons, 1994). Fishbein and colleagues (Fishbein, 1995; Institute of Medicine, 2002) proposed an integrative model based on constructs drawn from several health behavior theories or models, but this model has not yet been tested empirically for cancer screening behaviors. Noar and Zimmerman

(2005) and Curry and Emmons (1994) recommended that empirical data be used to compare theories to better understand what the best way is to conceptualize and measure constructs and the causal pathways that link these constructs to each other and to cancer screening behaviors.

INTERVENTIONS TO PROMOTE CANCER SCREENING

There is now an extensive body of research on interventions to promote cancer screening behaviors. A number of systematic reviews and meta-analyses have assessed the effects of interventions on the use of mammography (Bonfill, Marzo, Pladevall, Marti, & Emparanza, 2003; Legler et al., 2002; Mandelblatt & Yabroff, 1999; Ratner, Bottorff, Johnson, Cook, & Lovato, 2001; Snell & Buck, 1996; Stone et al., 2002; Wagner, 1998; Yabroff & Mandelblatt, 1999; Yabroff, O'Malley, Mangan, & Mandelblatt, 2001), Pap tests (Forbes, Jepson, & Martin-Hirsch, 2003; Snell & Buck, 1996; Stone et al., 2002; Tseng, Cox, Plane, & Hla, 2001), and colorectal cancer screening with FOBT or sigmoidoscopy (Peterson & Vernon, 2000; Snell & Buck, 1996; Stone et al., 2002; Vernon, 1997). The Task Force on Community Preventive Services (2005) also has reviewed and evaluated the published literature on interventions to promote breast, cervical, and colorectal cancer screening. We synthesize these findings here to identify effective strategies that promote the uptake of cancer screening behaviors.

Breast Cancer Screening With Mammography

Most intervention research has focused on increasing breast cancer screening with mammography, and a number of meta-analyses have been performed. All included patient-directed interventions (Bonfill et al., 2003; Legler et al., 2002; Ratner et al., 2001; Stone et al., 2002; Wagner, 1998; Yabroff & Mandelblatt, 1999; Yabroff et al., 2001), but only three analyzed provider-directed interventions (Mandelblatt & Yabroff, 1999; Snell & Buck, 1996; Stone et al., 2002). The typologies used by meta-analysts to classify mammography interventions varied, making comparisons difficult.

With a few exceptions, results of meta-analyses consistently showed that minimal interventions directed at patients (Bonfill et al., 2003; Stone et al., 2002; Wagner, 1998; Yabroff & Mandelblatt, 1999; Yabroff et al., 2001) or providers (Mandelblatt & Yabroff, 1999; Snell & Buck, 1996; Stone et al., 2002) are effective at increasing mammography screening (see Table 15.1). Results of meta-analyses also show that more intensive patient-directed interventions—including those using multiple strategies (e.g., letter plus phone call, letter plus voucher), those tailored to an individual's characteristics, and those based on theory—have reported larger intervention

TABLE 15.1

Summary of Effect Sizes From Meta-Analyses of Cancer Screening Interventions

Authors, publication year	Intervention categories	Number of studies/cases	Years included	Odds ratio	95% confidence interval	Effect size	95% confidence interval
Pap patient interventions							
Forbes, Jepson, & Martin-Hirsch, 2003	Invitations	35	1966–2000	No pooled estimate due to statistical heterogeneity.			
		19					
	Educational print	3		1.03	(0.75, 1.43)		
	Counseling	2		1.23	(1.07, 1.41)		
	Risk factor assessment	2		No pooled estimate due to statistical heterogeneity.			
Tseng, Cox, Plane, & Hla, 2001	Patient reminders	10	1966–2000				
	Patient reminders	10		1.64	(1.49, 1.80)		
	Patient reminders (low SES)	2		1.16	(0.99, 1.35)		
	Patient reminders (mixed SES)	8		2.02	(1.79, 2.28)		
Pap patient/provider interventions							
Snell & Buck, 1996	Patient or provider focused	150 cases[a]	1989–1994			0.83	(–1.7, 3.4)
		35 cases					
Stone et al., 2002	Organizational change	27	1966–1999				
		9		3.03[b]	(2.56, 3.58)		
	Patient financial incentive	3		2.82	(2.35, 3.38)		
	Patient reminder	16		1.74	(1.58, 1.92)		

(continues)

TABLE 15.1

Summary of Effect Sizes From Meta-Analyses of Cancer Screening Interventions (*Continued*)

Authors, publication year	Intervention categories	Number of studies/cases	Years included	Odds ratio	95% confidence interval	Effect size	95% confidence interval
	Provider education	10		1.72	(1.39, 2.13)		
	Patient education	14		1.53	(1.30, 1.81)		
	Provider reminder	17		1.37	(1.25, 1.51)		
	Provider feedback	3		1.1	(0.93, 1.31)		
Mammography patient interventions							
Bonfill, Marzo, Pladevall, Marti, & Emparanza, 2003	Invitation letter	14	1966–2000	1.66	(1.43, 1.92)		
	Letter + educational material	5		0.62	(0.32, 1.20)		
	Mailed educational materials	1		2.81	(1.96, 4.02)		
	Letter + phone call	1		2.53	(2.02, 3.18)		
	Invitation phone call	3		1.94	(1.70, 2.23)		
	Training activity + reminder	2		2.46	(1.72, 3.50)		
	Home visits	2		1.06	(0.80, 1.40)		
Legler et al., 2002	Access-enhancing[c]	38	1984–1997	2.3	(1.7, 3.1)	18.9[d]	(10.4, 27.4)
	Individual-directed in health care setting[e]	14		2.5	(1.9, 3.4)	17.6	(11.6, 24.0)
	Individual-directed in community setting[e]	15		1.3	(1.0, 1.6)	6.8	(1.8, 11.8)
	Community education	13		1.5	(1.2, 1.9)	9.7	(3.9, 15.6)
	Media campaign	14		1.3	(1.0, 1.8)	5.9	(0.3, 11.5)
	Social network	6		1.4	(1.0, 2.0)	5.8	(−0.2, 11.9)
		7					

Study / Comparison	No. of studies	Years	Effect	(95% CI)	Effect	(95% CI)
Ratner, Bottorff, Johnson, Cook, & Lovato, 2001						
Randomized studies only	31	1966–1997				
Publication year: recent (1990–1997) vs. older (1980–1989)	not provided		2.14	(1.19, 3.85)		
Age: older (50–65) vs. younger (35–45)	not provided		0.57	(0.32, 1.03)		
Clinic vs. community setting	not provided		0.45	(0.25, 0.80)		
Study design: posttest only	not provided		3.09	(1.50, 6.37)		
Study design: pre- and posttest	not provided					
Wagner, 1998	16	1985–1996	1.33	(0.73, 2.44)		
U.S. studies (reminder vs. none)	11		1.48			
Non-U.S. studies (reminder vs. none)	4		5.57			
U.S. studies (personalized vs. generic)	5		1.87			
Yabroff & Mandelblatt, 1999[f]	51	1980–1998				
Behavioral						
vs. usual care[g]	11				13.2	(4.7, 21.2)
Single intervention vs. active[g]	8				5.6	(0.6, 10.6)
Multiple interventions vs. active	6				13.0	(8.6, 17.4)
Cognitive						
Generic vs. usual care	7				1.1	(−2.4, 4.6)
Theory-based vs. usual care	4				23.6	(16.4, 30.1)
Theory-based vs. active static[h]	5				0.4	(−5.4, 6.2)
Theory-based vs. active interactive[h]	5				7.9	(2.3, 13.5)
Sociological						
vs. usual care	8				12.6	(7.4, 17.9)
Yabroff, O'Malley, Mangan, & Mandelblatt, 2001[f]	66	1980–2001				

TABLE 15.1
Summary of Effect Sizes From Meta-Analyses of Cancer Screening Interventions (Continued)

Authors, publication year	Intervention categories	Number of studies	Years included	Odds ratio	95% confidence interval	Effect size	95% confidence interval
Inreach—Behavioral[i]	Vouchers only vs. usual care[g]	2				45.2	(22.1, 68.2)
	Single intervention vs. usual care[g]	7				16.4	(9.2, 23.6)
	Single intervention vs. active[e]	6				4.6	(-0.3, 9.4)
	Multiple interventions vs. active	3				14.0	(8.7, 19.2)
Outreach—Behavioral[i]	Multiple interventions vs. active	3				18.7	(4.9, 32.4)
Inreach—Cognitive	Generic vs. usual care	6				1.4	(-3.4, 6.3)
	Theory-based vs. usual care	1				5.7	(-12.6, 24.0)
	Theory-based static vs. active[h]	5				3.5	(-0.5, 7.5)
	Theory-based interactive vs. active[h]	9				10.7	(6.8, 14.7)
Outreach—Cognitive	Generic vs. usual care	2				1.8	(-2.9, 26.5)
	Theory-based vs. usual care	4				12.7	(6.6, 18.8)
	Theory-based static vs. active	2				2.7	(-1.5, 6.8)
	Theory-based interactive vs. active	2				19.9	(10.6, 29.1)
Inreach—Cognitive and behavioral	Generic vs. usual care	1				-10.3	(-23.0, 2.4)
	Theory-based vs. usual care	2				14.0	(7.9, 20.2)
Outreach—Cognitive and behavioral	Generic vs. usual care	0					
	Theory-based vs. usual care	2				27.3	(14.7, 40.0)
	Theory-based vs. active	5				2.7	(-2.0, 7.4)

	Intervention	No. of studies/cases	Years	Estimate	(95% CI)
Inreach					
	Sociological vs. usual care/active	3		10.7	(3.4, 18.0)
Outreach					
	Sociological and behavioral	1		22.0	(14.1, 29.9)
	Sociological	5		9.1	(1.7, 13.3)
	Sociological and cognitive	3		3.2	(1.3, 5.1)
	Sociological, cognitive, and behavioral	4		12.3	(3.1, 21.4)
Mammography patient and provider interventions					
Mandelblatt & Yabroff, 1999[f]			1980–1998		
Behavioral					
	Provider-directed vs. usual care	21		13.2	(7.8, 18.4)
	Provider-directed vs. active	9		6.8	(4.8, 8.7)
	Provider- and patient-directed vs. usual care	8		20.5	(9.7, 31.3)
	Provider- and patient-directed vs. active	2			
Cognitive					
	Provider-directed vs. usual care	4		8.9	(3.1, 14.6)
	Provider- and patient-directed vs. usual care	4		18.6	(12.8, 24.4)
	Community-directed vs. usual care[j]	1		16.0	(7.3, 24.7)
Cognitive and behavioral					
	Provider-directed vs. usual care	3		9.6	(3.4, 15.8)
	Provider- and patient-directed vs. usual care/active	4		21.0	(8.8, 33.6)
	Community-directed vs. usual care[j]	5		16.1	(11.6, 20.7)
Sociological					
	vs. usual care/active	3		1.1	(−6.8, 9.0)
		4		13.1	(6.8, 19.3)
Snell & Buck, 1996	Patient- or provider-directed	150 cases[a] / 41 cases	1989–1994	22.3	(19.6, 25.1)
Stone et al., 2002		33	1966–1999		
	Patient financial incentive	2		2.74[b]	(1.78, 4.24)
	Organizational change	14		2.47	(1.97, 3.10)
	Patient reminder	29		2.31	(1.97, 2.70)

(continues)

TABLE 15.1
Summary of Effect Sizes From Meta-Analyses of Cancer Screening Interventions *(Continued)*

Authors, publication year	Intervention categories	Number of studies	Years included	Odds ratio	95% confidence interval	Effect size	95% confidence interval
	Provider education	15		1.99	(1.58, 2.51)		
	Provider feedback	4		1.76	(1.33, 2.15)		
	Provider reminder	21		1.63	(1.39, 1.92)		
	Patient education	26		1.31	(1.12, 1.52)		
FOBT patient and provider interventions							
Snell & Buck, 1996		150 cases[a]	1989–1994				
	FOBT patient- or provider-focused	46 cases				20.6	(18.9, 22.2)
Stone et al., 2002		19	1966–1999				
	Organizational change	7		17.6[b]	(12.3, 25.2)		
	Provider education	11		3.01	(1.98, 4.56)		
	Patient reminder	19		2.75	(1.90, 3.97)		
	Patient financial incentive	5		1.82	(1.35, 2.46)		
	Provider reminder	15		1.46	(1.15, 1.85)		
	Patient education	19		1.38	(0.84, 2.25)		
	Provider feedback	4		1.18	(0.98, 1.43)		
Multiple screening type (mamm, Pap, FOBT) patient interventions							
Snell & Buck, 1996		150 cases[a]	1989–1994				
	Patient-directed	50 cases				17.5	(16.0, 20.0)
	Patient- and provider-directed	25 cases				5.1	(1.0, 9.0)
	1 intervention	34 cases				24.5	(21.4, 27.6)
	2 interventions	12 cases				14.0	(11.4, 16.7)
	3 interventions	4 cases				-2.1	(-11.5, 7.3)

Multiple screening type provider interventions
Snell & Buck, 1996

	150 cases[a]	1989–1994	
Provider-directed[k]			
Manual reminders	75 cases	18.9	(17.0, 21.0)
Computer reminders	14 cases	21.1	(14.1, 28.0)
1 intervention	17 cases	8.8	(6.2, 11.4)
2 interventions	47 cases	13.6	(11.6, 15.6)
3 interventions	17 cases	24.9	(21.4, 28.5)
4 interventions	8 cases	68.3	(62.4, 74.2)
During visit	3 cases	-0.6	(-6.8, 5.7)
Outside visit	43 cases	12.2	(10.2, 14.3)
Combination of during and outside visit	6 cases	18.5	(13.8, 23.1)
	26 cases	33.8	(30.7, 36.8)

Note. Pap = Papanicolaou; SES = socioeconomic status; FOBT = fecal occult blood test; mamm = mammography.
[a]Snell reviewed 38 studies, some of which included multiple treatment groups. Each case is a comparison between a treatment and control group.
[b]Odds ratios provided by Stone et al. (2002) are adjusted for all remaining intervention methods as well as for study level differences such as study setting.
[c]Access-enhancing interventions include transportation to appointments, facilitated scheduling, mobile vans, vouchers, and reduced-cost mammograms.
[d]Legler et al. (2002) provided unadjusted difference estimates.
[e]Individual-directed interventions include in-person and/or telephone counseling, tailored and/or generic letters or reminders.
[f]These meta-analyses used the same classification system to categorize interventions: cognitive, behavioral, and sociological. Cognitive strategies provided information and education. Behavioral strategies used reminders, vouchers, or office-based systems as cues to engage in mammography. Sociological interventions focused on changing social norms or altering the structure of care delivery.
[g]Interventions could be compared against a usual care or an active control group (e.g., reminders in patients' charts).
[h]Interventions could be delivered through two modes: static (e.g., letters, videotapes) or interactive (e.g., telephone, in person).
[i]Yabroff, O'Malley, Mangan, and Mandelblatt (2001) examined whether outreach (i.e., delivered outside the health care setting) were as effective as inreach (i.e., delivered in the health care setting) interventions.
[j]Community-directed interventions attempted to educate large groups of individuals through media, newsletters, flyers, and posters.
[k]Provider-directed interventions include those taking place during the office visit (e.g., reminders) and outside of the office visit (e.g., chart audit with feedback).

effects compared with usual care or minimal interventions (Bonfill et al., 2003; Yabroff & Mandelblatt, 1999; Yabroff et al., 2001). Yabroff et al.'s (2001) meta-analysis found that theory-based interactive interventions (e.g., delivered by telephone or in person) were more effective than theory-based static interventions (e.g., letters, pamphlets).

Access-enhancing interventions (e.g., vouchers) were consistently associated with positive intervention effects. Both inreach (e.g., patient-directed interventions within a health care setting) and outreach (e.g., community-based interventions delivered outside a health care setting) strategies also were effective at increasing mammography screening (Legler et al., 2002; Yabroff et al., 2001), as were organizational change interventions (Stone et al., 2002). In general, outreach interventions showed smaller effects than inreach interventions (Legler et al., 2002; Mandelblatt & Yabroff, 1999; Yabroff et al., 2001).

Cervical Cancer Screening With the Pap Test

Four meta-analyses summarized intervention effects to increase cervical cancer screening with the Pap test (see Table 15.1; see also Forbes et al., 2003; Snell & Buck, 1996; Stone et al., 2002; Tseng et al., 2001). Snell and Buck's (1996) analysis that combined patient and provider interventions found no effect overall. In contrast, other meta-analyses (Forbes et al., 2003; Stone et al., 2002; Tseng et al., 2001) found positive intervention effects associated with most categories of patient or provider interventions. Most of the interventions to increase Pap testing involved education or reminders directed at patients or providers. The strongest effects were observed for interventions using patient financial incentives and for those labeled "organizational change," for instance, modification in the structure of health care delivery (Stone et al., 2002).

Colorectal Cancer Screening With the Fecal Occult Blood Test

To date, there have been only two meta-analyses of colorectal cancer screening, and both were of FOBT (see Table 15.1; see also Snell & Buck, 1996; Stone et al., 2002). Few published studies evaluate intervention efforts to promote colorectal cancer screening with sigmoidoscopy, although there are several randomized controlled trials (RCTs) currently in the field. Snell and Buck (1996) found an overall effect size of 20.6 for combined patient- and provider-directed FOBT interventions. Stone et al. (2002) reported a range of effect sizes from 1.18 for minimal interventions that gave only provider feedback on screening recommendation or performance to 17.6 for interventions that targeted organizational change (see Table 15.1). Patient reminders were more effective than provider reminders at increasing FOBT use; however, education targeted to providers was more effective than patient education (Stone et al., 2002). In contrast to Pap testing, patient financial incentives were somewhat less effective than several other intervention categories for FOBT (Stone et al., 2002).

Multiple Screening Tests

Snell and Buck (1996) computed pooled estimates across types of cancer screening behaviors and conducted subgroup analyses for different intervention categories. Patient- or provider-directed interventions showed large and similar effect size estimates (see Table 15.1). For patient-directed interventions, the effect size decreased as the number of interventions delivered increased. In contrast, for provider-directed interventions, the effect size increased with the number of interventions delivered, up to three. However, for both patient- and provider-directed interventions, there appeared to be a point after which increasing the number of interventions was not effective.

Summary of Interventions Across Cancer Screening Behaviors

Meta-analyses consistently showed that minimal interventions increased the uptake of all cancer screening behaviors (Bonfill et al., 2003; Mandelblatt & Yabroff, 1999; Stone et al., 2002; Tseng et al., 2001; Wagner, 1998). Larger effect sizes were observed when comparisons were made with usual care rather than with a minimal intervention comparison, a finding consistent with the effectiveness of minimal interventions. In general, interventions that used multiple strategies or tailored messaging, or those that were theory-based, showed larger effect sizes than usual care or minimal interventions.

Much less intervention research has focused on providers. Two meta-analyses found that interventions targeting both patients and providers were not more effective than provider-only interventions (Mandelblatt & Yabroff, 1999; Snell & Buck, 1996). It is unclear whether this lack of effect is because the intervention components did not complement each other; did not reach the target population; were not implemented as designed; or increased patient resistance to screening because of anxiety, misperceptions, or feeling harassed. An important limitation of provider-only interventions is that they do not reach persons who do not have access to health care or who do not present for care.

Researchers conducting meta-analyses should consider how methodological issues may affect conclusions about which cancer screening interventions are most effective. For example, the meta-analyses of mammography interventions had the most extensive and diverse typologies. Different typologies make it difficult to draw conclusions about the relative effectiveness of intervention categories other than those classified as minimal. Consensus about intervention typologies would enhance researchers' ability to draw conclusions from this body of work. Other important methodological issues are the inclusion and exclusion criteria, and the choice of effect size measure and how it is calculated.

Standardized reporting of methods and results from RCTs of cancer screening interventions also would enhance researchers' ability to synthesize and interpret the literature and to better estimate intervention effects. The Consolidated Standards for Reporting of Trials statement was developed to improve reporting of RCTs (Moher, Schulz, & Altman, 2001) and has been adapted for behavioral interventions (Davidson et al., 2003; Kaplan, Trudeau, & Davidson, 2004).

DIRECTIONS FOR FUTURE RESEARCH

Sallis et al. (2000) proposed a framework to classify research in the behavioral sciences that is relevant to understanding and intervening to reduce morbidity and mortality from chronic diseases. They proposed five research categories or phases that, if addressed, would provide a scientific evidence base for public health interventions. This framework is used to organize the discussion of future research directions.

Establish Links Between Behaviors and Health

Population-based screening for breast, cervical, and colorectal cancers is supported by scientific evidence of a reduction in morbidity or mortality. As yet, such evidence is lacking for prostate and lung cancers, although RCTs are in progress to evaluate the efficacy of screening with the prostate-specific antigen test and spiral computed tomography. As noted by Meissner, Smith, et al. (2004), behavioral research should be conducted concurrently with the development and evaluation of new screening tests as well as throughout the dissemination process once test efficacy is established. Such research may permit a better understanding of factors that facilitate or impede diffusion and also may inform communication efforts about the risks and benefits of screening and about changes in screening guidelines. In the mid-1990s, research on the psychosocial aspects of cancer genetic testing was conducted almost simultaneously with the discovery of genetic mutations for breast and colorectal cancers (e.g., see Lerman & Croyle, 1995). More recently, behavioral scientists have begun to examine psychosocial factors associated with the use of spiral computed tomography (Schnoll et al., 2003).

Develop Measures of the Behavior

As noted by Sallis et al. (2000, p. 295), "high-quality measures are essential for all stages of research," including "establishing the reliability and validity of extant measures, developing new measures, and field testing new tools," yet studies of measures development were least common among the five research phases. Rigorous and comprehensive evaluation of prevalence estimates, patterns of association with predictor variables, and intervention effects is impossible without clearly defined and consistent outcome measures that can be compared across studies (Vernon, Briss, Tiro, & Warnecke, 2004). In fact, a standard vocabulary is needed in many areas of cancer screening research (Bastani, Yabroff, Myers, & Glenn, 2004; Glasgow, Marcus, Bull, & Wilson, 2004; Pasick, Hiatt, & Paskett, 2004; Rimer, Briss, Zeller, Chan, & Woolf, 2004).

More attention needs to be directed to the effects on prevalence and intervention effect estimates (Clark et al., 2003; Legler et al., 2002; Vernon, Briss, et al., 2004) of different conceptual definitions (e.g., *initial, ever, recent, repeat screening*) and operational definitions (e.g., *recent* might be defined as in the past 12, 15, or 24 months) for the same behavioral outcome (e.g., mammography screening completion). Recent systematic reviews and meta-analyses have called attention to the problem of inconsistent definitions and measures across studies and the difficulty it poses in synthesizing results from intervention research; no one has systematically evaluated different definitions as a potential source of heterogeneity in study findings (Bonfill et al., 2003; Clark et al., 2003; Legler et al., 2002; Mandelblatt & Yabroff, 1999; Vernon, 1997). For behavioral research in cancer screening to progress, greater clarity and consistency is needed in definitions and measures.

Even if researchers could agree on definitions and measures for cancer screening behaviors, agreement does not ensure validity of self-reported information. Self-report of cancer screening behaviors requires respondents to recall autobiographical information, including the circumstances of a screening event, the frequency, the interval between each screening, and sometimes the date of the most recent test. Researchers know relatively little about the cognitive processes respondents use to answer survey questions about cancer screening or about how those processes affect the reliability and validity of their answers (e.g., see Warnecke et al., 1997; Vernon, Briss, et al., 2004). Cross-cutting the cognitive tasks are issues that result from the growing ethnic and cultural diversity in the United States, raising issues about question interpretation and data comparability (e.g., see Johnson et al., 1997). In cancer screening, for example, culture may affect how respondents understand issues such as screening intervals or preventive health care visits (Pasick, Stewart, Bird, & D'Onofrio, 2001). Thus, assuming questions are conceptually equivalent may produce misleading results (Johnson et al., 1997; Scheuch, 1993). Other cognitive tasks or processes, including judgment formation and response editing, have received little or no attention in cancer screening research (Vernon, Briss, et al., 2004). All of these processes may affect the accuracy of outcome measurement and may be differentially affected by culture.

Most investigators conduct qualitative studies, such as focus groups or structured interviews, as part of intervention development efforts, but results of those studies are less frequently published in the peer-reviewed literature. Further, there are very few reports on systematic attempts to evaluate sources of response error through research methods such as experimental manipulation of different versions of a question or through cognitive interviewing techniques (e.g., see Beatty & Willis, 2007; Warnecke et al., 1997). For example, through cognitive interviews and qualitative studies, investigators learned that survey respondents did not understand the difference between different types of endoscopy tests used to detect colorectal cancer (Vernon, Meissner, et al., 2004). More attention to integrating qualitative and quantitative research could enhance both the internal and the external validity of study findings (Steckler, McLeroy, Goodman, Bird, & McCormick, 1992).

Identify Influences on the Behavior

Most studies investigating factors that influence cancer screening behaviors are cross-sectional, and fewer studies prospectively measure hypothesized determinants (Jepson et al., 2000). As noted by Weinstein (2007), correlational designs are not adequate to test the predictive accuracy of cognitively oriented health behavior constructs or theories. To date, only a few studies have compared correlates and predictors in cross-sectional and longitudinal studies (Rauscher, Hawley, & Earp, 2005; McQueen et al., 2007). Thus, researchers know little about whether the same factors predict a target screening behavior over time.

Issues related to conceptualization and measurement of psychosocial variables used to predict screening (e.g., benefits and barriers, perceived risk) require attention because there is little consensus on how they should be defined and measured. Different labels are used for the same underlying construct, and different operational definitions are often used to measure the same construct.

A related area of inquiry that deserves attention is conceptualizing and measuring variables at an analytic level beyond the individual (e.g., neighborhood). Although group-level factors have been considered in epidemiologic studies of morbidity and mortality (e.g., see G. A. Kaplan, Everson, & Lynch, 2000), they have been less well studied in the area of cancer screening research. Multilevel approaches can help researchers conceptualize and understand screening as a product of individual characteristics and the social and physical environments (Meissner, Vernon, et al., 2004). Inclusion of group-level factors (e.g., see Haas et al., 2004) may help researchers understand initial uptake and trends in screening and provide new insights about factors that can be addressed through policy changes.

Evaluate Interventions to Change the Behavior

Despite the diversity of typologies, findings from the meta-analyses consistently showed that minimal patient- or provider-directed interventions were effective in increasing all three types of cancer screening behaviors. The consistency of this finding argues for making the comparison group in future intervention studies a minimal intervention group rather than a no-contact control. Only a few studies have compared the relative efficacy of minimal interventions or reminders using different delivery channels (Crane, Leakey, Ehrsam, Rimer, & Warnecke, 2000; Taplin et al., 2000; Vogt, Glass, Glasgow, La Chance, & Lichtenstein, 2003). Therefore, the optimal and least costly method for delivering a minimal cue (e.g., letter, telephone call) needs to be identified for cancer screening behaviors. If all channels are equally effective, more options would be available to health care systems.

Because minimal interventions, such as reminders, are less costly than more intensive interventions, such as telephone counseling or tailored print interventions, researchers may consider using a stepped or progressive approach in which a relatively brief and less expensive intervention is disseminated first and is followed by increasingly intensive and complex interventions for those who do not respond. This approach provides the ability to give not only the right content or type but also the right "dose" of an intervention to each person. With only a few exceptions (e.g., see Taplin et al., 2000), the effects of delivering stepped interventions of increasing intensity have not been evaluated in cancer screening research. In addition to being cost-effective, stepped interventions permit researchers to identify what worked and for whom.

In the area of cancer screening, channels to deliver tailored interventions have included print and telephone. With the exception of face-to-face counseling, telephone counseling is perhaps the most intensive form of a tailored intervention. Newer technologies such as the Internet or computerized interactive telephone counseling (e.g., see Friedman, 1998) may offer alternatives to more labor-intensive, person-delivered strategies, but these are only beginning to be evaluated. More research on tailored interventions that vary delivery channel and intensity (e.g., number of contacts, personalization) of the intervention messages is needed. Recently, behavioral scientists have focused on understanding how people react to tailored messages (e.g., perceived relevance) and how those reactions affect decision making (Kreuter & Wray, 2003). Researchers also do not know whether tailored interventions have longer lasting effects than minimal interventions after the intervention is withdrawn.

As screening diffuses in a population and personal screening histories become more diverse, interventions may need to take those differences into account (Pasick et al., 2004; Rakowski & Breslau, 2004). For example, one's past experience with a test may reinforce a screening behavior or negatively affect willingness to repeat it. Researchers are only beginning to evaluate interventions that target repeat or regular screening, and they do not yet know whether interventions that are effective at increasing initial or one-time screening also are effective at maintaining the behavior (e.g., see Clark et al., 2002).

With the exception of colorectal cancer, the cancers for which there is an evidence base adequate to recommend population-based screening occur in women. Thus, researchers have limited data about whether similar intervention strategies are equally effective at increasing cancer screening in men and women and whether there are gender differences in attitudes and expectations related to screening (e.g., see Wardle et al., 2003).

Although not a subject of this chapter, there is a growing body of intervention research on informed and shared decision making that focuses on outcomes such as decisional conflict or patient perceptions of their role in decision making, rather than on completion of a screening test (Briss et al., 2004). There also is little evidence on the cost-effectiveness of cancer screening interventions (Andersen, Urban, Ramsey, & Briss, 2004). The latter type of research is needed because it identifies financial as well as opportunity costs that can inform dissemination efforts, especially issues related to program implementation.

Translate Research Into Practice

RCTs are often considered the gold standard of evaluation design because they reduce measured and unmeasured confounding, may have unique strengths in supporting causal inference, and are easily understood. Nevertheless, RCTs can have important threats to both internal and external validity (e.g., see Britton et al., 1999; Victora, Habicht, & Bryce, 2004), and for many group-oriented approaches to increasing screening (e.g., laws, policies), they may not be feasible. Much of the current work on study quality focuses primarily on internal validity. More attention needs to be focused on external validity (Gartlehner, Hansen, Nissman, Lohr, & Carey, 2006) if interventions are to have significant potential for dissemination across populations and settings (Glasgow et al., 2004; Meissner, Vernon, et al., 2004). Glasgow et al. (2004) identified lessons learned from dissemination research and recommended that researchers, administrators, clinicians, and funding organizations collaborate and create policies to support research studies that translate research findings into health promotion practice.

CONCLUSION

To reduce morbidity and mortality from cancer in the general population, widespread use of efficacious screening tests is necessary. Behavioral interventions are one strategy to increase the use of cancer screening tests, but such interventions do not occur in a vacuum. Other factors also may increase screening; for example, the efforts of advocacy groups and professional organizations to increase awareness about colorectal cancer may result in policy changes that reduce barriers to colorectal cancer screening. As noted by Susser (1995), broad social movements are needed to stimulate and sustain change in health behavior at the population level, yet researchers still know relatively little about the best methods to bring about social change. Health promotion interventions at the individual or community level are one part of a social movement and may help to accelerate secular trends in cancer screening, but they alone do not explain them. At present, researchers know very little about factors that influence secular trends in cancer screening.

Screening is only part of a continuum of care that begins with prevention and extends to timely follow-up of abnormal test results and treatment of disease (Bastani et al., 2004). Over the past 2 decades, much has been learned about how to develop, implement, and evaluate behavioral interventions to promote cancer screening, and conceptual models and methods have evolved. As we look toward the next generation of cancer screening research, we see that efforts rest on a solid foundation and that the lessons learned from the past 2 decades have provided many insights with which to meet the challenges that lie ahead (Meissner, Smith, et al., 2004; Meissner, Vernon, et al., 2004).

REFERENCES

Aiken, L. S., West, S. G., Woodward, C. K., Reno, R. R., & Reynolds, K. D. (1994). Increasing screening mammography in asymptomatic women: Evaluation of a second-generation, theory-based program. *Health Psychology, 13,* 526–538.

Andersen, M. R., Urban, N., Ramsey, S., & Briss, P. A. (2004). Examining the cost-effectiveness of cancer screening promotion. *Cancer, 101*(Suppl. 5), 1229–1238.

Bastani, R., Yabroff, K. R., Myers, R. E., & Glenn, B. (2004). Lessons learned regarding interventions to improve follow-up of abnormal findings in cancer screening. *Cancer, 101*(Suppl. 5), 1188–1200.

Beatty, P. C., & Willis, G. B. (2007). Research synthesis: The practice of cognitive interviewing. *Public Opinion Quarterly, 71,* 287–311.

Bonfill, X., Marzo, M., Pladevall, M., Marti, J., & Emparanza, J. (2003). Strategies for increasing the participation of women in community breast cancer screening. *Cochrane Database of Systematic Reviews, 1.* Available from http://www.cochrane.org

Briss, P., Rimer, B., Reilley, B., Coates, R. C., Lee, N. C., Mullen, P., et al. (2004). Promoting informed decisions about cancer screening in communities and health care systems. *American Journal of Preventive Medicine, 26,* 67–80.

Britton, A., McKee, M., Black, N., McPherson, K., Sanderson, C., & Bain, C. (1999). Threats to applicability of randomised trials: Exclusions and selective participation. *Journal of Health Services Research & Policy, 4,* 112–121.

Clark, M. A., Rakowski, W., & Bonacore, L. B. (2003). Repeat mammography: Prevalence estimates and considerations for assessment. *Annals of Behavioral Medicine, 26*, 201–211.

Clark, M. A., Rakowski, W., Ehrich, B., Rimer, B. K., Velicer, W. F., Dube, C. E., et al. (2002). The effect of a stage-matched and tailored intervention on repeat mammography. *American Journal of Preventive Medicine, 22*, 1–7.

Crane, L. A., Leakey, T. A., Ehrsam, G., Rimer, B. K., & Warnecke, R. B. (2000). Effectiveness and cost-effectiveness of multiple outcalls to promote mammography among low-income women. *Cancer Epidemiology, Biomarkers & Prevention, 9*, 923–931.

Curry, S. J., & Emmons, K. M. (1994). Theoretical models for predicting and improving compliance with breast cancer screening. *Annals of Behavioral Medicine, 16*, 302–316.

Davidson, K. W., Goldstein, M., Kaplan, R. M., Kaufmann, P. G., Knatterud, G. L., Orleans, C. T., et al. (2003). Evidence-based behavioral medicine: What is it and how do we achieve it? *Annals of Behavioral Medicine, 26*, 161–171.

Fishbein, M. (1995). Developing effective behavior change interventions: Some lessons learned from behavioral research. *NIDA Research Monographs, 155*, 246–261.

Forbes, C., Jepson, R., & Martin-Hirsch, P. (2003). Interventions targeted at women to encourage the uptake of cervical screening. *Cochrane Database of Systematic Reviews, 4*. Available from http://www.cochrane.org

Friedman, R. H. (1998). Automated telephone conversations to assess health behavior and deliver behavioral interventions. *Journal of Medical Systems, 22*, 95–102.

Gartlehner, G., Hansen, R. A., Nissman, D., Lohr, K. N., & Carey, T. S. (2006). *Criteria for distinguishing effectiveness from efficacy trials in systematic reviews* (AHRQ Publication No. 06-0046). Rockville, MD: Agency for Healthcare Research and Quality.

Glasgow, R. E., Marcus, A. C., Bull, S. S., & Wilson, K. M. (2004). Disseminating effective cancer screening interventions. *Cancer, 101*(Suppl. 5), 1239–1250.

Haas, J. S., Phillips, K. A., Sonneborn, D., McCulloch, C. E., Baker, L. C., Kaplan, C. P., et al. (2004). Variation in access to health care for different racial/ethnic groups by the racial/ethnic composition of an individual's county of residence. *Medical Care, 42*, 707–714.

Hartman, K. E., Hall, S. A., Nanda, K., Boggess, J. F., & Zolnoun, D. (2002). *Cervical cancer: Screening.* Rockville, MD: Agency for Healthcare Research and Quality.

Hiatt, R. A., Klabunde, C., Breen, N., Swan, J., & Ballard-Barbash, R. (2002). Cancer screening practices from National Health Interview Surveys: Past, present, and future. *Journal of the National Cancer Institute, 94*, 1837–1846.

Hoffman-Goetz, L., Breen, N. L., & Meissner, H. (1998). The impact of social class on the use of cancer screening within three racial/ethnic groups in the United States. *Ethnicity & Disease, 8*, 43–51.

Humphrey, L. L., Helfand, M., & Chan, B. K. S. (2002). Breast cancer screening: A summary of the evidence for the U.S. Preventive Services Task Force. *Annals of Internal Medicine, 137*, 347–360.

Institute of Medicine. (2002). *Speaking of health: Assessing health communication strategies for diverse populations*. Washington, DC: National Academies Press.

Jepson, R., Clegg, A., Forbes, C., Lewis, R., Sowden, A., & Kleijnen, J. (2000). The determinants of screening uptake and interventions for increasing uptake: A systematic review. *Health Technologies Assessment, 4*, 1–133.

Johnson, T., O'Rourke, D., Chavez, N., Sudman, S., Warnecke, R. B., & Lacey, L. (1997). Social cognition and responses to survey questions in culturally diverse populations. In L. Lyberg, P. Biemer, M. Collins, E. de Leeuw, C. Dippo, N. Schwarz, & D. Trewin (Eds.), *Survey measurement and process quality* (pp. 97–113). New York: Wiley.

Kaplan, G. A., Everson, S. A., & Lynch, J. W. (2000). The contribution of social and behavioral research to an understanding of the distribution of disease: A multilevel approach. In B. D. Smedley & S. L. Syme (Eds.), *Promoting health: Intervention strategies from social and behavioral research* (pp. 37–80). Washington, DC: National Academies Press.

Kaplan, R. M., Trudeau, K. J., & Davidson, K. W. (2004). New policy on reports of randomized clinical trials. *Annals of Behavioral Medicine, 27*, 81.

Kreuter, M. W., & Wray, R. J. (2003). Tailored and targeted health communication: Strategies for enhancing information relevance. *American Journal of Health Behavior, 27*(Suppl. 3), 227–232.

Legler, J., Meissner, H. I., Coyne, C., Breen, N., Chollette, V., & Rimer, B. K. (2002). The effectiveness of interventions to promote mammography among women with historically lower rates of screening. *Cancer Epidemiology, Biomarkers & Prevention, 11*, 59–71.

Lerman, C., & Croyle, R. T. (1995). Genetic testing for cancer predisposition: Behavioral science issues. *Journal of the National Cancer Institute Monographs, 17*, 63–66.

Mandelblatt, J. S., & Yabroff, K. R. (1999). Effectiveness of interventions designed to increase mammography use: A meta-analysis of provider-targeted strategies. *Cancer Epidemiology, Biomarkers & Prevention, 8*, 759–767.

Manne, S., Markowitz, A., Winawer, S., Guillem, J., Meropol, N. J., Haller, D., et al. (2003). Understanding intention to undergo colonoscopy among intermediate-risk siblings of colorectal cancer patients: A test of a mediational model. *Preventive Medicine, 36*, 71–84.

McQueen, A., Vernon, S. W., Watts, B. G., Myers, R. E., Lee, E. S., & Tilley, B. C. (2007). Correlates and predictors of colorectal cancer screening among male automotive workers. *Cancer Epidemiology, Biomarkers & Prevention, 16*, 500–509.

Meissner, H. I., Breen, N., Klabunde, C. N., & Vernon, S. W. (2006). Patterns of colorectal screening uptake among men and women in the United States. *Cancer Epidemiology, Biomarkers & Prevention, 15*, 389–394.

Meissner, H. I., Smith, R. A., Rimer, B. K., Wilson, K. M., Rakowski, W., Vernon, S. W., et al. (2004). Promoting cancer screening: Learning from experience. *Cancer, 101*(Suppl. 5), 1107–1117.

Meissner, H. I., Vernon, S. W., Rimer, B. K., Wilson, K. M., Rakowski, W., Briss, P. A., et al. (2004). The future of research that promotes cancer screening. *Cancer, 101*(Suppl. 5), 1251–1259.

Moher, D., Schulz, K. F., & Altman, D. (2001). The CONSORT Statement: Revised recommendations for improving the quality of reports of parallel-group randomized trials. *Journal of the American Medical Association, 285*, 1987–1991.

Montano, D. E., & Taplin, S. H. (1991). A test of an expanded theory of reasoned action to predict mammography participation. *Social Science & Medicine, 32*, 733–741.

Noar, S. M., & Zimmerman, R. S. (2005). Health behavior theory and cumulative knowledge regarding health behaviors: Are we moving in the right direction? *Health Education Research: Theory & Practice, 20*, 275–290.

Pasick, R. J., Hiatt, R. A., & Paskett, E. D. (2004). Lessons learned from community-based cancer screening intervention research. *Cancer, 101*(Suppl. 5), 1146–1164.

Pasick, R. J., Stewart, S. L., Bird, J. A., & D'Onofrio, C. N. (2001). Quality of data in multiethnic health surveys. *Public Health Report, 116*(Suppl 1.), 223–243.

Pearlman, D. N., Rakowski, W., Ehrich, B., & Clark, M. A. (1996). Breast cancer screening practices among Black, Hispanic, and White women: Reassessing differences. *American Journal of Preventive Medicine, 12*, 327–337.

Peterson, S. K., & Vernon, S. W. (2000). A review of patient and physician adherence to colorectal cancer screening guidelines. *Seminars in Colon & Rectal Surgery, 11*, 58–72.

Pignone, M., Rich, M., Teutsch, S. M., Berg, A. O., & Lohr, K. N. (2002). Screening for colorectal cancer in adults at average risk: A summary of the evidence for the U.S. Preventive Services Task Force. *Annals of Internal Medicine, 137*, 132–131, 141.

Rakowski, W., & Breslau, E. S. (2004). Perspectives on behavioral and social science research on cancer screening. *Cancer, 101*(Suppl. 5), 1118–1130.

Ratner, P. A., Bottorff, J. L., Johnson, J. L., Cook, R., & Lovato, C. Y. (2001). A meta-analysis of mammography screening promotion. *Cancer Detection and Prevention, 25*, 147–160.

Rauscher, G. H., Hawley, S. T., & Earp, J. A. (2005). Baseline predictors of initiation vs. maintenance of regular mammography use among rural women. *Preventive Medicine, 40*, 822–830.

Rimer, B. K. (2002). Perspectives on intrapersonal theories of health behavior. In K. Glanz, B. K. Rimer, & F. M. Lewis (Eds.), *Health behavior and health education: Theory, research, and practice* (3rd ed., pp. 144–159). San Francisco: Jossey-Bass.

Rimer, B. K., Briss, P. A., Zeller, P. K., Chan, E. C., & Woolf, S. H. (2004). Informed decision making: What is its role in cancer screening? *Cancer, 101*(Suppl. 5), 1214–1228.

Sallis, J. F., Owen, N., & Fotheringham, M. J. (2000). Behavioral epidemiology: A systematic framework to classify phases of research on health promotion and disease prevention. *Annals of Behavioral Medicine, 22*, 294–298.

Scheuch, E. K. (1993). The cross-cultural use of sample surveys: Problems of comparability. *Historical Social Research, 18*, 104–138.

Schnoll, R. A., Bradley, P., Miller, S. M., Unger, M., Babb, J., & Cornfeld, M. (2003). Psychological issues related to the use of spiral CT for lung cancer early detection. *Lung Cancer, 39*, 315–325.

Snell, J. L., & Buck, E. L. (1996). Increasing cancer screening: A meta-analysis. *Preventive Medicine, 25*, 702–707.

Steckler, A., McLeroy, K. R., Goodman, R. M., Bird, S. T., & McCormick, L. (1992). Toward integrating qualitative and quantitative methods: An introduction. *Health Education Quarterly, 19*, 1–8.

Stone, E. G., Morton, S. C., Hulscher, M. E., Maglione, M. A., Roth, E. A., Grimshaw, J. M., et al. (2002). Interventions that increase use of adult immunization and cancer screening services: A meta-analysis. *Annals of Internal Medicine, 136*, 641–651.

Susser, M. (1995). The tribulations of trials—Intervention in communities. *American Journal of Public Health, 85*, 156–158.

Swan, J., Breen, N., Coates, R. J., Rimer, B. K., & Lee, N. C. (2003). Progress in cancer screening practices in the United States: Results from the 2000 National Health Interview Survey. *Cancer, 97*, 1528–1540.

Taplin, S. H., Barlow, W. E., Ludman, E., MacLehos, R., Meyer, D. M., Seger, D., et al. (2000). Testing reminder and motivational telephone calls to increase screening mammography: A randomized study. *Journal of the National Cancer Institute, 92*, 233–242.

Task Force on Community Preventive Services. (2005). Improving the use of breast, cervical and colorectal cancer screening. *Guide to community preventive services: Systematic reviews and evidence based recommendations.* Retrieved March 24, 2008, from http://www.thecommunityguide.org/cancer/screening/ca-screening.pdf

Tseng, D. S., Cox, E., Plane, M. B., & Hla, K. M. (2001). Efficacy of patient letter reminders on cervical cancer screening: A meta-analysis. *Journal of General Internal Medicine, 16*, 563–568.

Vernon, S. W. (1997). Participation in colorectal cancer screening: A review. *Journal of the National Cancer Institute, 89*, 1406–1422.

Vernon, S. W., Briss, P. A., Tiro, J. A., & Warnecke, R. B. (2004). Some methodologic lessons learned from cancer screening research. *Cancer, 101*(Suppl. 5), 1131–1145.

Vernon, S. W., Meissner, H., Klabunde, C., Rimer, B. K., Ahnen, D. J., Bastani, R., et al. (2004). Measures for ascertaining use of colorectal cancer screening in behavioral, health services, and epidemiologic research. *Cancer Epidemiology, Biomarkers & Prevention, 13*, 898–905.

Victora, C. G., Habicht, J. P., & Bryce, J. (2004). Evidence-based public health: Moving beyond randomized trials. *American Journal of Public Health, 94*, 400–405.

Vogt, T. M., Glass, A., Glasgow, R. E., La Chance, P. A., & Lichtenstein, E. (2003). The safety net: A cost-effective approach to improving breast and cervical cancer screening. *Journal of Women's Health, 12*, 789–798.

Wagner, T. H. (1998). The effectiveness of mailed patient reminders on mammography screening: A meta-analysis. *American Journal of Preventive Medicine, 14,* 64–70.

Wardle, J., Williamson, S., McCaffery, K., Sutton, S., Taylor, T., Edwards, R., & Atkin, W. (2003). Increasing attendance at colorectal cancer screening: Testing the efficacy of a mailed, psychoeducational intervention in a community sample of older adults. *Health Psychology, 22,* 99–105.

Warnecke, R. B., Sudman, S., Johnson, T. P., O'Rourke, D., Davis, A. M., & Jobe, J. B. (1997). Cognitive aspects of recalling and reporting health-related events: Papanicolaou smears, clinical breast examinations, and mammograms. *American Journal of Epidemiology, 146,* 982–992.

Weber, B. E., & Reilly, B. M. (1997). Enhancing mammography use in the inner city: A randomized trial of intensive case management. *Archives of Internal Medicine, 157,* 2345–2349.

Weinstein, N. D. (2007). Misleading tests of health behavior theories. *Annals of Behavioral Medicine, 33,* 1–10.

Whitman, S., Ansell, D., Lacey, L., Chen, E. H., Ebie, N., Dell, J., & Phillips, C. W. (1991). Patterns of breast and cervical cancer screening at three public health centers in an inner-city urban area. *American Journal of Public Health, 81,* 1651–1653.

Wilson, J. M. G., & Jungner, G. (1968). *Principles and practice of screening for disease.* Geneva, Switzerland: World Health Organization.

Yabroff, K. R., & Mandelblatt, J. S. (1999). Interventions targeted toward patients to increase mammography use. *Cancer Epidemiology, Biomarkers & Prevention, 8,* 749–757.

Yabroff, K. R., O'Malley, A., Mangan, P., & Mandelblatt, J. (2001). Inreach and outreach interventions to improve mammography use. *Journal of the American Medical Women's Association, 56,* 166–173, 188.

16

PSYCHOLOGICAL CONSEQUENCES OF CANCER SCREENING

ANNE MILES, JO WALLER, AND JANE WARDLE

The aim of cancer screening is to detect malignant disease at an early or premalignant stage and thereby increase the potential for effective interventions. In line with World Health Organization guidelines, most developed countries make breast, cervical, and colorectal screening available. However, the need to balance the benefits of screening against the harms is widely acknowledged. Certain forms of screening, such as for lung and prostate cancers, are less widely available because of the lack of strong evidence that they do more good than harm. But even when the balance of harms and benefits appears favorable (e.g., for cervical screening), concerns remain that screening may have adverse emotional and behavioral effects.

The negative consequences of screening may vary according to both test and person characteristics. The threat associated with a positive screening result depends partly on the particular screening technology being used. Early detection screening (e.g., mammography, fecal occult blood test [FOBT]) aims to identify early disease, and therefore a positive result immediately raises the prospect of cancer. Screening for precancerous conditions (e.g., Papanicolaou [Pap] test, sigmoidoscopy, colonoscopy), however, aims to detect signs of cellular changes that are potential precursors of oncogenic transformations (e.g., cytological changes in the cervical cells) rather than cancer per se. A positive result in this type of screening is therefore indicative of higher risk for future disease rather than current disease and is arguably less threatening. However, patients might still be distressed by the idea that an abnormality had been developing without them realizing, or they may believe that precancerous and cancerous outcomes are equivalent.

In addition to the characteristics of the test, the impact of screening is almost certainly moderated by the characteristics of the individual being screened. Some people may be particularly vulnerable to threatening information. As discussed earlier, in chapter 13, those with a monitoring attentional style are thought more likely to amplify health threats, to believe they are at risk for the specified illness, and to respond with increased levels of distress (Miller, Fang, Manne, Engstrom, & Daly, 1999). These reactions, in turn, may be modified by other person and situational factors, such as dispositional optimism (Andrykowski et al., 2002; Miller, Shoda, & Hurley, 1996).

In this chapter, we examine the evidence that cancer screening affects emotional well-being, worry about cancer, and health behaviors. Because of differences between them, breast, cervical, and colorectal screening are considered separately.

BREAST CANCER SCREENING

Breast screening is carried out primarily through mammography, which consists of a series of X-rays of the breasts looking for signs of abnormality such as asymmetries, areas of increased density or calcification, or any skin thickening that might be indicative of a tumor. Other forms of screening include the clinical breast examination (i.e., a manual examination carried out by a trained health professional) and breast self-examination (i.e., a manual examination carried out by the woman herself), but research into the psychological impact of these screenings has focused largely on mammography (cf. Chiarelli et al., 2003).

The process of mammography always has the potential to be stressful. The procedure itself may be uncomfortable or even painful, and there is usually a delay before women receive their results. In addition, a significant minority of women (7.4% in the United Kingdom, and 11%–13% in the United States) will be recalled for further investigation (Smith-Bindman et al., 2003) either because the mammogram is technically inadequate (e.g., yielding an unclear picture) or because of suspicious findings that require immediate investigation. Follow-up investigations can include a repeat mammogram (e.g., using different angles or magnification), a clinical examination, an ultrasound examination, or some form of biopsy. When the index of suspicion is high, samples of breast tissue will be taken for further analysis, with either a nonsurgical technique (i.e., fine-needle aspiration cytology or core biopsy) or an open biopsy, which involves the surgical removal of part or all of a breast lump for testing, resulting in a surgical scar.

Overall Impact of Breast Cancer Screening and the Effect of a Negative Screening Result

Using the crude index of psychiatric morbidity, Aro, Pilvikki Absetz, van Elderen, van der Ploeg, and van der Kamp (2000) found no evidence that screened populations differ from unscreened populations. Similarly, women in receipt of a negative result do not appear to experience adverse effects, whether measured in terms of psychiatric morbidity (Dean, Roberts, French, & Robinson, 1986) or with specially tailored instruments such as the Psychological Consequences Questionnaire (PCQ), which assesses the emotional, social, and physical impact of mammography (Cockburn, Staples, Hurley, & De Luise, 1994). Intriguingly, distress may even be reduced below population levels in women with negative findings, implying a beneficial emotional effect (Scaf-Klomp, Sanderman, van de Wiel, Otter, & van den Heuvel, 1997).

A major concern about all forms of screening is that negative results could lead to false reassurance, which could result in delay in presentation of any subsequent symptoms. Ramirez et al.'s (1999) review of this area concluded that there was insufficient evidence to judge whether there was a relationship between false negative results and delay in presentation, and little seems to have been published in the intervening years. More research is therefore needed to clarify this issue.

The Psychological Impact of False Positive Results

A *false positive* mammogram denotes a result that triggers recall for further investigations that ultimately do not result in a diagnosis of cancer. As previously noted, women may be recalled for a number of reasons, and therefore the information they are given about the likelihood of malignancy will almost certainly vary accordingly. They will also experience different lengths of delay before cancer is excluded.

Being recalled for further investigation of suspicious findings at mammography is remembered as an extremely stressful experience, even several years after the event (Schwartz, Woloshin, Fowler, & Welch, 2004). It raises anxiety at the time of the recall, with approximately half of women with suspicious mammograms reporting borderline or clinically significant anxiety (Lampic, Thurfjell, Bergh, & Sjoden, 2001). Transient anxiety would be expected, but there has been concern over whether anxiety levels return to normal once women are given a clear outcome. Although most of the research findings are reassuring when general measures of anxiety and psychiatric morbidity are used (Brett, Bankhead, Henderson, Watson, & Austoker, 2005;

Cockburn et al., 1994; Lampic et al., 2001), cancer-specific worries, including perceived personal risk for getting breast cancer, appear to remain raised for some time after a false positive result (Absetz, Aro, & Sutton, 2003; Aro et al., 2000; Brett & Austoker, 2001). For example, Gram, Lund, and Slenker (1990) found that more women in the false positive group were anxious about breast cancer 6 months after screening compared with women with negative results, those never invited for screening, or those who had been invited to screening but failed to attend. This adverse effect on cancer-specific worry has also been shown to persist for up to 3 years (Brett & Austoker, 2001).

However, evidence also suggests positive emotional effects following false positive results. Lampic et al. (2001) found lower depression scores among women who had received false positive results compared with clear results, both 3 and 12 months after attending for recall, with no differences in anxiety. They suggested that this could be a relief effect, although they noted that the differences between the two groups, although significant, were small.

The relationship between negative psychological consequences and the degree of mammographic suspicion has received limited attention, but the available research suggests an association. In a British study, worry about cancer was found to be greater among women requiring fine needle aspiration and surgical biopsy compared with a repeat mammogram or clinical breast examination (Ong & Austoker, 1997). Five months later, worries remained higher in women put on early recall or who had been given an open biopsy—that is, those with the highest levels of mammographic suspicion (Brett, Austoker, & Ong, 1998).

The differing results across studies of the long-term psychological impact of mammography appear to stem from assessing different aspects of psychological well-being. Measures of overall emotional distress tend to give reassuring findings, whereas measures of specific worries about cancer suggest a more protracted effect. This indicates either that specific concerns about cancer do not affect overall emotional well-being or that generic measures lack the specificity needed to detect adverse effects (Brodersen, Thorsen, & Cockburn, 2004). The degree of specificity required to assess impact may be quite high. Even the Psychological Consequences Questionnaire—which was developed to assess the impact of mammography—has been judged inadequate as a measure of the impact of abnormal mammograms. Consequently, a questionnaire that specifically assesses the latter has recently been developed (Brodersen, Thorsen, & Kreiner, 2007).

Impact of False Positive Screening Outcomes on Reattendance

In their review of the psychosocial effects of abnormal breast and cervical screening results, Paskett and Rimer (1995) raised the possibility that negative emotional effects may lead to a failure to comply with the follow-up and treatment of abnormalities or to reattend for subsequent screening rounds. There could also be a positive impact, because increases in cancer worry as a consequence of a false positive result might facilitate screening participation. A meta-analysis of prospective data showed that greater breast cancer worry was associated with a stronger likelihood of attending for mammography, indicating that worry facilitated, rather than inhibited, attendance (Hay, McCaul, & Magnan, 2006). However, research findings on the impact of abnormal mammograms on reattendance have been mixed. Studies with the strongest methodology—those using population samples, following up all participants initially identified, and using objective measures of screening outcome and attendance (from screening records)—have found either no association (O'Sullivan, Sutton, Dixon, & Perry, 2001) or higher reattendance among women with a false positive result (Pinckney, Geller, Burman, & Littenberg, 2003).

A recent meta-analysis of the effect of false positives on reattendance at breast screening suggests that inconsistent findings may be due to differences in geographic region (Brewer, Salz, & Lillie, 2007). This article showed that a false positive increased the chance of reattendance in the United States, led to a decrease in reattendance in Canada, but had no effect on reattendance in Europe. One possible explanation for the regional variation is that certain provider characteristics, rather than the receipt of a false positive result per se, determine the impact on reattendance. Differences in screening provision between the United States and Europe include the proportion of the population who get access to screening (higher in Europe), the proportion who experience a false positive mammogram (lower in Europe), and the interval between routine screens (longer in Europe; Miles, Cockburn, Smith, & Wardle, 2004). In their review of the impact of screening on health-promoting behaviors, Bankhead et al. (2003) suggested that the impact of false positives on reattendance at screening may reflect the length of time taken for diagnostic workup: When the workup takes longer, women may have a shorter time before their next invitation for routine screening and could be less likely to attend because it was perceived as unnecessary. However, that there are shorter intervals between screens in the United States yet higher rates of reattendance suggests this may not be the critical variable. Brewer et al. (2007) proposed that although the worry generated by a false positive may promote reattendance at mammography, if it causes a decrease in trust in the health care provider, this would have the reverse effect. The implication appears to be that a decrease in trust in health care might be more likely in public health care systems, although this variable has rarely been measured and this possibility remains to be explored.

The time taken to investigate abnormalities, and hence the speed with which people are informed of their abnormal result, could also be an important variable, although regional differences in this aspect of service delivery are harder to determine. Evidence to suggest this might be an important factor comes from a Canadian study of reattendance by Chiarelli et al. (2003), who found that false positives reduced reattendance in some centers but not in a screening center at which the screening service offered an integrated assessment service.

Interventions to Reduce Distress About Recalls

A number of intervention strategies to reduce distress at being recalled have been tried. One option is to raise women's awareness of the possibility of recall in advance, thereby normalizing the experience and giving some indication of the likely implications. Austoker and Ong (1994) found that women were less likely to be worried about recall if they had been warned about it in the initial appointment letter or leaflet. They also found that women reporting higher distress were more likely to express a desire for additional information about the reasons for recall, the length of the assessment appointment, and how to get more information. It is not surprising that the information they found most reassuring was that the majority of women recalled are found to have normal breasts.

Women themselves suggest that their anxiety could be reduced by cutting waiting times at all stages of the procedure (Ellman et al., 1989; Lampic et al., 2001). In a randomized controlled trial of the impact of a one-stop clinic that offered same-day reporting of diagnostic investigations, Dey et al. (2002) found that anxiety 24 hours after attendance was significantly lower in the one-stop group compared with a group attending a dedicated breast clinic where they did not receive an immediate diagnosis.

CERVICAL SCREENING

Cervical cancer screening currently relies on the cytological examination of a sample of cells from the cervix. Until recently, these were collected using the Pap test, but a new method known as liquid-based cytology has now been introduced. Although this test uses a similar procedure for collecting the cervical sample, the preparation of cells is different, resulting in a large reduction in inadequate results. The aim of cervical screening is to identify precancerous cell changes, classed as either low-grade squamous intraepithelial lesions (L-SIL) or high-grade squamous intraepithelial lesions (H-SIL). L-SIL may regress without treatment, and H-SIL can be treated successfully through excision or ablation, thereby preventing the development of invasive cancer.

Recently, tests have been developed for the high-risk types of human papillomavirus (HPV) that are now accepted as the primary causal agents in the etiology of cervical cancer (Bosch, Lorincz, Munoz, Meijer, & Shah,

2002). Testing for HPV is currently recommended in the United States for the management of women with mildly abnormal Pap results and is being considered as a primary screening tool elsewhere (Cox & Cuzick, 2006).

Prophylactic vaccinations against the two most common high-risk HPV types have also been developed and have shown high levels of efficacy in young women (The Future II Study Group, 2007; Paavonen et al., 2007). Our review focuses on the psychological sequelae of cytological screening, but we discuss some implications of HPV testing and vaccination at the end of the section.

Overall Impact of Cervical Screening and Effect of a Negative Result

As in the breast cancer literature, relatively few studies assess the psychological impact of introducing screening programs for cervical cancer. One early, very small ($N = 17$) qualitative study found that the receipt of a screening invitation was taken by some women as an indication that they had cancer and induced serious anxiety (Nathoo, 1988). However, no larger studies have tried to confirm this finding, and it could have been associated with the introduction of a new and unfamiliar screening technology. The overall psychological impact of an established cervical screening program is therefore unknown, although women's enthusiasm for the service indicates a favorable attitude.

Most women get a negative result at Pap screening, and the limited evidence available suggests that this has a beneficial effect. Women receiving a negative result have reported more positive feelings about their fertility, health, and cervical cancer risk than women receiving abnormal results (Wardle, Pernet, & Stephens, 1995). However, no studies have compared the psychological well-being of women receiving a negative Pap smear result with that of women who have not attended screening.

Psychological Impact of Positive Screening Results

Approximately 7% of women are recalled after a Pap test because an abnormality is detected (Wright, Cox, Massad, Twiggs, & Wilkinson, 2002). Women with H-SIL are invited for further investigation by colposcopy and may be offered one of a range of excision and ablation treatments to remove the affected cells. Management strategies vary for women with borderline or mild abnormalities, who are sometimes invited for immediate colposcopy or else given a shorter repeat Pap test interval (i.e., cytological surveillance).

Anxiety levels do not seem to be related to the seriousness of the initial screening result (Rogstad, 2002), although they may be affected by the recommended follow-up. Among women with mildly abnormal Pap results, those invited for colposcopy were found to be more anxious than those recommended to attend for a repeat Pap (Wardle et al., 1995). And overall, the anxiety scores of women awaiting colposcopy have been found to be elevated beyond those found in women awaiting surgery (Marteau, Kidd, & Cuddeford, 1996) and are exacerbated in women who have waited a long time for their result (Wardle et al., 1995). Although anxiety usually decreases immediately after colposcopy, it is unclear whether it returns to prescreening levels. One study found that anxiety remained raised in at least one fifth of women 1 week after colposcopy (Bell et al., 1995), but it is unclear how many of the women in this study were awaiting treatment when anxiety was assessed. In a study of longer term impact, Idestrӧm, Milsom, and Andersson-Ellstrӧm (2003) surveyed women 5 years after receiving two consecutive abnormal Pap results and a referral to colposcopy. They found no evidence of any residual anxiety, but it should be noted that the study did not use validated measures. Anxiety has also been shown to be sustained in women who are managed by cytological surveillance (Peters, Somerset, Baxter, & Wilkinson, 1999), although other studies have found that women receiving a Pap result recommending surveillance are less anxious than those referred for colposcopy (Jones, Singer, & Jenkins, 1996; Wardle et al., 1995).

Some evidence indicates that women with mildly abnormal results prefer immediate colposcopy over cytological surveillance (Jones et al., 1996). However, in a recent randomized trial testing the effect on psychological outcomes of giving women with mildly abnormal Pap results a choice of management, Kitchener et al. (2004) found that similar numbers of women chose colposcopy (56%) and surveillance (44%). The two groups showed an almost identical reduction in General Health Questionnaire (GHQ; Goldberg & Hillier, 1979) scores over 12 months. Those who opted for colposcopy tended to have higher anxiety at baseline, indicating that this might be a more appropriate management strategy for more anxious women. However, no evidence indicated that having a choice of management conferred better psychological outcomes or increased adherence to follow-up.

Women who are more anxious following a mildly abnormal Pap result are less likely to attend for follow-up (Kitchener et al., 2004), and noncompliance with colposcopy has been associated with prolonged anxiety, possibly because uncertainties about the initial abnormal result remain (Lerman et al., 1991). There is therefore a possibility that distress and nonattendance may be mutually reinforcing.

In addition to measuring generalized anxiety, studies have also measured screening-specific concerns. Women receiving an abnormal result report a number of areas of concern: medical procedures (including embarrassment and discomfort), beliefs or feelings about cervical cancer and changes to perception of self, worry about infectivity, and effect on sexual relationships and reproductive health (Bennetts et al., 1995; Shinn et al., 2004; Wardle et al., 1995; see also Rogstad, 2002, for a review). These sorts of worries have been found even among women who show no increase in generalized anxiety

(Wardle et al., 1995) and may be longer lasting than any increases in general anxiety (Ideström et al., 2003).

Impact of Positive Screening Outcomes on Reattendance and Other Health Behaviors

A systematic review of the impact of screening on health behaviors found that attendance at cervical screening was associated with higher attendance for subsequent screening and engagement in other health-promoting behaviors (Bankhead et al., 2003), but this may reflect the characteristics of the population who attend for screening. There seems to be a dearth of studies investigating the impact of an abnormal result on reattendance or on other health behaviors. The most obvious behavior of interest is smoking, because women who smoke are at greater risk for L-SIL, H-SIL, and cancer, and smoking cessation promotes regression of cervical lesions (Szarewski et al., 1996). Although attendance at cervical screening has been identified as a teachable moment, when women could be given smoking cessation advice, only one intervention study (McBride et al., 1999) has been carried out. The intervention had no effect, and the authors did not provide information about whether women with abnormal Pap smear results were more likely to quit. This is an important area for future research.

Compliance with recommended follow-up after an abnormal result is another concern. A recent review of this area has shown a variety of strategies, such as reminder letters, may help but that telephone counseling that addresses barriers to screening appears to be particularly effective (Bastani, Yabroff, Myers, & Glenn, 2004).

Interventions to Reduce Negative Psychological Impact of Abnormal Results

Given the immediate negative psychological impact of an abnormal result, and the large numbers of women who are affected, developing interventions to reduce confusion and anxiety has been an important focus of research. Many women express the need for more information about the meaning of the result and about what to expect at colposcopy, so educational interventions have been the most common. Wilkinson, Jones, and McBride (1990) found that an information leaflet sent with a personalized results letter reduced women's anxiety prior to medical consultation, although this made no difference to postconsultation anxiety levels. Freeman-Wang et al. (2001) found that women who were shown an educational video were significantly less anxious than those given only a leaflet prior to their see-and-treat colposcopy appointment. The efficacy of video over written information has been supported by another study (Greimel, Gappmayer-Locker, Girardi, &

Huber, 1997). A short booklet has been shown to be more effective than a leaflet in reducing anxiety, although a longer booklet was more effective at increasing knowledge (Marteau et al., 1996). Other studies have confirmed that increasing knowledge does not necessarily reduce anxiety (Somerset & Peters, 1998; Tomaino-Brunner, Freda, Damus, & Runowicz, 1998). However, there have also been negative findings, with one study finding that a leaflet showed no benefit (Howells et al., 1999) and others finding that counseling did not achieve any reduction in anxiety (Richardson et al., 1996; Wolfe, Doherty, Raju, Holtom, & Richardson, 1992).

One problem with information is whether it successfully provides what women want. A recent review of colposcopy leaflets in the United Kingdom found that many do not contain the key pieces of information that women want to receive (e.g., information about the cervix and the meaning of abnormal Pap test results, practical information about colposcopy, treatment and follow-up, time interval until test results, and the impact on future fertility; Byrom et al., 2003). Anxiety among women under cytological surveillance for mild abnormalities (i.e., not referred for immediate colposcopy) has also been examined, and one study developed an intervention for such women, again with no success, and anxiety remained high over the course of the study (Peters et al., 1999). The variability of these results may be related to the time at which they were carried out, the service context in which they were delivered, or the measures of outcome, but they highlight the need for a better framework within which to develop and test interventions.

Human Papillomavirus Testing and Vaccination

The introduction of HPV screening, either for the triage of women with borderline or mildly abnormal Pap results, on the one hand, or as a method of primary screening, on the other, may alter the psychological sequelae associated with cervical cancer screening. HPV is a sexually transmitted infection (STI) and, as such, has the potential to influence the meaning and emotional impact of an abnormal Pap result, once its causal role in the development of L-SIL and H-SIL is more widely understood.

Studies of other STIs have found that diagnosis is associated with feelings of stigma, shame, guilt, and anger (e.g., Gilmore & Somerville, 1994). Qualitative work that elicited women's responses to information about HPV and its link with cervical cancer found that participants were shocked and surprised to find that cervical abnormalities are caused by an STI. Although women were in favor of a test that could detect abnormalities at an early stage, they predicted that a positive result would be associated with feelings of anxiety, anger, and distress and would raise questions about who the infection came from (McCaffery et al., 2003). In another study, participants who were informed about the sexually transmitted nature of HPV reported greater anticipated stigma, shame, and anxiety when asked to imagine that they had tested positive for it (Waller, Marlow, & Wardle, 2007). These are issues that are rarely reported in the literature on Pap testing, and it is vital that the psychological impact of HPV testing is carefully monitored as it is introduced.

HPV vaccination is recommended for girls ages 11 to 12, with a catch-up campaign for women up to 26 years old (Kuehn, 2006). The vaccination protects against the two most common strains of HPV, which cause around 70% of cervical cancers. Cervical screening will still be necessary to detect L-SIL and H-SIL caused by the remaining high-risk HPV types, but once the vaccinated cohort reach screening age, there is expected to be a significant decrease in cervical abnormalities and the psychological consequences that accompany them.

What has been established is that knowledge of HPV is poor, with well under half of adults having heard of it (Tiro, Meissner, Kobrin, & Chollette, 2007). This lack of knowledge is likely to augment the anxiety and confusion experienced by women taking part in a screening program that is already fraught with confusing and poorly understood terminology (Wilkinson, Jones, & McBride, 1990).

COLORECTAL CANCER SCREENING

Several different techniques are in use for colorectal cancer (CRC) screening. FOBTs examine stool samples for blood loss, which can be an indication of cancer. Flexible sigmoidoscopy (FS) involves visual inspection of the distal bowel for bowel polyps and cancers. Colonoscopy is a more invasive examination that visualizes the whole bowel, and double-contrast barium enema enables X-rays of the bowel to be taken. These technologies have been available for many years but have only relatively recently been promoted vigorously, and many countries have only just introduced them, so research into the impact of CRC screening is therefore scant.

Overall Impact of Screening

One of the few studies of the impact of publicity about cancer screening was carried out in the context of FS screening. Publicity about screening appeared to be reassuring rather than alarming, with the group sent publicity about new CRC screening reporting less worry and lower subjective risk than the uninformed group, although the former did report a greater number of bowel symptoms (Wardle, Taylor, Sutton, & Atkin, 1999).

Little work has been conducted on worry associated with receiving an invitation to attend CRC screening. Although one study found that 10% to 20% of people reported severe worry on receipt of an invitation for FOBT screening (Lindholm, Berglund, Kewenter, & Haglind, 1997), the absence of preinvitation measures of worry and the lack of a control group make it difficult to assess whether such levels are significant.

To date, studies assessing the overall psychological impact of screening attendance have shown no adverse effects for FOBT, FS, or colonoscopy. As part of a large randomized controlled trial into the efficacy of screening using FOBT in the United Kingdom, psychiatric morbidity was assessed before and after screening and was found to be unchanged, although there was no unscreened control group (Parker, Robinson, Scholefield, & Hardcastle, 2002). In a comparison of screening attenders with age- and sex-matched control participants in Norway, there was no evidence of adverse effects of screening using FS up to 17 months after screening (Thiis-Evensen, Wilhelmsen, Hoff, Blomhoff, & Sauar, 1999). In a small Australian study into the impact of colonoscopy screening among average risk members of the population, health-related quality of life was assessed prior to colonoscopy and an average of 36 days after the procedure using the Medical Outcomes Study Short Form—36 (SF–36; Stewart, Hays, & Ware, 1988; Ware & Sherbourne, 1992). Prescreening quality-of-life scores did not significantly differ from population norms. Changes from before to after colonoscopy have shown clinically significant improvements in mental health, role limitations because of emotions, and vitality, although the absence of an unscreened control group limited the conclusion (Taupin, Chambers, Corbett, & Shadbolt, 2006).

However, the issue of content specificity of measures needs to be considered. In a qualitative study as part of the prostate, lung, colon, and ovarian screening study, McGovern et al. (2004) found health distress, fear of cancer, and death all emerged as concerns among people who had participated in screening, and they pointed out that these issues are rarely measured in generic health-related quality-of-life measures, such as the SF–36.

Approximately 75% of people attending for FS and 95% to 99% of those using FOBT in their prevalent (i.e., first) screen will have a negative result (Atkin et al., 2002; Levin, 2001). The impact of a negative result on perceived personal risk and complacency about health behaviors, such as diet, exercise, and smoking, has been highlighted as an important issue. Two studies have examined this, both finding broadly reassuring results. A report from the Telemark Study observed poorer improvements in smoking behavior and a greater increase in body mass index in the group who had a negative FS screening result compared with those who had polyps detected, but neither effect was statistically significant (Hoff et al., 2001). Similarly, no deterioration in the practice of a number of health behaviors was found following negative results in the UK FS Trial (Miles, Wardle, McCaffery, Williamson, & Atkin, 2003). However, in the latter study, the results letters emphasized the need to maintain a healthy lifestyle, which could have attenuated any negative impact. A more recent study, again from Norway, did find evidence for a certificate of health effect among people invited to attend for FS screening in comparison with an unscreened control group (Larsen, Grotmol, Almendingen, & Hoff, 2007). The screen-invited group reported greater weight gain 3 years later and smaller improvements in smoking, exercise, and fruit and vegetable consumption than the unscreened control group. The authors pointed to the need for patient education at screening to attenuate any complacency that might accompany the experience of colorectal screening.

One early study gave some concern that a negative FOBT could result in false reassurance, finding that patients having a negative test were less likely to say that they would see their doctor if they were to suffer rectal bleeding in the future (Mant et al., 1990). This worrying observation could be specific to the trial in which it was found, but it indicates that further research is needed in this area.

Psychological Impact of False Positive Fecal Occult Blood Test Results

Two studies have examined anxiety and worry among people with a positive FOBT result, although neither had a negative comparison group. As part of a randomized controlled trial in the United Kingdom, Parker et al. (2002) asked 100 people with false positive results to complete measures of anxiety at various points from arrival at the assessment clinic following notification of a positive FOBT result to 1 month after the results were known. Those testing positive were recalled for further assessment, including a digital rectal examination and rigid sigmoidoscopy, and were sent for colonoscopy 1 to 2 weeks later. Anxiety was highest after notification of a positive test and just before colonoscopy but fell the day after colonoscopy and remained low 1 month later, leading to the conclusion that receipt of a false positive FOBT screening test did not cause sustained anxiety. Differences between the false positive and negative groups on GHQ scores were not reported (Parker et al., 2002). Similar results were found in a retrospective study using a questionnaire and structured telephone interview to assess the impact of FOBT screening in Sweden. Worry was assessed on receipt of the invitation, on receipt of the screening result, and 1 year later. Sixty percent of people with false positive results reported severe worry following receipt of the initial positive result, but this decreased to 24% following a subsequent negative test (Lindholm et al., 1997).

One study that compared distress in patients receiving false positive and negative results found that 22% of false positive patients reported having been "quite" or "very" worried that their positive test may mean that they had cancer; 70% suspected the test might be a false alarm (Mant et al., 1990). However, the false positive and negative groups did not differ in terms of perceptions of whether the FOBT test was worthwhile.

Psychological Impact of Positive Screening Results in Flexible Sigmoidoscopy

FS screening aims to detect and remove adenomatous polyps. In the UK FS Trial, individuals found to have "higher risk" (i.e., either large or numerous) polyps were referred for colonoscopy, whereas those with "lower risk" polyps had their polyps removed during the sigmoidoscopy and were discharged. No adverse effects were found among people who had polyps detected compared with those with negative results using measures of general anxiety or bowel cancer worry, regardless of whether they had been sent for a colonoscopy (Wardle et al., 2003). In a study in Norway, people with polyps detected did not differ from those with no polyps detected on measures of anxiety, depression, and general well-being, either immediately after screening or 17 months postscreening (Thiis-Evensen et al., 1999). The one exception was slightly poorer levels of reported well-being among those with polyps at 3 months, although there was no difference between the groups at 17 months. The authors suggested that the reassuring results may be attributed to the clinicians' efforts to explain the significance of polyps, which attenuated any negative impact. No short-term impact on quality of life was observed as a result of the detection of adenomatous polyps as part of colonoscopy screening, although the sample size in this study was small ($N = 231$; Taupin et al., 2006).

Interventions to Reduce Negative Psychological Impact of Abnormal Results

Testing positive on an FOBT or at FS may lead to referral for colonoscopy, which can also be a source of anxiety. A number of U.S. studies have examined the impact of patient information, and the results suggest that providing additional information can increase knowledge of the procedure, although effects on anxiety have been mixed (Luck, Pearson, Maddern, & Hewett, 1999; Shaw, Beebe, Tomshine, Adlis, & Cass, 2001). The content of such materials will be critical in determining effects on anxiety, and further research is needed to identify the specific content that patients find reassuring and to establish whether there is any benefit in tailoring the information to people's information-processing style.

CONCLUSIONS AND FUTURE DIRECTIONS

The development of screening tests for early cancers or precancers has been one of the great advances against cancer. But at the same time, screening has the potential to cause distress by bringing people face to face with this much-feared disease. To determine the public health gain, the psychological costs of participating in screening for healthy adults, which may involve further investigations, have to be weighed against the life years saved for those with positive results. Fortunately, the results summarized in this review provide no evidence that participating in breast, cervical, or colorectal cancer screening has serious or long-term adverse psychological consequences. In addition, there is overwhelming public enthusiasm for screening, even among those who have experienced abnormal results (Schwartz et al., 2004).

In the short term, recall for further testing raises both cancer-related worry and general anxiety. Some degree of anxiety is inevitable, but it should be possible to minimize this through providing high-quality information both at the time of screening and along with the results. Shorter waiting times also help, and one-stop clinics that offer same-day reporting of diagnostic investigations are a good way of achieving this.

False positive results in mammography or FOBT screening do not appear to lead to long-term mood disturbances, but at least in the context of breast screening, cancer-specific worries and concerns can persist for months and possibly years. Although worries about cancer do not necessarily lead to generalized mood disturbances such as anxiety or depression, more work is needed to document the extent to which these worries impact daily life.

The opposite kind of emotional impact—a positive effect on mood—has rarely been investigated, although there are hints from some findings of lower-than-normal levels of anxiety among those with a clear result. Future research might profitably include some measures of screening benefits and of positive well-being to complement the emphasis on adverse effects.

The possibility that future use of screening services, responses to signs of an interval cancer, or practice of healthy behaviors might be compromised by either positive or negative screening findings has often been raised. One important behavior in the screening context is reattendance, because many forms of screening require not just a single test but repeated attendance on a regular basis. Further research is needed on the impact of false positive results on reattendance at screening, because existing findings have been mixed and vary regionally. However, at its worst, the impact appears to be small. If there is an adverse effect, then it is likely that improvements in the way that the mammography recall is handled could improve the situation. In addition, little work has been conducted on the impact of mammography screening on other health-promoting behaviors, such as diet and exercise (cf. Absetz et al., 2003), and more research could be done in this area.

Early detection tests can miss cancers, and new cancers can develop between tests (so-called interval cancers), so it is vital that a clear screening result does not inhibit subsequent recognition of early signs of cancer. The issue of false reassurance from a negative screening result has been extended to other health behaviors, with concerns that people might interpret a negative screening result as evidence that their poor health behaviors have not been detrimental and may be continued. The idea of screening participation as a teachable moment—either at the point of screening or when the results are given—has often been put forward. Few studies have tested this directly, but there are positive results (Baker & Wardle, 2002), suggesting that opportunities to enhance cancer prevention through behavior change are being missed.

Detecting premalignancy at screening is a desirable outcome from the point of view of the screening provider but raises questions about whether psychological interventions could be developed to reduce the adverse emotional impact. In the case of cervical screening, some evidence indicates that when follow-up is recommended, very anxious women should be offered immediate colposcopy rather than being monitored. Again, aspects of service delivery need to be examined to see whether they can be modified to help reduce anxiety. Attention also needs to be paid to the information given to women during screening and follow-up. Some individuals may be unclear what testing positive for premalignant conditions, such as cervical neoplasia or adenomatous polyps, actually means. Believing that one has been diagnosed with cancer rather than a precancerous condition is far more distressing, and the prevalence of such erroneous beliefs should be explored. Testing for HPV, particularly if it is introduced in primary screening, will identify women who are at increased risk for cervical cancer but who have not been treated because no lesions have developed. The risk status of these women is unclear, and the psychological impact of what might be long-term monitoring needs to be evaluated. More research is needed, particularly in the area of cervical screening, to find effective interventions to reduce distress associated with receipt of a positive result. In addition, the impact of a positive result on perceptions of future risk for cervical cancer remains to be explored.

False negatives might be important but have received little attention. Petticrew, Sowden, and Lister-Sharp's (2001) review of the psychological consequences of false negatives found that research was exclusively in the domain of antenatal screening, with no studies on cancer screening, and nothing appears to have been published since. Publicity surrounding false negatives on attitudes toward screening has been examined and results suggest that although awareness of false negatives undermines women's confidence in the screening program, intentions to have a Pap test in the future are unchanged (Houston, Lloyd, Drysdale, & Farmer, 2001), but more research on this issue is needed.

One underresearched issue is the moderating effect of environmental factors. For example, in a screening service with poor-quality staff, minimal information provision, no integration between screening and follow-up care, and a long wait for results, recall for further investigation is likely to cause more distress than in a dedicated service in which the staff are experienced at dealing with all possible screening outcomes. Tailoring information to the educational level and attentional style of its recipients is feasible now that computer methods make this economically practical. Evidence that matching information improves attendance at screening (Williams-Piehota, Pizarro, Schneider, Mowad, & Salovey, 2005) points to the value of this approach. However, there may be important differences in the kinds of initiatives that are considered within organized compared with opportunistic screening systems. Organized systems look toward systems factors to promote a more positive screening experience, whereas opportunistic programs take a more person-centered approach, modifying the service according to the coping abilities or understanding of each individual.

Public understanding of screening is an important issue. Breast and cervical screening have been offered for many years, and the public has grown familiar with them, including the fact that screening generates a certain number of false positive results (Schwartz et al., 2004). If people are aware that a recall is a fairly common event and most likely does not denote cancer, then they should be less upset than when the process was less well understood. In Great Britain in the 1980s, many women seemed to think that an abnormal Pap smear result meant that they had cancer (Posner & Vessey, 1988), but results appear to be better understood now. The implication of this is that findings from one screening service or one time period do not necessarily give a valid indication of the psychological impact of screening in another time or place.

In recent years, there has been a move away from the traditional public health model of screening, for which high uptake is the primary goal, toward a model of informed participation. Increasingly, individuals are being encouraged to make an informed choice about whether to undergo screening tests, on the basis of information about the costs and benefits involved (Raffle, 2001). Making information about the test and its possible outcomes explicit before participation could reduce the likelihood of misunderstanding and anxiety following results. However, it is also possible that the decision-making process would be associated with psychological sequelae that have not hitherto been investigated or that a greater public understanding of the inherent inaccuracies of screening might lead to an increase in population worry about cancer. These issues highlight the need for ongoing research to track differences in the psychological impact of screening across settings and over time.

REFERENCES

Absetz, P., Aro, A. R., & Sutton, S. R. (2003). Experience with breast cancer, pre-screening perceived susceptibility, and the psychological impact of screening. *Psycho-Oncology, 12*, 305–318.

Andrykowski, M. A., Carpenter, J. S., Studts, J. L., Cordova, M. J., Cunningham, L. L., Beacham, A., et al. (2002). Psychological impact of benign breast biopsy: A longitudinal, comparative study. *Health Psychology, 21*, 485–494.

Aro, A. R., Pilvikki Absetz, S., van Elderen, T. M., van der Ploeg, E., & van der Kamp, L. J. (2000). False-positive findings in mammography screening induces short-term distress—Breast cancer-specific concern prevails longer. *European Journal of Cancer, 36,* 1089–1097.

Atkin, W. S., Cooke, L., Cuzick, J., Edwards, R., Northover, J. M. A., & Wardle, J. (2002). Single flexible sigmoidoscopy screening to prevent colorectal cancer: Baseline findings of a UK multicentre randomised trial. *Lancet, 359,* 1291–3000.

Austoker, J., & Ong, G. (1994). Written information needs of women who are recalled for further investigation of breast screening: Results of a multicentre study. *Journal of Medical Screening, 1,* 238–244.

Baker, A. H., & Wardle, J. (2002). Increasing fruit and vegetable intake among adults attending colorectal cancer screening: The efficacy of a brief tailored intervention. *Cancer Epidemiology, Biomarkers & Prevention, 11,* 203–206.

Bankhead, C. R., Brett, J., Bukach, C., Webster, P., Stewart-Brown, S., Munafo, M., & Austoker, J. (2003). The impact of screening on future health-promoting behaviours and health beliefs: A systematic review. *Health Technology Assessments, 7,* 1–92.

Bastani, R., Yabroff, K. R., Myers, R. E., & Glenn, B. (2004). Interventions to improve follow-up of abnormal findings in cancer screening. *Cancer, 101,* 1188–1200.

Bell, S., Porter, M., Kitchener, H., Fraser, C., Fisher, P., & Mann, E. (1995). Psychological response to cervical screening. *Preventive Medicine, 24,* 610–616.

Bennetts, A., Irwig, L., Oldenburg, B., Simpson, J. M., Mock, P., Boyes, A., et al. (1995). PEAPS-Q: A questionnaire to measure the psychosocial effects of having an abnormal Pap smear. *Journal of Clinical Epidemiology, 48,* 1235–1243.

Bosch, F. X., Lorincz, A., Munoz, N., Meijer, C. J., & Shah, K. V. (2002). The causal relation between human papillomavirus and cervical cancer. *Journal of Clinical Pathology, 55,* 244–265.

Brett, J., & Austoker, J. (2001). Women who are recalled for further investigation for breast screening: Psychological consequences 3 years after recall and factors affecting re-attendance. *Journal of Public Health Medicine, 23,* 292–300.

Brett, J., Austoker, J., & Ong, G. (1998). Do women who undergo further investigation for breast screening suffer adverse psychological consequences? A multicentre follow-up study comparing different breast screening result groups five months after their last breast screening appointment. *Journal of Public Health Medicine, 20,* 396–403.

Brett, J., Bankhead, C., Henderson, B., Watson, E., & Austoker, J. (2005). The psychological impact of mammographic screening: A systematic review. *Psycho-Oncology, 14,* 917–938.

Brewer, N. T., Salz, T., & Lillie, S. E. (2007). Systematic review: The long-term effects of false-positive mammograms. *Annals of Internal Medicine, 146,* 502–510.

Brodersen, J., Thorsen, H., & Cockburn, J. (2004). The adequacy of measurement of short and long-term consequences of false-positive screening mammography. *Journal of Medical Screening, 11,* 39–44.

Brodersen, J., Thorsen, H., & Kreiner, S. (2007). Validation of a condition-specific measure for women having an abnormal screening mammography. *Value in Health, 10,* 294–304.

Byrom, J., Dunn, P. D., Hughes, G. M., Lockett, J., Johnson, A., Neale, J., & Redman, C. W. (2003). Colposcopy information leaflets: What women want to know and when they want to receive this information. *Journal of Medical Screening, 10,* 143–147.

Chiarelli, A. M., Moravan, V., Halapy, E., Majpruz, V., Mai, V., & Tatla, R. K. (2003). False-positive result and reattendance in the Ontario Breast Screening Program. *Journal of Medical Screening, 10,* 129–133.

Cockburn, J., Staples, M., Hurley, S. F., & De Luise, T. (1994). Psychological consequences of screening mammography. *Journal of Medical Screening, 1,* 7–12.

Cox, T., & Cuzick, J. (2006). HPV DNA testing in cervical cancer screening: From evidence to policies. *Gynecologic Oncology, 103,* 8–11.

Dean, C., Roberts, M. M., French, K., & Robinson, S. (1986). Psychiatric morbidity after screening for breast cancer. *Journal of Epidemiology and Community Health, 40,* 71–75.

Dey, P., Bundred, N., Gibbs, A., Hopwood, P., Baildam, A., Boggis, C., et al. (2002, March 2). Costs and benefits of a one stop clinic compared with a dedicated breast clinic: Randomised controlled trial. *BMJ, 324,* 507.

Ellman, R., Angeli, N., Christians, A., Moss, S., Chamberlain, J., & McGuire, P. (1989). Psychiatric morbidity associated with screening for breast cancer. *British Journal of Cancer, 60,* 781–784.

Freeman-Wang, T., Walker, P., Linehan, J., Coffey, C., Glasser, B., & Sherr, L. (2001). Anxiety levels in women attending colposcopy clinics for treatment for cervical intraepithelial neoplasia: A randomised trial of written and video information. *British Journal of Obstetrics and Gynaecology, 108,* 482–484.

The Future II Study Group. (2007). Quadrivalent vaccine against human papillomavirus to prevent high-grade cervical lesions. *New England Journal of Medicine, 356,* 1915–1927.

Gilmore, N., & Somerville, M. A. (1994). Stigmatization, scapegoating, and discrimination in sexually transmitted diseases: Overcoming "them" and "us." *Social Science & Medicine, 39,* 1339–1358.

Goldberg, D. P., & Hillier, V. F. (1979). A scaled version of the General Health Questionnaire. *Psychological Medicine, 9,* 139–145.

Gram, I. T., Lund, E., & Slenker, S. E. (1990). Quality of life following a false positive mammogram. *British Journal of Cancer, 62,* 1018–1022.

Greimel, E. R., Gappmayer-Locker, E., Girardi, F. L., & Huber, H. P. (1997). Increasing women's knowledge and satisfaction with cervical cancer screening. *Journal of Psychosomatic Obstetrics and Gynaecology, 18,* 273–279.

Hay, J. L., McCaul, K. D., & Magnan, R. E. (2006). Does worry about breast cancer predict screening behaviors? A meta-analysis of the prospective evidence. *Preventive Medicine, 42,* 401–408.

Hoff, G., Thiis-Evensen, E., Grotmol, T., Sauar, J., Vatn, M. H., & Moen, I. E. (2001). Do undesirable effects of screening affect all-cause mortality in flexible sigmoidoscopy programmes? Experience from the Telemark Polyp Study 1983–1996. *European Journal of Cancer Prevention, 10*, 131–137.

Houston, D. M., Lloyd, K., Drysdale, S., & Farmer, M. (2001). The benefits of uncertainty: Changes in women's perceptions of the cervical screening programme as a consequence of screening errors by Kent and Canterbury NHS Trust. *Psychology, Health & Medicine, 6*, 107–113.

Howells, R. E., Dunn, P. D., Isasi, T., Chenoy, R., Calvert, E., Jones, P. W., et al. (1999). Is the provision of information leaflets before colposcopy beneficial? A prospective randomised study. *British Journal of Obstetrics and Gynaecology, 106*, 528–534.

Ideström, M., Milsom, I., & Andersson-Ellström, A. (2003). Women's experience of coping with a positive Pap smear: A register-based study of women with two consecutive Pap smears reported as CIN 1. *Acta Obstetricia et Gynecologica Scandinavica, 82*, 756–761.

Jones, M. H., Singer, A., & Jenkins, D. (1996). The mildly abnormal cervical smear: Patient anxiety and choice of management. *Journal of the Royal Society of Medicine, 89*, 257–260.

Kitchener, H., Burns, S., Nelson, L., Myers, A., Fletcher, I., Desai, M., et al. (2004). A randomised controlled trial of cytological surveillance versus patient choice between surveillance and colposcopy in managing mildly abnormal cervical smears. *British Journal of Obstetrics and Gynaecology, 111*, 63–70.

Kuehn, B. M. (2006). CDC panel backs routine HPV vaccination. *Journal of the American Medical Association, 296*, 640–641.

Lampic, C., Thurfjell, E., Bergh, J., & Sjoden, P. O. (2001). Short- and long-term anxiety and depression in women recalled after breast cancer screening. *European Journal of Cancer, 37*, 463–469.

Larsen, I. K., Grotmol, T., Almendingen, K., & Hoff, G. (2007). Impact of colorectal cancer screening on future lifestyle choices: A three-year randomized controlled trial. *Clinical Gastroenterology and Hepatology, 5*, 477–483.

Lerman, C., Miller, S. M., Scarborough, R., Hanjani, P., Nolte, S., & Smith, D. (1991). Adverse psychologic consequences of positive cytologic cervical screening. *American Journal of Obstetrics and Gynecology, 165*, 658–662.

Levin, B. (2001). Overview of colorectal cancer screening in the United States. *Journal of Psychosocial Oncology, 19*, 9–19.

Lindholm, E., Berglund, B., Kewenter, J., & Haglind, E. (1997). Worry associated with screening for colorectal carcinomas. *Scandinavian Journal of Gastroenterology, 32*, 238–245.

Luck, A., Pearson, S., Maddern, G., & Hewett, P. (1999). Effects of video information on precolonoscopy anxiety and knowledge: A randomised trial. *Lancet, 354*, 2032–2035.

Mant, D., Fitzpatrick, R., Hogg, A., Fuller, A., Farmer, A., Verne, J., & Northover, J. (1990). Experiences of patients with false positive results from colorectal cancer screening. *British Journal of General Practice, 40*, 423–425.

Marteau, T. M., Kidd, J., & Cuddeford, L. (1996). Reducing anxiety in women referred for colposcopy using an information booklet. *British Journal of Health Psychology, 1,* 181–189.

McBride, C. M., Scholes, D., Grothaus, L. C., Curry, S. J., Ludman, E., & Albright, J. (1999). Evaluation of a minimal self-help smoking cessation intervention following cervical cancer screening. *Preventive Medicine, 29,* 133–138.

McCaffery, K. J., Forrest, S., Waller, J., Desai, M., Szarewski, A., & Wardle, J. (2003). Attitudes towards HPV testing: A qualitative study of beliefs among Indian, Pakistani, African Caribbean, and White British women in the UK. *British Journal of Cancer, 88,* 42–46.

McGovern, P. M., Gross, C. R., Krueger, R. A., Engelhard, D. A., Cordes, J. E., & Church, T. R. (2004). False-positive cancer screens and health-related quality of life. *Cancer Nursing, 27,* 347–352.

Miles, A., Cockburn, J., Smith, R. A., & Wardle, J. (2004). A perspective from countries using organized screening programs. *Cancer, 101,* 1201–1213.

Miles, A., Wardle, J., McCaffery, K., Williamson, S., & Atkin, W. (2003). The effects of colorectal cancer screening on health attitudes and practices. *Cancer Epidemiology, Biomarkers & Prevention, 12,* 651–655.

Miller, S. M., Fang, C. Y., Manne, S. L., Engstrom, P. F., & Daly, M. B. (1999). Decision making about prophylactic oophorectomy among at-risk women: Psychological influences and implications. *Gynecological Oncology, 75,* 406–412.

Miller, S. M., Shoda, Y., & Hurley, K. (1996). Applying cognitive-social theory to health-protective behavior: Breast self-examination in cancer screening. *Psychological Bulletin, 119,* 70–94.

Nathoo, V. (1988, April 9). Investigation of non-responders at a cervical cancer screening clinic in Manchester. *BMJ, 296,* 1041–1042.

Ong, G., & Austoker, J. (1997). Recalling women for further investigation of breast screening: Women's experiences at the clinic and afterwards. *Journal of Public Health Medicine, 19,* 29–36.

O'Sullivan, I., Sutton, S., Dixon, S., & Perry, N. (2001). False positive results do not have a negative effect on reattendance for subsequent breast screening. *Journal of Medical Screening, 8,* 145–148.

Paavonen, J., Jenkins, D., Bosch, F. X., Naud, P., Salmerón, J., Wheeler, C. M., et al. (2007). Efficacy of a prophylactic adjuvanted bivalent L1 virus-like-particle vaccine against infection with human papillomavirus Types 16 and 18 in young women: An interim analysis of a Phase III double-blind, randomised controlled trial. *Lancet, 369,* 2161–2170.

Parker, M. A., Robinson, M. H. E., Scholefield, J. H., & Hardcastle, J. D. (2002). Psychiatric morbidity and screening for colorectal cancer. *Journal of Medical Screening, 9,* 7–10.

Paskett, E. D., & Rimer, B. K. (1995). Psychosocial effects of abnormal Pap tests and mammograms: A review. *Journal of Women's Health, 4,* 73–82.

Peters, T., Somerset, M., Baxter, K., & Wilkinson, C. (1999). Anxiety among women with mild dyskaryosis: A randomized trial of an educational intervention. *British Journal of General Practice, 49*, 348–352.

Petticrew, M., Sowden, A., & Lister-Sharp, D. (2001). False-negative results in screening programs: Medical, psychological, and other implications. *International Journal of Technology Assessment in Health Care, 17*, 164–170.

Pinckney, R. G., Geller, B. M., Burman, M., & Littenberg, B. (2003). Effect of false-positive mammograms on return for subsequent screening mammography. *American Journal of Medicine, 114*, 120–125.

Posner, T., & Vessey, M. (1988). Psychosexual trauma of an abnormal cervical smear. *British Journal of Obstetrics and Gynaecology, 95*, 729.

Raffle, A. E. (2001). Information about screening—Is it to achieve high uptake or to ensure informed choice? *Health Expectations, 4*, 92–98.

Ramirez, A. J., Westcombe, A. M., Burgess, C. C., Sutton, S., Littlejohns, P., & Richards, M. A. (1999). Factors predicting delayed presentation of symptomatic breast cancer: A systematic review. *Lancet, 353*, 1127–1131.

Richardson, P. H., Doherty, I., Wolfe, C. D. A., Carman, N., Chamberlain, F., Holtom, R., & Raju, K. S. (1996). Evaluation of cognitive-behavioural counselling for the distress associated with an abnormal cervical smear result. *British Journal of Health Psychology, 1*, 327–338.

Rogstad, K. E. (2002). The psychological impact of abnormal cytology and colposcopy. *British Journal of Obstetrics and Gynaecology, 109*, 364–368.

Scaf-Klomp, W., Sanderman, R., van de Wiel, H. B., Otter, R., & van den Heuvel, W. J. (1997). Distressed or relieved? Psychological side effects of breast cancer screening in the Netherlands. *Journal of Epidemiology and Community Health, 51*, 705–710.

Schwartz, L. M., Woloshin, S., Fowler, F. J. J., & Welch, H. G. (2004). Enthusiasm for cancer screening in the United States. *Journal of the American Medical Association, 291*, 71–78.

Shaw, M. J., Beebe, T. J., Tomshine, P. A., Adlis, S. A., & Cass, O. W. (2001). A randomized, controlled trial of interactive, multimedia software for patient colonoscopy education. *Journal of Clinical Gastroenterology, 32*, 142–147.

Shinn, E., Basen-Engquist, K., Le, T., Hansis-Diarte, A., Bostic, D., Martinez-Cross, J., et al. (2004). Distress after an abnormal Pap smear result: Scale development and psychometric validation. *Preventive Medicine, 39*, 404–412.

Smith-Bindman, R., Chu, P. W., Miglioretti, D. L., Sickles, E. A., Blanks, R., Ballard-Barbash, R., et al. (2003). Comparison of screening mammography in the United States and the United Kingdom. *Journal of the American Medical Association, 290*, 2129–2137.

Somerset, M., & Peters, T. J. (1998). Intervening to reduce anxiety for women with mild dyskaryosis: Do we know what works and why? *Journal of Advanced Nursing, 28*, 563–570.

Stewart, A. L., Hays, R. D., & Ware, J. E., Jr. (1988). The MOS Short-Form General Health Survey: Reliability and validity in a patient population. *Medical Care, 26*, 724–735.

Szarewski, A., Jarvis, M. J., Sasieni, P., Anderson, M., Edwards, R., Steele, S. J., et al. (1996). Effect of smoking cessation on cervical lesion size. *Lancet, 347,* 941–943.

Taupin, D., Chambers, S. L., Corbett, M., & Shadbolt, B. (2006). Colonoscopic screening for colorectal cancer improves quality of life measures: A population-based screening study. *Health and Quality of Life Outcomes, 18,* 82–87.

Thiis-Evensen, E., Wilhelmsen, I., Hoff, G. S., Blomhoff, S., & Sauar, J. (1999). The psychologic effect of attending a screening program for colorectal polyps. *Scandinavian Journal of Gastroenterology, 34,* 103–109.

Tiro, J. A., Meissner, H. I., Kobrin, S., & Chollette, V. (2007). What do women in the U.S. know about human papillomavirus and cervical cancer? *Cancer Epidemiology, Biomarkers & Prevention, 16,* 288–294.

Tomaino-Brunner, C., Freda, M. C., Damus, K., & Runowicz, C. D. (1998). Can pre-colposcopy education increase knowledge and decrease anxiety? *Journal of Obstetric, Gynecologic, and Neonatal Nursing, 27,* 636–645.

Waller, J., Marlow, L. A. V., & Wardle, J. (2007). The association between knowledge of HPV and feelings of stigma, shame, and anxiety. *Sexually Transmitted Infections, 82,* 155–159.

Wardle, J., Pernet, A., & Stephens, D. (1995). Psychological consequences of positive results in cervical cancer screening. *Psychology and Health, 10,* 185–194.

Wardle, J., Taylor, T., Sutton, S., & Atkin, W. (1999, October 16). Does publicity about cancer screening raise fear of cancer? Randomised trial of the psychological effect of information about cancer screening. *BMJ, 319,* 1037–1038.

Wardle, J., Williamson, S., Sutton, S., Biran, A., Cuzick, J., & Atkin, W. (2003). Psychological impact of bowel cancer screening. *Health Psychology, 22,* 54–59.

Ware, J. E., Jr., & Sherbourne, C. D. (1992). The MOS 36-Item Short-Form health survey (SF–36): I. Conceptual framework and item selection. *Medical Care, 30,* 473–483.

Wilkinson, C., Jones, J. M., & McBride, J. (1990, February 17). Anxiety caused by abnormal result of cervical smear test: A controlled trial. *BMJ, 300,* 440.

Williams-Piehota, P., Pizarro, J., Schneider, T. R., Mowad, L., & Salovey, P. (2005). Matching health messages to monitor–blunter coping styles to motivate screening mammography. *Health Psychology, 24,* 58–67.

Wolfe, C., Doherty, I., Raju, K. S., Holtom, R., & Richardson, P. (1992). First steps in the development of an information and counselling service for women with an abnormal smear result. *European Journal of Obstetrics, Gynaecology, and Reproductive Biology, 45,* 201–206.

Wright, T. C., Jr., Cox, J. T., Massad, L. S., Twiggs, L. B., & Wilkinson, E. J. (2002). 2001 consensus guidelines for the management of women with cervical cytological abnormalities. *Journal of the American Medical Association, 287,* 2120–2129.

17

PSYCHOLOGICAL ISSUES IN GENETIC TESTING

CATHARINE WANG AND SUZANNE M. MILLER

In 2003, 50 years after the discovery of DNA's structure, scientists announced the completion of the human genome sequence. In honor of this landmark event, the vision for genomics research was presented in a report by Francis S. Collins and colleagues (F. S. Collins, Green, Guttmacher, & Guyer, 2003), in an effort to outline the implications and future directions of this area as it pertains not only to the biological and medical sciences but also to the social sciences. A major theme addressed in this report centers on the translation of genome-based knowledge into health benefits. Ultimately, the impact of the Human Genome Project on health will depend, in large part, on the extent to which genetic risk information is effectively communicated, so that it can be used to help people to make informed decisions about their surveillance, treatment, and preventive strategies, as well as their health behaviors.

To date, one of the best studied applications of the new genetic technologies has been in the area of hereditary cancer syndromes. Information about familial disease risk is typically conveyed during genetic counseling, with the goal of helping individuals make a high-quality decision about whether to undergo genetic testing; if they do decide to undergo testing, further counseling is required to help them make subsequent decisions about the appropriate preventive, management, and treatment options to pursue, given their mutational status and their personal preferences. The extent to which the use of genetic technologies is associated with beneficial effects for the individual thus hinges on a cascade of psychological reactions that range along a continuum, from the individual's response to, and comprehension of, the initial risk communication to the psychological issues that stem from being confronted by a sequence of complex decisions about one's health over the long term.

This chapter provides an overview of the psychological issues involved in genetic testing for hereditary cancer syndromes. These issues are organized around the evidence base in the following areas: (a) the psychosocial and background factors that predict genetic testing uptake; (b) the impact of genetic risk feedback on psychological responses, preventive and management decisions, and health behaviors; and (c) future directions, focusing on the design and evaluation of psychosocial interventions to facilitate information processing, decision making, and psychological and behavioral responses to genetic testing.

PREDICTORS OF GENETIC TESTING UPTAKE

Psychosocial Influences on Testing Decisions

Descriptive studies suggest that overall interest in and uptake of genetic testing is high but varies by the population studied. Testing rates for individuals from high-risk populations involved in genetic research studies have ranged from 55% to 93% (Biesecker et al., 2000; Evans, Maher, Macleod, Davies, & Craufurd, 1997; Lerman et al., 1996; Smith, West, Croyle, & Botkin, 1999). In contrast, studies with clinical populations, for which counseling and testing are often provided as a service, have documented lower range uptake rates: 18% to 58%. The lower rates observed in clinical settings may be attributed to the population being seen (i.e., individuals at lower risk for whom testing may not be appropriate) or the costs associated with testing, which can serve as a prohibitive barrier to uptake (Armstrong et al., 2000; S. Lee, Bernhardt, & Helzlsouer, 2002; E. A. Peterson, Milliron, Lewis, Goold, & Merajver, 2002).

Subjective reasons provided for undergoing genetic testing have been fairly consistent across cancer syndromes and center on such factors as (a) undergoing testing to make decisions about cancer treatment or prevention, (b) learning about one's cancer risk for a relative, and (c) reducing uncertainty about one's risk status (Hadley et al., 2003; Lerman, Seay, Balshem, & Audrain, 1995; Loader, Levenkron, & Rowley, 1998; Lynch et al., 1999). Reasons for declining testing are diverse and include practical concerns, such as fear of insurance discrimination, emotional impact on self and family, perceptions of inability to cope, and perceived absence of medical interventions. The cost of genetic testing is often identified as a reason for declining testing among those who are not offered the procedure free of charge as part of a research protocol.

Two individual difference factors—cognition and affect—appear to play an important role in genetic testing decisions (Miller, Shoda, & Hurley, 1996; Shoda et al., 1998). Several studies have identified two cognitive variables that consistently predict decisions to undergo genetic testing, notably higher perceived risk for cancer and greater perceived benefits of testing (Bosompra et al., 2000; Jacobsen, Valdimarsdottir, Brown, & Offit, 1997). Other studies have found that greater knowledge of testing and confidence in one's ability to cope with the test results are also associated with greater testing uptake (Codori et al., 1999; Lerman et al., 1996).

The role of affect has also been shown to be important in influencing testing decisions (Cameron & Reeve, 2006; Codori et al., 1999; Diefenbach, Schnoll, Miller, & Brower, 2000; Lerman, Schwartz, et al., 1997; Wang, Gonzalez, Janz, Milliron, & Merajver, 2007). For example, in a study of women from high-risk families, Lerman et al. (1997) found that cancer-specific distress predicted genetic testing to identify mutations on the BRCA1 and BRCA2 genes, which predispose women to hereditary breast and ovarian cancers. However, affect may also be significant because it influences other factors important in genetic testing decisions. For example, several studies suggest that a primary role of affect is as a moderator of the relationship between perceived risk and testing decisions (Codori et al., 1999; Shiloh & Ilan, 2005). Thus, the effect of perceived risk on test uptake depends on how worried or distressed the individual is about developing cancer or being a mutation carrier.

Apart from cognitions and affect, certain values and goals that impact the meaning of the situation for the individual, such as spiritual faith and religious identity, have been identified as important in testing decisions. For example, the greater the individual's spiritual faith or religious identity, the lower the interest in and uptake of genetic testing (Bowen, Singal, Eng, Crystal, & Burke, 2003; Schwartz et al., 2000). Results of qualitative studies are consistent with these findings (Harris, Parrott, & Dorgan, 2004). Thus, individuals with stronger religious or spiritual faith appear to be deterred from testing, but the reasons are not yet well understood.

Interpersonal and Demographic Influences on Testing Decisions

Interpersonal and demographic factors that have been associated with decisions to undergo genetic testing include familial structure, race, and ethnicity. Because genetic information is based in a familial context, it is not surprising that interpersonal factors are associated with genetic testing decisions. For example, the type of family structure appears to influence testing decisions. Those individuals who report greater cohesiveness or closeness in the family are more likely to undergo BRCA1 and BRCA2 genetic testing (Biesecker et al., 2000; Loader et al., 1998). Family support has also been associated with greater intentions and uptake of genetic testing (Glanz, Grove, Lerman, Gotay, & Le Marchand, 1999). In contrast, those with greater perceptions of family-related guilt (i.e., anticipated feelings of guilt if a relative has a mutation but they themselves do not) are less likely to undergo genetic testing (Thompson et al., 2002).

Because an individual's genetic test result has direct implications for his or her family members, researchers have begun to explore the familial communication patterns that occur around the disclosure of test results. Several studies have demonstrated that communication and disclosure of genetic information is most frequently directed at first-degree relatives and spouses (Claes et al., 2003; Hughes et al., 2001; Patenaude et al., 2006; Smith, Zick, Mayer, & Botkin, 2002). Moreover, women are more frequently informed of test results than men are, although gender may be less important in disclosure than feelings of closeness among the family members in question (Mellon, Berry-Bobovski, Gold, Levin, & Tainsky, 2006; Patenaude et al., 2006).

Certain barriers to communication and disclosure between relatives may affect the extent to which genetic risk feedback is disseminated to family members. Most notably, reports of communication difficulties are more likely when there is greater emotional distance between relatives, larger family rifts, and greater age gaps between siblings (Claes et al., 2003; Hughes et al., 2002; McGivern et al., 2004). These barriers need to be addressed in family communication studies to better understand how to facilitate and encourage communication when structural barriers are prominent.

Finally, differences in the uptake of genetic counseling and testing for BRCA1 and BRCA2 appear to vary across racial and ethnic groups. For example, African Americans with a family history of breast or ovarian cancer are less likely to undergo BRCA1 and BRCA2 counseling compared with Caucasian women, after controlling for probability of carrying a mutation, socioeconomic characteristics, risk perceptions and worry, attitudes, and primary care physician recommendations (Armstrong, Micco, Carney, Stopfer, & Putt, 2005). Several factors may contribute to these disparities, including greater concerns about racial discrimination, confidentiality of test results, and the risks and limitations of genetic testing on the part of African American women (Donovan & Tucker, 2000; Peters, Rose, & Armstrong, 2004). Decisions to decline genetic testing among African American women have been found to be associated not only with lack of knowledge of breast cancer genetics but also with greater concerns about stigmatization (Thompson et al., 2002).

Although differences in knowledge and attitudes toward genetic testing raise concerns about the willingness of diverse racial and ethnic groups to use genetic services (Singer, Antonucci, & Van Hoewyk, 2004), overall uptake of BRCA1 and BRCA2 testing among African American women has ranged between 52% and 61% in studies in which genetic testing is offered without cost (Hughes, Fasaye, LaSalle, & Finch, 2003; Thompson et al., 2002). These uptake rates are consistent with rates observed in BRCA1 and BRCA2 studies with other populations for which the cost of testing is included as a part of the research protocol (Biesecker et al., 2000; Lerman et al., 1996; Smith et al., 1999). It remains to be determined whether genetic testing rates would differ between ethnic groups in the context of clinical or population-based settings in which participants are required to pay for testing, either out of pocket or through their insurance company.

IMPACT OF GENETIC RISK INFORMATION

Psychological Responses

Initially, significant concerns were raised about the potential negative psychological consequences of undergoing genetic testing for BRCA1 and BRCA2 and other cancer syndromes. However, the evidence for adverse psychosocial responses to genetic risk feedback has been minimal to date (Braithwaite, Emery, Walter, Prevost, & Sutton, 2004; Meiser, 2005). Levels of elevated distress or anxiety have tended to be short term (Croyle, Smith, Botkin, Baty, & Nash, 1997; van Roosmalen et al., 2004). Moreover, differences in psychological responses that do emerge between carriers and non-carriers following genetic testing are generally attributable to a decline in distress among individuals who receive a true negative test result (i.e., negative for a prior mutation identified in the family) rather than to an increase in distress among those who receive a positive test result (Lerman et al., 1996; Schwartz et al., 2002). The emergence of negative psychological reactions to testing feedback may be outweighed, in part, by the psychological benefit of clarifying risk uncertainty that is provided by receiving testing results. Indeed, several studies have identified uncertainty reduction as a central motivator for undergoing genetic testing (Braithwaite, Sutton, & Steggles, 2002; Croyle, Dutson, Tran, & Sun, 1995; Tessaro, Borstelmann, Regan, Rimer, & Winer, 1997), which is consistent with this line of reasoning.

Nonetheless, certain subgroups of individuals have been found to express high levels of anxiety at testing (Bonadona et al., 2002), such as BRCA1 and BRCA2 carriers who have already had breast cancer (Dorval et al., 2000). Psychological responses to genetic information appear to vary as a function of both individual difference and medical factors, such as underestimating distress responses following testing (poorer response; Dorval et al., 2000), prior personal experience with cancer (better response; Croyle et al., 1997), and more recent diagnosis (poorer response; Bonadona et al., 2002; van Roosmalen et al., 2004). This last finding is not surprising, given the psychological salience of a recent diagnosis and the fact that genetic test results can have implications for decisions about subsequent medical treatments (Schwartz et al., 2003). An individual's dispositional coping style also appears to be an important moderator of responses to genetic information (Grosfeld, Lips, Beemer, & ten Kroode, 2000; Shoda et al., 1998).

Preventive and Risk Reduction Decisions

Prophylactic mastectomy and oophorectomy are surgical options available for BRCA1 and BRCA2 mutation carriers, which have been demonstrated to significantly reduce the risk for breast and ovarian cancer (Rebbeck et al., 2002, 2004). Actual uptake rates for prophylactic mastectomy have been lower than initially anticipated, especially among unaffected carriers. One to 2 years following BRCA1 and BRCA2 testing, uptake of prophylactic mastectomy among unaffected carriers ranges from 0% to 9% (Botkin et al., 2003; Claes et al., 2005; Lerman et al., 2000). In contrast, rates of prophylactic mastectomy are higher in studies that report on a mix of affected and unaffected BRCA1 and BRCA2 mutation carriers (15%–25%; Lynch et al., 2006; Scheuer et al., 2002) or studies examining affected carriers only (35%; Meijers-Heijboer et al., 2003).

Predictors of prophylactic mastectomy uptake among BRCA1 and BRCA2 carriers include younger age, family history, and parenthood (i.e., having children; Meijers-Heijboer et al., 2000; Scheuer et al., 2002; Unic, Verhoef, Stalmeier, & Van Daal, 2000). Greater psychological distress and awareness of the genetic nature of cancer in the family for a longer period of time are also associated with decisions to opt for surgery (Lodder et al., 2002).

The uptake of prophylactic oophorectomy has been much higher than for prophylactic mastectomy (Botkin et al., 2003; Lerman et al., 2000). Among unaffected BRCA1 and BRCA2 carriers, rates among U.S.-based studies have ranged from 13% to 46% (Botkin et al., 2003; Lerman et al., 2000; Schwartz et al., 2003), whereas rates in the United Kingdom, Belgium, and the Netherlands have ranged from 31% to 75% (Claes et al., 2005; Meijers-Heijboer et al., 2000; Watson et al., 2004). U.S. and European studies examining either a mix of affected and unaffected carriers or affected carriers only have found prophylactic oophorectomy rates to range from 50% to 65% (Lynch et al., 2006; Meijers-Heijboer et al., 2003; Scheuer et al., 2002).

Perceived risk for ovarian cancer, perceived benefits of surgery, cancer anxiety, and uncertainty reduction are all factors that are associated with interest in and intentions to undergo prophylactic oophorectomy (Fang et al., 2003; Hurley, Miller, Costalas, Gillespie, & Daly, 2001; Meiser et al., 1999). Further, positive genetic test results, perceived risk, and family history of ovarian cancer predict prophylactic oophorectomy uptake (Schwartz et al., 2003). Mutation carriers are also more likely to undergo prophylactic oophorectomy if they are older and have had a prior breast cancer diagnosis (Meijers-Heijboer et al., 2000; Scheuer et al., 2002). Psychosocial interventions that enhance genetic counseling for BRCA1 and BRCA2 by focusing on helping participants anticipate and plan for their reactions to test outcomes have demonstrated greater information seeking and uptake of prophylactic oophorectomy at 6 months follow-up compared with control conditions in which general health information is provided (Miller, Roussi, et al., 2005).

Screening Behaviors

Mammography screening rates among BRCA1 and BRCA2 mutation carriers range from 68% to 95% (Botkin et al., 2003; Claes et al., 2005; Lerman et al., 2000; Tinley et al., 2004). Although mammography screening over time increased for both carriers and noncarriers in one study, 29% of carrier women in that same study did not obtain a single mammogram by 2 years posttesting (Botkin et al., 2003), suggesting that rates of screening among this population are suboptimal. Among women who learn they are not at elevated breast cancer risk, what is more commonly observed is a decline in mammography adherence (Lerman et al., 2000; Schwartz, Rimer, Daly, Sands, & Lerman, 1999). These findings raise concerns that noncarriers may be experiencing a false sense of reassurance about their risk, which is negatively affecting screening adherence.

Screening for ovarian cancer among BRCA1 and BRCA2 carriers has been relatively low and likely reflects the uncertainties related to the efficacy of available tests, with rates between 14% and 29% (Lerman et al., 2000; Tinley et al., 2004). In the year following a positive BRCA1 and BRCA2 test result, transvaginal ultrasound rates increased from 16% to 40% and CA125 blood test rates increased from 12% to 43% (Schwartz et al., 2003).

The impact of genetic testing on colorectal cancer screening has been more encouraging. Colonoscopy screening among unaffected individuals who were identified as mutation carriers for hereditary nonpolyposis colorectal cancer ranged from 71% to 100% within 1 to 2 years following genetic testing (V. Collins, Meiser, Gaff, St. John, & Halliday, 2005; Halbert et al., 2004; Johnson, Trimbath, Petersen, Griffin, & Giardiello, 2002). However, the low adherence rate among noncarriers in need of screening continues to raise concerns about the potential false sense of reassurance individuals may be experiencing following a negative test result (Johnson et al., 2002).

Lifestyle Behaviors

Some studies have examined the potential utility of incorporating genetic information into interventions to motivate changes in health behaviors such as smoking (Audrain et al., 1997; Lerman, Gold, et al., 1997; McBride et al., 2002). Incorporating biomarker feedback about genetic susceptibility to lung cancer has a beneficial impact on quit attempts made by smokers (Audrain et al., 1997). Moreover, this effect is more pronounced for smokers who are in the preparation stage of readiness to quit smoking—defined as planning to quit in the next 30 days and a quit attempt in the past 12 months. Smokers in the preparation stage are also more likely to reduce the number of cigarettes smoked compared with smokers not in the preparation stage at baseline (Lerman, Gold, et al., 1997).

Unfortunately, there is inconsistency around the extent to which biomarker feedback impacts actual quit rates. One study found a positive impact of biomarker feedback on actual quit rates (McBride et al., 2002), in contrast to two studies that found no differences in smoking cessation between individuals who received genetic feedback versus those who did not (Audrain et al., 1997; Lerman, Gold, et al., 1997). Methodological differences between the studies (e.g., how *smoking cessation* is defined) may partially account for the differences observed. Finally, the McBride et al. (2002) study also found that 6-month quit rates were higher for those identified at low genetic risk compared with those identified at high genetic risk (23% vs. 17%, respectively), suggesting that additional research is needed to better understand the process by which genetic feedback may (or may not) influence health behaviors.

Some preliminary evidence is emerging about the use of chemoprevention (i.e., tamoxifen) and complementary medicine following BRCA1 and BRCA2 testing. Among unaffected carriers, only 12.3% of women had used tamoxifen and 9.9% had used raloxifene (Metcalfe et al., 2005). Moreover, 58.3% of women reported that their doctors had not provided them with sufficient information about tamoxifen to consider its use, raising concerns about whether women are making informed decisions about the use of chemoprevention. One year following genetic testing, initiation of complementary medicine use for cancer prevention (including exercise, vitamins, special diet, etc.) is greater among those who are mutation carriers (DiGianni, Rue, Emmons, & Garber, 2006), suggesting that high-risk women might implement behavioral changes upon learning their carrier status. These results highlight the potential benefits of learning one's risk status for motivating change in general health behaviors.

SUMMARY AND FUTURE DIRECTIONS

Recent advances in genomic medicine provide an unprecedented opportunity to forge new ground in translational research by building on findings from biological, social, and behavioral research to inform clinical and public health practice. Research to date has shed light on some of the key motivators and barriers underlying individuals' decisions regarding the uptake of genetic testing for hereditary cancer syndromes. Moreover, a wealth of data is accumulating on the impact of genetic risk feedback, not only on psychological well-being but also on decision making pertaining to prevention and risk reduction options.

Drawing on existing knowledge, future research efforts should clarify how psychosocial interventions can be designed and evaluated to facilitate information processing, decision making, and psychological and behavioral responses to genetic testing. One innovative approach to facilitating information processing is to consider the ways in which information can be customized to address the specific characteristics of individuals (Kreuter & Strecher, 1995). Information can be tailored a number of ways to facilitate understanding, including by assessing and addressing demographic background, information-processing styles, and coping styles (Miller, Fang, Diefenbach, & Bales, 2001). Although readily used in interventions to modify health behaviors, tailored approaches have been used in only one study to date to improve knowledge and risk comprehension in the context of hereditary cancer syndromes. Skinner et al. (2002) tailored precounseling print information to various individual characteristics, including preferences for the amount and format of information. Compared with women who were provided with nontailored print material, those who received tailored print material showed greater improvements in knowledge and in the accuracy of their risk perceptions. Further research is needed to explore the benefits of tailoring to improve knowledge, risk comprehension, and decision making in the context of hereditary cancer syndromes.

To date, several communication channels have been used to deliver interventions to improve patients' understanding of risk information and to facilitate informed decision making about genetic testing. For example, researchers have used existing telephone service programs such as the National Cancer Institute's Cancer Information Service to deliver theory-based enhanced educational interventions that are efficacious in helping women better understand their cancer risk and to act on the appropriate risk assessment option for them personally (e.g., whether to have genetic testing; Miller, Fleisher, et al., 2005). Others have focused on developing information packets, videos, and interactive CD-ROMs that can be used in conjunction with genetic counseling to supplement and enhance genetic counseling outcomes such as knowledge and understanding of risk, psychological distress, and informed decision making about genetic testing (Cull et al., 1998; Green et al., 2004; Mancini et al., 2006; S. K. Peterson et al., 2006; Wang, Gonzalez, Milliron, Strecher, & Merajver, 2005). Overall, these studies provide evidence for the beneficial impact of educational supplements on increasing knowledge, improving satisfaction with information provided, and decreasing counseling time. However, the extent to which these strategies influence decision-making processes and outcomes are not yet well understood. For example, Green et al. (2004) did not find a difference in testing uptake between women who viewed a CD-ROM program compared with those who did not, whereas Wang et al. (2005) did find differences, with CD-ROM viewers being significantly less likely to undergo genetic testing compared with nonviewers. A greater understanding of the impact of education supplements on testing decisions is necessary to ensure that women are making informed decisions about testing.

Further research is also needed to clarify demographic differences in the use of genetic testing—especially between racial and ethnic groups, as well as between individuals of varied socioeconomic levels. Prior research in the area of genetic testing for hereditary cancer syndromes has been conducted with populations that are relatively homogenous (i.e., Caucasian, well-educated, high socioeconomic status), thus greatly limiting the generalizability of study findings. The need for replication of prior work among other populations is vital, especially because underserved populations may face unique barriers to access that may preclude them from using genetic testing. Barriers to access to genetic services include lack of knowledge of genetic testing, unavailability of relevant information (e.g., culturally and linguistically appropriate), and cost barriers—all of which may further magnify health disparities among underserved populations (Beene-Harris, Wang, & Bach, 2007; Institute of Medicine, 2005). The innovative efforts that are beginning to be undertaken to increase knowledge and access to genetic testing among underserved populations—such as the development of culturally and linguistically appropriate materials for patient education and recruitment into hereditary clinics—are examples of approaches that may help to overcome some of these barriers (Baty, Kinney, & Ellis, 2003; R. Lee et al., 2005; Thompson et al., 2004).

Studies are also needed to address the difficulties in communicating genetic risk information to family members. In part, the difficulties stem from relatives' misunderstanding of test results. For example, one study found that 20% of relatives have a hard time understanding the meaning of a positive test result (Costalas et al., 2003). Moreover, the same study also noted that approximately 20% of the BRCA1 and BRCA2 carriers reported being upset at conveying test results to family members, and over half of the family members reported that they were upset upon hearing the positive test result. These findings suggest that problems may arise because an individual carrier is ill prepared to deal with family members' emotional reactions to test feedback.

The prevalence of communication difficulties suggests a critical need for interventions to help individuals anticipate, plan for, and develop strategies for discussing testing results with key family members. These types of interventions may be especially warranted for male mutation carriers, who have reported feeling conflicted between the duty to warn children of their risk and the duty not to harm children by causing emotional distress (Hallowell et al., 2005) and thus may be in greater need of professional support when communicating test results to family members. Although interventions have been developed to provide communication skills training to help individuals effectively convey genetic test results to family members (e.g., Daly et al., 2001), little is known about the effectiveness of these interventions in addressing the barriers to communicating among family members.

Clearly, one of the key motivators for providing genetic risk information to individuals is to prompt the uptake of available lifestyle behaviors to prevent and control risk (Marteau & Lerman, 2001). However, it remains unclear whether and under what circumstances genetic risk information motivates behavior change and the circumstances under which behavioral efforts are undermined. For example, some studies have demonstrated that beliefs about disease controllability are lower if a genetic cause is emphasized (Senior, Marteau, & Peters, 1999). Other studies incorporating genetic biomarkers in smoking interventions have found an increase in short-term depression among those identified at increased susceptibility (Lerman, Gold, et al., 1997), which may undermine future behavioral change such as quit attempts. These data underscore the need to examine how genetic information influences both cognitive and affective processing systems and, subsequently, health behaviors. Research in this area is especially pressing, as family history assessment is increasingly being incorporated into public health interventions targeting a wide range of health behaviors, such as smoking, alcohol use, diet, and physical activity (Guttmacher, Collins, & Carmona, 2004).

As advances in genomic discoveries continue and increase at an unprecedented pace, so do the psychological issues being faced by all those professions involved. Continued efforts to understand and examine these issues from the psychosocial perspective will help to enhance the effective translation of genetic information into health benefits. Accordingly, the necessity of transdisciplinary collaborations is especially pertinent for the full vision of genomic medicine to be realized.

REFERENCES

Armstrong, K., Calzone, K., Stopfer, J., Fitzgerald, G., Coyne, J., & Weber, B. (2000). Factors associated with decisions about clinical BRCA1/2 testing. *Cancer Epidemiology, Biomarkers & Prevention, 9,* 1251–1254.

Armstrong, K., Micco, E., Carney, A., Stopfer, J., & Putt, M. (2005). Racial differ-ences in the use of BRCA1/2 testing among women with a family history of breast or ovarian cancer. *Journal of the American Medical Association, 293,* 1729–1736.

Audrain, J., Boyd, N. R., Roth, J., Main, D., Caparaso, N. E., & Lerman, C. (1997). Genetic susceptibility testing in smoking-cessation treatment: One-year out-comes of a randomized trial. *Addictive Behaviors, 22,* 741–751.

Baty, B. J., Kinney, A. Y., & Ellis, S. E. (2003). Developing culturally sensitive can-cer genetics communication aids for African Americans. *American Journal of Medical Genetics: Part A, 118,* 146–155.

Beene-Harris, R. Y., Wang, C., & Bach, J. V. (2007). Barriers to access: Results from focus groups to identify genetic service needs in the community. *Community Genetics, 10,* 10–18.

Biesecker, B. B., Ishibe, N., Hadley, D. W., Giambarresi, T. R., Kase, R. G., Lerman, C., & Struewing, J. P. (2000). Psychosocial factors predicting BRCA1/BRCA2 testing decisions in members of hereditary breast and ovarian cancer families. *American Journal of Medical Genetics, 93,* 257–263.

Bonadona, V., Saltel, P., Desseigne, F., Mignotte, H., Saurin, J., Wang, Q., et al. (2002). Cancer patients who experienced diagnostic genetic testing for cancer susceptibility: Reactions and behavior after the disclosure of a positive test result. *Cancer Epidemiology, Biomarkers & Prevention, 11,* 97–104.

Bosompra, K., Flynn, B. S., Ashikaga, T., Rairikar, C. J., Worden, J. K., & Solomon, L. J. (2000). Likelihood of undergoing genetic testing for cancer risk: A population-based study. *Preventive Medicine, 30,* 155–166.

Botkin, J. R., Smith, K. R., Croyle, R. T., Baty, B. J., Wylie, J. E., Dutson, D., et al. (2003). Genetic testing for BRCA1 mutation: Prophylactic surgery and screen-ing behavior in women 2 years posttesting. *American Journal of Medical Genetics: Part A, 118,* 201–209.

Bowen, D. J., Singal, R., Eng, E., Crystal, S., & Burke, W. (2003). Jewish identity and intentions to obtain breast cancer screening. *Cultural Diversity and Ethnic Minor-ity Psychology, 9,* 79–87.

Braithwaite, D., Emery, J., Walter, F., Prevost, A. T., & Sutton, S. (2004). Psycho-logical impact of genetic counseling for familial cancer: A systematic review and meta-analysis. *Journal of the National Cancer Institute, 96,* 122–133.

Braithwaite, D., Sutton, S., & Steggles, N. (2002). Intention to participate in pre-dictive genetic testing for hereditary cancer: The role of attitude toward uncer-tainty. *Psychology and Health, 17,* 761–772.

Cameron, L. D., & Reeve, J. (2006). Risk perceptions, worry, and attitudes about genetic testing for breast cancer susceptibility. *Psychology and Health, 21,* 211–230.

Claes, E., Evers-Kiebooms, G., Boogaerts, A., Decruyenaere, M., Denayer, L., & Legius, E. (2003). Communication with close and distant relatives in the con-text of genetic testing for hereditary breast and ovarian cancer in cancer patients. *American Journal of Medical Genetics: Part A, 116,* 11–19.

Claes, E., Evers-Kiebooms, G., Decruyenaere, M., Denayer, L., Boogaerts, A., Philippe, K., & Legius, E. (2005). Surveillance behavior and prophylactic surgery after predictive testing for hereditary breast/ovarian cancer. *Behavioral Medicine, 31,* 93–105.

Codori, A., Peterson, G. M., Miglioretti, D. L., Larkin, E. K., Bushey, M. T., Young, C., et al. (1999). Attitudes toward colon cancer gene testing: Factors predicting test uptake. *Cancer Epidemiology, Biomarkers & Prevention, 8,* 345–351.

Collins, F. S., Green, E. D., Guttmacher, A. E., & Guyer, M. S. (2003, April 24). A vision for the future of genomics research: A blueprint for the genomic era. *Nature, 422,* 835–847.

Collins, V., Meiser, B., Gaff, C., St. John, D. J., & Halliday, J. (2005). Screening and preventive behaviors one year after predictive genetic testing for hereditary non-polyposis colorectal carcinoma. *Cancer, 104,* 273–281.

Costalas, J. W., Itzen, M., Malick, J., Babb, J. S., Bove, B., Godwin, A. K., & Daly, M. B. (2003). Communication of BRCA1 and BRCA2 results to at-risk relatives: A cancer risk assessment program's experience. *American Journal of Medical Genetics: Part C. Seminars in Medical Genetics, 119,* 11–18.

Croyle, R. T., Dutson, D. S., Tran, V. T., & Sun, Y. (1995). Need for certainty and interest in genetic testing. *Women's Health: Research on Gender, Behavior, and Policy, 1,* 329–339.

Croyle, R. T., Smith, K. R., Botkin, J. R., Baty, B., & Nash, J. (1997). Psychological responses to BRCA1 mutation testing: Preliminary findings. *Health Psychology, 16,* 63–72.

Cull, A., Miller, H., Porterfield, T., Mackay, J., Anderson, E. D. C., Steel, C. M., & Elton, R. A. (1998). The use of videotaped information in cancer genetic counseling: A randomized evaluation study. *British Journal of Cancer, 77,* 830–837.

Daly, M. B., Barsevick, A., Miller, S. M., Buckman, R., Costalas, J., Montgomery, S., & Bingler, R. (2001). Communicating genetic test results to the family: A six-step, skills-building strategy. *Family and Community Health, 24,* 13–26.

Diefenbach, M. A., Schnoll, R. A., Miller, S. M., & Brower, L. (2000). Genetic testing for prostate cancer: Willingness and predictors of interest. *Cancer Practice, 8,* 82–86.

DiGianni, L. M., Rue, M., Emmons, K., & Garber, J. E. (2006). Complementary medicine use before and 1 year following genetic testing for BRCA1/2 mutations. *Cancer Epidemiology, Biomarkers & Prevention, 15,* 70–75.

Donovan, K. A., & Tucker, D. C. (2000). Knowledge about genetic risk for breast cancer and perceptions of genetic testing in a sociodemographically diverse sample. *Journal of Behavioral Medicine, 23,* 15–36.

Dorval, M., Patenaude, A. F., Schneider, K. A., Kieffer, S. A., DiGianni, L., Kalkbrenner, K. J., et al. (2000). Anticipated versus actual emotional reactions to disclosure of results of genetic tests for cancer susceptibility: Findings from p53 and BRCA1 testing programs. *Journal of Clinical Oncology, 18,* 2135–2145.

Evans, D. G. R., Maher, E. R., Macleod, R., Davies, D. R., & Craufurd, D. (1997). Uptake of genetic testing for cancer predisposition. *Journal of Medical Genetics, 34,* 746–748.

Fang, C. Y., Miller, S. M., Malick, J., Babb, J., Engstrom, P. F., & Daly, M. B. (2003). Psychosocial correlates of intention to undergo prophylactic oophorectomy among women with a family history of ovarian cancer. *Preventive Medicine, 37,* 424–431.

Glanz, K., Grove, J., Lerman, C., Gotay, C., & Le Marchand, L. (1999). Correlates of intentions to obtain genetic counseling and colorectal cancer gene testing among at-risk relatives from three ethnic groups. *Cancer Epidemiology, Biomarkers & Prevention, 8,* 329–336.

Green, M. J., Peterson, S. K., Baker, M. W., Harper, G. R., Friedman, L. C., Rubinstein, W. S., & Mauger, D. T. (2004). Effect of a computer-based decision aid on knowledge, perceptions, and intentions about genetic testing for breast cancer susceptibility. *Journal of the American Medical Association, 292,* 442–452.

Grosfeld, F. J. M., Lips, C. J. M., Beemer, F. A., & ten Kroode, H. F. J. (2000). Who is at risk for psychological distress in genetic testing programs for hereditary cancer disorders? *Journal of Genetic Counseling, 9,* 253–266.

Guttmacher, A. E., Collins, F. S., & Carmona, R. H. (2004). The family history—More important than ever. *New England Journal of Medicine, 351,* 2333–2336.

Hadley, D. W., Jenkins, J., Dimond, E., Nakahara, K., Grogan, L., Liewehr, D. J., et al. (2003). Genetic counseling and testing in families with hereditary nonpolyposis colorectal cancer. *Archives of Internal Medicine, 163,* 573–582.

Halbert, C. H., Lynch, H., Lynch, J., Main, D., Kucharski, S., Rustgi, A. K., & Lerman, C. (2004). Colon cancer screening practices following genetic testing for hereditary nonpolyposis colon cancer (HNPCC) mutations. *Archives of Internal Medicine, 164,* 1881–1887.

Hallowell, N., Ardern-Jones, A., Eeles, R., Foster, C., Lucassen, A., Moynihan, C., & Watson, M. (2005). Men's decision-making about predictive BRCA1/2 testing: The role of family. *Journal of Genetic Counseling, 14,* 207–217.

Harris, T. M., Parrott, R., & Dorgan, K. A. (2004). Talking about human genetics within religious frameworks. *Health Communication, 16,* 105–116.

Hughes, C., Fasaye, G., LaSalle, V. H., & Finch, C. (2003). Sociocultural influences on participation in genetic risk assessment and testing among African American women. *Patient Education and Counseling, 51,* 107–114.

Hughes, C., Lerman, C., Schwartz, M., Peshkin, B. N., Wenzel, L., Narod, S., et al. (2002). All in the family: Evaluation of the process and content of sisters' communication about BRCA1 and BRCA2 genetic test results. *American Journal of Medical Genetics, 107,* 143–150.

Hughes, C., Lynch, H., Durham, C., Snyder, C., Lemon, S., Narod, S., et al. (2001). Communication of BRCA1/2 test results in hereditary breast cancer families. *Cancer Research Therapy and Control, 8,* 51–59.

Hurley, K. E., Miller, S. M., Costalas, J. W., Gillespie, D., & Daly, M. B. (2001). Anxiety/uncertainty reduction as a motivation for interest in prophylactic oophorectomy in women with a family history of ovarian cancer. *Journal of Women's Health & Gender-Based Medicine, 10,* 189–199.

Institute of Medicine. (2005). *Implications of genomics for public health: Workshop summary.* Washington, DC: National Academies Press.

Jacobsen, P. B., Valdimarsdottir, H. B., Brown, K. L., & Offit, K. (1997). Decision-making about genetic testing among women at familial risk for breast cancer. *Psychosomatic Medicine, 59,* 459–466.

Johnson, K. A., Trimbath, J. D., Petersen, G. M., Griffin, C. A., & Giardiello, F. M. (2002). Impact of genetic counseling and testing on colorectal cancer screening behavior. *Genetic Testing, 6,* 303–306.

Kreuter, M. W., & Strecher, V. J. (1995). Changing inaccurate perceptions of health risk: Results from a randomized trial. *Health Psychology, 14,* 56–63.

Lee, R., Beattie, M., Crawford, B., Mak, J., Stewart, N., Komaromy, M., et al. (2005). Recruitment, genetic counseling, and BRCA testing for underserved women at a public hospital. *Genetic Testing, 9,* 306–312.

Lee, S., Bernhardt, B. A., & Helzlsouer, K. J. (2002). Utilization of BRCA1/2 genetic testing in the clinical setting. *Cancer, 94,* 1876–1885.

Lerman, C., Gold, K., Audrain, J., Lin, T. H., Boyd, N. R., Orleans, C. T., et al. (1997). Incorporating biomarkers of exposure and genetic susceptibility into smoking cessation treatment: Effects on smoking-related cognitions, emotions, and behavior change. *Health Psychology, 16,* 87–99.

Lerman, C., Hughes, C., Croyle, R. T., Main, D., Durham, C., Snyder, C., et al. (2000). Prophylactic surgery decisions and surveillance practices one year following BRCA1/2 testing. *Preventive Medicine, 31,* 75–80.

Lerman, C., Narod, S., Schulman, K., Hughes, C., Gomez-Caminero, A., Bonney, G., et al. (1996). BRCA1 testing in families with hereditary breast–ovarian cancer: A prospective study of patient decision making and outcomes. *Journal of the American Medical Association, 275,* 1885–1892.

Lerman, C., Schwartz, M. D., Lin, T. H., Hughes, C., Narod, S., & Lynch, H. T. (1997). The influence of psychological distress on use of genetic testing for cancer risk. *Journal of Consulting and Clinical Psychology, 65,* 414–420.

Lerman, C., Seay, J., Balshem, A., & Audrain, J. (1995). Interest in genetic testing among first-degree relatives of breast cancer patients. *American Journal of Medical Genetics, 57,* 385–392.

Loader, S., Levenkron, J. C., & Rowley, P. T. (1998). Genetic testing for breast–ovarian cancer susceptibility: A regional trial. *Genetic Testing, 2,* 305–313.

Lodder, L. N., Frets, P. G., Trijsburg, R. W., Meijers-Heijboer, E. J., Klijn, J. G. M., Seynaeve, C., et al. (2002). One year follow-up of women opting for presymptomatic testing for BRCA1 and BRCA2: Emotional impact of the test outcome and decisions on risk management (surveillance or prophylactic surgery). *Breast Cancer Research and Treatment, 73,* 97–112.

Lynch, H. T., Snyder, C., Lynch, J. F., Karatoprakli, P., Trowonou, A., Metcalfe, K., et al. (2006). Patient responses to the disclosure of BRCA mutation tests in hereditary breast–ovarian cancer families. *Cancer Genetics and Cytogenetics, 165,* 91–97.

Lynch, H. T., Watson, P., Tinley, S., Snyder, C., Durham, C., Lynch, J., et al. (1999). An update on DNA-based BRCA1/BRCA2 genetic counseling in hereditary breast cancer. *Cancer Genetics and Cytogenetics, 109,* 91–98.

Mancini, J., Nogues, C., Adenis, C., Berthet, P., Bonadona, V., Chompret, A., et al. (2006). Impact of an information booklet on satisfaction and decision-making about BRCA genetic testing. *European Journal of Cancer, 42*, 871–881.

Marteau, T. M., & Lerman, C. (2001, April 28). Genetic risk and behavioural change. *BMJ, 322*, 1056–1059.

McBride, C. M., Bepler, G., Lipkus, I. M., Lyna, P., Samsa, G., Albright, J., et al. (2002). Incorporating genetic susceptibility feedback into a smoking cessation program for African-American smokers with low income. *Cancer Epidemiology, Biomarkers & Prevention, 11*, 521–528.

McGivern, B., Everett, J., Yager, G. G., Baumiller, R. C., Hafertepen, A., & Saal, H. M. (2004). Family communication about positive BRCA1 and BRCA2 genetic test results. *Genetics in Medicine, 6*, 503–509.

Meijers-Heijboer, E. J., Brekelmans, C. T. M., Menke-Pluymers, M., Seynaeve, C., Baalbergen, A., Burger, C., et al. (2003). Use of genetic testing and prophylactic mastectomy and oophorectomy in women with breast or ovarian cancer from families with a BRCA1 or BRCA2 mutation. *Journal of Clinical Oncology, 21*, 1675–1681.

Meijers-Heijboer, E. J., Verhoog, L. C., Brekelmans, C. T. M., Seynaeve, C., Tilanus-Linthorst, M. M. A., Wagner, A., et al. (2000). Presymptomatic DNA testing and prophylactic surgery in families with a BRCA1 or BRCA2 mutation. *Lancet, 355*, 2015–2020.

Meiser, B. (2005). Psychological impact of genetic testing for cancer susceptibility: An update of the literature. *Psycho-Oncology, 14*, 1060–1074.

Meiser, B., Butow, P., Barratt, A., Friedlander, M., Gattas, M., Kirk, J., et al. (1999). Attitudes toward prophylactic oophorectomy and screening utilization in women at increased risk of developing hereditary breast/ovarian cancer. *Gynecologic Oncology, 75*, 122–129.

Mellon, S., Berry-Bobovski, L., Gold, R., Levin, N., & Tainsky, M. A. (2006). Communication and decision-making about seeking inherited cancer risk information: Findings from female survivor-relative focus groups. *Psycho-Oncology, 15*, 193–208.

Metcalfe, K. A., Snyder, C., Seidel, J., Hanna, D., Lynch, H. T., & Narod, S. (2005). The use of preventive measures among healthy women who carry a BRCA1 or BRCA2 mutation. *Familial Cancer, 4*, 97–103.

Miller, S. M., Fang, C. Y., Diefenbach, M. A., & Bales, C. B. (2001). Tailoring psychosocial interventions to the individual's health information-processing style: The influence of monitoring versus blunting in cancer risk and disease. In A. Baum & B. L. Anderson (Eds.), *Psychosocial interventions for cancer* (pp. 343–362). Washington, DC: American Psychological Association.

Miller, S. M., Fleisher, L., Roussi, P., Buzaglo, J. S., Schnoll, R., Slater, E., et al. (2005). Facilitating informed decision making about breast cancer risk and genetic counseling among women calling the NCI's Cancer Information Service. *Journal of Health Communication, 10*(Suppl. 1), 119–136.

Miller, S. M., Roussi, P., Daly, M. B., Buzaglo, J. S., Sherman, K., Godwin, A. K., et al. (2005). Enhanced counseling for women undergoing BRCA1/2 testing: Impact on subsequent decision making about risk reduction behaviors. *Health Education and Behavior, 32,* 654–667.

Miller, S. M., Shoda, Y., & Hurley, K. (1996). Applying cognitive-social theory to health-protective behavior: Breast self-examination in cancer screening. *Psychological Bulletin, 119,* 70–94.

Patenaude, A. F., Dorval, M., DiGianni, L. S., Schneider, K. A., Chittenden, A., & Garber, J. E. (2006). Sharing BRCA1/2 test results with first-degree relatives: Factors predicting who women tell. *Journal of Clinical Oncology, 24,* 700–706.

Peters, N., Rose, A., & Armstrong, K. (2004). The association between race and attitudes about predictive genetic testing. *Cancer Epidemiology, Biomarkers & Prevention, 13,* 361–365.

Peterson, E. A., Milliron, K. J., Lewis, K. E., Goold, S. D., & Merajver, S. D. (2002). Health insurance and discrimination concerns and BRCA1/2 testing in a clinic population. *Cancer Epidemiology, Biomarkers & Prevention, 11,* 79–87.

Peterson, S. K., Pentz, R. D., Blanco, A. M., Ward, P. A., Watts, B. G., Marani, S. K., et al. (2006). Evaluation of a decision aid for families considering p53 genetic counseling and testing. *Genetics in Medicine, 8,* 226–233.

Rebbeck, T. R., Friebel, T., Lynch, H. T., Neuhausen, S. L., van't Veer, L., Garber, J. E., et al. (2004). Bilateral prophylactic mastectomy reduces breast cancer risk in BRCA1 and BRCA2 mutation carriers: The PROSE study group. *Journal of Clinical Oncology, 22,* 1055–1062.

Rebbeck, T. R., Lynch, H. T., Neuhausen, S. L., Narod, S. A., van't Veer, L., Garber, J. E., et al. (2002). Prophylactic oophorectomy in carriers of BRCA1 or BRCA2 mutations. *New England Journal of Medicine, 346,* 1616–1622.

Scheuer, L., Kauff, N., Robson, M., Kelly, B., Barakat, R., Satagopan, J., et al. (2002). Outcome of preventive surgery and screening for breast and ovarian cancer in BRCA mutation carriers. *Journal of Clinical Oncology, 20,* 1260–1268.

Schwartz, M. D., Hughes, C., Roth, J., Main, D., Peshkin, B. N., Isaacs, C., et al. (2000). Spiritual faith and genetic testing decisions among high-risk breast cancer probands. *Cancer Epidemiology, Biomarkers & Prevention, 9,* 381–385.

Schwartz, M. D., Kaufman, E., Peshkin, B. N., Isaacs, C., Hughes, C., DeMarco, T., et al. (2003). Bilateral prophylactic oophorectomy and ovarian cancer screening following BRCA1/2 mutation testing. *Journal of Clinical Oncology, 21,* 4034–4041.

Schwartz, M. D., Peshkin, B. N., Hughes, C., Main, D., Isaacs, C., & Lerman, C. (2002). Impact of BRCA1/BRCA2 mutation testing on psychologic distress in a clinic-based sample. *Journal of Clinical Oncology, 20,* 514–520.

Schwartz, M. D., Rimer, B. K., Daly, M., Sands, C., & Lerman, C. (1999). A randomized trial of breast cancer risk counseling: The impact on self-reported mammography use. *American Journal of Public Health, 89,* 924–926.

Senior, V., Marteau, T. M., & Peters, T. J. (1999). Will genetic testing for predisposition for disease result in fatalism? A qualitative study of parents' responses to neonatal screening for familial hypercholesterolaemia. *Social Science & Medicine, 48,* 1857–1860.

Shiloh, S., & Ilan, S. (2005). To test or not to test? Moderators of the relationship between risk perceptions and interest in predictive genetic testing. *Journal of Behavioral Medicine, 28,* 467–479.

Shoda, Y., Mischel, W., Miller, S. M., Diefenbach, M., Daly, M. B., & Engstrom, P. F. (1998). Psychological interventions and genetic testing: Facilitating informed decisions about BRCA1/2 cancer susceptibility. *Journal of Clinical Psychology in Medical Settings, 5,* 3–17.

Singer, E., Antonucci, T., & Van Hoewyk, J. (2004). Racial and ethnic variations in knowledge and attitudes about genetic testing. *Genetic Testing, 8,* 31–43.

Skinner, C. S., Schildkraut, J. M., Berry, D., Calingaert, B., Marcom, P. K., Sugerman, J., et al. (2002). Pre-counseling education materials for BRCA testing: Does tailoring make a difference? *Genetic Testing, 6,* 93–105.

Smith, K. R., West, J. A., Croyle, R. T., & Botkin, J. R. (1999). Familial context of genetic testing for cancer susceptibility: Moderating effect of siblings' test results on psychological distress one to two weeks after BRCA1 mutation testing. *Cancer Epidemiology, Biomarkers & Prevention, 8,* 383–392.

Smith, K. R., Zick, C. D., Mayer, R. N., & Botkin, J. R. (2002). Voluntary disclosure of BRCA1 mutation test results. *Genetic Testing, 6,* 89–92.

Tessaro, I., Borstelmann, N., Regan, K., Rimer, B. K., & Winer, E. (1997). Genetic testing for susceptibility to breast cancer: Findings from women's focus groups. *Journal of Women's Health, 6,* 317–327.

Thompson, H. S., Valdimarsdottir, H. B., Duteau-Buck, C., Guevarra, J., Bovbjerg, D. H., Richmond-Avellaneda, C., et al. (2002). Psychosocial predictors of BRCA counseling and testing decisions among urban African-American women. *Cancer Epidemiology, Biomarkers & Prevention, 11,* 1579–1585.

Thompson, H. S., Wahl, E., Fatone, A., Brown, K., Kwate, N. O., & Valdimarsdottir, H. (2004). Enhancing the readability of materials describing genetic risk for breast cancer. *Cancer Control, 11,* 245–253.

Tinley, S. T., Houfek, J., Watson, P., Wenzel, L., Clark, M. B., Coughlin, S., & Lynch, H. T. (2004). Screening adherence in BRCA1/2 families is associated with primary physicians' behavior. *American Journal of Medical Genetics: Part A, 125,* 5–11.

Unic, I., Verhoef, L. C. G., Stalmeier, P. F. M., & Van Daal, W. A. J. (2000). Prophylactic mastectomy or screening in women suspected to have the BRCA1/2 mutation: A prospective pilot study of women's treatment choices and medical and decision-analytic recommendations. *Medical Decision Making, 20,* 251–262.

van Roosmalen, M. S., Stalmeier, P. F. M., Verhoef, L. C. G., Hoekstra-Weebers, J. E. H. M., Oosterwijk, J. C., Hoogerbrugge, N., et al. (2004). Impact of BRCA1/2 testing and disclosure of a positive test result on women affected and unaffected with breast or ovarian cancer. *American Journal of Medical Genetics: Part A, 124,* 346–355.

Wang, C., Gonzalez, R., Janz, N. K., Milliron, K. J., & Merajver, S. D. (2007). The role of cognitive appraisal and worry in BRCA1/2 testing decisions among a clinic population. *Psychology and Health, 22,* 719–736.

Wang, C., Gonzalez, R., Milliron, K., Strecher, V. J., & Merajver, S. D. (2005). Genetic counseling for BRCA1/2: A randomized controlled trial of two strategies to facilitate the education and counseling process. *American Journal of Medical Genetics: Part A, 134,* 66–73.

Watson, M., Foster, C., Eeles, R., Eccles, D., Ashley, S., Davidson, R., et al. (2004). Psychosocial impact of breast/ovarian (BRCA1/2) cancer-predictive genetic testing in a UK multi-centre clinical cohort. *British Journal of Cancer, 91,* 1787–1794.

V

TERTIARY PREVENTION: TREATING CLINICAL CANCER

TERTIARY PREVENTION: TREATING CLINICAL CANCER

Part V, on tertiary prevention, presents the substantial body of research that has been conducted on the psychosocial issues that emerge in response to a cancer diagnosis and cancer treatment. In chapter 18, Baile, Aaron, and Parker review research on oncologist–patient–family communication and document the progress that has been made in establishing an evidence base for breaking bad news to cancer patients about diagnosis, prognosis, and transition to palliative and end-of-life care. Morrow, Roscoe, Mustian, Hickok, Ryan, and Matteson, in chapter 19, review research on the efficacy of adjuvant behavioral alternatives to pharmacologic agents in reducing the adverse side effects of cancer treatment. In chapter 20, Meyerowitz and Oh detail the nature and severity of the emotional, cognitive, and social effects experienced by cancer patients during and shortly after primary treatment, and they review research on behavioral interventions to mitigate these effects. Schover, in chapter 21, describes the sexual dysfunctions experienced by cancer patients, reviews behavioral interventions designed to treat these dysfunctions and notes methodological limitations of research in this area. Chapter 22, by Given, Sherwood, and Given, reviews the literature on family caregivers of patients undergoing cancer treatment, focusing on the adverse emotional and physical effects of caregiving, the skills needed for successful caregiving, and the effects of the experience on caregivers themselves. The chapter also reviews research on interventions designed to enhance caregiver well-being and assist caregivers in providing care.

18
PRACTITIONER–PATIENT COMMUNICATION IN CANCER DIAGNOSIS AND TREATMENT

WALTER F. BAILE, JOANN AARON, AND PATRICIA A. PARKER

The patient-centered model has replaced the clinician-centered model as the most appropriate way of providing comprehensive cancer care (Levy, 1998; Tobias & Hamilton, 2002). This approach acknowledges the importance of relationship building with the patient and family, endorses shared decision making as a key component of treatment, and emphasizes clinician self-understanding and addressing of patient concerns and information needs. Interpersonal and communication skills are essential in achieving these goals and are associated with important other outcomes for the patient, the family, and the medical team. These goals and objectives of clinical care have directed attention toward better understanding of the oncologist–patient–family communication in the context of the medical encounter and finding improved ways to scientifically study the relationship and to translate findings into practical recommendations for clinical practice and the education of oncology trainees. Although research on communication has also been conducted in other medical settings, in this chapter we highlight the most important practitioner–patient communication issues in oncology and describe key research findings. We also offer suggestions for needed future work in this area.

THE SCIENTIFIC STUDY OF COMMUNICATION

Studying communication is very complex because the scientific investigation of a number of dimensions of communication is open to varying approaches and methodologies. In addition, many studies are done on small groups of patients with different types of cancer or at different stages of disease, which makes it difficult to identify a coherent body of literature and compare findings across studies. Recently, new methodologies that involve direct observation of medical visits, video and audio recording of doctor–patient interactions, and coding by impartial observers of dialogue and affective behaviors promise to bring a more scientific focus to the study of this area (Baile & Aaron, 2005).

Unique Aspects of the Communication Issues With Cancer Patients

The majority of studies on practitioner–patient communication have focused on primary care or general internal medicine settings. Although many of these findings may be applicable to oncology, several unique elements are not present in many other medical settings. First, cancer is a life-threatening illness, with a 50% 5-year survival rate. Although recent treatments have increased the hope for, if not cure of, at least the arrest of the disease, the diagnosis of cancer results in significant fear, uncertainty, and commitment to often arduous, expensive, and complex treatments. Because of reimbursement issues, medical visits have become shorter; however, the desires of patients for information have increased (Tattersall, Butow, & Clayton, 2002). Patients regard their oncologists as one of the most important sources of psychological support (Davis Williams, Parle, Redman, & Turner, 2004; Molleman et al., 1984) yet oncologists receive almost no training in the communication and the interpersonal dimensions of patient care (Hoffman et al., 2004). Communication research in oncology has begun to change this landscape by demonstrating the association of good communication skills with enhanced patient satisfaction, improved coping, compliance with treatment, increased patient knowledge, enhanced accrual to clinical trials, better transition of patients from curative to palliative treatment, and decreased oncologist stress and burnout (Baile & Aaron, 2005; Ong, Visser, Lammes, & de Haes, 2000; Roberts, Cox, Reintgen, Baile, & Gibertinin, 1994).

Communication Skills

Communication between cancer patients and their health care practitioners is a multidimensional concept and involves both the content of dialogue and its affective component (i.e., what happens emotionally to the practitioner and patient during the encounter), as well as nonverbal behaviors. Clinicians in oncology need to have basic communication skills (e.g., engaging the patient, using open-ended questions) and specific skills to handle high-stakes encounters (e.g., breaking bad news, discussing prognosis, discussing transition to palliative care). In the next sections, we describe several points on the cancer continuum in which specific skills are required.

Breaking Bad News

Giving bad news is a frequent and significant communication challenge for oncologists. A typical oncologist in practice may give bad news as many as 20,000 times over the course of a career. Increased cancer survival now means communicating with the patient not only information regarding the state of the disease and its response to a multitude of treatments over time but also adverse information related to potentially irreversible side effects, complications of the illness, the treatment, and diminished prospects for the future. This process is made difficult by several factors. Oncologists are rarely trained in techniques for giving bad news (Baile, Lenzi, Parker, Buckman, & Cohen, 2002). Physicians often experience negative emotions such as anxiety and fear of being blamed when they must tell patients that treatment has not worked (Buckman, 1984; Wallace, Hlubocky, & Daugherty, 2006). They may react to patient emotion by offering false hope, providing premature reassurance, or omitting important information from the disclosure (Baile et al., 2002; Maguire, 1999). Moreover, patients may process information through a repertoire of coping strategies or styles called *denial* or *blunting* (Miller, 1987). This may include avoiding asking questions, being overly optimistic about the outcome, and distorting information to put it in a better light.

Diagnostic Disclosure and Discussions About Prognosis

Today in North America and many Western countries, there is open disclosure regarding the presence of cancer, although physicians often do not discuss the prognosis unless the patient asks. The reluctance to truthfully disclose a terminal prognosis persists in southern Europe, including Italy and Spain (Mitchell, 1998; Surbone, 2008). For patients, however, not discussing the diagnosis may engender feelings of isolation, anxiety, lack of autonomy or control, psychological abandonment, mistrust, suspicion, and a sense of betrayal. Open discussion of the diagnosis decreases uncertainty, improves participation in decisions about care, allows access to psychological support, encourages self-care, and permits the patient to begin planning for the future (Arber & Gallagher, 2003).

In current North American medical practice, clinicians and medical ethicists have strongly argued that for patients to make informed treatment decisions, they must have an understanding of their disease and its underlying prognosis, that is, *open awareness*. With such information in hand, patients can then make informed medical decisions (Gordon & Daugherty, 2003). Reports in the literature suggest that although honest disclosure can have a negative emotional impact in the short term, most cancer survivors adjust well over time. Gratitude, peace of mind, positive attitude, reduced anxiety, and better adjustment are some of the benefits that patients report from having been told about their diagnosis of cancer (Coughlin, 2008). Because uncertainty is a major cause of emotional distress for patients, relief from uncertainty can, in itself, be therapeutic (Girgis & Sanson-Fisher, 1998), and some believe that over time, patients achieve a psychosocial objective correlative of order within the context of chaos theory (Mishel, 1990).

Although most physicians in Western countries tell their patients that they have cancer, information about prognosis is less commonly presented. This often occurs despite the fact that patients often desire this information and that it has been demonstrated that if patients are actively encouraged to ask questions, prognosis is the one area in which patients increase their question asking (Butow, Dowsett, Hagerty, & Tattersall, 2002). An ethical dilemma exists in that physicians and their patients with advanced cancers have a tendency to overestimate the probability of their long-term survival, which can lead to a belief that the purpose of the treatment options offered is to cure them (Gordon & Daugherty, 2003). To guide realistic treatment decisions, accurate prognostication is key. However, statistics, which apply to groups, drive prognostics, and individuals can vary greatly in their responses to treatment. Clearly, additional research is required in the area of prognosis. Some still argue that humanistic principles should permit practitioners to temporize believing that a respect for autonomy need not imply that all information is given all of the time (Arber & Gallagher, 2003; Helft, 2005), an approach that is at odds with the dictates of informed consent. Many specialists in palliative care have, for example, adopted a conditional approach to disclosing terminal prognoses, indicated by use of terms such as *titrated*, or through the delivery of graduated dosages of truth. It is important to note, however, despite a commitment to open awareness, doctors and nurses retain control over medical information and its disclosure, which actuates ambiguity and uncertainty surrounding how open health care professionals should be (Arber & Gallagher, 2003).

When bad news is given tactfully, honestly, and in a supportive fashion, the patient's experience of the conversation is less stressful. Friedrichsen and Strang (2003) reported on the patients' perception of "supporting" and "fortifying" of physician statements conveying the intention of helping the patients through the course of the cancer; sentences such as "there is nothing more to do" were perceived as "abandoning" and meaning that no further support would be provided.

Not being told about the severity of their condition or not having the opportunity to express their fears and concerns may lead patients to believe that nothing can be done to help them or to misunderstand their disease (Fallowfield & Jenkins, 1999). However, patients who are told bad news bluntly by a practitioner who is trying to quickly complete the difficult task of sharing bad news will likely feel extremely frightened and unsupported (Bedell, Graboys, Bedell, & Lown, 2004). Loge, Kaasa, and Hytten (1997) surveyed 497 cancer patients regarding their experience of receiving their cancer diagnosis. Significant predictors of patient satisfaction with the conversation included perceiving the physicians as personally interested, being able to understand the information given, being informed in the proper environment (i.e., a doctor's office), and having more time invested in discussing the information (Loge et al., 1997). Although the majority of patients wish to have complete and accurate information regarding their condition, many patients feel that the news is forced on them unless their right to have the news given according to their preferences is acknowledged by the physician (e.g., "Are you the type of person who wants to know all the details about your condition?").

In a study by Parker et al. (2001), the highest-rated elements of communication included the doctor being up-to-date on the latest research on the patient's cancer, informing the patient about the best treatment options and taking time to answer all his or her questions, being honest about the severity of the condition, using simple and clear language, giving the news directly, and giving full attention to the patient. Cancer type did not predict patients' preferences. It is important for the physician to elicit the patient's perspective on his or her condition because many incorrect beliefs can be clarified to the patient's benefit.

Transition to Palliation and End-of-Life Care

For practitioners, communicating with dying patients is often complicated by countertransference issues surrounding their personal fear of dying combined with the historic tendency in Western medicine to focus on cure. Physicians who are too blunt can shatter hope for patients (Wenrich et al., 2001), leaving them feeling that they have been abandoned, whereas physicians who present bad news in an unhurried, honest, balanced, and empathic fashion have been shown to elicit greater satisfaction with communication of the news (Baile & Aaron, 2005; Ellis & Tattersall, 1999). Patients also differ in how much information they want and how quickly they want to receive it (Wenrich et al., 2001). American physicians fear that the revelation of a grim prognosis may psychologically damage patients' hopes and may diminish their will to survive through a form of prophecy. This is consistent with a Western cultural assumption that one needs hope to battle cancer. Physicians are also uncomfortable with putting odds on longevity, recurrence, and cure, because they do not know when nor how individual patients will die (Gordon & Daugherty, 2003). In one study, hope was a constant theme of the respondents.

Despite the severity of the situation, people could still feel hope, the nature of which changed with time. At the beginning of their disease, patients hoped for successful treatment, whereas later they hoped for a little more time with their children, for instance (Adelbratt & Strang, 2000).

Patients facing death have a myriad of concerns: leaving children and other loved ones behind, decrements in socially based aspects of one's identity (Byock, 1996), the end of being able to fulfill normal roles, fear of burdening loved ones (Singer, Martin, & Kelner, 1999), loss of control, deterioration in personal appearance, needing help with intimate personal care and routine activities of daily living, worries about mental awareness (Steinhauser et al., 2000), pain, management of symptoms, quality of life, dignity (Chochinov et al., 2002), achieving a sense of completion, having a good death, and abandonment. In fact, many patients are grateful for the opportunity to talk about questions of death, although they often have few opportunities because they find that the staff is afraid of, or uncomfortable with talking about, death and dying (Adelbratt & Strang, 2000), which exacerbates feelings of isolation and separation.

Breaking Bad News: Guidelines and Strategies

Various strategies or guidelines have been proposed for having bad news consultations with patients (Baile, Glober, Lenzi, Beale, & Kudelka, 1999; Buckman, 1984). The use of a specific strategy may more reliably result in the understanding and appropriate response to these and similar patients' doubts and fears. There have been some general guidelines and recommendations for how bad news interviews should be conducted (Baile et al., 2000; Blanchard, Labrecque, Ruckdeschel, & Blanchard, 1988; Buckman, 1984; Fallowfield, Jenkins, & Beveridge, 2002; Loge et al., 1997; Parker et al., 2001); however, these recommendations have most frequently taken the form of practical advice formulated on the basis of anecdotal experiences or opinions with little empirical foundation (Girgis & Sanson-Fisher, 1995). Two approaches (Baile et al., 2000; Girgis & Sanson-Fisher, 1995) are outlined briefly in Table 18.1, which shows some subtle differences between these approaches and also many common elements. For example, each of these strategies recommends giving the news in an appropriate setting (i.e., quiet place, with uninterrupted time), assessing the patient's understanding of his or her illness, providing the information the patient wants, allowing the patient to express his or her emotions and responding appropriately, summarizing the information provided, and coming up with a plan for the next step(s). Additional research is needed to empirically support these techniques. It is important to note that research also suggests that the structure and content of the consultation influence the patient's ability to remember what has been said in several ways: (a) Patients usually recall facts provided at the start of a consultation more readily than

TABLE 18.1
Breaking Bad News: Strategies

Girgis and Sanson-Fisher (1995)	Baile et al. (1999)
1. Give bad news in a quiet, private place.	S = Get the setting right.
2. Allow sufficient uninterrupted time for the initial consultation.	P = Understand the patient's perception of the illness.
3. Assess patient's understanding and emotional status.	I = Obtain an invitation to impart information.
4. Provide information simply and honestly.	K = Provide knowledge and education.
5. Encourage patients to express their feelings.	E = Respond to the patient's emotions with empathy, that is, through responses and gestures.
6. Respond to patients' feelings with empathy.	S = Provide a summary strategy; that is, respond to questions and discuss treatment options; provide information about support services and willingness to answer questions at a future date.
7. Provide a broad time frame for the prognosis.	
8. Avoid conveying that nothing more can be done.	
9. Arrange a time to review the situation.	
10. Discuss treatment options.	
11. Offer assistance in telling others.	
12. Provide information about support services.	
13. Document the information given to the patient.	

those given later; (b) topics deemed most relevant and important to the patient (which might not be those considered most pertinent to the doctor) are recalled most accurately; (c) the greater the number of statements made by a doctor, the smaller the mean percentage recalled by the patient; and (d) items that patients do manage to recall do not decay over time as do other memories (Fallowfield & Jenkins, 1999).

COMMUNICATION AND TREATMENT DECISION MAKING

Promoting patient involvement in decision making is a core concept in patient-centered oncology. Communication is essential to the decision-making process.

Information Needs

An area that has received significant empirical attention is in identifying cancer patients' information needs. *Information needs* or *information desires* is the degree to which patients want detailed information about their cancer and the type of information they desire. Patients' information needs and preferences may be related to information about their disease status (e.g., the diagnosis, the extent of the disease) and information about treatment options or plans (e.g., the best way to manage the disease).

Many patients actively seek out information and identify acquiring information as a priority. In several studies, information seeking has been found to have beneficial effects on increased compliance, increased patient satisfaction, improved quality of life, and reduced distress (Butow, Maclean, Dunn, Tattersall, & Boyer, 1997; Mills & Sullivan, 1999; Parker et al., 2001; Siminoff, Ravdin, Colabianchi, & Sturm, 2000). Mills and Sullivan (1999), for example, identified six key functions of information for patients: to gain control, reduce anxiety, improve compliance, create realistic expectations, promote self-care and participation, and generate feelings of safety and security. In a study by Butow et al. (1997), out of 12 specific information and support topics listed, patients expressed the greatest need for information. Of the three highest ranking topics, 97% of patients wanted more feedback on what is happening to the cancer, 88% expressed a desire for increased information on the likely future of their illness, and 91% wished for more information about their illness. Patient needs immediately after the first consultation shifted to an emphasis on support. Of the three highest ranking topics for supportive communications, 63% of patients wanted more assurance that they would be looked after, 59% wished for greater reassurance and hope, and 59% expressed an increased need to talk about their worries and fears (Butow et al., 1997). Lobb et al. (2002) found that 83% of the women they interviewed wanted as much information as possible, whereas 16% wanted limited information; further, 91% wanted to know their prognosis before beginning adjuvant treatment, whereas 63% wanted their oncologist to ask them whether they wanted to know their prognosis. Lobb et al. concluded that women should be given information in a staged manner that allows them the opportunity to confirm their diagnosis and prognosis and formulate questions and that emotional support is vital when prognosis is being discussed (Jenkins, Fallowfield, & Saul, 2001). In addition, patients' information needs may change at different points on the disease and treatment trajectory. It is often difficult for practitioners to accurately estimate or provide the amount or type of information that patients want, and patients may be dissatisfied with the amount or type of information they receive (Lobb, Butow, Kenny, & Tattersall, 1999; Schofield, Juraskova, & Butow, 2003; Silliman, Dukes, Sullivan, & Kaplan, 1998; Wright, Holcombe, & Salmon, 2004). For example, in a study by Lobb et al. (1999), prognostic information that was rated as most important by women with early-stage breast cancer included knowing the probability of cure, disease stage, and chance of curative treatment and receiving 10-year survival figures comparing receipt and nonreceipt of adjuvant therapy. Probability of cure and disease stage were also identified as high priority needs in another study of women with early-stage breast cancer (Degner et al., 1997).

Research has attempted to characterize these different information styles in a variety of ways. One of these is monitoring and blunting (Miller, 1987; Miller, Brody, & Summerton, 1988). Monitors actively seek information, whereas blunters avoid or distract themselves from information (Ong et al., 1999; Parker et al., 2001). Thus, patients' information style may greatly affect their communication preferences and how they interact with their health care practitioners. This is an area that warrants additional study and has implications for how patients adjust to their cancer experience.

Participation Styles in Decision Making

Participation style in decision making is the degree to which patients want to be involved in the decision-making process related to their cancer. Studies of patients' desire to participate in treatment decisions have yielded conflicting results, largely depending on how *participation in decision making* is defined. This can range from the patient actively engaging in the decision-making process to the patient making the ultimate decision (Guadagnoli & Ward, 1998). The desire to participate in treatment decisions is associated with locus of control, which describes how an individual tends to attribute control. Patients with an internal locus of control seek information to control their own destinies, whereas those with an external locus of control tend to passively accept their lot (Webber, 1990).

Influence of Culture, Ethnicity, and Language on Communication

Developing awareness about cross-cultural practices regarding cancer disclosure issues allows the clinician to become more sensitive to the expectations of culturally and individually diverse cancer patients. When discussing diagnoses and treatment options with patients from different cultures, physicians must consider how to balance a commitment to frank discussion and a respect for the cultural values of the patient (Hern, Koenig, Moore, & Marshall, 1998). In general, patients whose dominant culture is derived from a Western philosophy subscribe to certainty, predictability, control, and obtainable outcomes (Mishel, 1990). This has engendered an approach that fosters self-determination and autonomy in making treatment decisions (Gordon & Daugherty, 2003). Western cultural assumptions exist about what is good and just in medical care. The Western patient-centered society deems it of vital importance to keep patients fully informed, so they can make accurate assessments about their health (Hern et al., 1998).

However, patients in Italy, China, and Japan (Gordon & Daugherty, 2003); Spain (Mitchell, 1998); Tanzania (Harris & Templeton, 2001); and Korean Americans and Mexican Americans believe that there is a positive value inherent in nondisclosure of diagnosis and of a terminal prognosis (Gordon & Daugherty, 2003; Mitchell, 1998). In the family-centered model of medical decision making, such as that found for Mexican Americans and Korean Americans, Ethiopian refugees, and in Italy, autonomy is seen as isolating (Gordon & Daugherty, 2003; Mitchell, 1998). Thus, it is essential to assess and consider patients' cultural beliefs when communicating with them about their cancer.

Communicating With the Patient's Family

Families can be an important resource for patients in helping them to make better decisions about their care (Ballard-Reisch & Letner, 2003). Some believe that patient-centered approaches emphasizing patient autonomy in medical decision making should be shifted to family-centered approaches, as most decision making in health care situations is carried out in the context of family care and obligation. Health care professionals are valued when they establish a structured and ongoing dialogue with family members about treatment goals, plans of care, and expectations regarding patient outcomes (Given, Given, & Kozachik, 2001). Caregivers report that specific and tailored direction is supportive and reduces the uncertainty they experience as they provide care (Given et al., 2001). However, some argue that families should not be allowed to preempt honest communication with the patient for the sake of sparing him or her from the reality of his or her illness. The patient can even be made to feel as though there is a "conspiracy" of silence among family members, which may thwart his or her end-of-life goals (Baile et al., 2002). Thus, one must ultimately check with the patient to determine his or her desires about what level of involvement in making decisions caretakers should occupy.

Communication and Informed Consent

Traditionally, informed consent has been applied to treatment, which unlike diagnosis, is considered to be invasive and thus liable to breach patient autonomy. The technological boom in medicine in recent decades has led to the realization that diagnosis, too, may be invasive (e.g., in cardiac catheterization) and that it, too, requires informed consent because it may breach patient autonomy (Rudnick, 2002). However, the physicians surveyed in one study said they were accustomed to communicating bad news verbally, in a highly individualized fashion, and the researchers found that the written nature of the form caused great difficulty for physicians who were accustomed to the flexibility and nonaccountability of verbal discussion (Taylor & Kelner, 1987). Unfortunately, in some cases, the importance of informed consent generally drives the decision to give all information relevant to the patient regarding his or her medical condition. If patients are not given necessary information, then there may be negligence claims in the future (Arber & Gallagher, 2003). Rudnick (2002) suggested that informed consent should be sought before, not after, the diagnosis has been established, so as to avoid the patient's inference that the established diagnosis is bad news.

COMMUNICATION SKILLS INTERVENTIONS

Recent research has underscored the importance of communication skills training for cancer clinicians. Other research has explored the best way to accomplish this.

Training Practitioners in Communication Skills

Poor communication between practitioners and patients is associated with poor health outcomes, patient dissatisfaction, the propensity to sue for medical malpractice (Beckman & Frankel, 2003), uncertainty and denial, anxiety and depression, and a problematic psychological adjustment to cancer (Ong et al., 2000). Some believe that effective communication between doctor and patient is a core clinical skill that should be taught with the same rigor as other basic medical sciences (Kurtz & Silverman, 1996). Underlying this belief is a growing body of research and guidelines acknowledging that practitioners do not have to be born with excellent communication skills but rather can learn them as they practice the various other aspects of medicine (Lee, Back, Block, & Stewart, 2002).

Practitioners specializing in cancer acknowledge that insufficient training in communication and management skills is a major factor contributing to their stress, lack of job satisfaction, and emotional burnout (Fallowfield & Jenkins, 1999; Penson, Dignan, Canellos, Picard, & Lynch, 2000). Unfortunately, few oncologists or nurses have received adequate formal education in communication skills using methods likely to promote change, confidence, and competence (Fallowfield & Jenkins, 1999; Hoffman et al., 2004; Penson et al., 2000). However, good practitioner–patient communication is associated with adherence to drug regimens and diets, pain control, resolution of physical and functional symptoms, control of blood sugar and hypertension, and good psychological functioning (Fallowfield & Jenkins, 1999; Penson et al., 2000). Additionally, Ong et al. (2000) found that patients' satisfaction was predicted by doctors' socioemotional behaviors and affective tone. Explicit communication of doctors' negative affect resulted in less patient satisfaction.

Communication is also a vital conduit for providing support, and family communication has been shown to influence both patient and family adaptation to illness. Less satisfactory reallocation of roles, more role conflict and role strain, less family cohesion, and greater family conflict have been found to result from poor communication (Heiney, 1988).

Reviewing the communication literature, Cegala and Broz (2003) found a lack of overall coherence and focus, with a lack of consistency about what a communication skill is. Moreover, they found that little effort has been made to provide an overarching framework for organizing practitioner communication skills, although some scholars have proposed instituting a classification scheme that distinguishes between information exchange and relational development. Additionally, the vast majority (80%) of practitioner–patient communication studies involved primary care physicians (i.e., family medicine physicians, general internists, or pediatricians). The 20% of studies reviewed in the context of oncology revealed that the majority of oncologists and other health professionals who deal with cancer patients did not receive adequate training in communicating with patients, particularly with respect to breaking bad news and handling strong, emotionally charged interview contexts (Baile et al., 1999; Cegala & Broz, 2003).

Beckman and Frankel (2003) believed that the first task in teaching effective practitioner–cancer patient communication is defining and distributing a comprehensive evidenced-based curriculum. Second, to teach this curriculum, faculty or local practitioners who embrace the curriculum and use it in practice must be recruited. Third, anchoring the curriculum in evidence-supported behaviors promotes effective interventions and focuses clinical controversies on the spectrum of naturally occurring communication styles that arise in the course of working with patients. The fourth element of a successful communication program is longitudinal reinforcement (Beckman & Frankel, 2003). Given a well-developed and broadly endorsed curriculum, the next building block to a successful communication program is creating environments that maximize the opportunity to learn, practice, and internalize the curriculum. Longitudinal learning programs, using a cohesive faculty, results in more meaningful incorporation of curricular elements into learner practice styles (Beckman & Frankel, 2003).

Various approaches to training practitioners in dealing with cancer patients have been instituted. One approach is *Oncotalk* (Back, Arnold, Tulsky, Baile, & Fryer-Edwards, 2003), a communication skills program built around evidence-based educational techniques. In an intensive 4-day retreat focused on communication at the end of life, medical oncology fellows are exposed to didactic material that incorporates specific interviewing skills. They then interview standardized patients while they are observed by trained facilitators, who act as coaches in helping them recognize and deal with obstacles and challenges in the encounter. The curriculum encompasses basic communication skills such as how to respond to emotional concerns and affect, giving bad news, conducting a family conference, managing the transition from curative to palliative therapy, and responding to requests for futile treatments (Back et al., 2003; Back, Li, & Sales, 2005). Results from analysis of audiotaped recordings with standardized patients have shown that medical oncology fellows can improve their skills significantly in giving bad news and transitioning the patient to palliative care (Back et al., 2007). More recently, societies such as the American Society of Clinical Oncology have developed and adopted specialized curricula for communicating with older cancer patients (Beckman & Frankel, 2003).

Other approaches that have been used to enhance the communication skills of practitioners include (a) a skills-based approach used to design structured training activities for teaching communication skills (Wagner, Lentz, & Heslop, 2002); (b) development of an innovative assessment instrument to facilitate curricular mapping of palliative care education (Meekin, Klein, Fleischman, & Fins, 2000); (c) efforts to enhance residents' knowledge, skills, and attitudes needed for effective palliative care (Fins & Nilson, 2000); (d) listening to the patient and responding with care as a model for teaching communication skills and to frame the practitioner–patient relationship around trust and respect (DiBartola, 2001); and (e) the use of serial standardized patient assessments for determining the acquisition of core clinical skills (Prislin, Giglio, Lewis, Ahearn, & Radecki, 2000). For excellent reviews on issues related to improving communication with cancer patients, see Maguire (1999) and a recent article by Baile and Aaron (2005).

Training Patients in Communication Skills

The majority of intervention studies have been directed at improving communication through health care providers and have most commonly emphasized the teaching of specific communication skills that may help providers interact better with their patients. Although the provider's role is essential, the provider–patient communication process is reciprocal and interactive, and the patient also has an essential role in the communication. Although less common than interventions for providers, a number of interventions have been designed to help cancer patients navigate their health care and improve communication with their providers. The goals of these interventions have varied across studies and have included outcomes such as increasing patients' question asking in the consultation (Butow, Dunn, Tattersall, & Jones, 1994; Clayton et al., 2003; Ford, Fallowfield, Hall, & Lewis, 1995), increasing recall of the information discussed in the consultation (Hogbin & Fallowfield, 1989; McHugh et al., 1995), increasing patient satisfaction (Damian & Tattersall, 1991; Tattersall, Butow, Griffin, & Dunn, 1994), improving patients' psychological adjustment (Deutsch, 1992; McHugh et al., 1995; North, Cornbleet, Knowles, & Leonard, 1992), and acquiring specific skills such as breaking bad news and discussing end-of-life issues (Back et al., 2007).

Although the literature stresses the importance of active patient participation to achieve efficacious changes in health-related behavior, it rarely occurs (Webber, 1990). Patients with cancer continue to lack practical information regarding their illness and report low levels of awareness and use of patient services. Barriers to patient education include the lack of coordination of educators, educators who are poorly prepared for their task, the low priority given to patient education by administrators (Webber, 1990), the belief that it is the physician's responsibility to determine what information patients should be given, limitations in the patient's ability to understand the information given or the realities of their illness, a lack of time, and unwillingness to share the power of decision making with the patient (Webber, 1990). In light of increasing concerns about the cost of health care, there is good reason to devote more attention to the effects of training patients in provision skills. Training patients to present information to their doctors effectively and efficiently may have the potential to reduce interview time while maintaining or even enhancing health care quality (Cegala & Broz, 2003). A meta-analysis of 49 studies calculated that psychoeducational interventions (e.g., providing information and teaching skills to reduce pain) reduced hospital stays by 1.25 days. Preoperative education has also been shown to hasten recovery and reduce patient anxiety (Webber, 1990), which has been stimulated by research suggesting that patients' active participation in their health care leads to greater satisfaction, increased compliance, and better health outcomes (Cegala & Broz, 2003).

FUTURE DIRECTIONS IN PRACTITIONER–PATIENT COMMUNICATION RESEARCH

Future research into patient communication skills training should examine ways of maximizing instructional effectiveness and ease of dissemination without increasing costs (Cegala & Broz, 2003). The challenge to educators is thus to find cost-effective and timely ways to deliver a complex mix of interesting and high-quality information and expertise to a large and diverse patient population while still tailoring the content to individual needs and situations. The Princess Margaret Hospital (PMH) computer-based patient education program, described by Jones, Nyhof-Young, Friedman, and Catton (2001), was developed to address this need and was aimed toward those dealing with cancer. The program provides comprehensive medical information and support through an interactive Intranet Web site containing information about cancer (i.e., the Oncology Interactive Education Series), library resources, Internet links, information about PMH services, and a hospital calendar of events. Preliminary evaluation results have provided valuable direction for ongoing program development and suggest that the program is easy to use; informative; and enjoyable for patients, families, volunteers, and health professionals (Jones et al., 2001).

Additional intervention studies are needed that simultaneously focus on both the practitioner and the patient. For example, educational intervention studies aimed at both patients and physicians could be developed and evaluated to examine both sides of the practitioner–patient communication, which may improve the interaction. Future studies should also more closely examine the role of culture, language, and ethnicity on the communication.

SUMMARY AND CONCLUSION

Because of the complexities facing patients with a diagnosis of cancer, the need for communication with health care practitioners—particularly the treating physician(s)—is of utmost importance. Not only do patients have to deal with a myriad of treatment decisions, fear of recurrence, fear of death, fear of isolation and loss of control, but they also have to deal with practitioners without the ability to provide a cogent prognosis. Patients with cancer have great needs for information, but it is well known that they often do not feel that the information they receive is adequate. This discrepancy is fed, in part, by physicians' lack of training in communication. Research shows, however, that communication skills can be learned by physicians and patients alike; as more research is done in the area of oncology communication, new ways of educating patients and physicians will continue to be developed.

REFERENCES

Adelbratt, S., & Strang, P. (2000). Death anxiety in brain tumour patients and their spouses. *Palliative Medicine, 14*, 499–507.

Arber, A., & Gallagher, A. (2003). Breaking bad news revisited: The push for negotiated disclosure and changing practice implications. *International Journal of Palliative Nursing, 9*, 166–172.

Back, A. L., Arnold, R. M., Baile, W. D. F., Fryer-Edwards, K. A., Alexander, S. C., Barley, G. C., & Tulsky, J. A. (2007). Efficacy of communication skills training for giving bad news and discussing transitions to palliative care. *Archives of Internal Medicine, 167*, 453–460.

Back, A. L., Arnold, R. M., Tulsky, J. A., Baile, W. F., & Fryer-Edwards, K. A. (2003). Teaching communication skills to medical oncology fellows. *Journal of Clinical Oncology, 21*, 2433–2466.

Back, A. L., Li, Y. F., & Sales, A. E. (2005). Impact of palliative care case management on resource use by patients dying of cancer at a Veterans Affairs medical center. *Journal of Palliative Medicine, 8,* 26–35.

Baile, W. F., & Aaron, J. (2005). Patient–physician communication in oncology: Past, present, and future. *Current Opinions in Oncology, 17,* 331–335.

Baile, W. F., Buckman, R., Lenzi, R., Glober, G., Beale, E. A., & Kudelka, A. P. (2000). SPIKES—A six-step protocol for delivering bad news: Application to the patient with cancer. *Oncologist, 5,* 302–311.

Baile, W. F., Glober, G. A., Lenzi, R., Beale, E. A., & Kudelka, A. P. (1999). Discussing disease progression and end-of-life decisions. *Oncology, 13,* 1021–1031.

Baile, W. F., Lenzi, R., Parker, P. A., Buckman, R., & Cohen, L. (2002). Oncologists' attitudes toward and practices in giving bad news: An exploratory study. *Journal of Clinical Oncology, 20,* 2189–2196.

Ballard-Reisch, D. S., & Letner, J. A. (2003). Centering families in cancer communication research: Acknowledging the impact of support, culture, and process on client–provider communication in cancer management. *Patient Education and Counseling, 50,* 61–66.

Beckman, H. B., & Frankel, R. M. (2003). Training practitioners to communicate effectively in cancer care: It is the relationship that counts. *Patient Education and Counseling, 50,* 85–89.

Bedell, S. E., Graboys, T. B., Bedell, E., & Lown, B. (2004). Words that harm, words that heal. *Archives of Internal Medicine, 164,* 1365–1368.

Blanchard, C. G., Labrecque, M. S., Ruckdeschel, J. C., & Blanchard, E. B. (1988). Information and decision-making preferences of hospitalized adult cancer patients. *Social Science & Medicine, 27,* 1139–1145.

Buckman, R. (1984, May 26). Breaking bad news: Why is it still so difficult? *BMJ, 288,* 1597–1599.

Butow, P. N., Dowsett, S., Hagerty, R., & Tattersall, M. H. N. (2002). Communicating prognosis to patients with metastatic disease: What do they really want to know? *Supportive Care in Cancer, 10,* 161–168.

Butow, P. N., Dunn, S. M., Tattersall, M. H., & Jones, Q. J. (1994). Patient participation in the cancer consultation: Evaluation of a question prompt sheet. *Annals of Oncology, 5,* 199–204.

Butow, P. N., Maclean, M., Dunn, S. M., Tattersall, M. H. N., & Boyer, M. J. (1997). The dynamics of change: Cancer patients' preferences for information, involvement, and support. *Annals of Oncology, 8,* 857–863.

Byock, I. R. (1996). The nature of suffering and the nature of opportunity at the end of life. *Clinics in Geriatric Medicine, 12,* 237–252.

Cegala, D. J., & Broz, S. L. (2003). Provider and patient communication skills training. In T. L. Thompson, A. Dorsey, K. Miller, & R. Parrott (Eds.), *Handbook of health communication* (pp. 95–119). Mahwah, NJ: Erlbaum.

Chochinov, H. M., Hack, T., Hassard, T., Kristjanson, L. J., McClement, S., & Harlos, M. (2002). Dignity in the terminally ill: A cross-sectional, cohort study. *Lancet, 360,* 2026–2030.

Clayton, J., Butow, P., Tattersall, M., Chye, R., Noel, M., Davis, J. M., & Glare, P. (2003). Asking questions can help: Development and preliminary evaluation of a question prompt list for palliative care patients. *British Journal of Cancer, 89*, 2069–2077.

Coughlin, S. S. (2008). Surviving cancer or other serious illnesses: A review of individual and community resources. *CA: A Cancer Journal of Clinicians, 58*, 60–64.

Damian, D., & Tattersall, M. H. (1991). Letters to patients: Improving communication in cancer care. *Lancet, 338*, 923–925.

Davis, C., Williams, P., Parle, M., Redman, S., & Turner, J. (2004). Assessing the support needs of women with early breast cancer in Australia. *Cancer Nursing, 27*, 169–174.

Degner, L. F., Kristjanson, L. J., Bowman, D., Sloan, J. A., Carriere, K. C., O'Neil, J., et al. (1997). Information needs and decisional preferences in women with breast cancer: The patient–physician relationship. *Journal of the American Medical Association, 277*, 1485–1492.

Deutsch, G. (1992). Improving communication with oncology patients: Taping the consultation. *Clinical Oncology, 4*, 46–47.

DiBartola, L. M. (2001). Listening to patients and responding with care: A model for teaching communication skills. *Journal on Quality Improvement, 27*, 315–323.

Ellis, P. M., & Tattersall, M. H. N. (1999). How should doctors communicate the diagnosis of cancer to patients? *Annals of Medicine, 31*, 336–341.

Fallowfield, L., & Jenkins, V. (1999). Effective communication skills are the key to good cancer care. *European Journal of Cancer, 35*, 1592–1597.

Fallowfield, L., Jenkins, V. A., & Beveridge, H. A. (2002). Truth may hurt but deceit hurts more: Communication in palliative care. *Palliative Medicine, 16*, 297–303.

Fins, J. J., & Nilson, E. G. (2000). An approach to educating residents about palliative care and clinical ethics. *Academic Medicine, 75*, 662–665.

Ford, S., Fallowfield, L., Hall, A., & Lewis, S. (1995). The influence of audiotapes on patient participation in the cancer consultation. *European Journal of Cancer, 31*, 2264–2269.

Friedrichsen, M. J., & Strang, P. M. (2003). Doctors' strategies when breaking bad news to terminally ill patients. *Journal of Palliative Medicine, 6*, 565–574.

Girgis, A., & Sanson-Fisher, R. W. (1995). Breaking bad news: Consensus guidelines for medical practitioners. *Journal of Clinical Oncology, 13*, 2449–2456.

Girgis, A., & Sanson-Fisher, R. W. (1998). Breaking bad news: I. Current best advice for clinicians. *Behavioral Medicine, 24*, 53–59.

Given, B. A., Given, C. W., & Kozachik, S. (2001). Family support in advanced cancer. *CA: A Cancer Journal for Clinicians, 51*, 213–231.

Gordon, E. J., & Daugherty, C. K. (2003). "Hitting you over the head": Oncologists' disclosure of prognosis to advanced cancer patients. *Bioethics, 17*, 142–168.

Guadagnoli, E., & Ward, P. (1998). Patient participation in decision-making. *Social Science & Medicine, 47*, 329–339.

Harris, S. R., & Templeton, E. (2001). Who's listening? Experiences of women with breast cancer in communicating with physicians. *The Breast Journal, 7*, 444–449.

Heiney, S. (1988). Assessing and intervening with dysfunctional families. *Oncology Nursing Forum, 15*, 585–590.

Helft, P. R. (2005). Necessary collusion: Prognostic communication with advanced cancer patients. *Journal of Clinical Oncology, 23*, 3146–3150.

Hern, H. E. J., Koenig, B. A., Moore, L. J., & Marshall, P. A. (1998). The difference that culture can make in end-of-life decision making. *Cambridge Quarterly of Healthcare Ethics, 7*, 27–40.

Hoffman, M., Ferri, J., Sison, C., Roter, D., Schapira, L. & Baile, W. F. (2004). Teaching communication skills: An AACE survey of oncology training programs. *Journal of Cancer Education, 19*, 220–224.

Hogbin, B., & Fallowfield, L. (1989). Getting it taped: The "bad news" consultation with cancer patients. *British Journal of Hospital Medicine, 41*, 330–333.

Jenkins, V., Fallowfield, L., & Saul, J. (2001). Information needs of patients with cancer: Results from a large study in UK cancer centers. *British Journal of Cancer, 84*, 48–51.

Jones, J. M., Nyhof-Young, J., Friedman, A., & Catton, P. (2001). More than just a pamphlet: Development of an innovative computer-based education program for cancer patients. *Patient Education and Counseling, 44*, 271–281.

Kurtz, S. M., & Silverman, J. D. (1996). The Calgary–Cambridge Referenced Observation Guides: An aid to defining the curriculum and organizing the teaching in communication training programmes. *Medical Education, 30*, 83–89.

Lee, S. J., Back, A. L., Block, S. D., & Stewart, S. K. (2002). Enhancing physician–patient communication. *Hematology*, 464–483.

Levy, M. (1998). Doctor–patient communication: The lifeline to comprehensive care. *American Society of Clinical Oncology*, 195–202.

Lobb, E. A., Butow, P. N., Kenny, D. T., & Tattersall, M. H. (1999). Communicating prognosis in early breast cancer: Do women understand the language used? *Medical Journal of Australia, 171*, 290–294.

Lobb, E. A., Butow, P. N., Meiser, B., Barratt, A., Gaff, C., Young, M. A., et al. (2002). Tailoring communication in consultations with women from high risk breast cancer families. *British Journal of Cancer, 87*, 502–508.

Loge, J. H., Kaasa, S., & Hytten, K. (1997). Disclosing the cancer diagnosis: The patients' experiences. *European Journal of Cancer, 33*, 878–882.

Maguire, P. (1999). Improving communication with cancer patients. *European Journal of Cancer, 35*, 1415–1422.

McHugh, P., Lewis, S., Ford, S., Newlands, E., Rustin, G., Coombes, C., et al. (1995). The efficacy of audiotapes in promoting psychological well-being in cancer patients: A randomised, controlled trial. *British Journal of Cancer, 71*, 388–392.

Meekin, S. A., Klein, J. E., Fleischman, A. R., & Fins, J. J. (2000). Development of a palliative education assessment tool for medical student education. *Academic Medicine, 75*, 986–992.

Miller, S. M. (1987). Monitoring and blunting: Validation of a questionnaire to assess styles of information seeking under threat. *Journal of Personality and Social Psychology, 52,* 345–353.

Miller, S. M., Brody, D. S., & Summerton, J. (1988). Styles of coping with threat: Implications for health. *Journal of Personality and Social Psychology, 54,* 142–148.

Mills, M. E., & Sullivan, K. (1999). The importance of information giving for patients newly diagnosed with cancer: A review of the literature. *Journal of Clinical Nursing, 8,* 631–642.

Mishel, M. H. (1990). Reconceptualization of the uncertainty in illness theory. *Image: The Journal of Nursing Scholarship, 22,* 256–262.

Mitchell, J. L. (1998). Cross-cultural issues in the disclosure of cancer. *Cancer Practice, 6,* 153–160.

Molleman, E., Krabbendam, P. J., Annyas, A. A., Koops, H. S., Sleijfer, D. T., & Vermey, A. (1984). The significance of the doctor–patient relationship in coping with cancer. *Social Science & Medicine, 18,* 475–480.

North, N., Cornbleet, M. A., Knowles, G., & Leonard, R. C. (1992). Information giving in oncology: A preliminary study of tape-recorder use. *British Journal of Clinical Psychology, 31*(Pt. 3), 357–359.

Ong, L. M. L., Visser, M. R. M., Lammes, F. B., & de Haes, J. C. (2000). Doctor–patient communciation and cancer patients' quality of life and satisfaction. *Patient Education and Counseling, 41,* 145–156.

Ong, L. M. L., Visser, M. R., van Zuuren, F. J., Rietbroek, R. C., Lammes, F. B., & de Haes, J. C. (1999). Cancer patients' coping styles and doctor–patient communication. *Psycho-Oncology, 8,* 155–166.

Parker, P. A., Baile, W. F., de Moor, C., Lenzi, R., Kudelka, A. P., & Cohen, L. (2001). Breaking bad news about cancer: Patients' preferences for communication. *Journal of Clinical Oncology, 19,* 2049–2056.

Penson, R. T., Dignan, F. L., Canellos, G. P., Picard, C. L., & Lynch, T. J. J. (2000). Burnout: Caring for the caregivers. *Oncologist, 5,* 425–434.

Prislin, M. D., Giglio, M., Lewis, E. M., Ahearn, S., & Radecki, S. (2000). Assessing the acquisition of core clinical skills through the use of serial standardized patient assessments. *Academic Medicine, 75,* 480–483.

Roberts, C. S., Cox, C. E., Reintgen, D. S., Baile, W. F., & Gibertinin, M. (1994). Influence of physician communication on newly diagnosed breast patients' psychologic adjustment and decision-making. *Cancer, 74,* 336–341.

Rudnick, A. (2002). Informed consent to breaking bad news. *Nursing Ethics, 9,* 61–66.

Schofield, P. E., Juraskova, I., & Butow, P. N. (2003). How oncologists discuss complementary therapy use with their patients: An audio-tape audit. *Support Care Cancer, 11,* 348–355.

Silliman, R. A., Dukes, K. A., Sullivan, L. M., & Kaplan, S. H. (1998). Breast cancer care in older women: Sources of information, social support, and emotional health outcomes. *Cancer, 83,* 706–711.

Siminoff, L. A., Ravdin, P., Colabianchi, N., & Sturm, C. M. (2000). Doctor–patient communication patterns in breast cancer adjuvant therapy discussions. *Health Expectations, 3,* 26–36.

Singer, P. A., Martin, D. K., & Kelner, M. (1999). Quality end-of-life care: Patients' perspectives. *Journal of the American Medical Association, 281,* 163–168.

Steinhauser, K. E., Christakis, N. A., Clipp, E. C., McNeilly, M., McIntyre, L., & Tulsky, J. A. (2000). Factors considered important at the end of life by patients, family, physicians, and other care providers. *Journal of the American Medical Association, 284,* 2476–2482.

Surbone, A. (2008). Cultural aspects of communication in cancer care. *Supportive Care in Cancer, 16,* 235–240.

Tattersall, M. H. N., Butow, P. N., & Clayton, J. M. (2002). Insights from cancer patient communication research. *Hematology/Oncology Clinics of North America, 16,* 731–743.

Tattersall, M. H. N., Butow, P. N., Griffin, A. M., & Dunn, S. M. (1994). The take-home message: Patients prefer consultation audiotapes to summary letters. *Journal of Clinical Oncology, 12,* 1305–1311.

Taylor, K. M., & Kelner, M. (1987). Informed consent: The physician's perspective. *Social Science & Medicine, 24,* 135–143.

Tobias, J. S., & Hamilton, R. D. (2002). Prospective clinical trials as a model for patient-centered care. *Annals of Oncology, 13,* 1695–1696.

Wagner, P. J., Lentz, L., & Heslop, S. D. M. (2002). Teaching communication skills: A skills-based approach. *Academic Medicine, 77,* 1164.

Wallace, J. A., Hlubocky, F. J., & Daugherty, C. K. (2006). Emotional responses of oncologists when disclosing prognostic information to patients with terminal disease: Results of quantitative data from a mailed survey to ASCO members. *Journal of Clinical Oncology, 24*(Suppl. 18, Pt. 1), 8520.

Webber, G. C. (1990). Patient education: A review of the issues. *Medical Care, 28,* 1089–1103.

Wenrich, M. D., Curtis, J. R., Shannon, S. E., Carline, J. D., Ambrozy, D. M., & Ramsey, P. G. (2001). Communicating with dying patients within the spectrum of medical care from terminal diagnosis to death. *Archives of Internal Medicine, 161,* 2623–2624.

Wright, E. B., Holcombe, C., & Salmon, P. (2004, April 10). Doctors' communication of trust, care, and respect in breast cancer: Qualitative study. *BMJ, 328,* 864.

19

BEHAVIORAL INTERVENTIONS FOR SIDE EFFECTS RELATED TO CANCER AND CANCER TREATMENTS

GARY R. MORROW, JOSEPH A. ROSCOE, KAREN M. MUSTIAN,
JANE T. HICKOK, JULIE L. RYAN, AND SARA MATTESON

Increasing numbers of people diagnosed with cancer are surviving their disease. This longevity comes with a price for the survivors, who frequently experience harsh, life-altering side effects during and after treatment. The principal methods of managing the side effects of cancer treatment and cancer are pharmacologic. Over the past 2 decades, however, substantial research has shown that behavioral techniques are beneficial in controlling cancer treatment–related side effects and the pain and emotional effects of cancer. Continued research of behavioral interventions for cancer treatment- and cancer-related issues is important because of the numerous advantages of behavioral treatments and the well-documented strong association between psychology and physiology (Abramson, Seligman, & Teasdale, 1978; Kirsch, 1997; Rotter, 1966).

Behavioral treatments have several assets that contribute to their usefulness. They are cost-effective and noninvasive; accepted by the patient; require little training; and can be implemented by psychologists, nurses, physicians, social workers, and others (Redd, 1994). These interventions also have few side effects (Morrow & Hickok, 1993), which is not the case with antiemetic medication or other drugs. Furthermore, behavioral techniques empower patients to assume control over an aspect of their care, thereby enhancing patient feelings of self-efficacy and control (Molassiotis, Yung, Yam, Chan, & Mok, 2002). Indeed, at a time when people may feel that their lives and bodies are out of their own control regarding what and when substances are put into their bodies, interventions that are not based on chemicals or drugs have a great deal to offer the patient.

NAUSEA AND VOMITING

A great deal of research has focused on chemotherapy-induced nausea and vomiting (NV), which are experienced by up to 76% (nausea) and 36% (vomiting) of patients (Grunberg et al., 2004; Hickok et al., 2003). Antiemetic medications, including 5-hydroxytryptamine-3 receptor antagonists, help alleviate nausea to some degree and are quite effective in alleviating vomiting (Hickok, Roscoe, Morrow, Bole, et al., 2005). Unfortunately, antiemetics have their own side effects (Raynov, 2001), and NV persist as frequently reported troublesome side effects of chemotherapy (Roscoe, Morrow, Hickok, & Stern, 2000). These side effects can impede the ability to maintain adequate nutrition and can lead to dehydration, fatigue, and a reduction in quality of life (Osoba et al., 1997; Roscoe, Morrow, et al., 2000). Patients may postpone, refuse, or cease chemotherapy because of fear of these side effects, potentially decreasing their chance for survival (Burish & Tope, 1992; Klastersky, Schimpff, & Senn, 1999). Controlling these side effects is critical to the overall health of the individual, and initial endeavors to curtail side effects of chemotherapy with behavioral methods have focused largely on NV (Redd, 1994).

The great variation in the frequency and severity of chemotherapy-induced NV cannot be accounted for by pharmacologic properties of the chemotherapeutic agents or physiologic characteristics of patients (Roscoe, Hickok, & Morrow, 2000). Patients' expectations about developing NV were postulated to account for some of this variance, and numerous studies have shown a positive relationship between patients' expectations for the development of NV because of chemotherapy and the subsequent occurrence of these side effects (Montgomery, 2000; Roscoe et al., 2004; Shelke et al., 2008). These results suggest that patients' expectancies related to nausea development are significant predictors of, and likely contributing factors to, treatment-related nausea.

The concept that expectancy may be related to the occurrence of cancer treatment–related side effects (i.e., a potential mediator) is similar to the ideas put forth in self-regulation (Wrosch, Scheier, Miller, Schulz, & Carver, 2003) and cognitive-emotional processing approaches to well-being and development of new behaviors (S. M. Miller, Shoda, & Hurley, 1996). These studies provide a broad conceptual basis that supports the idea that behavioral interventions that target or enhance the belief in the efficacy of the intervention or in the individuals' ability to successfully use the intervention are ideal for the treatment of chemotherapy-related nausea.

One such intervention that might delay or prevent conditioned side effects of treatment (Burish & Tope, 1992) is progressive muscle relaxation (PMR), in which one learns to relax by tensing and releasing specific muscle groups in a progressive manner (Morrow & Hickok, 1993). Patients who practice PMR have significantly less nausea during and immediately after chemotherapy (Burish & Lyles, 1981) and experience a reduced duration of NV (Molassiotis et al., 2002). PMR has a significant effect size in controlling nausea (Luebbert, Dahme, & Hasenbring, 2001). Relaxation is often combined with guided imagery (i.e., focused attention designed to elicit specific physiological responses and attain specific health goals). Imagery mentally addresses all sensory modalities such that both psychological and physiological responses are generated as if an actual external stimulus had been presented (Sodergren, 1992). Guided imagery visualizing quiet scenes (Redd, 1994) and imagery that is patient-specific and tailored around meaningful images patients have of their symptoms or disease are both beneficial (Eller, 1999; Van Fleet, 2000). Patients who receive a combined intervention of relaxation plus guided imagery have a reduced incidence of nausea during chemotherapy; lower incidence, duration, and severity of postchemotherapy nausea; shorter duration of posttreatment vomiting (Burish, Carey, Krozely, & Greco, 1987); and a more positive experience with chemotherapy than patients who receive antiemetic treatment alone (Troesch, Rodehaver, Delaney, & Yanes, 1993).

Other interventions include hypnosis, or suggestive therapy (Bakke, Purtzer, & Newton, 2002; DuHamel, Redd, & Vickberg, 1999; Elkins, Marcus, Palamara, & Stearns, 2004; Montgomery, David, Winkel, Silverstein, & Bovbjerg, 2002), systematic desensitization (Morrow & Dobkin, 1988), biofeedback (Morrow & Hickok, 1993), wristbands (Roscoe et al., 2003), and electrical stimulation at the wrist (Dundee, Yang, & McMillan, 1991). Another commonly reported and unfortunate consequence of chemotherapy is anticipatory nausea and vomiting (ANV). Anticipatory nausea is reported by 25% to 30% of patients at the fourth treatment cycle, and anticipatory vomiting develops in up to 20% of patients (Aapro, Molassiotis, & Olver, 2005). These pretreatment side effects rarely occur in the absence of posttreatment difficulties, suggesting that the mechanisms behind ANV may be explained by a learning model in which an unconditioned response (e.g., nausea) that results from the unconditioned stimulus (e.g., chemotherapy drugs) can be elicited by a conditioned stimulus (e.g., sights, sounds, and smells of the clinic) that is present at the same time as (i.e., paired with) the unconditioned stimulus. Over time, a conditioned response (NV) can eventually be elicited by the conditioned stimulus. Behavioral interventions are especially appropriate to address ANV, a conditioned response (Morrow & Hickok,

1993; Redd, 1994), and are best implemented prior to the complete development of the undesired conditioned response. Many of the same interventions that are effective in controlling NV have been used with success for ANV (Eller, 1999; Vasterling, Jenkins, Tope, & Burish, 1993) and systematic desensitization (Morrow et al., 1992).

No single mode of delivery of these behavioral interventions is universally effective or flawless. One-on-one instruction (i.e., clinician to patient) of these strategies allows the clinician to tailor them to the individual patient preferences and is more effective than instruction by audiotapes (Morrow, 1984), but audiotapes allow for independent practice after live intervention (Burish & Tope, 1992) and are cost-effective (Morrow & Hickok, 1993). The needs, resources, abilities, psychological history, and condition of the patient and treatment setting must be considered when choosing how to implement these interventions (Van Fleet, 2000).

FATIGUE

Unlike NV, there are few effective interventions for chemotherapy-induced fatigue. The specific causes of cancer-related fatigue (CRF) are not yet known, but potential causes include depression, pain, sleep problems, anemia, and medication side effects. Although anemia and depression associated with CRF can be treated, this success does not alleviate the problem completely, and nothing addresses the entire CRF spectrum (Berger, 2003).

There have been limited studies on behavioral interventions for the alleviation of chemotherapy-induced fatigue. Relaxation has been shown to reduce fatigue (Oyama, Kaneda, Katsumata, Akechi, & Ohsuga, 2000), but meta-analysis of the data available in the literature shows that relaxation training had no effect (Luebbert et al., 2001). More promising effects have been found with exercise. Cancer patients and survivors participating in exercise programs report less fatigue than those who do not exercise (Mustian et al., 2007). Finally, psychotherapy interventions offer some hope for patients suffering cancer treatment–related fatigue (Spiegel, Bloom, & Yalom, 1981). In light of this success of behavioral interventions in alleviating fatigue and the pervasiveness of this side effect of cancer treatment, continued studies in this area are warranted.

The literature is much less developed regarding the side effects and the behavioral management of radiation than those of chemotherapy. This discrepancy may be because the side effects from radiation are specific to the treatment site, whereas side effects from the systemic treatment of any cancer with chemotherapy are more universal. A multitude of unpleasant radiation treatment effects are documented in the literature, with fatigue being one of the most commonly experienced side effects (Jereczek-Fossa, Marsiglia,

& Orecchia, 2002). The cause and prevalence rate of radiation-induced fatigue are not well understood (Smets et al., 1998), but it is known to accumulate during the course of treatment and gradually abate over time (Hickok, Roscoe, Morrow, Mustian, et al., 2005; Irvine, Vincent, Graydon, & Bubela, 1998; Morrow et al., 2007). Few pharmacological interventions have proven to be helpful at alleviating this fatigue (Jereczek-Fossa, Marsiglia, & Orecchia, 2001).

One such empowering action is to increase the knowledge base of patients undergoing radiation to better prepare them for treatment and potential side effects (Kim, Roscoe, & Morrow, 2002). These results stress the important effects that can be obtained when patients are well informed and prepared for their treatment experience; that is, their ability to cope with radiation is enhanced by removing ambiguity from the treatment, and they have confidence to focus on solving problems rather than worrying about uncertainties. There has also been some experimental research regarding behavioral methods of alleviating radiation-induced fatigue (Decker, Cline-Elsen, & Gallager, 1992; Graydon, Bubela, Irvine, & Vincent, 1995; Irvine et al., 1998; Jacobsen & Thors, 2003; Mock et al., 1997).

PAIN

Pain is a subjective phenomenon, the intensity of which is affected by physical factors (e.g., efficacy of analgesic medications) and psychological factors (e.g., anxiety, perceived controllability, self-efficacy, symptom preoccupation; Ahles & Martin, 1992; Main & Spanswick, 1991). These psychological factors, which are interrelated and related to the physical factors, can be conceptualized as components of an expectancy schema and have the potential to influence pain indirectly through the medium of expectancy. Evidence indicates that beliefs can substantially impact the pain experience and the effectiveness of interventions for pain, including the efficacy of inert placebo medications (Roscoe et al., 2006). Thoughts and expectations can be converted into physiological reality (N. E. Miller, 1989), and the placebo response is a powerful pain management tool (Wall, 1993). In addition, self-efficacy, coping methods (Bachiocco, Morselli, & Carli, 1993), and learning about the relevant experiences of others (Turk & Feldman, 1992) all predict pain levels. For these reasons, cognitive behavior interventions may be especially effective in diminishing pain associated with cancer and its treatment.

Few controlled studies have examined the use of nonpharmacological interventions for cancer pain (Syrjala, Donaldson, Davis, Kippes, & Carr, 1995), but they include a myriad of strategies. PMR has a significant effect size for pain management (Sloman, Brown, Aldana, & Chee, 1994), and exercise has reduced pain severity (Dimeo, Stieglitz, Novelli-Fischer, Fetscher, & Keul,

1999; Given et al., 2002; Syrjala, Cummings, & Donaldson, 1992; Syrjala et al., 1995). Evidence also supports the use of hypnosis for pain control in cancer patients (Montgomery, David, Winkel, Silverstein, & Bovbjerg, 2002; Montgomery, Weltz, Seltz, & Bovbjerg, 2002). Devine's (2003) meta-analysis of 25 studies of many types of interventions indicated that a moderate but statistically significant alleviation of pain was achieved across all studies.

RACIAL/ETHNIC DISPARITY

Much of the effort that has gone into investigating and developing effective means to control side effects experienced by individuals undergoing treatment for cancer has been done in Europe (Wengstrom, Haggmark, Strander, & Forsberg, 1999). Racial and ethnic data are often not provided in these studies, but some information regarding socioeconomic status of the participants (e.g., highest level of education attained) has been reported. Most subjects studied have had at least some college education (Given et al., 2002; Syrjala et al., 1995). This information gives a rough idea of the patients to whom the findings might be generalized. Review articles tend not to mention this type of demographic information at all. Thus, little is known about whether and how different cultural and ethnic groups differ in their side effect profile, the expression of emotional or physical distress, or coping styles. Some investigators are purposely modifying their recruitment strategies and accruing substantial numbers of non-Caucasian patients in their studies (Mishel et al., 2002), perhaps signaling a shift in perspective and focus that will provide more information and understanding of the needs of diverse patient groups.

SPECULATION ON COMMON MECHANISMS

A key aspect of both the development and the management of treatment side effects is patient expectations. Patient expectancy may be a common mechanism influencing the outcome of treatments for a wide range of disorders (Benedetti, 2002; Chvetzoff & Tannock, 2003; Di Blasi, Harkness, Ernst, Georgiou, & Kleijnen, 2001; Mondloch, Cole, & Frank, 2001), including chemotherapy and radiation for cancer. A number of theories (Abramson et al., 1978; Kirsch, 1997; Rotter, 1966; Stewart-Williams, 2004) explain, and data support, the close connection between psychological and physiological states in the general medical literature. In one theory, Kirsch (1997) proposed that expectations directly affect both physiological and psychological outcomes. The exact mechanism by which these response expectancies operate remains a mystery, but they are self-confirming, account for the placebo effect, and may involve aspects of treatment that cannot be attributed to physical effect of pharmacological interventions (e.g., attention by health care providers, credibility of the treatment). Several studies have confirmed this theory by demonstrating, for example, the impact of patient expectations in the development of postsurgical disability (Gidron, McGrath, & Goodday, 1995) and pain (Roscoe et al., 2004).

The concept of expectancy also plays a prominent role in psychological theories of behavior and cognition. The locus of control theory (Rotter, 1966) and social learning theory (Abramson et al., 1978) incorporate expectations as influences on perceptions of control and the ability to cope. One's sense of personal efficacy is thought to greatly determine the behavior that follows. Thus, individuals who believe they can cope with challenges will behave in an active, solution-oriented way that is consistent with this belief as opposed to someone who believes he or she is unable to deal with the situation at hand. These expectations are a significant predictor of behaviors and impact both physiological and psychological outcomes by influencing coping responses, attitudes, and motivation (Scheier & Carver, 1992).

Expectations are also factors in schema theory (Thorndyke & Hayes Roth, 1979), a model of how people organize and plan action (G. A. Miller, Galanter, & Pribram, 1960). *Schemas* are cognitive structures that contain the elements of both expectancy and efficacy and are unique to the individual, modifiable by experience, and specific to what is being perceived (Rumelhart, 1984). Thus, information such as sensory data is interpreted through a relevant schema, causing an individual expecting to experience a symptom (e.g., nausea, fatigue) to be more likely to interpret sensations as that symptom than an individual not expecting to experience the symptom. To carry this example further, an appraisal of expected nausea creates a corresponding level of anxiety. A feedback loop creating an increase in expected nausea level may occur if the anxiety generated has a negative impact on successful implementation of the management strategy. Expectation, therefore, can act as a mediator between the actual sensory stimulus and the symptom experience.

Because of this close connection between psychology and physiology, behavioral techniques are useful in controlling side effects of cancer treatment (Molassiotis et al., 2002). Behavioral interventions applied during cancer treatment target and modify maladaptive beliefs and behaviors and foster the development of adaptive ones (Morrow & Bellg, 1994). Several recent studies support the key role of patient expectancy in cancer treatment side effect outcome, which is in keeping with the close psychology–physiology connection (Montgomery, 2000). Data gathered from a multicenter clinical trial indicate that breast cancer patients who thought it was *very likely* they would have severe nausea from chemotherapy were 5 times more likely to experience severe nausea than those who thought its occurrence would be *very unlikely* (Roscoe et al., 2004). Another study of breast cancer patients undergoing chemotherapy revealed a significant ($p < .01$) relation between patient expectation and severity of side effects (Stein & Jacobsen, 1998). A significant positive relationship ($p < .05$) between patients' pretreatment expectations for nausea and its subsequent development was also demonstrated in a homogeneous group of 29 female cancer patients receiving platinum-containing chemotherapy as inpatients and in 81 subjects with any of a variety of cancers (Roscoe, Hickok, & Morrow, 2000). Response expectancy has also been shown to influence the occurrence of anticipatory nausea (Matteson, Roscoe, Hickok, & Morrow, 2002).

SUMMARY

Behavioral interventions offer a viable alternative to pharmacologic agents for the relief of cancer treatment–related side effects and the pain and emotional effects of cancer. The documented strong association between psychology and physiology and the numerous advantages of behavioral treatments position this type of intervention for success. A potential common mechanism involved in this association between psychology and physiology is patient expectancy, which is part of several behavioral theories. Patient expectancy significantly affects the occurrence, severity, and duration of some of the key side effects of radiation and chemotherapy treatments (e.g., nausea, vomiting, fatigue) and the pain and emotional stress of cancer itself. Behavioral interventions that have been used to successfully ameliorate these problems include PMR, guided imagery, hypnosis, cognitive distraction, systematic desensitization, biofeedback, acupressure wristbands, exercise, psychotherapy, and support groups. More research into the nuances of behavioral interventions and how individual patients' needs can be most successfully met is needed to add to the success of cancer treatments and patients' quality of life.

REFERENCES

Aapro, M. S., Molassiotis, A., & Olver, I. (2005). Anticipatory nausea and vomiting. *Supportive Care in Cancer, 13,* 117–121.

Abramson, L. Y., Seligman, M. E., & Teasdale, J. D. (1978). Learned helplessness in humans: Critique and reformulation. *Journal of Abnormal Psychology, 87,* 49–74.

Ahles, T. A., & Martin, J. B. (1992). Cancer pain: A multidimensional perspective. *Hospice Journal, 8,* 25–48.

Bachiocco, V., Morselli, A. M., & Carli, G. (1993). Self-control expectancy and postsurgical pain: Relationships to previous pain, behavior in past pain, familial pain tolerance models, and personality. *Journal of Pain and Symptom Management, 8,* 205–214.

Bakke, A. C., Purtzer, M. Z., & Newton, P. (2002). The effect of hypnotic-guided imagery on psychological well-being and immune function in patients with prior breast cancer. *Journal of Psychosomatic Research, 53*, 1131–1137.

Benedetti, F. (2002). How the doctor's words affect the patient's brain. *Evaluation & The Health Professions, 25*, 369–386.

Berger, A. (2003). Treating fatigue in cancer patients. *The Oncologist, 8*, 10–14.

Burish, T. G., Carey, M. P., Krozely, M. G., & Greco, F. A. (1987). Conditioned side effects induced by cancer chemotherapy: Prevention through behavioral treatment. *Journal of Consulting and Clinical Psychology, 55*, 42–48.

Burish, T. G., & Lyles, J. N. (1981). Effectiveness of relaxation training in reducing adverse reactions to cancer chemotherapy. *Journal of Behavioral Medicine, 4*, 65–78.

Burish, T. G., & Tope, D. M. (1992). Psychological techniques for controlling the adverse side effects of cancer chemotherapy: Findings from a decade of research. *Journal of Pain and Symptom Management, 7*, 287–301.

Chvetzoff, G., & Tannock, I. (2003). Placebo effects in oncology. *Journal of the National Cancer Institute, 95*, 19–29.

Decker, T. W., Cline-Elsen, J., & Gallager, M. (1992). Relaxation therapy as an adjunct in radiation oncology. *Journal of Clinical Psychology, 48*, 388–393.

Devine, E. C. (2003). Meta-analysis of the effect of psychoeducational interventions on pain in adults with cancer. *Oncology Nursing Forum, 30*, 75–89.

Di Blasi, Z., Harkness, E., Ernst, E., Georgiou, A., & Kleijnen, J. (2001). Influence of context effects on health outcomes: A systematic review. *Lancet, 357*, 757–762.

Dimeo, F. C., Stieglitz, R. D., Novelli-Fischer, U., Fetscher, S., & Keul, J. (1999). Effects of physical activity on the fatigue and psychologic status of cancer patients during chemotherapy. *Cancer, 85*, 2273–2277.

DuHamel, K. N., Redd, W. H., & Vickberg, S. M. (1999). Behavioral interventions in the diagnosis, treatment and rehabilitation of children with cancer. *Acta Oncologica, 38*, 719–734.

Dundee, J. W., Yang, J., & McMillan, C. (1991). Non-invasive stimulation of the P6 (NeiGuan) antiemetic acupuncture point in cancer chemotherapy. *Journal of the Royal Society of Medicine, 84*, 210–212.

Elkins, G., Marcus, J., Palamara, L., & Stearns, V. (2004). Can hypnosis reduce hot flashes in breast cancer survivors? A literature review. *American Journal of Clinical Hypnosis, 47*, 29–42.

Eller, L. S. (1999). Guided imagery interventions for symptom management. *Annual Review of Nursing Research, 17*, 57–84.

Gidron, Y., McGrath, P. J., & Goodday, R. (1995). The physical and psychosocial predictors of adolescents' recovery from oral surgery. *Journal of Behavioral Medicine, 18*, 385–399.

Given, B., Given, C. W., McCorkle, R., Kozachik, S., Cimprich, B., Rahbar, M. H., & Wojcik, C. (2002). Pain and fatigue management: Results of a nursing randomized clinical trial. *Oncology Nursing Forum, 29*, 949–956.

Graydon, J. E., Bubela, N., Irvine, D., & Vincent, L. (1995). Fatigue-reducing strategies used by patients receiving treatment for cancer. *Cancer Nursing, 18*, 23–28.

Grunberg, S. M., Deuson, R. R., Mavros, P., Geling, O., Hansen, M., Cruciani, G., et al. (2004). Incidence of chemotherapy-induced nausea and emesis after modern antiemetics. *Cancer, 100*, 2261–2268.

Hickok, J. T., Roscoe, J. A., Morrow, G. R., Bole, C. W., Zhao, H., Hoelzer, K. L., et al. (2005). 5-hydroxytryptamine-receptor antagonists versus prochlorperazine for control of delayed nausea caused by doxorubicin: A URCC CCOP randomised controlled trial. *Lancet Oncology, 6*, 765–772.

Hickok, J. T., Roscoe, J. A., Morrow, G. R., King, D. K., Atkins, J. N., & Fitch, T. R. (2003). Nausea and emesis remain significant problems of chemotherapy despite prophylaxis with 5-hydroxytryptamine-3 antiemetics: A University of Rochester James P. Wilmot Cancer Center Community Clinical Oncology Program Study of 360 cancer patients treated in the community. *Cancer, 97*, 2880–2886.

Hickok, J. T., Roscoe, J. A., Morrow, G. R., Mustian, K. M., Okunieff, P., & Bole, C. W. (2005). Frequency, severity, clinical course, and correlates of fatigue in 372 patients during five weeks of radiotherapy (RT) for cancer. *Cancer, 104*, 1772–1778.

Irvine, D. M., Vincent, L., Graydon, J. E., & Bubela, N. (1998). Fatigue in women with breast cancer receiving radiation therapy. *Cancer Nursing, 21*, 127–135.

Jacobsen, P. B., & Thors, C. L. (2003). Fatigue in the radiation therapy patient: Current management and investigations. *Seminars in Radiation Oncology, 13*, 372–380.

Jereczek-Fossa, B. A. M., Marsiglia, H. R., & Orecchia, R. (2001). Radiotherapy-related fatigue: How to assess and how to treat the symptom. A commentary. *Tumori, 87*, 147–152.

Jereczek-Fossa, B. A. M., Marsiglia, H. R., & Orecchia, R. (2002). Radiotherapy-related fatigue. *Critical Reviews in Oncology/Hematology, 41*, 317–325.

Kim, Y., Roscoe, J. A., & Morrow, G. R. (2002). The effects of information and negative affect on severity of side effects from radiation therapy for prostate cancer. *Supportive Care in Cancer, 10*, 416–421.

Kirsch, I. (1997). Response expectancy theory and application: A decennial review. *Applied & Preventive Psychology, 6*, 69–79.

Klastersky, J., Schimpff, S. C., & Senn, H. J. (1999). *Supportive care in cancer* (2nd ed.). New York: Marcel Dekker.

Luebbert, K., Dahme, B., & Hasenbring, M. (2001). The effectiveness of relaxation training in reducing treatment-related symptoms and improving emotional adjustment in acute non-surgical cancer treatment: A meta-analytical review. *Psycho-Oncology, 10*, 490–502.

Main, C. J., & Spanswick, C. C. (1991). Pain: Psychological and psychiatric factors. *British Medical Bulletin, 47*, 732–742.

Matteson, S., Roscoe, J., Hickok, J., & Morrow, G. R. (2002). The role of behavioral conditioning in the development of nausea. *American Journal of Obstetrics and Gynecology, 185*, 239–243.

Miller, G. A., Galanter, E., & Pribram, K. H. (1960). *Plans and the structure of behavior*. New York: Holt, Rinehart & Winston.

Miller, N. E. (1989). Placebo factors in treatment: Views of a psychologist. In M. Shepherd & N. Sartorius (Eds.), *Non-specific aspects of treatment* (pp. 39–51). Toronto, Canada: Huber.

Miller, S. M., Shoda, Y., & Hurley, K. (1996). Applying cognitive-social theory to health-protective behavior: Breast self-examination in cancer screening. *Psychology Bulletin, 119*, 70–94.

Mishel, M. H., Belyea, M., Germino, B. B., Stewart, J. L., Bailey, D. E., Jr., Roberston, C., & Mohler, J. (2002). Helping patients with localized prostate carcinoma manage uncertainty and treatment side effects: Nurse-delivered psychoeducational intervention over the telephone. *Cancer, 94*, 1854–1866.

Mock, V., Dow, K. H., Meares, C. J., Grimm, P. M., Dienemann, J. A., Haisfield, W., et al. (1997). Effects of exercise on fatigue, physical functioning, and emotional distress during radiation therapy for breast cancer. *Oncology Nursing Forum, 24*, 991–1000.

Molassiotis, A., Yung, H. P., Yam, B. M. C., Chan, F. Y. S., & Mok, T. S. (2002). The effectiveness of progressive muscle relaxation training in managing chemotherapy-induced nausea and vomiting in Chinese breast cancer patients: A randomized controlled trial. *Supportive Care in Cancer, 10*, 237–246.

Mondloch, M. V., Cole, D. C., & Frank, J. W. (2001). Does how you do depend on how you think you'll do? A systematic review of the evidence for a relation between patients' recovery expectations and health outcomes. *Canadian Medical Association Journal, 165*, 174–179.

Montgomery, G. H. (2000). Pre-infusion expectations predict post-treatment nausea during repeated adjuvant chemotherapy infusions for breast cancer. *British Journal of Health Psychology, 5*, 105–119.

Montgomery, G. H., David, D., Winkel, G., Silverstein, J. H., & Bovbjerg, D. H. (2002). The effectiveness of adjunctive hypnosis with surgical patients: A meta-analysis. *Anesthesia & Analgesia, 94*, 1639–1645.

Montgomery, G. H., Weltz, C., Seltz, M., & Bovbjerg, D. H. (2002). Brief pre-surgery hypnosis reduces distress and pain in excisional breast biopsy patients. *International Journal of Clinical and Experimental Hypnosis, 50*, 15–30.

Morrow, G. R. (1984). Appropriateness of taped versus live relaxation in the systematic desensitization of anticipatory nausea and vomiting in cancer patients. *Journal of Consulting and Clinical Psychology, 52*, 1098–1099.

Morrow, G. R., Asbury, R., Hammon, S., Dobkin, P., Caruso, L., Pandya, K., & Rosenthal, S. (1992). Comparing the effectiveness of behavioral treatment for chemotherapy-induced nausea and vomiting when administered by oncologists, oncology nurses, and clinical psychologists. *Health Psychology, 11*, 250–256.

Morrow, G. R., & Bellg, A. J. (1994). Behavioral science in translational research and cancer control. *Cancer, 74*, 1409–1417.

Morrow, G. R., & Dobkin, P. L. (1988). Anticipatory nausea and vomiting in cancer patients undergoing chemotherapy treatment: Prevalence, etiology, and behavioral interventions. *Clinical Psychology Review, 8*, 517–556.

Morrow, G. R., & Hickok, J. T. (1993). Behavioral treatment of chemotherapy-induced nausea and vomiting. *Oncology, 7*, 83–89, 93–94.

Morrow G. R., Roscoe J. A., Kaufman, M. E., Bole, C., Figuero-Moseley, C., Hofman, M., & Mustian, K. M. (2007). Cancer-related fatigue as a late effect: Severity in relation to diagnosis, therapy, and related symptoms. In P. Rubin, L. S. Constine, L. B. Marks, & P. Okuneiff (Eds.), *Medical radiology: Vol. 1. Late effects on normal tissues of cancer* (pp. 91–99). Berlin, Germany: Springer Publishing Company.

Mustian, K. M., Morrow, G. R., Carroll, J. K., Figueroa-Moseley, C. D., Jean-Pierre, P., & Williams, G. C. (2007). Integrative nonpharmacologic behavioral interventions for the management of cancer-related fatigue. *The Oncologist, 12*, 52–67.

Osoba, D., Zee, B., Warr, D., Latreille, J., Kaizer, L., & Pater, J. (1997). Effect of postchemotherapy nausea and vomiting on health-related quality of life: The Quality of Life and Symptom Control Committees of the National Cancer Institute of Canada Clinical Trials Group. *Supportive Care in Cancer, 5*, 307–313.

Oyama, H., Kaneda, M., Katsumata, N., Akechi, T., & Ohsuga, M. (2000). Using the bedside wellness system during chemotherapy decreases fatigue and emesis in cancer patients. *Journal of Medical Systems, 24*, 173–182.

Raynov, J. (2001). Antiemetics: Side effects and reactions. *Archive of Oncology, 9*, 151–153.

Redd, W. H. (1994). Behavioral intervention for cancer treatment side effects. *Acta Oncologica, 33*, 113–117.

Roscoe, J. A., Bushunow, P., Morrow, G. R., Hickok, J. T., Kuebler, P. J., Jacobs, A., & Banerjee, T. K. (2004). Patient expectation is a strong predictor of severe nausea after chemotherapy: A University of Rochester Community Clinical Oncology Program study of patients with breast carcinoma. *Cancer, 101*, 2701–2708.

Roscoe, J. A., Hickok, J. T., & Morrow, G. R. (2000). Patient expectations as predictor of chemotherapy-induced nausea. *Annals of Behavioral Medicine, 22*, 121–126.

Roscoe, J. A., Jean-Pierre, P., Shelke, A. R., Kaufman, M. E., Bole, C., & Morrow, G. R. (2006). The role of patients' response expectancies in side effect development and control. *Current Problems in Cancer, 30*, 40–98.

Roscoe, J. A., Morrow, G. R., Hickok, J. T., Bushunow, P. W., Pierce, H. I., Flynn, P. J., et al. (2003). The efficacy of acupressure and acustimulation wrist bands for the relief of chemotherapy-induced nausea and vomiting: A URCC CCOP multicenter study. *Journal of Pain and Symptom Management, 26*, 731–742.

Roscoe, J. A., Morrow, G. R., Hickok, J. T., & Stern, R. M. (2000). Nausea and vomiting remain a significant clinical problem: Trends over time in controlling chemotherapy-induced nausea and vomiting in 1,413 patients treated in community clinical practices. *Journal of Pain and Symptom Management, 20*, 113–121.

Rotter, J. B. (1966). Generalized expectancies for internal versus external control of reinforcement. *Psychological Monographs, 80,* 1–28.

Rumelhart, D. E. (1984). Schemata and the cognitive system. In R. S. Wyer Jr. & T. K. Srull (Eds.), *Handbook of social cognition: Vol. 1. Basic processes* (pp. 161–186). Hillsdale, NJ: Erlbaum.

Scheier, M. F., & Carver, C. S. (1992). Effects of optimism on psychological and physical well-being: Theoretical overview and empirical update. *Cognitive Therapy and Research, 16,* 201–228.

Shelke, A. R., Roscoe, J. A., Morrow, G. R., Colman, L. K., Banerjee, T. K., & Kirshner, J. J. (2008). Effect of a nausea expectancy manipulation on chemotherapy-induced nausea: A University of Rochester Cancer Center Community Clinical Oncology Program study. *Journal of Pain and Symptom Management, 35,* 381–387.

Sloman, R., Brown, P., Aldana, E., & Chee, E. (1994). The use of relaxation for the promotion of comfort and pain relief in persons with advanced cancer. *Contemporary Nurse, 3,* 6–12.

Smets, E. M., Visser, M. R., Willems-Groot, A. F., Garssen, B., Oldenburger, F., van Tienhoven, G., & de Haes, J. C. (1998). Fatigue and radiotherapy: A. Experience in patients undergoing treatment. *British Journal of Cancer, 78,* 899–906.

Sodergren, K. M. (1992). Guided imagery. In M. Snyder (Ed.), *Independent nursing interventions* (pp. 103–124). New York: Wiley.

Spiegel, D., Bloom, J. R., & Yalom, I. (1981). Group support for patients with metastatic cancer: A randomized outcome study. *Archives of General Psychiatry, 38,* 527–533.

Stein, K. D., & Jacobsen, P. B. (1998). Expectancies, perceived control, and severity of physical side effects of adjuvant chemotherapy for breast cancer. *Psychosomatic Medicine, 60,* 121.

Stewart-Williams, S. (2004). The placebo puzzle: Putting together the pieces. *Health Psychology, 23,* 198–206.

Syrjala, K. L., Cummings, C., & Donaldson, G. W. (1992). Hypnosis or cognitive behavioral training for the reduction of pain and nausea during cancer treatment: A controlled clinical trial. *Pain, 48,* 137–146.

Syrjala, K. L., Donaldson, G. W., Davis, M. W., Kippes, M. E., & Carr, J. E. (1995). Relaxation and imagery and cognitive–behavioral training reduce pain during cancer treatment: A controlled clinical trial. *Pain, 63,* 189–198.

Thorndyke, P. W., & Hayes Roth, B. (1979). The use of schemata in the acquisition and transfer of knowledge. *Cognitive Psychology, 11,* 82–106.

Troesch, L. M., Rodehaver, C. B., Delaney, E. A., & Yanes, B. (1993). The influence of guided imagery on chemotherapy-related nausea and vomiting. *Oncology Nursing Forum, 20,* 1179–1185.

Turk, D. C., & Feldman, C. S. (1992). Facilitating the use of noninvasive pain management strategies with the terminally ill. *Hospice Journal, 8,* 193–214.

Van Fleet, S. (2000). Relaxation and imagery for symptom management: Improving patient assessment and individualizing treatment. *Oncology Nursing Forum, 27,* 501–510.

Vasterling, J., Jenkins, R. A., Tope, D. M., & Burish, T. G. (1993). Cognitive distraction and relaxation training for the control of side effects due to cancer chemotherapy. *Journal of Behavioral Medicine, 16,* 65–80.

Wall, P. D. (1993). Pain and the placebo response. *Ciba Foundation Symposium, 174,* 187–211.

Wengstrom, Y., Haggmark, C., Strander, H., & Forsberg, C. (1999). Effects of a nursing intervention on subjective distress, side effects, and quality of life of breast cancer patients receiving curative radiation therapy: A randomized study. *Acta Oncologica, 38,* 763–770.

Wrosch, C., Scheier, M., Miller, G., Schulz, R., & Carver, C. (2003). Adaptive self-regulation of unattainable goals: Goal disengagement, goal reengagement, and subjective well-being. *Personality and Social Psychology Bulletin, 29,* 1494–1508.

20
PSYCHOSOCIAL RESPONSE TO CANCER DIAGNOSIS AND TREATMENT

BETH E. MEYEROWITZ AND SINDY OH

Over the past 3 decades, psychological and medical researchers have made enormous strides in understanding the emotional and psychosocial responses of individuals who are diagnosed with and treated for cancer. This literature has developed through three overlapping and interrelated phases. Initially, interview and questionnaire studies focused on describing the distress and disruption associated with cancer diagnosis and treatment. This line of research was designed to provide the patient and the health care team with an empirically based sense of common responses and concerns that would allow them to be prepared for likely outcomes and to identify reactions that were not within normal limits. Equally as valuable, these studies confirmed the importance of considering quality, as well as length, of survival in cancer care, a perspective that now is widely accepted, thanks to patient advocates and psychosocial research. As more became known about the psychosocial experiences of individuals with cancer, researchers became interested in understanding variations in responses: Why did some patients appear to have ongoing difficulties, whereas others seemed to return to prediagnostic quality of life fairly quickly? Thus, in the second phase, researchers attempted to identify personal, social, and cancer-related predictors of adjustment following the diagnosis of cancer. With knowledge of common difficulties and of characteristics and resources of patients who might be at high risk for psychosocial problems, researchers were able to develop treatment programs. The third phase of research has involved testing the efficacy of psychosocial interventions in cancer care.

We review the literature directed at describing, predicting, and treating psychosocial responses to cancer diagnosis and treatment in adults. Some relevant issues—such as treatment-specific side effects, psychosexual dysfunction, survivorship issues, and familial support—are covered in other chapters of this volume. We focus on the general distress and disruption experienced by adult patients during and shortly after primary treatment. We are not able to describe all of the research in this area but have provided examples of some of the key references in the field.

A note of caution about this literature is necessary. Although there is a vast body of psychosocial research, the participants do not fully represent the population of patients. Upper-middle-class, non-Hispanic White women, particularly women with early-stage breast cancer, make up a disproportionate share of research respondents in both questionnaire and treatment outcome studies (Andersen, 2002; Rehse & Pukrop, 2003; Sheard & Maguire, 1999). Ethnic minorities, low-income patients, patients with cancers at certain sites, and patients with poor prognoses are seriously underrepresented. When men are studied, the focus has tended to be on physical and functional domains rather than on emotions and relationships (Meyerowitz & Hart, 1995). Thus, until these biases are remedied, care must be taken in generalizing these research results.

DESCRIPTION OF PSYCHOSOCIAL REACTIONS TO THE DIAGNOSIS AND TREATMENT OF CANCER

The diagnosis and treatment of cancer affect patients' lives in multiple domains. It has been widely accepted that a comprehensive description requires a multidimensional and subjective assessment by the patient, whenever possible (Aaronson et al., 1991; Sneeuw et al., 1999). Most studies gather these data through administering questionnaires, either generic questionnaires targeted to important aspects of quality of life or questionnaires developed specifically to assess components of quality of life among individuals with cancer. The domains of response to the diagnosis and treatment of cancer listed in the sections that follow are not orthogonal. Difficulties in one area can exacerbate problems in another area, making it hard to identify underlying processes and possible causal relations.

Emotions and Mood

Distress, negative affect, and depressed mood are among the most common reactions to receiving a diagnosis of, and treatment for, cancer (Kornblith,

1998; Shapiro, Lopez, Schwartz, Braden, & Kurker, 2001). On average, close to one quarter of cancer patients appear to experience depression, with rates ranging from approximately 1% to 50% on the basis of disease stage, cancer site, time since diagnosis, other disease-related variables, and study methods (Bottomley, 1998a; McDaniel, Musselman, Porter, Reed, & Nemeroff, 1995). Several studies also found an increased relative risk for suicide, particularly among men with cancer, as compared with population norms (Filiberti & Ripamonti, 2002). Clinical levels of anxiety have been identified in 30% to 40% of newly diagnosed patients in some studies but have been far less common in other studies (Bottomley, 1998b; Epping-Jordan et al., 1999). Burgess et al. (2005) found that breast cancer survivors were approximately twice as likely as the general female population to experience depression, anxiety, or both in the months immediately after diagnosis. For women who remained in remission, prevalence rates dropped by 1 year postdiagnosis, to reach levels similar to women in the general population. Subclinical levels of depression and anxiety are common responses to the diagnosis and treatment of cancer (Kornblith, 1998). Feelings of sadness, loss, vulnerability, agitation, and grief, typically at moderate levels, are nearly universal. In addition to increased levels of negative affect, patients also may experience decreased levels of positive affect, leading to mild to moderate anhedonia.

The wide variation in prevalence estimates across studies can be explained in part by the difficulty inherent in diagnosing mood disorders in individuals with cancer (McDaniel et al., 1995; Newport & Nemeroff, 1998). It is not always clear when appropriate levels of sadness and grief cross the threshold to psychiatric disorders. Moreover, several diagnostic criteria for mood disorders—fatigue, loss of appetite, poor concentration—are symptoms commonly associated with cancer and its treatments (McDaniel et al., 1995).

Thoughts and Fears

Upon learning of the diagnosis, many patients experience difficulty remembering and processing complex information, which can impair their ability to make informed decisions about their treatment. In addition, several cancer-related fears and concerns arise, such as fears of pain or disfigurement, creating a burden for one's family, and death. Perhaps the most common fear for individuals completing successful primary treatment is fear of recurrence. Almost all patients report that at least on occasion, they worry about a life-threatening cancer recurrence and the need for additional treatment that such a diagnosis would cause (Lee-Jones, Humphris, Dixon, & Hatcher, 1997). In light of the wide range of disfiguring and disruptive physical effects of treatments, it is not surprising that body image is also a common area of concern for patients. In some cases, relative dissatisfaction with body image is associated with more disfiguring treatments (Moyer, 1997). In other cases, however, body image does not appear to bear a direct relation to cancer treatments and may instead represent a more global self-appraisal (Perez, Skinner, & Meyerowitz, 2002). Perceived threats to one's sense of masculinity or femininity may lead to concerns, regardless of whether these changes are visible to others. Although relatively few patients meet diagnostic criteria for posttraumatic stress disorder, many experience hyperalertness and intrusive thoughts (Cordova et al., 1995; Epping-Jordan et al., 1999). Moreover, periodic reminders such as medical exams or minor aches and pains can cause fear long after remission (Schag et al., 1993).

In addition to assessing fears, there has been an increasing awareness of the importance of considering changes in outlook associated with being diagnosed with cancer. Most patients report that they are forever changed by having been diagnosed with cancer. In some cases, these changes are directly related to the disfigurement and dysfunction caused by treatments. Patients also frequently experience an increased sense of vulnerability about their bodies and their health (Giedzinska, Meyerowitz, Ganz, & Rowland, 2004) and a disruption in their views of the world as a safe and benign place (Cordova, Cunningham, Carlson, & Andrykowski, 2001a). This recognition of the impermanence of life can lead to rethinking one's values and goals, which in turn, can stimulate benefit finding and personal growth (Bower et al., 2005).

Social Well-Being

Most individuals who are diagnosed with cancer report that their close family relationships remain strong and supportive and, in some cases, become closer as a result of the cancer experience. An exception is marriages that were seriously troubled prior to the diagnosis, such that the stresses of cancer can cause further deterioration in the relationship (Kornblith, 1998). Patients do report increased strain in some less intimate relationships with extended family, friends, acquaintances, and colleagues. These problems can take the form of oversolicitous concern, insensitivity, avoidance, or outright discrimination (Hoffman, 1989; Meyerowitz, Yarkin-Levin, & Harvey, 1997).

Even for strong relationships, however, there appear to be areas in which difficulties occur. Sexual dysfunction and dissatisfaction are common (see chap. 21, this volume), as is difficulty communicating about cancer. Poor communication can result from the patient's own avoidance, from the patient's desire to protect loved ones from the cancer experience, from family members' responses that constrain discussion about cancer concerns, and from family members' unsupportive behaviors (Cordova, Cunningham, Carlson, & Andrykowski, 2001b; Helgeson & Cohen, 1996; Kayser, Sormanti, & Strainchamps, 1999; Manne & Glassman, 2000).

PREDICTION OF PSYCHOSOCIAL REACTIONS
TO THE DIAGNOSIS AND TREATMENT OF CANCER

For the most part, distress and disruption associated with cancer diagnosis and treatment abate within 1 to 2 years for survivors who remain disease free. However, some individuals continue to experience reductions in quality of life, and for many others, selected domains continue to be troublesome. Many studies have attempted to elucidate factors that are associated with variations in postdiagnostic quality of life (see reviews by Compas & Luecken, 2002; Glanz & Lerman, 1992; Kornblith, 1998; Ronson & Body, 2002; Spencer, Carver, & Price, 1998). Helgeson, Snyder, and Seltman (2004) recommended two general groupings of predictors, internal–personal resources and external–social resources, and documented that these sets of variables can distinguish between groups of breast cancer patients who experience distinct trajectories of functioning. Personal and social characteristics that predate the cancer diagnosis also can be predictive of psychosocial responses. Finally, a comprehensive understanding requires placing these personal and social predictors in the context of the disease, treatment, and resources available in the medical setting.

Personal, Social, and Disease-Related Characteristics

For the most part, research on the personal, social, and disease-related characteristics that predict postdiagnostic adjustment has been descriptive and atheoretical. These characteristics do not tend to be amenable to change and are studied primarily to identify individuals who are at increased risk for difficulties during or after cancer treatments. This information can be helpful in preparing patients and medical personnel and in targeting populations for intervention.

Most studies that have identified personal characteristics find that older age, higher income, and more education are associated with less distress (Epping-Jordan et al., 1999; Parker, Baile, de Moor, & Cohen, 2003; Schnoll & Harlow, 2001). Younger age, however, is associated with fewer physical problems and more rapid physical recovery (Helgeson et al., 2004). Those studies that have considered ethnicity have reported few differences in overall quality of life, although comparisons among groups have identified differences in specific quality of life domains (Giedzinska et al., 2004; Spencer et al., 1999). It is not surprising that a history of psychiatric problems and neuroticism prior to cancer has been linked to an increased risk for poor adjustment (Glanz & Lerman, 1992; Ronson & Body, 2002).

The most frequently studied characteristics of the social context in the psychosocial oncology literature are marital status and living situation, with most research indicating that unmarried individuals and those who live alone are more likely to report distress and dysphoria (Burgess et al., 2005; Parker et al., 2003; Rodrigue & Park, 1996). Although it is rarely studied, some data suggest that preexisting, noncancer-related stressors in patients' lives may exacerbate postdiagnostic difficulties (Meyerowitz, Formenti, Ell, & Leedham, 2000).

Many studies have considered characteristics of the disease and treatment as possible predictors of psychosocial responses. In addition to the obvious physical effects (discussed elsewhere in this volume), disease site and stage play a major role in determining the type of treatment the patient will receive and the likelihood of recovery. When survivors remain disease free following initial treatment, most individuals show improvement over time (Helgeson et al., 2004) and, after time, do not differ from norms on standardized measures of quality of life and emotional disturbance (Burgess et al., 2005; Ganz, Rowland, Desmond, Meyerowitz, & Wyatt, 1998). However, those patients who experience disease progression or metastatic recurrences are at high risk for distress (Oh et al., 2004; Schnoll & Harlow, 2001). In addition to specific disease-related characteristics, the extent to which the patient faces practical barriers to obtaining medical care can predict ongoing difficulties. For example, problems with transportation, child care, and taking time off from work for treatment have been linked to greater depression in low-income, Latina patients with cervical cancer (Meyerowitz et al., 2000).

Personal, Social, and Disease-Related Resources

Literature on the types of resources that predict adjustment following a cancer diagnosis has made substantial theoretical and clinical contributions. Through investigations with patients facing cancer, researchers have sought to understand the basic mechanisms by which individuals adjust to uncontrollable, life-threatening events. This research also has identified factors that predict optimal recovery, leading to suggestions for therapeutic interventions.

It is beyond the scope of this chapter to provide a comprehensive review of the theoretical underpinnings of this body of research. In general terms, models based on stress and coping theories and on emotional–cognitive processing theories assume that psychological recovery from a life-threatening trauma such as cancer requires regaining a sense of the world as a controllable and safe place (Schmidt & Andrykowski, 2004; Stanton & Snider, 1993). By engaging in active behavioral, emotional, and cognitive coping efforts and by maintaining expectations for positive outcomes, individuals are able to recover. It is in the context of these theories that personal, social, and medical resources have been considered as predictors of adjustment. For example, according to the social-cognitive processing model, a diagnosis of cancer disrupts patients' views of the world and of themselves (Creamer, Burgess, & Pattison, 1992). This threat to preexisting mental schemas, can lead to emotional distress and to periods of uncontrollable intrusive thoughts and hyper-arousal alternating with avoidance as the patient attempts to assimilate and adjust to the threatening information (Cordova et al., 2001b). Adjustment requires that the new information be approached actively and processed cognitively in a social environment that allows for unconstrained emotional expression (Lepore & Helgeson, 1998; Schmidt & Andrykowski, 2004).

A large body of literature has considered personal resources—particularly coping and expectations—as predictors of adjustment. Consistent with theoretical models, high levels of approach-oriented coping with, and unconstrained emotional expression about, cancer-related stressors are generally associated with less distress and better adjustment, whereas avoiding cancer-related stressors and giving up on life's goals predict high distress (Compas & Luecken, 2002; Cordova et al., 2003; Epping-Jordan et al., 1999; Stanton et al., 2000; Stanton & Snider, 1993). The likelihood of engaging in active coping efforts is increased when individuals believe that these efforts will be successful. For example, optimism, a generalized tendency to expect positive outcomes, has been found to be a significant predictor of low distress cross-sectionally and, in some studies, of decreasing distress over time (Carver et al., 1993; Epping-Jordan et al., 1999; Stanton & Snider, 1993). According to these studies, the association between optimism and lower distress was mediated by high levels of active coping and acceptance and low levels of avoidant coping. Disease-specific positive expectations for control and self-efficacy, in contrast to feelings of helplessness and hopelessness in the face of cancer, also have empirical support as predictors of positive outcomes (Bekkers, van Knippenberg, van den Borne, & van Berge-Henegouwen, 1996; Helgeson et al., 2004).

Social support, which has been studied extensively as a resource for cancer patients, is routinely associated with better adjustment. However, as Helgeson and Cohen (1996) reviewed, a comprehensive understanding of the role of social support requires consideration of the interaction between type and source of support. Patients seem to benefit most from emotional support, especially from friends and family. Stanton et al. (2000) found that better physical health and less distress were reported by women who expressed their emotions about breast cancer in social contexts that were receptive. Conversely, unsupportive behaviors from loved ones—including criticism, avoidance, and constraint on emotional expression—are associated with greater distress and more avoidance and intrusive thoughts (Cordova et al., 2001b; Helgeson et al., 2004; Lepore & Helgeson, 1998). For example, Manne and Glassman (2000) found that avoidance of thoughts and feelings about cancer was associated with both perceptions of unsupportive spousal behaviors and patient distress and that avoidance mediated the relationship between those variables. Instrumental support, the provision of practical help, is useful from any source, but only to the extent that it is needed. When the social network takes over handling tasks that the patient can perform without difficulty, a sense of loss of control and dependence can be fostered. Informational support appears to be helpful when offered by the medical team; however, having family and friends provide information and instruction has not been associated with better outcomes (Helgeson & Cohen, 1996).

The medical environment in which cancer is diagnosed and treated provides the opportunity for resources that aid in adjustment. Allowing patients access to information and a role in decision making, to the extent that they desire such involvement, has consistently been associated with fewer difficulties. However, pressure to make major decisions can increase distress and the sense of uncontrollability for patients with a more physician-centric approach to decision making (Glanz & Lerman, 1992). Being offered the opportunity to be involved is more important to patients, data suggest, than actually making decisions about treatment.

TREATING PSYCHOSOCIAL REACTIONS TO THE DIAGNOSIS AND TREATMENT OF CANCER

Clinicians and researchers have developed and tested a wide range of psychosocial interventions for cancer patients and survivors. In some cases, these treatments have been based on the research on predictors of quality of life previously described, and in other cases, the development of interventions has placed less emphasis on previous empirical findings. Overall, general qualitative and quantitative reviews of the psychosocial treatment literature have concluded that interventions have a modest to moderate beneficial effect for individuals with early-stage disease (Compas, Haaga, Keefe, Leitenberg, & Williams, 1998; Fawzy, Fawzy, Arndt, & Pasnau, 1995; Iacovino & Reesor, 1997; Meyer & Mark, 1995; Rehse & Pukrop, 2003; Ross, Boesen, Dalton, & Johansen, 2002). In their meta-analyses, Meyer and Mark (1995) found effect sizes ranging from .19 to .28 across outcome measurement categories, and Rehse and Pukrop (2003) obtained an overall effect size of .31. However, one meta-analysis of group interventions for women with metastatic breast cancer did not find substantial or long-lasting effects for either psychological outcomes or survival (Edwards, Hailey, & Maxwell, 2005). The high degree of heterogeneity in approach and methods across studies makes it difficult to draw generalizable conclusions (Andersen, 2002; Owen, Klapow, Hicken, & Tucker, 2001; Sheard & Maguire, 1999). A more refined analysis requires specific documentation of the nature and timing of the intervention, whom and for what problems it is designed to help, and how it is likely to achieve its goals. Some meta-analyses have addressed these concerns by limiting their reviews to specific outcome measures (Sheard & Maguire, 1999), conceptual elements (Graves, 2003), intervention types (Luebbert, Dahme, & Hasenbring, 2001), or patient populations (Edwards et al., 2005).

A few caveats are necessary before summarizing the literature. Most studies have biased samples. In addition, participation rates tend to be fairly low (Clark, Bostwick, & Rummans, 2003). Patient self-selection through consent to participate and nonrandom attrition due to physical limitations, disease progression, or death further bias much of this research. Although patient self-selection biases may have external validity, in that only patients interested and able to participate are likely to take part in practice, they complicate interpretation of findings. Problems are exacerbated by the small sample sizes in most studies, which make it impossible to control for possible confounds or to test for interaction effects. Small sample sizes also may contribute to Type II error, such that significant effects may be masked by insufficient power or large within-treatment variance. Interpretation is further complicated by the omission in many studies of details about participant recruitment, treatment design, analytic strategy, and other methodological details.

Types of Interventions

Interventions for cancer patients have used a variety of approaches, including foci on providing education and information, enhancing social support and communication, increasing emotional expression, training in coping skills, and managing stress (Blake-Mortimer, Gore-Felton, Kimerling, Turner-Cobb, & Spiegel, 1999; Fawzy et al., 1995; Meyer & Mark, 1995). These interventions have varied in terms of number of sessions, timing relative to the diagnosis of cancer, training and background of the therapist, and length of follow-up (Andersen, 2002; Owen et al., 2001; Ross et al., 2002; Sheard & Maguire, 1999). Outcome measures are not always standardized and are not always directly linked to the focus of the intervention (see chap. 7, this volume). It is not surprising, therefore, that it has been difficult to make meaningful comparisons of the efficacy of interventions across studies or to draw empirically based conclusions about optimal treatment methods (Iacovino & Reesor, 1997; Sheard & Maguire, 1999). However, using standard criteria for empirically supported interventions, Compas et al. (1998) concluded that both cognitive behavior and coping skills interventions, which teach and encourage approach coping and stress management, and supportive–expressive interventions, which encourage emotional disclosure in a supportive social environment, were possibly efficacious.

A few attempts have been made to distinguish among intervention strategies. For example, several reviews have considered the relative merits of individual versus group interventions, and some have found advantages for group approaches (Blake-Mortimer et al., 1999; Fawzy & Fawzy, 1998; Graves, 2003; Sheard & Maguire, 1999). Although group interventions can be more cost-effective and, for some people, more useful, there are many logistic problems that can limit their acceptance. Groups are difficult to schedule and are not preferred by some patients and thus require many more patients to reach enrollment goals in studies (Edgar, Rosberger, & Collet, 2001; Goodwin et al., 2000). In addition to distinguishing between treatment modalities, it is likely that there are differential effects, depending on the selection of treatment components and of outcome measures. Graves (2003) conducted a meta-analysis to compare interventions that included treatment components drawn from social cognitive theories with those that did not. She found that there were larger effect sizes for some, but not all, outcomes for interventions that included components for enhancing self-efficacy, outcome expectations, and self-regulation. Sheard and Maguire (1999) presented results from two meta-analyses, one considering anxiety as the outcome measure and the other considering depression outcomes. They concluded that effects for anxiety were more robust than those for depression.

Possible Moderators and Mediators

For the most part, these studies have not attempted to identify moderating variables. They have tended to be inclusive, enrolling participants without consideration of their apparent need for psychosocial treatment and without testing for differential effects based on personal, social, or medical characteristics. When level of distress is considered, however, most studies find that it moderates treatment effects (Ross et al., 2002). For example, McLachlan et al. (2001) conducted a randomized trial of the value of providing the health care team with patient self-assessments for use in targeting interventions. They found that only those patients who were moderately or severely depressed prior to enrollment were significantly more likely to benefit than the control group. Helgeson, Cohen, Schulz, and Yasko (2000) found that patients with breast cancer who had insufficient social support benefited from peer discussion groups; however, peer discussion was harmful for patients who had high levels of support. Stanton et al. (2005) recently documented in a randomized trial that an empirically and theoretically based peer-modeling videotape accelerated recovery of energy during the immediate posttreatment phase for breast cancer survivors who were less prepared for reentry. In one of the few intervention studies designed for African American women, Taylor et al. (2003) randomized women with nonmetastatic breast cancer to an 8-week support group or an assessment-only group. The support group was effective in improving mood and psychological functioning for women who had greater baseline distress or lower income.

There have been few systematic efforts to determine the mechanisms by which interventions have their effects. Treatments rarely test theory-based models (Owen et al., 2001). Most treatments are multidimensional, with several components that cannot be separated either conceptually or empirically. Moreover, few studies use true control groups but rather have comparison groups that differ from the active intervention in many ways. Thus, it is often not possible to determine which elements are effective, nor what might mediate any benefits. By providing multimodal assessments based on empirically supported models of adjustment to cancer, researchers can avoid some of the shortcomings. For example, Andersen et al. (2004) randomly assigned women with regional breast cancer to an intervention (vs. an assessment-only condition) that was carefully structured to address and measure a range of conceptually relevant processes. They found significant effects for the intervention on multiple measures of psychological, social, and physiological functioning, with some measures showing benefits especially for women with high initial cancer stress. They also were able to examine the interrelations among domains of response.

CONCLUSION AND RECOMMENDATIONS FOR FUTURE RESEARCH

In this chapter, we have reviewed three overlapping literatures that provide descriptive, correlational, and experimental findings regarding quality of life and adjustment following the diagnosis of cancer in adults. Despite methodological difficulties, these studies, taken together, have provided extremely valuable information for patients, their families, and their health care providers. Patients and their caregivers now can know what to expect following a diagnosis of cancer and can determine when responses are not within normal limits. They can anticipate areas in which problems may continue and instances in which patients could benefit from help. They can identify resources that might be useful to patients and can choose from among several interventions that have been demonstrated to be helpful, especially for individuals in greatest need of help. The literature to date clearly demonstrates the feasibility and desirability of integrating psychosocial research into the medical care of cancer patients. With this information, the face of cancer care has changed for patients.

The field has reached the point in the state of the science at which multidimensional conceptual models should be guiding work that moves beyond simple description and prediction to focus on identifying moderating variables and mediating pathways. Researchers need to know whether widely accepted findings generalize to understudied populations and apply across the recovery trajectory. Researchers also need to understand the mechanisms of action whereby cognitive and emotional processing, personal attributes, active coping, and successful interventions have their effects. The field also should examine the possibility of moderated mediation to determine whether these mechanisms are universal or differ on the basis of individual, sociocultural, or disease characteristics.

These issues can be addressed fully only when psychological functioning is studied in the broader biopsychosocial context. It is clear that the social environment plays a central role in patient adjustment, but less is known about how loved ones cope with the stress of cancer themselves and how their own attributes and coping strategies might interact with those of the patient. What, for example, predicts whether a spouse will be socially receptive or constraining in dealing with the patient? It is perhaps even more important to ensure that psychological functioning is placed in the context of biological functioning. There is strong evidence to demonstrate that psychological stress leads not only to emotional and cognitive disruptions but also to changes in cortisol levels and to immune system downregulation (Kiecolt-Glaser & Glaser, 1999; Luecken & Compas, 2002). These physical changes can, in turn, lead to greater psychological difficulties and, potentially, to poorer cancer outcomes (see chap. 28, this volume). Future research will need to consider the multiple, bidirectional pathways among biological, psychological, and social functioning.

REFERENCES

Aaronson, N. K., Meyerowitz, B. E., Bard, M., Bloom, J. R., Fawzy, F. I., Feldstein, M., et al. (1991). Quality of life research in oncology. *Cancer, 67,* 839–843.

Andersen, B. L. (2002). Biobehavioral outcomes following psychological interventions for cancer patients. *Journal of Consulting and Clinical Psychology, 70,* 590–610.

Andersen, B. L., Farrar, W. B., Golden-Kreutz, D. M., Glaser, R., Emery, C. F., Crespin, T. R., et al. (2004). Psychological, behavioral, and immune changes after a psychological intervention: A clinical trial. *Journal of Clinical Oncology, 22,* 3570–3580.

Bekkers, M. J. T. M., van Knippenberg, F. C. E., van den Borne, H. W., & van Berge-Henegouwen, G. P. (1996). Prospective evaluation of psychosocial adaptation to stoma surgery: The role of self-efficacy. *Psychosomatic Medicine, 58,* 183–191.

Blake-Mortimer, J., Gore-Felton, C., Kimerling, R., Turner-Cobb, J. M., & Spiegel, D. (1999). Improving the quality and quantity of life among patients with cancer: A review of the effectiveness of group psychotherapy. *European Journal of Cancer, 35,* 1581–1586.

Bottomley, A. (1998a). Anxiety and the adult cancer patient. *European Journal of Cancer Care, 7,* 217–224.

Bottomley, A. (1998b). Depression in cancer patients: A literature review. *European Journal of Cancer Care, 7,* 181–191.

Bower, J. E., Meyerowitz, B. E., Desmond, K. A., Bernaards, C. A., Rowland, J. H., & Ganz, P. A. (2005). Perceptions of positive meaning and vulnerability following breast cancer: Predictors and outcomes among long-term breast cancer survivors. *Annals of Behavioral Medicine, 29,* 236–245.

Burgess, C., Ramirez, A., Cornelius, V., Love, S., Graham, J., & Richards, M. (2005, March 26). Depression and anxiety in women with early breast cancer: Five year observational cohort study. *BMJ*, *330*, 702.

Carver, C. S., Pozo, C., Harris, S. D., Noriega, V., Scheier, M. F., Robinson, D. S., et al. (1993). How coping mediates the effect of optimism on distress: A study of women with early stage breast cancer. *Journal of Personality and Social Psychology*, *65*, 375–390.

Clark, M. M., Bostwick, J. M., & Rummans, T. A. (2003). Group and individual treatment strategies for distress in cancer patients. *Mayo Clinic Proceedings*, *78*, 1538–1543.

Compas, B. E., Haaga, D. A. F., Keefe, F. J., Leitenberg, H., & Williams, D. A. (1998). Sampling of empirically supported psychological treatments from health psychology: Smoking, chronic pain, cancer, and bulimia nervosa. *Journal of Consulting and Clinical Psychology*, *66*, 89–112.

Compas, B. E., & Luecken, L. (2002). Psychological adjustment to breast cancer. *Current Directions in Psychological Science*, *11*, 111–114.

Cordova, M. J., Andrykowski, M. A., Kenady, D. E., McGrath, P. C., Sloan, D. A., & Redd, W. H. (1995). Frequency and correlates of PTSD-like symptoms following treatment for breast cancer. *Journal of Consulting and Clinical Psychology*, *63*, 981–986.

Cordova, M. J., Cunningham, L. L. C., Carlson, C. R., & Andrykowski, M. A. (2001a). Posttraumatic growth following breast cancer: A controlled comparison study. *Health Psychology*, *20*, 176–185.

Cordova, M. J., Cunningham, L. L. C., Carlson, C. R., & Andrykowski, M. A. (2001b). Social constraints, cognitive processing, and adjustment to breast cancer. *Journal of Consulting and Clinical Psychology*, *69*, 706–711.

Cordova, M. J., Giese-Davis, J., Golant, M., Kronnenwetter, C., Chang, V., McFarlin, S., & Spiegel, D. (2003). Mood disturbance in community cancer support groups: The role of emotional suppression and fighting spirit. *Journal of Psychosomatic Research*, *55*, 461–467.

Creamer, M., Burgess, P., & Pattison, P. (1992). Reaction to trauma: A cognitive processing model. *Journal of Abnormal Psychology*, *101*, 452–459.

Edgar, L., Rosberger, Z., & Collet, J.-P. (2001). Lessons learned: Outcomes and methodology of a coping skills intervention trial comparing individual and group formats for patients with cancer. *International Journal of Psychiatry in Medicine*, *31*, 289–304.

Edwards, A. G. K., Hailey, S., & Maxwell, M. (2005). Psychological interventions for women with metastatic breast cancer. *The Cochrane Database of Systematic Reviews*, *2*. Available from http://www.cochrane.org

Epping-Jordan, J. E., Compas, B. E., Osowiecki, D. M., Oppedisano, G., Gerhardt, C., Primo, K., & Krag, D. N. (1999). Psychological adjustment in breast cancer: Processes of emotional distress. *Health Psychology*, *18*, 315–326.

Fawzy, F. I., & Fawzy, N. W. (1998). Group therapy in the cancer setting. *Journal of Psychosomatic Research*, *45*, 191–200.

Fawzy, F. I., Fawzy, N. W., Arndt, L. A., & Pasnau, R. O. (1995). Critical review of psychosocial interventions in cancer care. *Archives of General Psychiatry, 52,* 100–113.

Filiberti, A., & Ripamonti, C. (2002). Suicide and suicidal thoughts in cancer patients. *Tumori, 88,* 193–199.

Ganz, P. A., Rowland, J. H., Desmond, K. A., Meyerowitz, B. E., & Wyatt, G. E. (1998). Life after breast cancer: Understanding women's health-related quality of life and sexual functioning. *Journal of Clinical Oncology, 16,* 501–514.

Giedzinska, A. S., Meyerowitz, B. E., Ganz, P. A., & Rowland, J. H. (2004). Health-related quality of life in a multiethnic sample of breast cancer survivors. *Annals of Behavioral Medicine, 28,* 39–51.

Glanz, K., & Lerman, C. (1992). Psychosocial impact of breast cancer: A critical review. *Annals of Behavioral Medicine, 14,* 204–212.

Goodwin, P. J., Leszcz, M., Quirt, G., Koopmans, J., Arnold, A., Dohan, E., et al. (2000). Lessons learned from enrollment in the BEST study—A multicenter, randomized trial of group psychosocial support in metastatic breast cancer. *Journal of Clinical Epidemiology, 53,* 47–55.

Graves, K. D. (2003). Social cognitive theory and cancer patients' quality of life: A meta-analysis of psychosocial intervention components. *Health Psychology, 22,* 210–219.

Helgeson, V. S., & Cohen, S. (1996). Social support and adjustment to cancer: Reconciling descriptive, correlational, and intervention research. *Health Psychology, 15,* 135–148.

Helgeson, V. S., Cohen, S., Schulz, R., & Yasko, J. (2000). Group support interventions for women with breast cancer: Who benefits from what? *Health Psychology, 19,* 107–114.

Helgeson, V. S., Snyder, P., & Seltman, H. (2004). Psychological and physical adjustment to breast cancer over 4 years: Identifying distinct trajectories of change. *Health Psychology, 23,* 3–15.

Hoffman, B. (1989). Cancer survivors at work: Job problems and illegal discrimination. *Oncology Nursing Forum, 16,* 39–43.

Iacovino, V., & Reesor, K. (1997). Literature on interventions to address cancer patients' psychosocial needs: What does it tell us? *Journal of Psychosocial Oncology, 15,* 47–71.

Kayser, K., Sormanti, M., & Strainchamps, E. (1999). Women coping with cancer: The influence of relationship factors on psychosocial adjustment. *Psychology of Women Quarterly, 23,* 725–739.

Kiecolt-Glaser, J. K., & Glaser, R. (1999). Psychoneuroimmunology and cancer: Fact or fiction? *European Journal of Cancer, 35,* 1603–1607.

Kornblith, A. B. (1998). Psychosocial adaptation of cancer survivors. In J. C. Holland (Ed.), *Psycho-oncology* (pp. 223–254). New York: Oxford University Press.

Lee-Jones, C., Humphris, G., Dixon, R., & Hatcher, M. B. (1997). Fear of cancer recurrence—A literature review and proposed cognitive formulation to explain exacerbation of recurrence fears. *Psycho-Oncology, 6,* 95–105.

Lepore, S. J., & Helgeson, V. S. (1998). Social constraints, intrusive thoughts, and mental health after prostate cancer. *Journal of Social and Clinical Psychology, 17*, 89–106.

Luebbert, K., Dahme, B., & Hasenbring, M. (2001). The effectiveness of relaxation training in reducing treatment-related symptoms and improving emotional adjustment in acute non-surgical cancer treatment: A meta-analytical review. *Psycho-Oncology, 10*, 490–502.

Luecken, L. J., & Compas, B. E. (2002). Stress, coping, and immune function in breast cancer. *Annals of Behavioral Medicine, 24*, 336–344.

Manne, S., & Glassman, M. (2000). Perceived control, coping efficacy, and avoidance coping as mediators between spouses' unsupportive behaviors and cancer patients' psychological distress. *Health Psychology, 19*, 155–164.

McDaniel, J. S., Musselman, D. L., Porter, M. R., Reed, D. A., & Nemeroff, C. B. (1995). Depression in patients with cancer. *Archives of General Psychiatry, 52*, 89–99.

McLachlan, S.-A., Allenby, A., Matthews, J., Wirth, A., Kissane, D., Bishop, M., et al. (2001). Randomized trial of coordinated psychosocial interventions based on patient self-assessments versus standard care to improve the psychosocial functioning of patients with cancer. *Journal of Clinical Oncology, 19*, 4117–4125.

Meyer, T. J., & Mark, M. M. (1995). Effects of psychosocial interventions with adult cancer patients: A meta-analysis of randomized experiments. *Health Psychology, 14*, 101–108.

Meyerowitz, B. E., Formenti, S. C., Ell, K. O., & Leedham, B. (2000). Depression among Latina cervical cancer patients. *Journal of Social and Clinical Psychology, 19*, 352–371.

Meyerowitz, B. E., & Hart, S. (1995). Women and cancer: Have assumptions about women limited our research agenda? In A. L. Stanton & S. J. Gallant (Eds.), *The psychology of women's health: Progress and challenges in research and application* (pp. 51–84). Washington, DC: American Psychological Association.

Meyerowitz, B. E., Yarkin-Levin, K., & Harvey, J. (1997). On the nature of cancer patients' social interactions. *Journal of Personal and Interpersonal Loss, 2*, 49–69.

Moyer, A. (1997). Psychosocial outcomes of breast-conserving surgery versus mastectomy: A meta-analytic review. *Health Psychology, 16*, 284–298.

Newport, D. J., & Nemeroff, C. B. (1998). Assessment and treatment of depression in the cancer patient. *Journal of Psychosomatic Research, 45*, 215–237.

Oh, S., Heflin, L., Meyerowitz, B. E., Desmond, K. A., Rowland, J. H., & Ganz, P. A. (2004). Quality of life of breast cancer survivors after a recurrence: A follow-up study. *Breast Cancer Research and Treatment, 87*, 45–57.

Owen, J. E., Klapow, J. C., Hicken, B., & Tucker, D. C. (2001). Psychosocial interventions for cancer: Review and analysis using a three-tiered outcomes model. *Psycho-Oncology, 10*, 218–230.

Parker, P. A., Baile, W. F., de Moor, C., & Cohen, L. (2003). Psychosocial and demographic predictors of quality of life in a large sample of cancer patients. *Psycho-Oncology, 12*, 183–193.

Perez, M. A., Skinner, E. C., & Meyerowitz, B. E. (2002). Sexuality and intimacy following radical prostatectomy: Patient and partner perspectives. *Health Psychology, 21,* 288–293.

Rehse, B., & Pukrop, R. (2003). Effects of psychosocial interventions on quality of life in adult cancer patients: Meta analysis of 37 published controlled outcome studies. *Patient Education and Counseling, 50,* 179–186.

Rodrigue, J. R., & Park, T. L. (1996). General and illness-specific adjustment to cancer: Relationship to marital status and quality. *Journal of Psychosomatic Research, 40,* 29–36.

Ronson, A., & Body, J.-J. (2002). Psychosocial rehabilitation of cancer patients after curative care. *Support Care Cancer, 10,* 281–291.

Ross, L., Boesen, E. H., Dalton, S. O., & Johansen, C. (2002). Mind and cancer: Does psychosocial intervention improve survival and psychological well-being? *European Journal of Cancer Care, 38,* 1447–1457.

Schag, C. A. C., Ganz, P. A., Polinsky, M. L., Fred, C., Hirji, K., & Petersen, L. (1993). Characteristics of women at risk for psychosocial distress in the year after breast cancer. *Journal of Clinical Oncology, 11,* 783–793.

Schmidt, J. E., & Andrykowski, M. A. (2004). The role of social and dispositional variables associated with emotional processing in adjustment to breast cancer: An Internet-based study. *Health Psychology, 23,* 259–266.

Schnoll, R. A., & Harlow, L. L. (2001). Using disease-related and demographic variables to form cancer-distress risk groups. *Journal of Behavioral Medicine, 24,* 57–74.

Shapiro, S. L., Lopez, A. M., Schwartz, G. E., Braden, C. J., & Kurker, S. F. (2001). Quality of life and breast cancer: Relationship to psychosocial variables. *Journal of Clinical Psychology, 57,* 501–519.

Sheard, T., & Maguire, P. (1999). The effect of psychological interventions on anxiety and depression in cancer patients: Results of two meta-analyses. *British Journal of Cancer, 80,* 1770–1780.

Sneeuw, K. C. A., Aaronson, N. K., Sprangers, M. A. G., Detmar, S. B., Wever, L. D. V., & Schornagel, J. H. (1999). Evaluating the quality of life of cancer patients: Assessment by patients, significant others, physicians, and nurses. *British Journal of Cancer, 81,* 87–94.

Spencer, S. M., Carver, C. S., & Price, A. A. (1998). Psychological and social factors in adaptation. In J. C. Holland (Ed.), *Psycho-oncology* (pp. 211–222). New York: Oxford University Press.

Spencer, S. M., Lehman, J. M., Wynings, C., Arena, P., Carver, C. S., Antoni, M. H., et al. (1999). Concerns about breast cancer and relations to psychosocial well-being in a multiethnic sample of early-stage patients. *Health Psychology, 18,* 159–168.

Stanton, A. L., Danoff-Burg, S., Cameron, C. L., Bishop, M., Collins, C. A., Kirk, S. B., et al. (2000). Emotionally expressive coping predicts psychological and physical adjustment to breast cancer. *Journal of Consulting and Clinical Psychology, 68,* 875–888.

Stanton, A. L., Ganz, P. A., Kwan, L., Meyerowitz, B. E., Bower, J. E., Krupnick, J. L., et al. (2005). Outcomes from the Moving Beyond Cancer psychoeducational randomized, controlled trial with breast cancer patients. *Journal of Clinical Oncology, 23,* 6009–6018.

Stanton, A. L., & Snider, P. R. (1993). Coping with a breast cancer diagnosis: A prospective study. *Health Psychology, 12,* 16–23.

Taylor, K. L., Lamdan, R. M., Siegel, J. E., Shelby, R., Moran-Klimi, K., & Hrywna, M. (2003). Psychological adjustment among African-American breast cancer patients: One-year follow-up results of a randomized psychoeducational group intervention. *Health Psychology, 22,* 316–323.

21

REDUCTION OF PSYCHOSEXUAL DYSFUNCTION IN CANCER PATIENTS

LESLIE R. SCHOVER

Sexual dysfunction is one of the more common and persistent side effects of cancer treatment, particularly for survivors of pelvic malignancies or breast cancer. Knowledge of the impact of cancer and its treatments on sexuality has increased greatly in the past 25 years, but there still is no evidence-based, cost-effective behavioral interventions that could readily be disseminated in oncology treatment settings. Most men and women treated for cancer still do not get enough information to anticipate the sexual consequences and do not have access to medical or psychosocial elements of sexual rehabilitation.

IMPACT OF CANCER TREATMENT ON SEXUAL FUNCTION

Cancer and its treatments contribute to sexual dysfunction in many different ways, because each cancer site and its treatment options are unique. Cancer treatment frequently damages the hormonal, neurological, and vascular systems involved in the sexual response. Psychological factors in cancer-related sexual problems include disruption of body image, exacerbation of relationship stress, stigmatization, and negative beliefs about sex. The physiological damage to sexual function is often so profound that psychological factors are not directly causal in the sexual dysfunction, but rather moderate distress about the physical symptoms determines whether someone resumes sexual activity or influences whether medical help is sought for a sexual dysfunction. When a cancer survivor is in a relationship, both partners' sexual attitudes impact the ultimate outcome of sexual rehabilitation. Psychological factors may help explain why some men or women manage to stay sexually functional under difficult circumstances. For example, women at high risk for inherited breast and ovarian cancer may have both ovaries removed surgically for cancer prevention and are advised not to use estrogen replacement. About half subsequently experience vaginal dryness, pain with intercourse, reduced sexual desire, and difficulty reaching orgasm (Robson et al., 2003). It is not known what factors distinguish the women who do not report these problems because considerably more research has examined the physiological factors than the psychosocial ones.

Despite the varying factors that lead to sexual dysfunction, the problems common in men and women are similar across cancer sites and treatments. For both genders, typical dysfunctions include loss of desire for sex and difficulty feeling arousal and pleasure. Erectile dysfunction (ED) is the other frequent complaint for men, and sexual changes related to sudden menopause—reduced vaginal expansion and lubrication, and consequent pain during sexual activity—are common for women. Difficulty achieving orgasm is less common for men than for women and is often secondary to having sex with little erotic desire or arousal. Premature ejaculation is not associated with cancer treatment (Schover, Evans, & von Eschenbach, 1987).

Importance of Research in Defining Sexual Outcomes After Cancer

Sexual problems after cancer are most common and severe when the tumor and its treatment affect the reproductive system directly, for example, after prostate or vulvar cancer. Perhaps this seems obvious, but a number of pieces of conventional wisdom about sexual function after cancer have not been supported by research. For example, breast conservation (i.e., lumpectomy and radiation) or reconstruction does not produce any better sexual outcomes than mastectomy alone, whether measured in terms of frequency of sex, overall sexual satisfaction, or rates of sexual problems (Ganz et al., 2002; Schover et al., 1995). Mastectomy is only inferior in terms of women's ratings of their physical attractiveness (Schover, 1994).

Indeed, in women with breast cancer, as well as other malignancies, it is now clear that cancer treatments causing sudden ovarian failure in premenopausal women are the most likely to cause sexual dysfunction (Ganz et al., 2003). Regardless of whether both ovaries are removed surgically, are damaged beyond recovery by chemotherapy, or are within the target area of radiation therapy, ovarian failure can result in severe problems with vaginal dryness and pain during sexual activity. Sexual problems are also common after surgery that removes erotically sensitive areas such as the breast or clitoris, or (as is common after pelvic radiation) damage the vagina's ability to expand and lubricate with sexual arousal.

Initial reports after nerve-sparing radical prostatectomy indicated that 86% of men recovered erections sufficient for intercourse 18 months later (Walsh, Marschke, Ricker, & Burnett, 2000). Several recent large, detailed surveys of prostate cancer survivors paint a different picture. Overall, 75% to 85% of men have long-term ED after radical prostatectomy. Even after bilateral nerve sparing, less than 20% of men can achieve firm, reliable erections unaided by pills, injections, or mechanical devices at an average of 4 to 5 years after radical prostatectomy (Potosky et al., 2004; Schover et al., 2002). Results after treatment with radiation therapy are little better. Even with newer types of external beam radiotherapy that use computers to shape the target area and avoid damaging normal tissue, or with brachytherapy (i.e., the implantation of radioactive seeds or rods in the prostate), the great majority of men end up with ED (Cooperberg et al., 2003; Potosky et al., 2004; Schover et al., 2002). Erectile function is at its worst right after nerve-sparing prostatectomy, with possible recovery of erections over the next 1 to 2 years. After radiation therapy, however, erectile function may be normal initially but decline steadily over several years. If more demonstration of the sexual morbidity of prostate cancer treatment were needed, a prospective study of 31,742 nonphysician health professionals, ages 53 to 90, found that the 2,109 men who had been diagnosed with prostate cancer were 10 to 15 times more likely than men of comparable age to have ED (Bacon et al., 2003).

Methodological Problems in Research on Cancer-Related Sexual Dysfunction

Methodological problems still limit knowledge of the prevalence and causes of sexual dysfunction after cancer. It is important to compare cancer survivors with healthy samples matched in age and noncancer health status, and for women, menopausal status and rates of hormone replacement therapy. An important gender difference is that although ED increases consistently with both aging and ill health, sexual dysfunction is more common in young women, with vaginal dryness the only problem that increases with age.

Having a healthy comparison group does not help in understanding how to remediate cancer-related sexual problems, however. Another common problem is that many surveys are cross-sectional, asking patients to recall changes in sexual function from before cancer treatment. Retrospective questions can create biases in memory and attribution, so that preexisting problems are blamed on cancer. In the Netherlands, 58 women followed prospectively during the 1st year after treatment for early-stage gynecological cancer were compared with 220 similar women surveyed in a cross-sectional design at a mean of 4 years of follow-up (Leenhouts et al., 2002). The women surveyed retrospectively reported resuming sex at later intervals after their cancer treatment, probably reflecting a negative recall bias. However, men's retrospective recall of ED before prostate cancer diagnosis is quite accurate when compared with data collected prospectively (Legler, Potosky, Gilliland, Eley, & Stanford, 2000; Schover et al., 2002). Memory of the presence versus the absence of a problem such as ED may be more reliable than recall of sexual frequency years previously.

To understand the influence of psychological factors such as depression, feeling unattractive, negative beliefs about sexuality, or posttraumatic stress on postcancer sexual function, researchers must conduct prospective studies of patients with the same cancer site and treatment, assessing the psychological variables of interest as well as sexual function at a pretreatment baseline and continuing assessment periodically after treatment. Samples need to be large enough to provide adequate power for multivariate statistical analyses or modeling. The duration of follow-up needs to be sufficient to assess sexual function once it stabilizes after acute effects of cancer treatment have resolved. No study currently in the literature meets such criteria.

Assessment of Sexual Function After Cancer

Many published studies have another important methodological shortcoming—using idiosyncratic measures of sexual function rather than validated questionnaires. A number of self-report questionnaires with good reliability and validity assess sexual function. Although some have been developed for specific populations of cancer patients or survivors, they are not necessarily superior to the more generic inventories. In choosing a questionnaire, one must weigh the need for very specific information against the burden of asking patients or research participants to fill out a longer instrument, particularly if repeated assessments will be conducted. Whether the target population is male or female, it is important to assess problems across the dimensions of desire, arousal, orgasm, and pain rather than assuming that problems are restricted to one aspect of sexual functioning such as erections or orgasm. Even when men have ED after prostate cancer, low sexual desire, pain, and difficulty reaching orgasm are also common and troublesome (Schover et al., 2002). Men who have more advanced prostate cancer and have hormonal therapy to eliminate circulating androgens have profound impairment in their ability to feel desire and arousal (Schover et al., 2002). In women, apparent loss of desire for sex may in fact be secondary to anticipatory anxiety about pain with sexual activity.

Both the International Index of Erectile Dysfunction (Rosen, Capelleri, & Gendrano, 2002; Rosen et al., 1997), and the Female Sexual Function Index (Rosen et al., 2000) are brief, have been developed with extensive psychometric research and a variety of comparison samples, and have been used internationally. They have the disadvantage, however, of generating very low scores for people who are not active with a sexual partner.

Because sexual behavior is so private, assessment almost always relies on self-report (by either questionnaire, diary, or structured interview). When self-report questionnaires are administered by computer, more high-risk sexual behaviors have been reported, but it is unclear whether this represents greater accuracy in responding or a tendency to overreport stigmatized behavior under these conditions (Schroder, Carey, & Vanable, 2003). Studies do not find any clear superiority for diaries over self-report questionnaires in assessing sexual practices or frequency (Schroder et al., 2003). An innovative data collection method that has not yet been used in sex research is ecological momentary assessment (Stone & Schiffman, 2002). It is appealing to try to find physiological markers of sexual function, but reliable assessment modalities are difficult to find (Padma-Nathan, 2000).

THE NEED FOR BEHAVIORAL TECHNIQUES IN SEXUAL REHABILITATION AFTER CANCER

Despite the obvious need for interventions that would prevent and remediate the sexual dysfunction that cancer survivors experience, research on using psychotherapeutic approaches is scarce. Very few studies were published in the 1980s, when behavioral sex therapy was recognized as an effective intervention (Heiman & LoPiccolo, 1983). A group intervention was found to be superior to usual care in promoting a return to sexual activity after gynecologic cancer (Capone, Westie, & Good, 1979), and a structured group had a positive impact on the sexuality of women recently treated with mastectomy (Christensen, 1983). Schover et al. (1987) published a retrospective review of sex therapy consultations over 4 years in a major cancer center. Of 384 individuals or couples, 73% were seen only once or twice. Of the index patients seen, 308 were men and 76 were women. Most men sought help for ED, whereas women typically had a combination of loss of desire and vaginal dryness with dyspareunia. Follow-up data on outcome were available for only 118 cases. The therapist rating of improvement was *somewhat to much better* for 63% of this group. Patients were more likely to benefit from counseling if they were younger, were not depressed, and did not have conflicted relationships.

The entire field of behavior therapy for sexual dysfunction has seen little innovation in techniques or new outcome research in the past 25 years (Schover & Leiblum, 1994). Very few trials have examined the efficacy of an intervention for postcancer sexual dysfunction. One randomized trial with 76 postmenopausal breast cancer survivors found that a special session with a nurse practitioner followed by telephone contacts was superior to usual care in resolving hot flashes, vaginal dryness, or urinary stress incontinence (Ganz et al., 2000). The nurse assessed symptoms and applied treatment algorithms such as prescribing medication or advising on the use of vaginal lubricants. A three-session peer-counseling intervention, including a detailed written workbook, also produced significant improvement in hot flashes, overall distress, and sexual function in 48 African American breast cancer survivors (Schover et al., 2006). Brotto et al. (2008) have piloted a three-session cognitive behavior and mindfulness intervention that produced significant improvement in sexual function in 22 survivors of gynecologic cancer. Canada, Neese, Sui, and Schover (2005) also found significant gains in sexual function and satisfaction in men who participated in a three-session sex therapy program with their partners. Such inexpensive, brief interventions provide an excellent model for sexual rehabilitation after cancer and should be tested further to evaluate their effectiveness and dissemination into a variety of health care settings.

A model integrating sex therapy and medical intervention would be especially useful in treating loss of desire for sex. One of the most common sexual problems seen in both male and female cancer survivors, low desire, is often multifactorial. Risk factors include lingering posttreatment fatigue, pain, or nausea; distracting cognitions about feeling unattractive or stigmatized after cancer; medication side effects; mild depression; and relationship conflict exacerbated by cancer treatment. In men, loss of desire for sex is often linked to the frustration and low self-esteem that accompany ED (Latini et al., 2002). Women who have dyspareunia come to dread and avoid sex. Although sex therapy has been less effective for treating desire disorders than for some other dysfunctions, outcomes are still reasonably good (Hawton, Catalan, & Fagg, 1992; Schover & LoPiccolo, 1982). Researchers could develop and evaluate treatments for cancer survivors that address the risk factors and incorporate techniques already proven effective in treating desire disorders.

With the advent of more convenient ways to replace testosterone, prescribing androgen therapy for low sexual desire in both men and women has become very popular. Results are often disappointing, however. After bone marrow transplant, a minority of men have elevated luteinizing hormone levels combined with testosterone levels in the slightly low to low normal range. It is unclear whether this subtle hormone abnormality causes sexual problems. A trial of the testosterone patch in 35 such survivors failed to document positive changes in mood or sexual function (Howell et al., 2001). However, a combination of testosterone with sildenafil was helpful to 8 men with ED and severely low circulating androgen levels after bone marrow transplant (Chatterjee, Kottaridis, McGarrigle, & Linch, 2002). Testosterone replacement is a viable option for young male cancer survivors with levels of testosterone that are clinically abnormal, but older, sedentary men with testosterone that is in the bottom end of the normal range are far less likely to benefit and may run the risk of promoting prostate cancer by taking extra hormones (Institute of Medicine, 2004).

Testosterone replacement as a remedy for the impact of ovarian failure on sexual desire and arousal is also controversial. Not only are testosterone levels not related to sexual desire in breast cancer survivors (Greendale, Petersen, Zibecchi, & Ganz, 2001; Speer et al., 2005), but in a randomized trial, transdermal testosterone was not helpful in women cancer survivors with low desire (Barton et al., 2007). Giving women testosterone in patch form after both ovaries have been removed only boosts desire and arousal significantly if high doses are used to raise circulating levels of the hormone above normal (Shifren et al., 2000). Unfortunately, higher circulating testosterone levels are a risk factor for breast cancer in both postmenopausal and premenopausal women (Schover, 2007). Women with higher testosterone are also more likely to have a breast cancer recurrence after treatment for localized disease (Micheli et al., 2007). Not only women treated for breast cancer but also women positive for mutations for inherited breast cancer, with histories of Hodgkin's disease, radiation therapy to the chest area in childhood, or some types of sarcoma, are at high risk for future breast tumors—a risk that unfortunately appears to increase with exposure to estrogens and androgens (Kenney et al., 2004). Thus, regardless of whether testosterone replacement could be effective in treating low sexual desire, it carries significant risks for most of the women with cancer-related ovarian failure who might benefit.

CONCLUSIONS

To improve individuals' and couples' satisfaction with sexual rehabilitation after cancer and to increase rates of adherence to medical treatments for ED or ovarian failure, mental health professionals should develop collaborative treatment programs with urologists, gynecologists, and other oncology specialists. Unfortunately, insurance reimbursement is poor for mental health care in general and especially for sexual counseling. If researchers in academic medical centers could conduct randomized trials of behaviorally enhanced sexual rehabilitation versus medical treatments alone, they might be able to convince insurers of its cost-effectiveness. Components of behavior therapy that could potentially enhance sexual outcomes and should be tested include

- assessment of sexual problems in both partners that could be interfering with successful resumption of sex rather than a focus solely on the cancer survivor,

- traditional sex therapy techniques of sensate focus and communications training,
- behavioral marital therapy techniques to increase expression of affection,
- use of decision aids to help individuals or couples choose among the available medical treatments (inclusion of both partners in these decisions may be particularly valuable),
- behavioral analysis when a medical treatment is not producing a satisfactory outcome, and
- role play and cognitive rehearsal for single survivors who are reluctant to try dating.

To be successful in the long term, sexual rehabilitation treatment programs must address the full spectrum of sexual function and relationship concerns. Restoring a satisfying sex life may also have positive impact on overall happiness and quality of life.

REFERENCES

Bacon, C. G., Mittleman, M. A., Kawachi, I., Giovannucci, E., Glasser, D. B., & Rimm, E. B. (2003). Sexual function in men older than 50 years of age: Results from the Health Professionals Follow-Up Study. *Annals of Internal Medicine, 139,* 161–168.

Barton, D. L., Wender, D. B., Sloan, J. A., Dalton, R. J., Balcueva, E. P., Atherton, P. J., et al. (2007). Randomized controlled trial to evaluate transdermal testosterone in female cancer survivors with decreased libido: North Center Cancer Treatment Group Protocol N02C3. *Journal of the National Cancer Institute, 99,* 672–679.

Brotto, L. A., Heiman, J. R., Goff, B., Greer, B., Lentz, G. M., Swisher, E., et al. (2008). A psychoeducational intervention for sexual dysfunction in women with gynecologic cancer. *Archives of Sexual Behavior, 37,* 317–329.

Canada, A. L., Neese, L., Sui, D., & Schover, L. R. (2005). A pilot intervention to enhance sexual rehabilitation for couples after treatment for localized prostate cancer. *Cancer, 104,* 2689–2700.

Capone, M. A., Westie, K. S., & Good, R. S. (1979). Sexual rehabilitation of the gynecologic cancer patient: An effective counseling model. *Frontiers of Radiation Therapy and Oncology, 14,* 123–129.

Chatterjee, R., Kottaridis, P. D., McGarrigle, H. H., & Linch, D. C. (2002). Management of erectile dysfunction by combination therapy with testosterone and sildenafil in recipients of high-dose therapy for haematological malignancies. *Bone Marrow Transplantation, 29,* 607–610.

Christensen, D. N. (1983). Postmastectomy couple counseling: An outcome study of a structured treatment protocol. *Journal of Sex and Marital Therapy, 9,* 266–275.

Cooperberg, M. R., Koppie, T. M., Lubeck, D. P., Ye, J., Grossfeld, G. D., Mehta, S. S., et al. (2003). How potent is potent? Evaluation of sexual function and bother in men who report potency after treatment for prostate cancer: Data from CaPSURE. *Urology, 61,* 190–196.

Ganz, P. A., Desmond, K. A., Leedham, B., Rowland, J. H., Meyerowitz, B. E., & Belin, T. R. (2002). Quality of life in long-term, disease-free survivors of breast cancer: A follow-up study. *Journal of the National Cancer Institute, 94,* 39–49.

Ganz, P. A., Greendale, G. A., Petersen, L., Zibecchi, L., Kahn, B., & Belin, T. R. (2000). Managing menopausal symptoms in breast cancer survivors: Results of a randomized controlled trial. *Journal of the National Cancer Institute, 92,* 1054–1064.

Ganz, P. A., Greendale, G. A., Petersen, L., Zibecchi, L., Kahn, B., & Bower, J. E. (2003). Breast cancer in younger women: Reproductive and late health effects of treatment. *Journal of Clinical Oncology, 21,* 4184–4198.

Greendale, G. A., Petersen, L., Zibecchi, L., & Ganz, P. A. (2001). Factors related to sexual function in postmenopausal women with a history of breast cancer. *Menopause, 8,* 111–119.

Hawton, K., Catalan, J., & Fagg, J. (1992). Low sexual desire: Sex therapy results and prognostic factors. *Behaviour Research and Therapy, 29,* 217–224.

Heiman, J. R., & LoPiccolo, J. (1983). Clinical outcome of sex therapy: Effects of daily vs. weekly treatment. *Archives of General Psychiatry, 40,* 443–449.

Howell, S. J., Radford, J. A., Adams, J. E., Smets, E. M., Warburton, R., & Shalet, S. M. (2001). Randomized placebo-controlled trial of testosterone replacement in men with mild Leydig cell insufficiency following cytotoxic chemotherapy. *Clinical Endocrinology, 55,* 315–324.

Institute of Medicine. (2004). *Testosterone and aging: Clinical research directions.* Washington, DC: National Academies Press.

Kenney, L. B., Yasui, Y., Inskip, P. D., Hammond, S., Neglia, J. P., Mertens, A. C., et al. (2004). Breast cancer after childhood cancer: A report from the Childhood Cancer Survivor Study. *Annals of Internal Medicine, 141,* 590–597.

Latini, D. M., Penson, D. F., Colwell, H. H., Lubeck, D. P., Mehta, S. S., Henning, J. M., & Lue, T. F. (2002). Psychological impact of erectile dysfunction: Validation of a new health-related quality of life measure for patients with erectile dysfunction. *Journal of Urology, 168,* 2086–2091.

Leenhouts, G. H., Kylstra, W. A., Everaerd, W., Hahn, D. E., Schultz, W. C., van de Wiel, H. B., & Heintz, A. P. (2002). Sexual outcomes following treatment for early-stage gynecological cancer: A prospective and cross-sectional multi-center study. *Journal of Psychosomatic Obstetrics and Gynaecology, 23,* 123–132.

Legler, J., Potosky, A. L., Gilliland, F. D., Eley, J. W., & Stanford, J. L. (2000). Validation study of retrospective recall of disease-targeted function: Results from the Prostate Cancer Outcomes Study. *Medical Care, 48,* 847–857.

Micheli, A., Meneghini, E., Secreto, G., Berrino, F., Venturelli, E., Cavalleri, A., et al. (2007). Plasma testosterone and prognosis of postmenopausal breast cancer patients. *Journal of Clinical Oncology, 25,* 2685–2690.

Padma-Nathan, H. (2000). Diagnostic and treatment strategies for erectile dysfunction: The Process of Care model. *International Journal of Impotence Research, 12*(Suppl. 4), 119–121.

Potosky, A. L., Davis, W. W., Hoffman, R. M., Stanford, J. L., Stephenson, R. A., Penson, D. F., & Harlan, L. C. (2004). Five-year outcomes after prostatectomy or radiotherapy for prostate cancer: The Prostate Cancer Outcomes Study. *Journal of the National Cancer Institute, 96*, 1358–1367.

Robson, M., Hensley, M., Barakat, R., Brown, C., Chi, D., Poynor, E., & Offit, K. (2003). Quality of life in women at risk for ovarian cancer who have undergone risk-reducing oophorectomy. *Gynecologic Oncology, 89*, 281–287.

Rosen, R. C., Brown, C., Heiman, J., Leiblum, S., Meston, C., Shabsigh, R., et al. (2000). The Female Sexual Function Index (FSFI): A multidimensional self-report instrument for the assessment of female sexual function. *Journal of Sex and Marital Therapy, 26*, 191–208.

Rosen, R. C., Capelleri, J. C., & Gendrano, N., III. (2002). The International Index of Erectile Function (IIEF): A state-of-the-science review. *International Journal of Impotence Research, 14*, 226–244.

Rosen, R. C., Riley, A., Wagner, G., Osterloh, I. H., Kirkpatrick, J., & Mishra, A. (1997). The International Index of Erectile Function (IIEF): A multidimensional scale for assessment of erectile dysfunction. *Urology, 49*, 822–830.

Schover, L. R. (1994). Sexuality and body image in younger women with breast cancer. *Journal of the National Cancer Institute Monograph, 16*, 177–182.

Schover, L. R. (2007). Androgen therapy for loss of desire in women: Is the benefit worth the breast cancer risk? *Fertility and Sterility.* Advance online publication. Retrieved April 11, 2008. doi:10.1016/j.fertnstert.2007.05.057

Schover, L. R., Evans, R. B., & von Eschenbach, A. C. (1987). Sexual rehabilitation in a cancer center: Diagnosis and outcome in 384 consultations. *Archives of Sexual Behavior, 16*, 445–461.

Schover, L. R., Fouladi, R. T., Warneke, C. L., Neese, L., Klein, E. A., Zippe, C., & Kupelian, P. A. (2002). Defining sexual outcomes after treatment for localized prostate cancer. *Cancer, 95*, 1773–1778.

Schover, L. R., Jenkins, R., Sui, D., Adams, J. H., Marion, M. S., & Jackson, K. (2006). Randomized trial of peer counseling on reproductive health in African-American breast cancer survivors. *Journal of Clinical Oncology, 24*, 1620–1626.

Schover, L. R., & Leiblum, S. R. (1994). The stagnation of sex therapy. *Journal of Psychology and Human Sexuality, 6*, 5–10.

Schover, L. R., & LoPiccolo, J. (1982). Treatment effectiveness for dysfunctions of sexual desire. *Journal of Sex and Marital Therapy, 8*, 179–197.

Schover, L. R., Yetman, R. J., Tuason, L. J., Meisler, E., Esselstyn, C. B., Hermann, R. E., et al. (1995). Comparison of partial mastectomy with breast reconstruction on psychosocial adjustment, body image, and sexuality. *Cancer, 75*, 54–64.

Schroder, K. E. E., Carey, M. P., & Vanable, P. A. (2003). Methodological challenges in research on sexual risk behavior: II. Accuracy of self-reports. *Annals of Behavioral Medicine, 26*, 104–123.

Shifren, J. L., Braunstein, G. D., Simon, J. A., Casson, P. R., Buster, J. E., Redmond, G. P., et al. (2000). Transdermal testosterone treatment in women with impaired sexual function after oophorectomy. *New England Journal of Medicine, 343,* 682–688.

Speer, J. J., Hillenberg, B., Sugrue, D. P., Blacker, C., Kresge, C. L., Decker, V. B., et al. (2005). Study of sexual functioning determinants in breast cancer survivors. *Breast Journal, 11,* 440–447.

Stone, A. A., & Schiffman, S. (2002). Capturing momentary, self-report data: A proposal for reporting guidelines. *Annals of Behavioral Medicine, 24,* 235–243.

Walsh, P. C., Marschke, P., Ricker, D., & Burnett, A. L. (2000). Patient-reported urinary continence and sexual function after anatomic radical prostatectomy. *Urology, 55,* 58–61.

22

FAMILY CARE DURING CANCER CARE

BARBARA A. GIVEN, PAULA R. SHERWOOD, AND CHARLES W. GIVEN

Care for individuals with cancer is increasingly complex because of more aggressive treatment protocols with denser dosing and shorter intense dose intervals. Family members are expected to actively participate in helping the patient achieve treatment goals and manage side effects, while coping with their own emotional responses to the patient's diagnosis. Cancer and cancer-related treatment may alter family functioning, occupational and social roles, and communication patterns at multiple time points across the cancer care trajectory from the diagnosis to treatment to survivorship (B. Given & Given, 1992; Kurtz, Kurtz, Given, & Given, 2005; Northouse, Mood, Templin, Mellon, & George, 2000).

Family caregiving is defined as the provision of unpaid aid or assistance and care by one or more family members to another family member with cancer. This care goes beyond the usual family activities, such as cooking or household chores, that are a part of normal daily life. The purpose of this chapter is to review literature about the needs, roles, and concerns of family caregivers providing care to patients undergoing cancer treatment. We present implications for practice and recommendations for research, and we use references mostly from studies of caregivers of patients with cancer, rather than using the general caregiver literature. At times, we used general literature to supplement the cancer-specific research. For intervention research, we focused on randomized clinical trials.

CONCEPTUAL FRAMEWORKS

Conceptual frameworks have not been widely used to describe the family care of cancer patients, and it is often difficult to understand what theory or conceptualization underlies interventions being implemented. The frameworks most often described are those of stress and coping built on the work of Lazarus (1966) and Folkman (1997). Within this approach, caregiver responses to the care situation are dictated by a balance between care demands and resources available to meet demands (Sherwood, Given, Dorrenbos, & Given, 2004; Sherwood et al., 2007). This approach suggests that coping skills are central to adaptation to stress. The difficulty with this framework is that task variation or decision-making requirements of caregivers are largely absent. Consideration of course of illness and treatment change over time is absent as well. It is important that conceptual models be developed and clearly articulated.

CAREGIVER RESPONSES

Conceptual models help us understand how family members respond to the stress of providing care. In turn, those stress responses are the basis for designing intervention to improve the emotional and physical health of family caregivers.

Impact of Providing Care on Caregivers' Emotional Well-Being

Family members of patients with cancer who assume the role of caregiver often experience emotional distress. Caregiver burden is an initial emotional reaction to care—one in which care demands are outweighed by available resources to meet demands, resulting in caregiver distress (Sherwood, Given, Given, et al., 2004). "Burden" is a multidimensional concept that grows from the imbalance between the social, psychological, and economic consequences that permeate a care situation and caregivers' coping strategies to meet demands. Caregivers who are unable to apply effective coping strategies to care demands may develop burden, which if sustained, may lead to depression (B. Given et al., 2004; Kozachik et al., 2001; Sherwood, Given, Given, et al., 2004; Sherwood, Given, Given, & von Eye, 2005). Caregiver burden is a negative reaction specific to the demands of care. Disruption of daily activities, competing demands, and physical care demands have all been shown to result in caregiver burden (Kurtz et al., 2005; Pinquart & Sörensen, 2004).

Caregiver depression is considered to be a secondary or long-term mood disturbance that may develop as a result of providing care (Clyburn, Stones, Hadjistavropoulos, & Tuokko, 2000; Fortinsky, Kercher, & Burant, 2002; Harris, Godfrey, Partridge, & Knight, 2001; Kurtz et al., 2005). Caregiver depression may emerge as a consequence of sustained burden and may be manifested by feelings of loneliness, sadness, isolation, fearfulness, and being easily bothered (Sherwood et al., 2005). Caregiver depression may be less dependent on recent changes in the patient's status and more dependent on whether the caregiver is able to use coping mechanisms to alleviate burden before it progresses to depression (Northouse et al., 2000; Sherwood et al., 2005).

Impact of Providing Care on Caregivers' Physical Well-Being

More than a decade ago, investigators began to report negative physical consequences as a result of providing care (B. Given & Given, 1992; C. Given et al., 1993; Kurtz, Given, Kurtz, & Given, 1994; Kurtz, Kurtz, Given, & Given, 2004). General populations of caregivers have also been shown to be at risk for fatigue and sleep disturbances, lower immune functioning, altered response to influenza shots, slower wound healing, higher blood pressure, and altered lipid profiles (Carter, 2002, 2006; Kiecolt-Glaser et al., 1995, 2003; Vitaliano, Zhang, & Scanlan, 2003).

Impact of Providing Care on Caregivers' Roles

Negative consequences for the caregiver (such as increased burden) can arise as caregivers seek to balance caregiving with work, family, and leisure activities (Pavalko & Woodbury, 2000; Stephens, Townsend, Martire, & Druley, 2001). Cameron, Franche, Cheung and Stewart (2002) found that regardless of amount of care provided, when caregivers were unable to participate in valued activities and interests, they became more distressed. Providing care can also have a negative effect on caregivers' work roles (Grunfeld et al., 2004). Caregivers must adapt employment obligations to manage and meet care demands (C. J. Bradley, Given, Given, & Kozachik, 2004; Cameron et al., 2002), which may result in missed days, interruptions at work, leaves of absence, and reduced productivity. For some caregivers, however, employment provides respite and serves as a buffer to distress (Hayman et al., 2001; Sherwood et al., 2005).

Positive Responses to Providing Care

Although providing care may result in negative emotional and physical consequences for caregivers, it can also engender satisfaction and meaning.

It is important to consider that both negative and positive consequences of providing care may exist simultaneously (Pinquart & Sörensen, 2004). Positive consequences, such as rewards, self-esteem, support, uplifts, and satisfaction, may provide a buffer to the negative effects of caregiving (Kurtz et al., 2004; Nijboer, Tempelaar, Triemstra, van den Bos, & Sanderman, 2001; Pinquart & Sörensen, 2004). Unfortunately, researchers know little about how interventions directed to caregivers affect positive outcomes.

Recommendations for Research

Studies should examine how the use of risk assessments for caregivers identifies individuals at risk for negative outcomes. Intervention studies are needed that target at-risk caregivers and that distinguish between those who are depressed and those who are burdened. Research is also needed to better describe and understand the impact of variations in caregiver health depending on variations in hours, types of care needed, and duration of the demanded care tasks.

Longitudinal randomized trials need to be designed to alleviate caregiver distress on two levels. One approach is to assist caregivers to perform the needed care tasks related to skill building, problem solving, decision making, and priority setting specific to the tasks and activities of care. The second approach should be directed toward caregivers' emotional needs, stress reduction, time management, burden, depression and anxiety management, consideration of their own health maintenance, and chronic disease management. Researchers need to determine the appropriate intervention and outcome for each care situation and realize that caregivers need assistance in both dimensions.

This research would be most beneficial if it considered type, stage, and trajectory of cancer and sought to determine how positive and negative reactions vary throughout the care situation. Research is needed to identify the effect of the patient's mental and cognitive status on caregiver outcomes and to design interventions to minimize negative caregiver response to patients' dysfunction (Phillips & Bernhard, 2003). Studies are needed that take into consideration type, stage, and trajectory of cancer to determine how positive and negative reactions vary throughout the care situation. An inception cohort of caregivers is needed to examine variation in care demands that extend from diagnosis to palliation to determine whether there is a logical progression in the depth of complexity and judgment required for tasks of caregiving across the disease trajectory.

RISK FACTORS FOR NEGATIVE IMPACT ON FAMILY CAREGIVERS

Patient- and illness-related variables, such as the stage of the cancer treatment protocol, symptom experience, and degree of disability, dictate the patient's functional status (or ability to perform activities of daily living), which in turn predicts care needs (B. Given & Sherwood, 2006; C. Given, Given, Azzouz, Stommel, & Kozachik, 2000; Kurtz et al., 1995, 2004). Severity of functional impairment (e.g., activities of daily living and personal care) has been consistently shown to increase care demands and restrict other caregiver roles, thereby affecting caregiver distress (Breitbart, Gibson, & Tremblay, 2002; Jepson, McCorkle, Adler, Nuamah, & Lusk, 1999; Nijboer et al., 2000; Pinquart & Sörensen, 2003; Stommel, Given, Given, & Collins, 1995). Researchers have reported that the presence of neuropsychiatric and cognitive symptoms such as agitation, dysphoria, irritability, delusions, depression, inappropriate behavior, violence, and apathy (Calhoun, Beckham, & Bosworth, 2002; Fillit, Gutterman, & Brooks, 2000; Sherwood et al., 2006) may be difficult for caregivers of persons with neurologic sequelae. In fact, managing cognitive and neuropsychiatric sequelae may produce higher levels of caregiver distress than assisting with impaired physical functioning (Pinquart & Sörensen, 2004). Furthermore, caregivers report that other family members are less likely to assist with care demands resulting from changes in the patient's cognitive or neuropsychiatric status than those resulting from changes in the patient's functional status (Breitbart et al., 2002; Sherwood, Given, Dorrenbos, & Given, 2004).

As the number and/or severity of symptoms increase, the patient's physical activities are limited and the patient becomes more dependent on the caregiver for assistance; thus, the caregiver's distress can increase (Andrews, 2001; E. Bradley, Prigerson, et al., 2004; Kurtz et al., 2004; Morita, Chihara, & Kashiwagi, 2002; Weitzner, McMillan, & Jacobsen, 1999). Even though patient symptoms and functional abilities improve, caregivers report that they continue to provide assistance and be on call (Nijboer et al., 2000; Northouse et al., 2000). Caregivers center their life activities on care, adjusting their schedules and relinquishing valued personal activities (B. Given et al., 2004; Kurtz et al., 2004). When care is over, transition back to previous roles may be gradual and difficult.

Gender has been shown to be differentially related to caregiver distress. Overall, caregiving is reported to be more stressful for women (i.e., wives and daughters) than for men (i.e., husbands and sons; B. Given & Sherwood, 2006; Nijboer et al., 2000; Northouse et al., 2000). Age has also been related to caregiver distress (B. Given et al., 2004; Nijboer et al., 2000). Low personal and household incomes, loss of income, out-of-pocket costs, and limited financial resources can place caregivers at risk for negative outcomes (Hayman et al., 2001; Nijboer et al., 2000; Stephens et al., 2001). Finally, caregivers' own physical and emotional health may place them at risk for negative reactions to providing care. Caregiver depression may be associated with those who experience loss of physical strength or have a physical health problem (Nijboer, Triemstra, Tempelaar, Sanderman, & van den Bos, 1999).

Preexisting discordance among family members may be aggravated and affect the care process, decision making, and caregiver's role in response to the challenges of cancer care (Northouse, Kershaw, Mood, & Schafenacker, 2004; Northouse, Templin, & Mood, 2001). The quality of prior relationships and family functioning may be a form of social support (Nijboer et al., 1999) and influence care responsibilities. Among caregivers in less mutually satisfying relationships, patients' symptoms burden restricted caregivers' routine activities, which in turn caused negative responses in the caregivers (B. Given et al., 2004; Nijboer et al., 2000; Northouse et al., 2004).

The very nature of the caregiver–patient relationship may affect caregivers' risk for developing distress. For example, wives, husbands, daughters, and sons approach the practice of caregiving in different ways (Manne, Babb, Pinover, Horwitz, & Ebbert, 2004; Northouse, Templin, Mood, & Oberst, 1998; Pinquart & Sörensen, 2004). Husbands tend to focus on caregiving tasks while continuing their own activities and interests, and they have fewer expectations that the needs for care will interfere with their usual activities. Wives, however, give priority to their husband's needs and tend to focus attention on the interpersonal aspects of caregiving, considering their own needs to be secondary.

Spouse caregivers appear to be at risk for caregiver distress because they live with the patient, provide the most extensive and comprehensive care, maintain their role longer, and tolerate greater levels of patient disability (B. Given, Given, & Kozachik, 2001; Kurtz et al., 2004). In addition, spouse caregivers may have to assume other role responsibilities for financial and household activities vacated by the individual with cancer. Spouses may have stronger established patterns of decision making, which can facilitate the care experience. Adult children and other nonspousal caregivers may experience more lifestyle adjustment and exhibit lower levels of well-being (Coristine, Crooks, Grunfeld, Stonebridge, & Christie, 2003). The impact of caregiving and its associated distresses on marital relationships such as divorce or separation have not been well described.

Caregiver optimism may be related to how family members perceive the care situation and, in turn, relates to the experience of burden (Gaugler et al., 2005; Northouse et al., 2004) and postbereavement depressive symptoms (Kurtz, Kurtz, Given, & Given, 1997). Caregivers with higher levels of mastery regarding the care situation have more positive responses to care (Moody & McMillan, 2003) because they may have available coping strategies to meet care demands (Gitlin, Corcoran, Winter, Boyce, & Hauck, 2001; Szabo & Strang, 1999). Higher levels of caregiver mastery have been associated with problem-focused coping strategies (rather than emotion-focused coping; Li, Seltzer, & Greenberg, 1999) and lower stress response to providing care (Bookwala & Schulz, 1998; Nijboer et al., 2001; Yates & Stetz, 1999).

CAREGIVER SKILLS AND NEEDS

Caregivers require a variety of knowledge, skills, and judgment to perform care tasks. Caregivers need to enhance assistance role acquisition and to feel prepared to take on complex care responsibilities (Scherbring, 2002). Care demands include physical care, nutrition, emotional and social support, spiritual support, symptom management, housekeeping, transportation, and financial assistance. Caring for patients changes over time and can include providing direct care, performing complex monitoring tasks, interpreting patient symptoms, assisting with decision making, and providing emotional support and comfort. Each form of care involvement demands different skills and knowledge, organizational capacities, and social and psychological strengths (Schumacher, Stewart, Archbold, Dodd, & Dibble, 2000).

Monitoring, Surveillance, Direct Care, and Coordination of Care Skills

Family members interact with the health care system to obtain needed information, services, and equipment, as well as to negotiate with family and friends to enlist and mobilize support. Caregivers become involved in accessing resources, coordinating care, and negotiating with the health care system for care needs.

Caregivers' involvement in direct and indirect care changes over time in response to the stage of cancer and cancer treatment. Changes in treatment protocols as well as changes in patient conditions, such as disease progression, recurrence, or palliative care, often necessitate reallocations of care tasks. Caregivers must be able to adapt to changes in the amount, level, and intensity of care demands and change in nature of tasks. Change requires adapting to different schedules, altering routines, and accommodating other roles. Pasacreta, Barg, Nuamah, and McCorkle (2000) found that the perception of burden did not worsen when tasks of care and level of involvement increased in intensity. It may not be the amount of care itself but the change in care demands (either increased or decreased) that result in caregiver distress (C. Given et al., 1993; Sherwood et al., 2005). Guidance and information from a health care provider regarding how to organize, prioritize, and adjust care to the dynamics of cancer treatment is valuable for family members.

Information is needed not only about physical tasks of care activities but also regarding how to manage patients' emotional needs such as depression, anxiety, or anger. The results of the National Cancer Institute's (2003) focus groups with caregivers revealed that caregivers need information in the following areas: how to prepare for medical visits, how to search for related cancer topics on the Internet, how to seek and reconcile different medical opinions about what the patient is likely to experience physically and emotionally, and how the caregiver can best support the patient at each stage of the disease. Caregivers also expressed the need for information on the emotional experience of caregiving, their own self-care, the importance of networking with other caregivers, the importance of seeking support, warning signs of stress and medical risks, and general financial and insurance information. A lack of information and the uncertainties in disease and care expectations add to caregiver distress (Northouse et al., 2000).

Recommendations for Research

To better understand the effects of care on family caregivers and on patient outcomes, caregiver roles, responsibilities, knowledge, and skills need to be more rigorously explored and defined. Little is known about what skills caregivers perform well and what areas cause the greatest degree of distress for caregivers. This knowledge would help to target intervention early for those caregivers at risk for distress.

There is very little research to suggest how variations in amount and type of caregiver interaction within a formal cancer-related health care system affects the responsibilities and perceived burden and depression faced by family caregivers. Interventions must include professional or formal caregivers and family caregivers as partners in care. Family members offer unique and vital skills and resources and should be engaged as a part of the patient's plan of care.

INTERVENTION STRATEGIES TO IMPROVE FAMILY CAREGIVER HEALTH

A few randomized trials of interventions have examined how to enhance caregiver well-being, and even fewer have studied how to assist them in providing care. The following sections focus primarily on randomized clinical trials from 1990 to 2005 involving caregivers of patients with cancer.

Educational Interventions

Only a few intervention programs have reported the effects of providing education on improved caregiver outcomes (Barg, Pasacreta, Nuamah, & Robinson, 1998; Kozachik et al., 2001; Pasacreta & McCorkle, 2000). Grimm, Zawacki, Mock, Krumm, and Frink (2000) documented the importance of cancer education to meet the psychosocial needs of caregivers of patients undergoing bone marrow transplantation. They found correlations between caregivers' mood and satisfaction of informational needs across treatment time points over 12 months. Wells, Hepworth, Murphy, Wujcik, and Johnson (2003) examined whether continued access to information following a baseline pain education program would increase knowledge and positive beliefs about cancer pain management, thus resulting in improved pain control. Both patients and caregivers showed a long-term improvement in knowledge and beliefs. Ferrell, Grant, Chan, Ahn, and Ferrell (1995) implemented a pain education program for older family caregivers that included information on assessment, pharmacologic (in particular pain education), and nonpharmacologic interventions. The program was effective in improving caregiver knowledge and attitudes.

Interventions Aimed at Social Support

Studies on interventions to increase support for family caregivers have lagged far behind those provided for patients, despite research that shows that spouses of cancer patients have significantly less social support than patients (Northouse et al., 2000). Focus on the family as a part of the patient's therapeutic plan of care is largely absent from interventional research. Despite the increased likelihood of caregivers with lower levels of social support experiencing caregiver distress (Goldstein et al., 2004), there are limited interventions aimed solely at increasing and improving social support. This is an important avenue for future research.

Developing Problem-Solving Skills

Toseland, Blanchard, and McCallion (1995) and Blanchard, Toseland, and McCallion (1996) implemented a randomized trial (Coping with Cancer) using a psychosocial six-session problem-solving intervention aimed at spouses of persons with cancer. Toseland et al. (1995) found little change in depression for either distressed caregivers or the entire sample of caregivers in the intervention group. Cameron, Shin, Williams, and Stewart (2004) evaluated a brief problem-solving intervention for caregivers of individuals with advanced cancer (Homecare Guide for Advanced Cancer) and reported improvements in emotional tension, confidence, and positive problem solving skills.

Psychoeducational Interventions

The majority of cancer caregiver intervention studies have used a psychoeducational intervention that emphasizes the provision of information, problem-solving skills, and a psychological and counseling approach to decrease caregiver distress. Kozachik et al. (2001) described the results of a 10-contact, 20-week psychoeducational intervention for caregivers and patients that focused on symptom management, patient education, coordination of resources, emotional support, and caregiver preparation aimed at both assisting the caregiver in providing care and alleviating caregiver distress. The intervention had a positive effect on reducing caregiver depression.

A 6-hour psychoeducational program that addressed symptom management, psychosocial support, and resource identification for caregivers with less than 6 months experience in the role was implemented by Barg et al. (1998). The most difficult issues for caregivers included, among other psychosocial issues, simply not knowing what to do in their new role. The number of caregivers who reported being well informed and confident about caregiving increased in those receiving the intervention.

Northouse et al. (2002) implemented a family-based psychoeducational program, five sessions over 5 months, for caregivers of women with breast cancer, focused on communicating openly, providing mutual support, involving the family, thinking optimistically, sharing fears and negative thoughts, reducing uncertainty, managing symptoms, maintaining hope, dealing with stress, and learning coping effectiveness. Family members were helped to manage demands of illness and obtain information, and they were taught self-care strategies. This intervention led to higher reported satisfaction among family members.

Jepson et al. (1999) examined changes in the psychosocial status of caregivers of patients with cancer in a seven-contact, 4-week intervention. An oncology clinical nurse specialist led an intervention, focusing on helping caregivers monitor problems, manage symptoms, improve self-care, and coordinate resources. Caregivers' psychosocial well-being improved at 3 months and remained unchanged at 6 months. Among caregivers with physical problems, the psychosocial status in the intervention group declined at 3 months but improved at 6 months.

A psychoeducational support group intervention led by psychologists that focused on partners of women with breast cancer was carried out by Bultz, Speca, Brasher, Geggie, and Page (2000). The sessions provided partners with information on the medical and psychosocial aspects of breast cancer and helped partners deal with individual concerns, fears, anxieties, and feelings. Patients whose partners received the intervention reported less mood disturbance, greater confidant support, and increased marital satisfaction at 3 months.

Home Health Care Interventions

A few intervention studies have focused on care delivery approaches such as a home health care intervention to impact caregiver outcomes (Smeenk et al., 1998). The intervention improved caregiver quality of life at 1 week and 4 weeks after hospital discharge. Enhanced coordination, cooperation, and support to the caregiver also occurred.

Recommendations for Research

Interventions to assist cancer patients and their families to increase their preparedness to deal with the care process, including care acquisition, symptom control, and indirect care to the patient should be designed and tested. Research questions should address whether caregiver distress affects caregiver decision making, judgment, and ability to provide patient care and should examine caregiver behavior and choices. Improving caregiver preparedness and providing adequate formal support may lead to fewer patient hospital readmissions, fewer interruptions in treatment cycles, shorter periods of patient work loss, and better patient and caregiver mental health. More randomized trials are needed to substantiate the role of programs in enhancing caregiver skills as well as minimizing caregiver distress (Pasacreta et al., 2000).

BEREAVEMENT

Overall, home-based family caregivers are positive about their experience at the end of life, and previous studies have reported greater caregiver satisfaction and reductions in caregiver anxiety for those who received hospice over conventional care. Teno et al. (2004) found that family members of patients receiving hospice services were more satisfied with quality of care than those who died within an institution. Hauser and Kramer (2004) also spoke to caregiving experiences during palliative care. However, C. J. Bradley, Given, et al. (2004) looked at length of hospice enrollment of caregivers and found that 17% were enrolled for 3 or fewer days. Caregivers with fewer days of hospice were at increased risk for major depressive disorder (24% met this criteria, compared with 9% with longer hospice stays). The short stay may not allow time for counseling, alleviation of pain, or spiritual care. C. J. Bradley, Given, et al. suggested that earlier hospice enrollment and support to the family might help reduce the risk for major depression.

Rabow, Hauser, and Adams (2004) identified five areas of burdens at the end of life for family caregivers: family time and logistics, physical tasks, financial costs, emotional burden, and mental and physical health risks. They suggested that providers promote excellent communication with family, encourage appropriate advanced care planning, encourage home care support, provide empathy for family relationships, and attend to grief. The care transactions during the end of life are critical because roles, tasks, and needs differ at each stage and may require different caregiver time demands, skills, and decisions. Information and educational interventions are key, as are counseling and support groups. Strategies for problem-solving interventions are mentioned, but end-of-life interventions are not listed.

It is also important to remember that for caregivers, the effects of providing care do not abruptly cease at the end of the cancer patient's life, despite the paucity of systematic studies that examine the bereavement needs of caregivers of persons with cancer. Bereavement may be a critical time for caregivers—It comes at the end of a time of intense caregiving and attention. Suddenly, isolation may set in and caregivers may have an increased risk for depression, substance abuse, and sleep disturbances. Schulz et al. (2003) reported that some Alzheimer's disease caregivers with high depression when the patient was alive improved in the year after the patient's death; death was a relief. Risk factors for complicated grief include previous psychiatric illness, treatment of multiple losses, and lower levels of social support. Bernard and Guarnaccia (2003) found that older age among caregivers predicted better bereavement for husbands and daughters of women with breast cancer. Coristine et al. (2003) reported that caregivers of persons with advanced breast cancer were exhausted from caregiving at the time of patients' death but were recovering 3 to 12 months later. Some expressed regret that other family members disagreed with caregiver decisions. These few studies highlight the need to follow caregivers after the patient's death and evaluate their coping and psychological status.

CONCLUSION

In summary, multiple studies have described the negative responses of family members to caring for persons with cancer (such as burden and depression), as well as research identifying some of the factors that place caregivers at risk for negative responses (such as the patient's functional status and the caregiver's sociodemographic and personality characteristics). However, intervention research to provide support to family caregivers and moderate distress as caregivers go through the cancer experience with their family members is limited and without consistent outcomes.

Researchers have given limited attention to the nature of the knowledge and skills of the caregiver and to personality factors or dispositions of caregivers and then planning interventions with those factors in mind. The interventions studies summarized in this chapter are randomized clinical trials that included support groups and psychoeducational and problem-solving approaches. Unfortunately, most of the intervention studies did not consider potential confounding or risk variables such as prior family relationships, cultural variation, caregiver health status, stage of disease, hours of care, or competing caregiver role demands. In addition, little detail was provided about the intervention design used in the studies, thus adaptation into clinical practice is limited. Few studies described the nature of care tasks of the caregiver or skills required, so it is not known whether caregivers were effectively managing symptoms, providing emotional support, providing direct care, monitoring patient status, or performing a combination of these tasks. The literature also is not clear about how care tasks vary by diagnosis, treatment modality, stage of disease, or as the patient's condition deteriorates. Outcomes and effects of interventions are limited in providing future direction for research, thus much research in this area is needed.

The value added by family members to patients' outcomes in terms of the duration and depth of the symptoms experienced, the dimensions in the quality of life that are maintained during treatment, and caregiver outcomes through survivorship deserve careful documentation. When providers recognize the value of early and continued family care and can more accurately identify the situations and circumstances surrounding families' capacities to deliver needed patient care, untoward hospitalizations and emergency department visits and improved quality of life for patients will be more widely recognized. Balancing the achievement of outcomes against the impact that providing this care has on family members is the ultimate goal for family cancer care.

REFERENCES

Andrews, S. (2001). Caregiver burden and symptom distress in people with cancer receiving hospice care. *Oncology Nursing Forum, 28,* 1469–1474.

Barg, F., Pasacreta, J., Nuamah, R., & Robinson, K. (1998). A description of a psychoeducational intervention for family caregivers of cancer patients. *Journal of Family Nursing, 4,* 394–413.

Bernard, L., & Guarnaccia, C. (2003). Two models of caregiver strain and bereavement adjustment: A comparison of husband and daughter caregivers of breast cancer hospice patients. *Gerontologist, 43,* 808–816.

Blanchard, C., Toseland, R., & McCallion, P. (1996). The effects of a problem solving intervention with spouses of cancer patients. *Journal of Psychosocial Oncology, 14,* 1–21.

Bookwala, J., & Schulz, R. (1998). The role of neuroticism and mastery in spouse caregivers' assessment of and response to a contextual stressor. *The Journals of Gerontology: Series B. Psychological Sciences and Social Sciences, 53,* 155–164.

Bradley, C. J., Given, B., Given, C., & Kozachik, S. (2004). Physical, economic, and social issues confronting patients and families. In C. Yarbro, M. Frogge, & M. Goodman (Eds.), *Cancer nursing: Principles and practice* (6th ed., pp. 1694–1711). Boston: Jones and Bartlett.

Bradley, E., Prigerson, H., Carlson, M., Cherlin, E., Johnson-Hurzeler, R., & Kasl, S. (2004). Depression among surviving caregivers: Does length of hospice enrollment matter? *American Journal of Psychiatry, 161,* 2257–2262.

Breitbart, W., Gibson, C., & Tremblay, A. (2002). The delirium experience: Delirium recall and delirium-related distress in hospitalized patients with cancer, their spouses/caregivers, and their nurses. *Psychosomatics, 43,* 183–194.

Bultz, B., Speca, M., Brasher, P., Geggie, P., & Page, S. (2000). A randomized controlled trial of a brief psychoeducational support group for partners of early stage breast cancer patients. *Psycho-Oncology, 9,* 303–313.

Calhoun, P., Beckham, J., & Bosworth, H. (2002). Caregiver burden and psychological distress in partners of veterans with chronic posttraumatic stress disorder. *Journal of Traumatic Stress, 15,* 205–212.

Cameron, J., Franche, R., Cheung, A., & Stewart, D. (2002). Lifestyle interference and emotional distress in family caregivers of advanced cancer patients. *Cancer, 94,* 521–527.

Cameron, J., Shin, J., Williams, D., & Stewart, D. (2004). A brief problem-solving intervention for family caregivers to individuals with advanced cancer. *Journal of Psychosomatic Research, 57,* 137–143.

Carter, P. (2002). Caregivers' descriptions of sleep changes and depressive symptoms. *Oncology Nursing Forum, 29,* 1277–1283.

Carter, P. (2006). A brief behavioral sleep intervention for family caregivers of persons with cancer. *Cancer Nursing, 29,* 95–103.

Clyburn, L., Stones, M., Hadjistavropoulos, T., & Tuokko, H. (2000). Predicting caregiver burden and depression in Alzheimer's disease. *The Journals of Gerontology: Series B. Psychological Sciences and Social Sciences, 55,* 2–13.

Coristine, M., Crooks, D., Grunfeld, E., Stonebridge, C., & Christie, A. (2003). Caregiving for women with advanced breast cancer. *Psycho-Oncology, 12,* 709–719.

Ferrell, B. R., Grant, M., Chan, J., Ahn, C., & Ferrell, B. A. (1995). The impact of cancer pain education on family caregivers of elderly patients. *Oncology Nursing Forum, 22,* 1211–1218.

Fillit, H., Gutterman, E., & Brooks, R. (2000). Impact of donepezil on caregiving burden for patients with Alzheimer's disease. *International Psychogeriatrics, 12,* 389–401.

Folkman, S. (1997). Positive psychological states and coping with severe stress. *Social Science and Medicine, 45,* 1207–1221.

Fortinsky, R., Kercher, K., & Burant, C. (2002). Measurement and correlates of family caregiver self-efficacy for managing dementia. *Aging and Mental Health, 6,* 153–160.

Gaugler, J. E., Hanna, N., Linder, J., Given, C. W., Tolbert, V., Kataria, R., & Regine, W. F. (2005). Cancer caregiving and subjective stress: A multi-site, multi-dimensional analysis. *Psycho-Oncology, 14,* 771–785.

Gitlin, L., Corcoran, M., Winter, L., Boyce, A., & Hauck, W. (2001). A randomized controlled trial of a home environmental intervention: Effect on efficacy and upset in caregivers and on daily function of persons with dementia. *Gerontologist, 41,* 4–14.

Given, B., & Given, C. (1992). Patient and family caregiver reaction to new and recurrent breast cancer. *Journal of the American Medical Women's Association, 47,* 201–212.

Given, B., Given, C., & Kozachik, S. (2001). Family support in advanced cancer. *CA: A Cancer Journal for Clinicians, 51,* 213–231.

Given, B., & Sherwood, P. (2006). Family care for the older person with cancer. *Seminars in Oncology Nursing, 22*, 43–50.

Given, B., Wyatt, G., Given, C., Sherwood, P., Gift, A., DeVoss, D., & Rahbar, M. (2004). Burden and depression among caregivers of patients with cancer at the end of life. *Oncology Nursing Forum, 31*, 1105–1115.

Given, C., Given, B., Azzouz, F., Stommel, M., & Kozachik, S. (2000). Comparison of changes in physical functioning of elderly patients with new diagnoses of cancer. *Medical Care, 38*, 482–493.

Given, C., Stommel, M., Given, B., Osuch, J., Kurtz, M., & Kurtz, J. (1993). The influence of the cancer patient's symptoms, functional states on patient's depression, and family caregiver's reaction and depression. *Health Psychology, 12*, 277–285.

Goldstein, N., Concato, J., Fried, T., Kasl, S., Johnson-Hurzeler, R., & Bradley, E. (2004). Factors associated with caregiver burden among caregivers of terminally ill patients with cancer. *Journal of Palliative Care, 20*, 38–43.

Grimm, P., Zawacki, K., Mock, V., Krumm, S., & Frink, B. (2000). Caregiver responses and needs: An ambulatory bone marrow transplant model. *Cancer Practice, 8*, 120–128.

Grunfeld, E., Coyle, D., Whelan, T., Clinch, J., Reyno, L., Earle, C., et al. (2004). Family caregiver burden: Results of a longitudinal study of breast cancer patients and their principal caregivers. *Canadian Medical Association Journal, 170*, 1795–1801.

Harris, J., Godfrey, H., Partridge, F., & Knight, R. (2001). Caregiver depression following traumatic brain injury: A consequence of adverse effects on family members? *Brain Injury, 15*, 223–238.

Hauser, J. M., & Kramer, B. J. (2004). Family caregivers in palliative care. *Clinics in Geriatric Medicine, 20*, 671–688.

Hayman, J., Langa, K., Kabeto, M., Katz, S., DeMonner, S., Chernew, M., et al. (2001). Estimating the cost of informal caregiving for elderly patients with cancer. *Journal of Clinical Oncology, 19*, 3219–3225.

Jepson, C., McCorkle, R., Adler, D., Nuamah, I., & Lusk, E. (1999). Effects of home care on caregivers' psychological status. *Image: Journal of Nursing Scholarship, 31*, 115–120.

Kiecolt-Glaser, J. K., Marucha, P. T., Gravenstein, S., Malarkey, W. B., Mercado, A. B., & Glaser, R. (1995). Slowing of wound healing by psychological distress. *Lancet, 346*, 1194–1196.

Kiecolt-Glaser, J. K., Preacher, K. J., MacCallum, R. C., Atkinson, C., Malarkey, W. B., & Glaser, R. (2003). Chronic stress and age-related increases in the proinflammatory cytokine IL-6. *Proceedings of the National Academy of Sciences of the United States of America, 100*, 9090–9095.

Kozachik, S., Given, C., Given, B., Pierce, S., Azzouz, F., Rawl, S., & Champion, V. L. (2001). Improving depressive symptoms among caregivers of patients with cancer: Results of a randomized clinical trial. *Oncology Nursing Forum, 28*, 1149–1157.

Kurtz, M., Given, B., Kurtz, J., & Given, C. (1994). The interaction of age, symptoms, and survival status on physical and mental health of patients with cancer and their families. *Cancer, 74*(Suppl. 7), 2071–2078.

Kurtz, M., Kurtz, J., Given, C., & Given, B. (1995). Relationship of caregiver reactions and depression to cancer patients' symptoms, functional states, and depression—A longitudinal view. *Social Science and Medicine, 40*, 837–846.

Kurtz, M., Kurtz, J., Given, C., & Given, B. (1997). Predictors of postbereavement depressive symptomatology among family caregivers of cancer patients. *Supportive Care for Cancer, 5*, 53–60.

Kurtz, M., Kurtz, J., Given, C., & Given, B. (2004). Depression and physical health among family caregivers of geriatric patients with cancer—A longitudinal view. *Medical Science Monitor, 10*, 447–456.

Kurtz, M., Kurtz, J., Given, C., & Given, B. (2005). A randomized, controlled trial of a patient/caregiver symptom control intervention: Effects on depressive symptomatology of caregivers of cancer patients. *Journal of Pain and Symptom Management, 30*, 112–122.

Lazarus, R. (1966). *Psychological stress and the coping process*. New York: McGraw-Hill.

Li, L., Seltzer, M., & Greenberg, J. (1999). Change in depressive symptoms among daughter caregivers: An 18-month longitudinal study. *Psychology and Aging, 14*, 206–219.

Manne, S., Babb, J., Pinover, W., Horwitz, E., & Ebbert, J. (2004). Psychoeducational group intervention for wives of men with prostate cancer. *Psycho-Oncology, 13*, 37–46.

Moody, L., & McMillan, S. (2003). Dyspnea and quality of life indicators in hospice patients and their caregivers. *Health and Quality of Life Outcomes, 1*, 9.

Morita, T., Chihara, S., & Kashiwagi, T. (2002). Family satisfaction with inpatient palliative care in Japan. *Palliative Medicine, 16*, 185–193.

National Cancer Institute. (2003). *After cancer treatment ends—The impact on caregivers and families. Report of focus groups with caregivers and oncology social workers*. Bethesda, MD: Author.

Nijboer, C., Tempelaar, R., Triemstra, M., van den Bos, G., & Sanderman, R. (2001). The role of social and psychological resources in caregivers of cancer patients. *Cancer, 89*, 1029–1039.

Nijboer, C., Triemstra, M., Tempelaar, R., Mulder, M., Sanderman, R., & van den Bos, G. (2000). Patterns of caregiver experiences among partners of cancer patients. *The Gerontologist, 40*, 738–746.

Nijboer, C., Triemstra, M., Tempelaar, R., Sanderman, R., & van den Bos, G. (1999). Determinants of caregiving experiences and mental health of partners of cancer patients. *Cancer, 86*, 577–588.

Northouse, L., Kershaw, T., Mood, D., & Schafenacker, A. (2004). Effects of a family intervention on the quality of life of women with recurrent breast cancer and their family caregivers. *Psycho-Oncology, 14*, 478–491.

Northouse, L., Mood, D., Templin, T., Mellon, S., & George, T. (2000). Couples' patterns of adjustment to colon cancer. *Social Science and Medicine, 50*, 271–284.

Northouse, L., Templin, T., & Mood, D. (2001). Couples' adjustment to breast disease during the first year following diagnosis. *Journal of Behavioral Medicine, 24*, 115–136.

Northouse, L., Templin, T., Mood, D., & Oberst, M., (1998). Couples' adjustment to breast cancer and benign breast disease: A longitudinal analysis. *Psycho-Oncology*, *7*, 37–48.

Northouse, L., Walker, J., Schafenacker, A., Mood, D., Mellon, S., Galvin, E., et al. (2002). A family-based program of care for women with recurrent breast cancer and their family members. *Oncology Nursing Forum*, *29*, 1411–1419.

Pasacreta, J., Barg, F., Nuamah, I., & McCorkle, R. (2000). Participant characteristics before and 4 months after attendance at a family caregiver cancer education program. *Cancer Nursing*, *23*, 295–303.

Pasacreta, J., & McCorkle, R. (2000). Cancer care: Impact of interventions on caregiver outcomes. In J. Fitzpatrick & J. Goeppinger (Eds.), *Annual review of nursing research* (Vol. 19, pp. 127–148). New York: Springer Publishing Company.

Pavalko, E., & Woodbury, W. (2000). Social roles as process: Caregiving careers and women's health. *Journal of Health and Social Behavior*, *41*, 91–105.

Phillips, K., & Bernhard, J. (2003). Adjuvant breast cancer treatment and cognitive function: Current knowledge and research directions. *Journal of the National Cancer Institute*, *95*, 190–197.

Pinquart, M., & Sörensen, S. (2003). Associations of stressors and uplifts of caregiving with caregiver burden and depressed mood: A meta-analysis. *The Journals of Gerontology: Series B. Psychological Sciences and Social Sciences*, *58*, 112–128.

Pinquart, M., & Sörensen, S. (2004). Associations of caregiver stressors and uplifts with subjective well-being and depressive mood: A meta-analytic comparison. *Aging Mental Health*, *8*, 438–449.

Rabow, M., Hauser, J., & Adams, J. (2004). Supporting family caregivers at the end of life: "They don't know what they don't know." *Journal of the American Medical Association*, *291*, 483–491.

Scherbring, M. (2002). Effect of caregiver perception of preparedness on burden in an oncology population. *Oncology Nursing Forum*, *29*, 70–76.

Schulz, R., Mendelsohn, A. B., Haley, W., Mahoney, D., Allen, R. S., Zhang, S., et al. (2003). End-of-life care and the effects of bereavement on family caregivers of persons with dementia. *New England Journal of Medicine*, *349*, 1936–1942.

Schumacher, K., Stewart, B., Archbold, P., Dodd, M., & Dibble, S. (2000). Family caregiving skill: Development of the concept. *Research in Nursing and Health*, *23*, 191–203.

Sherwood, P., Given, B., Dorrenbos, A., & Given, C. (2004). Forgotten voices: Lessons from bereaved caregivers of persons with a brain tumor. *International Journal of Palliative Nursing*, *10*, 67–75.

Sherwood, P., Given, B., Given, C., Schiffman, R., Murman, D., & Lovely, M. (2004). Caregivers of persons with a brain tumor: A conceptual model. *Nursing Inquiry*, *11*, 43–53.

Sherwood, P., Given, B., Given, C., Schiffman, R., Murman, D., Lovely, M., et al. (2006). Predictors of distress in caregivers of persons with a primary malignant brain tumor. *Research in Nursing and Health*, *29*, 105–120.

Sherwood, P., Given, B., Given, C., Schiffman, R., Murman, D., von Eye, A., et al. (2007). Identifying caregivers in need of intervention: The role of caregiver mastery in neuro-oncology. *Journal of Nursing Scholarship, 39*, 249–255.

Sherwood, P., Given, C., Given, B., & von Eye, A. (2005). Caregiver burden and depression: Analysis of common caregiver outcomes. *Journal of Aging and Health, 17*, 125–147.

Smeenk, F., de Witte, L., van Haastregt, J., Schipper, R., Viezemans, H., & Crebolder, H. (1998). Transmural care of terminal cancer patients: Effects of the quality of life of direct caregivers. *Nursing Research, 47*, 129–136.

Stephens, M., Townsend, A., Martire, L., & Druley, J. (2001). Balancing parent care with other roles: Interrole conflict of adult daughter caregivers. *The Journals of Gerontology: Series B. Psychological Sciences and Social Sciences, 56*, 24–34.

Stommel, M., Given, B., Given, C., & Collins, C. (1995). The impact of frequency of care activities on the division of labor between primary caregivers and other care providers. *Research and Aging, 17*, 412–433.

Szabo, A., & Strang, V. (1999). Experiencing control in caregiving. *Image: Journal of Nursing Scholarship, 31*, 71–75.

Teno, J. M., Clarridge, B. R., Casey, V., Welch, L. C., Wetle, T., Shield, R., & Mor, V. (2004). Family perspectives on end-of-life care at the last place of care. *Journal of the American Medical Association, 29*, 88–93.

Toseland, R., Blanchard, C., & McCallion, P. (1995). A problem solving intervention for caregivers of cancer patients. *Social Science in Medicine, 40*, 517–528.

Vitaliano, P., Zhang, J., & Scanlan, J. (2003). Is caregiving hazardous to one's physical health? A meta-analysis. *Psychological Bulletin, 129*, 946–972.

Weitzner, M., McMillan, S., & Jacobsen, P. (1999). Family caregiver quality of life: Differences between curative and palliative cancer treatment settings. *Journal of Pain and Symptom Management, 17*, 418–428.

Wells, N., Hepworth, J., Murphy, B., Wujcik, D., & Johnson, R. (2003). Improving cancer pain management through patient and family education. *Journal of Pain and Symptom Management, 25*, 344–356.

Yates, P., & Stetz, K. M. (1999). Families' awareness of and response to dying. *Oncology Nursing Forum, 26*, 113–120.

VI

QUATERNARY PREVENTION: CANCER SURVIVORSHIP

QUATERNARY PREVENTION: CANCER SURVIVORSHIP

The quaternary prevention of cancer, the subject of Part VI, is a relatively new area that has emerged with the increasing number of cancer survivors. Alfano and Rowland, in chapter 23, describe the psychological and economic effects experienced by adult cancer survivors and review studies of interventions designed to alleviate adverse effects. They also highlight the factors associated with positive psychological and spiritual effects. Chapter 24, by Casillas and Ganz, details the physical late and chronic effects of cancer treatment and notes the need for future research to better characterize the medical and psychosocial needs of survivors in relation to late-occurring morbidities. Kazak, Alderfer, and Rodriguez, in chapter 25, describe the neurocognitive deficits and impairments in psychological and social functioning among childhood cancer survivors and review the available research on interventions for this population. The authors also describe findings on the psychological impact of childhood cancer on parents, siblings, and family functioning. Chapter 26, by Northouse, Mellon, Harden, and Schafenacker, reviews the literature on the family experiences of adult survivors. In chapter 27, Demark-Wahnefried and Aziz review research on the prevalence of lifestyle changes on the part of cancer survivors to promote health and prevent disease, focusing especially on tobacco use, physical activity, and diet. They also summarize findings on behavioral interventions designed to promote the initiation and maintenance of lifestyle changes among survivors.

23

THE EXPERIENCE OF SURVIVAL FOR PATIENTS: PSYCHOSOCIAL ADJUSTMENT

CATHERINE M. ALFANO AND JULIA H. ROWLAND

Both the research literature and clinical experience suggest that there are five domains that must be negotiated and addressed as part of comprehensive recovery after cancer and that have behavioral implications: (a) ongoing medical follow-up and health planning, (b) the persistent physical effects of cancer and its treatment, (c) altered social and interpersonal relationships, (d) residual psychological and spiritual effects of illness, and (e) the practical implications of having had cancer on issues such as employment and insurance. In this chapter, we review the research on the psychological and spiritual and the socioeconomic effects of illness among adults treated for cancer, focusing on studies conducted after the conclusion of primary treatment. In each section, we highlight the findings relative to a specific chronic or late effect, along with information on interventions to address these as available.

It is noteworthy that findings regarding the psychological, spiritual, and economic effects of cancer on survivors rely heavily on research conducted among largely White, urban or suburban, middle-class samples of women treated for breast cancer. Although there are a number of practical reasons for this (Rowland, 1994), it leads to a general caveat about the generalizability of this body of research to survivors of other cancers or from more diverse ethnocultural or socioeconomic backgrounds. Furthermore, survivorship studies in general (with the exception of those conducted among prostate cancer survivors) have also tended to exclude large samples of older survivors, leaving researchers with limited information on this important segment of our survivor population. This is a particularly troubling gap in researchers' knowledge base, given that approximately half of today's survivors are age 75 or older. This number is expected to grow in the years to come, with the dissemination of effective cancer screening and treatment and the aging population.

PSYCHOLOGICAL AND SPIRITUAL EFFECTS OF ILLNESS

Previous research points to four key types of problems that disrupt the psychological and spiritual health of cancer survivors, including distress, anxiety, depression, and impaired quality of life; fears of recurrence; posttraumatic stress disorder and stress syndromes; and poor body image. In addition to or sometimes concurrent with these problems, many cancer survivors also report positive changes after cancer. The literature on each of these effects is reviewed in the sections that follow.

Distress, Anxiety, Depression, and Quality of Life

Many survivors of cancer show rates of psychological distress, anxiety, depression, and quality of life (QOL) that are similar to those seen in healthy, population-based samples (Kattlove & Winn, 2003), with some important exceptions. Although approximately 80% of cancer survivors function very well after the first 1 to 2 years after treatment, a subset show poor adjustment and may be in need of psychiatric treatment (Kornblith, 1998).

Estimates of the prevalence of depression in cancer survivors vary from 0% to 38% for major depression and from 0% to 58% for depression spectrum syndromes (Massie, 2004). Depression is more common in survivors of oropharyngeal (22%–57%), pancreatic (33%–50%), breast (1.5%–46.0%), and lung (11%–44%) cancers and is less common in colon cancer (13%–25%), gynecological cancers (12%–23%), and lymphoma (8%–19%; Massie, 2004). Estimates of the prevalence of mood disorder, using instruments with validated cutoff scores, are 22% to 47% (breast cancer), 14% to 31% (acute leukemia), 18% to 22% (Hodgkin's disease), 18% (testicular cancer), and 16% (bone marrow transplant; Kornblith, 1998). Increased psychological distress consisting of anxious or depressive symptoms that does not meet full diagnostic criteria for a mood disorder has been found in survivors of Hodgkin's disease, acute leukemia, breast cancer, bone marrow transplant, colorectal cancer, prostate cancer, and lung cancer (Kornblith, 1998). Prevalence estimates vary because of measurement issues (e.g., instrument, timing, sample characteristics), and clinical interviews generally find much lower rates. More than

30 years ago, Weisman and Worden (1976) first identified risk factors for continued vulnerability to high emotional distress after cancer with poorer coping and resolutions and greater mood disturbance. Vulnerability was defined by a subgroup of patients with past regrets in life, marital problems, pessimism, poor self-esteem, and perceived lack of social support. For the most part, these factors have continued to predict poorer adjustment in studies. Factors that consistently predict psychosocial adjustment, well-being, and QOL in cancer patients across cancer sites include a past history of depression, persistent medical sequelae of cancer and treatment or comorbid physical problems, poor social support, low economic resources, psychological factors (e.g., coping style, personality), and length of time since treatment, although less consistently (Ronson & Body, 2002). Men may have poorer psychosocial adaptation to cancer, possibly because of poor social support or less adaptive coping responses resulting from health-related schemas that are part of the masculine gender role (Nicholas, 2000). Other researchers have proposed that survivor coping, social support, and sexual partner understanding may deteriorate with time and account for impaired QOL later in survivorship (Holzner et al., 2001).

In contrast, several factors are associated with successful adaptation to cancer: particular cancer treatments; perceived social support, especially from the spouse or partner; those with a positive, active coping style, religiosity, high optimism, and emotional expressivity; finding positive meaning; and maintaining normal life roles (Kneier, 2003; Spencer, Carver, & Price, 1998).

Fear of Recurrence

Fear of recurrence, one of the most universal and durable legacies of surviving cancer, is prevalent in cancer survivors across disease sites, ranging from 5% to 89% of survivors (Kornblith et al., 1998; Ronson & Body, 2002). Fear of recurrence has been ranked as the single largest concern of breast cancer survivors (Spencer et al., 1999) and ovarian and other gynecologic cancer survivors (Kattlove & Winn, 2003). For survivors of breast or ovarian cancers, these fears can be compounded by concerns about the risk for other family members being diagnosed with the disease (Hamilton, 1999). Fears of recurrence, death, pain, and suffering have been reported across ethnic groups in breast cancer survivors and were often more anxiety-provoking than were fears of dying (Ashing-Giwa et al., 2004). Fear of recurrence has varied inconsistently by treatment. Breast cancer survivors treated with chemotherapy report greater fear of recurrence than those not treated with chemotherapy (with lower staged cancers); however, those treated with breast-conserving treatment report equivalent levels of fear to those treated with mastectomy (Kornblith & Ligibel, 2003). Both symptom distress and fear of recurrence are predictive of the appraisal of cancer as stressful (Bowman, Deimling,

Smerglia, Sage, & Kahana, 2003). Across cancers, fear of recurrence has been correlated with psychological distress and overall adjustment, and tends to decrease with the passage of time (Ronson & Body, 2002). At its extreme, fear of recurrence may be a marker of more serious distress secondary to cancer.

Posttraumatic Stress Disorder and Stress Syndromes

Posttraumatic stress disorder (PTSD) is characterized by persistent re-experiencing of the trauma, avoidant behaviors, and increased arousal. There has been some controversy as to whether a diagnosis of cancer constitutes a traumatogenic stressor, because it is not a discrete event, and thus, whether a label of PTSD is diagnostically appropriate (Neel, 2000; Schmitt, Singer, & Schwarz, 2003; Smith, Redd, Peyser, & Vogl, 1999). However, the American Psychiatric Association's (2000; 4th ed., text rev.) *Diagnostic and Statistical Manual of Mental Disorders* lists diagnosis of a life-threatening illness as a potentially traumatic event partially responsible for the development of PTSD symptoms. PTSD-like manifestations have been repeatedly shown to develop in the context of cancer (Smith et al., 1999), including cognitive avoidance; emotional reactivity; hypervigilance; sleep disruption; difficulty concentrating; intrusive thoughts related to surgery, chemotherapy effects, and fear of recurrence; and physical reactions such as heart palpitations or nausea in response to these thoughts (Cordova & Andrykowski, 2003). PTSD symptomatology has been associated with poorer QOL, especially in social functioning and mental health (Cordova & Andrykowski, 2003).

Estimates of PTSD prevalence range from 3% to 35%, depending on assessment method and time since treatment (Gurevich, Devins, & Rodin, 2002; Kangas, Henry, & Bryant, 2002; Schmitt et al., 2003; Smith et al., 1999), and are more similar to estimates of PTSD after trauma than to lower national prevalence rates (Kornblith & Ligibel, 2003). Although a small number of cancer patients may meet full criteria for PTSD, subclinical syndromes are more common (Cordova & Andrykowski, 2003). Almost 50% of cancer survivors may report some cancer-related PTSD symptoms (Kornblith, 1998). PTSD symptomatology appears to decrease over time (Neel, 2000), declining considerably within 3 months postdiagnosis or posttreatment (Kangas et al., 2002). However, symptom resolution does not always occur (Gurevich et al., 2002), and some survivors report significant PTSD symptoms even 20 years after cancer treatment (Kornblith et al., 2003).

Body Image

Body image has been frequently assessed in studies of the psychosocial impact of cancer because of the significant risk for scarring and disfigurement associated with treatment for the most common cancers. This is particularly true for studies of breast cancer survivors, given the integral role of breasts in feelings of femininity and attractiveness for many women. Studies of breast cancer survivors have shown significantly better body image among women treated with breast-conserving surgeries (e.g., lumpectomy) compared with women treated with mastectomy (average effect size = .40; Moyer, 1997), who may continue to have significant body image disturbances, as much as 8 years postsurgery (Kornblith, 1998). However, as many as 25% of women treated with breast-conserving surgery may have significant body image problems as well (Sneeuw et al., 1992). A second line of research has shown a consistent pattern of better body image among women who have breast reconstruction surgery versus those with mastectomy alone (Al-Ghazal, Fallowfield, & Blamey, 2000; Nano et al., 2005; Roth, Lowery, Davis, & Wilkins, 2005; Rowland & Massie, 2004). However, women pursuing breast reconstruction may be at higher risk for problems with body image, as they tend to be younger and to place a higher value on their breasts (Nissen et al., 2001; Rowland et al., 2000). Body image concerns have been associated with poor psychosocial adjustment and decreased sexual activity and functioning across cancers (Ganz, Desmond, Belin, Meyerowitz, & Rowland, 1999; Kornblith, 1998). Body image concerns affect all ethnic groups but may be greater for African Americans (Giedzinska, Meyerowitz, Ganz, & Rowland, 2004), Latinas, and Caucasians (Ashing-Giwa et al., 2004) and lesser for older women (Ashing-Giwa et al., 2004). Body image has been studied to a lesser extent in other cancers and has been associated with adjustment and sexual health in gynecologic cancer survivors (Stead, 2003) and those who had surgical amputation to treat cancer (Shell & Miller, 1999).

Breast cancer patients frequently gain weight potentially related to adjuvant chemotherapy, onset of menopause, decreased physical activity, reduced metabolism rates, or depressive symptoms and abnormal eating, and these women rarely return to their prediagnosis weight levels (Chlebowski, Aiello, & McTiernan, 2002). In addition to associations with poorer prognosis and medical comorbidities (Chlebowski et al., 2002), this weight gain may be a source of increased anxiety (Knobf, Mullen, Xistris, & Moritz, 1983) and decreased QOL (Kornblith et al., 1993) in breast cancer survivors.

Positive Effects

The positive and negative sequelae of cancer coexist (Cordova & Andrykowski, 2003). That is, cancer survivors may concurrently report both decrements in functioning and positive changes. Furthermore, these positive changes are greater than, and likely different from, positive changes reported by healthy peers, a finding also reported by others (Tomich & Helgeson, 2004). Reviews of QOL in breast cancer survivors have reported several positive sequelae of cancer, including renewed vigor in one's approach to life, more positive social experiences, improved view of the self, positive life changes, and improved outlook on life (Shapiro et al., 2001); positive impacts on diet and exercise behaviors (Ganz et al., 2002); greater appreciation of life, reprioritization of values, strengthened character, and increased self-confidence (Kornblith & Ligibel, 2003); greater satisfaction with religious concerns and strengthened spirituality (Ganz et al., 2002); and stronger interpersonal relationships (Kornblith & Ligibel, 2003; Shapiro et al., 2001). Indeed, not only do the majority of breast cancer survivors (77%) report satisfactory marital adjustment after cancer, but over half (58%) report a strengthening of the marriage attributed to having had cancer (Kornblith & Ligibel, 2003).

Several variables are associated with greater posttraumatic growth after breast cancer, including the perceived degree of threat posed by cancer, time since diagnosis, and the extent to which the woman had discussed her experience with others (Cordova & Andrykowski, 2003), as well as distress; however, directionality may vary by race/ethnicity. More distress predicts less positive reframing among Hispanic survivors but more positive reframing among non-Hispanic White survivors (Culver, Arena, Antoni, & Carver, 2002). Breast cancer survivors report that cancer changes their lives through an increased sense of both vulnerability and meaning, with African American survivors reporting finding greater meaning (Giedzinska et al., 2004).

Interventions

The majority of interventions developed to date to alleviate the psychosocial burden of cancer rely heavily on the use of support groups (Meyer & Mark, 1995; Newell, Sanson-Fisher, & Savolainen, 2002; Rehse & Pukrop, 2003; Sheard & Maguire, 1999). This is important, given that researchers also know that relatively few cancer patients or survivors avail themselves of mental health services in general or support group interventions specifically. In their population-based sample, Hewitt and Rowland (2002) found that although mental health service use was reported as higher for cancer survivors than for individuals without a cancer history, use for both groups was low (7.2% vs. 5.7%). Barriers to support group participation may be both practical (e.g., limited access because of distance from home, lack of transportation, or lack of available group; inappropriateness of group membership or focus for personal needs) and psychological (e.g., fear of stigma associated with use; lack of perceived usefulness of the group; lack of encouragement or support to attend, especially from significant others; Grande, Myers, & Sutton, 2005). Many of these barriers are remediable with support, outreach, education, and the application of new technologies that permit access for those who are in remote locales or homebound (Lieberman et al., 2003). Online Internet-based cancer support groups avoid pitfalls of traditional cancer support groups while providing additional advantages such as 24-hour accessibility from the convenience of home; anonymity; and the potential to equalize communication by removing age, gender, and social status, with the exception that low-income survivors may not have Internet access. A further limitation to interpretation of the intervention research is that, with rare exceptions (e.g., Mishel et al., 2005; Stanton et al., 2005), few of these studies were designed specifically to target the posttreatment period of adaptation.

Distress, Anxiety, Depression, and Quality of Life

Substantial literature examines psychosocial interventions to prevent and treat psychological distress and mood disturbance and improve QOL in people with cancer. Although psychosocial interventions have reported multiple positive effects in cancer survivors, the magnitudes of the effects have generally been small (Kornblith & Ligibel, 2003). Authors of reviews and meta-analyses have had difficulty evaluating intervention studies both because manuscripts lack sufficient detail to evaluate the effectiveness of the intervention and because studies are fraught with methodological limitations and are thus excluded from reviews (Newell et al., 2002). For these reasons, the results of reviews and meta-analyses of psychological treatments in cancer survivors are inconsistent. Some find that only weak conclusions can be drawn about their effectiveness (Newell et al., 2002) or that the data are equivocal (Fisch, 2004). Reviews provide information on the specific attributes of interventions that may result in successful outcomes. Group therapy, education, structured and unstructured counseling, and cognitive behavior therapy delivered by trained staff show the best evidence for medium- and long-term psychological benefits (Newell et al., 2002; Sheard & Maguire, 1999). The appropriate intervention likely depends on the targeted outcome: Psychological interventions that include components of social-cognitive theory (i.e., self-efficacy for change, outcome expectations, and self-regulation) have shown a stronger effect on global affect, depression, social domains, physical outcomes, and specific QOL outcomes but not on anxiety, coping, or physical outcomes (Graves, 2003; Sheard & Maguire, 1999).

One important caveat to the generally null results of reviews and meta-analyses is that most studies were designed to prevent distress and were not limited to only those who were already clinically anxious or depressed. Effect sizes are much higher in the trials that screened participants for distress and included only those who were at risk for, or had, significant distress (Ross, Boesen, Dalton, & Johansen, 2002; Sheard & Maguire, 1999). It is interesting that unlike for other populations, no studies document a benefit of treating depression in cancer survivors with a combination of antidepressant medication and psychotherapy (Fisch, 2004).

Fear of Recurrence

It is surprising that few studies have reported on interventions to address fear of recurrence specifically, with the exception of Mishel et al. (2005). They have developed an uncertainty management intervention that has demonstrated improvements in cognitive reframing, cancer knowledge, patient–health care provider communication, and diverse coping skills among older breast cancer survivors (Mishel et al., 2005). Although other interventions that effectively reduce distress and improve a sense of well-being might be expected to result in decreased worry about disease recurrence, this remains to be tested.

Posttraumatic Stress Disorder and Stress Syndromes

Stress reduction is a component of many successful interventions in cancer survivors (Andersen, 2002; Cordova & Andrykowski, 2003; Gurevich et al., 2002; Kangas, Henry, & Bryant, 2002). These few studies involved cognitive behavior, educational, supportive, and expressive therapeutic techniques and most showed positive effects on overall adjustment and reductions in PTSD symptoms. More research is needed in this area, discerning factors that affect the meaning of the illness and perceived life threat that may mediate distress (Gurevich et al., 2002). Cordova and Andrykowski (2003) suggested viewing cancer as a psychosocial transition and developing interventions such as cognitive behavior and supportive–expressive therapies that target both reduction of posttraumatic stress and promotion of posttraumatic growth (Cordova & Andrykowski, 2003). Others caution, however, that focus on benefit finding without addressing the negative side of the cancer experience may lead to further distress (Tomich & Helgeson, 2004; Wortman, 2004).

Body Image

Despite the research identifying body image as an important concern for cancer survivors, research on interventions to improve body image in survivors is sparse. Psychosocial interventions in cancer survivors tend to focus on general distress instead but, to the extent that they help improve self-esteem more broadly, may improve body image by proxy. However, several intervention studies are currently under way that look specifically at body image as an outcome. One promising intervention is physical activity. Preliminary cross-sectional research has shown that breast cancer survivors who exercise regularly posttreatment report better body image than do sedentary breast cancer survivors, specifically in sexual attractiveness and body conditioning (i.e., stamina, strength, and agility; Pinto & Trunzo, 2004). Further, breast cancer survivors participating in a 12-week exercise program reported improved body image (i.e., with regard to body conditioning and weight concerns) compared with control participants (Pinto, Clark, Maruyama, & Feder, 2003). It is not known whether physical activity may alleviate a woman's concerns about her treatment-related scars, how these improvements in body image might relate to improvements in sexual functioning, or how physical activity may improve body image in survivors of other cancers. Manne, Girasek, and Ambrosino (1994) conducted a study of the impact of a popular American Cancer Society program, Look Good . . . Feel Better, and their findings suggest at least short-term benefit on women's appearance concerns. Unknown is whether these body image–enhancing skills are retained by women and what impact this brief intervention, now available for teens and men undergoing cancer treatment, may have on longer term psychosocial outcomes.

Effects of Psychosocial Interventions on Survival

Despite the considerable body of literature documenting the psychological and social benefits of a variety of psychosocial interventions in cancer survivors, three recent reviews and a meta-analysis have found no consistent survival benefit of psychological intervention (Andersen et al., 2004; Chow, Tsao, & Harth, 2004; Goodwin, 2004; Smedslund & Ringdal, 2004). However, the lack of benefit may be due to the small number of trials, small trial sizes, or inadequate follow-up time, because the studies that have found a survival effect have included longer follow-up time (Chow et al., 2004). The three purported mechanisms for a survival benefit are (a) increased social support; (b) stress reduction, resulting in better adoption of health behaviors or increased adherence to medical treatment; and (c) stress reduction interacting with neuroendocrine or immune factors that improve disease outcomes (Andersen et al., 2004; Goodwin, 2004).

SOCIOECONOMIC EFFECTS OF ILLNESS

In addition to its psychosocial cost, cancer demands a significant economic toll on most survivors. A number of changes over the past 20 years in how cancer care is delivered in the United States have resulted in a growing economic burden on patients and families. These include the shift toward outpatient treatment, greater use of multimodal treatment approaches (e.g., combinations of drugs; combined use of surgery, chemotherapy, radiation, hormonal therapy), and restructuring of reimbursement systems that do not align with cancer care coverage (e.g., inadequate outpatient care recapture, poor oral medication coverage, lack of reimbursement for health promotion visits; Lipscomb, Donaldson, & Hiatt, 2004). At the same time, with many cancers diagnosed at an earlier stage and lengthening prospects for survival, more cancer survivors will be in, and continue to function in, the workplace. The aging of the population, governmental policies (e.g., Social Security) that favor people working beyond age 65, and the lack of mandatory retirement in a number of key industries will contribute to this trend (Main, Nowels, Cavender, Etschmaier, & Steiner, 2005).

Employment After Cancer

Research suggests that the employability of cancer survivors is mixed. A report summarizing the results of 10 studies involving over 1,900 survivors assessed from 1986 to 1999 found 62% returned to work (Spelten, Sprangers, & Verbeek, 2002). Short, Vasey, and Tunceli (2005), following survivors diagnosed between 1997 and 1999, found that of those who were employed at diagnosis, 73% returned to work within 1 year and 84%, by 4 years. Bradley and Bednarek (2002), who interviewed 253 long-term survivors in 1999, found that 67% were still employed 5 to 7 years later. In this study, survivors who had stopped working stated they did so because they had retired (54%), were in poor health or disabled (24%), their business closed (9%), they quit (4%), or some other reason (9%). Women with breast cancer employed after their diagnosis worked more hours (i.e., between 3 and 4 additional hours per week) and had higher wages and earnings relative to a noncancer control group (Bradley, Bednarek, & Neumark, 2002a, 2002b).

For a distinct subset of survivors, cancer is a disabling event, especially when survivors' performance is compared with that of their peers (Chirikos, Russell-Jacobs, & Jacobsen, 2002; Yabroff, Lawrence, Clauser, Davis, & Brown, 2004). In addition to frank disability or lowered productivity, other factors that may cause a survivor to leave the workforce are diminished taste for work and increased value of leisure time (both potential consequences of the reprioritizing that cancer prompts), as well as increased time required for health maintenance (Bradley, Neumark, Bednarek, & Schenk, 2005; Grossman, 1972).

Many cancer survivors still may find themselves trapped in jobs they do not like (i.e., job lock) for fear of losing employment and its associated health benefits, whereas others may be forced to leave the workforce because of disability. Unwanted changes in their job or roles, and changes in their relationships with workers and employers, may also present problems (Maunsell, Brisson, Dubois, Lauzier, & Fraser, 1999). These attitudinal challenges can be problematic if special accommodation is needed for a survivor to remain on the job. Although a supportive work environment may facilitate labor market retention (Bouknight, Bradley, & Luo, 2006), it is clear that manual labor is negatively associated with return to work (Satariano & DeLorenze,

1996; Spelten et al., 2002). This latter risk factor may adversely affect more survivors from racial and ethnic minorities and those from low income, as they are more likely to be employed in physically demanding jobs. At least one study has shown that African American women with breast cancer are at higher risk for nonemployment soon after treatment for their illness (Bradley et al., 2005).

Interventions

We are unaware of any specific trials of interventions to improve cancer survivors' ability to remain in, or return to, the workforce posttreatment, nor are details of employment status and functioning routinely incorporated as an outcome in QOL studies (Steiner, Cavender, Main, & Bradley, 2004). However, a number of the interventions previously described would be expected to enhance work performance, in particular those that enabled survivors to better manage fatigue, cope with stress, and reduce symptoms of anxiety and depression. In addition, a recent self-management program designed by Cimprich et al. (2005) includes elements that would allow a survivor to target coping strategies geared to enhance adaptation to work-related stressors. A number of educational materials (e.g., National Cancer Institute's Facing Forward; National Coalition for Cancer Survivorship's Toolbox and Almanac), programs (e.g., Cancer Care teleconference series; Memorial Sloan Kettering Cancer Center's Post-Treatment Resource Program), and not-for-profit advocacy agencies (e.g., The Center for Patient Partnerships at the University of Wisconsin Law School, Cancer Legal Resource Center) are available to help survivors understand and successfully navigate employment issues after cancer. The President's Cancer Panel as well as the Institute of Medicine, in their cancer survivorship reports (Hewitt, Greenfield, & Stovall, 2005; Hewitt, Weiner, & Simone, 2003; President's Cancer Panel, 2004), emphasized the need for all survivors to routinely and as needed receive information on counseling with respect to their employment rights at the time of diagnosis. Implementation of this recommendation would be an excellent first step toward reducing unwanted consequences of cancer on employment outcomes.

FUTURE DIRECTIONS

Analysis of the literature on the psychological and spiritual and the socioeconomic effects of cancer after the conclusion of primary treatment points toward several promising avenues for targeting future studies. Specific recommendations are presented here for furthering knowledge and improving practice using both descriptive and intervention studies.

Describing the Terrain of Recovery

Despite the considerable research identifying the long-term and late effects of cancer, there are many obvious holes in researchers' knowledge that point toward future descriptive efforts. Future work must identify the complex interplay between psychosocial and physical sequelae of cancer in survivors from diverse racial/ethnic or socioeconomic backgrounds, in older populations, and in those with cancers other than breast cancer, including determining risk and protective factors in these diverse groups. Studies should use screening instruments with clinically valid cutoffs to determine subgroups of survivors who are in need of intervention. Ongoing national efforts to widely implement screening for distress in survivorship populations will help bring attention to those in need of help. Future work should also focus on identifying those survivors who are doing well to understand the factors that might promote positive adaptation, rehabilitation, and posttraumatic growth. Studies should focus attention on the uptake of healthy lifestyle behaviors in survivorship, including how healthy behaviors may influence second cancers, comorbidities, and survival. Studies of the economic effects of cancer in survivors have just begun to identify the wide array of implications at the individual, family, and societal levels. Much more work in this area is needed to determine the effects of continued employment, return to work, or disability in cancer survivors. Finally, longitudinal studies in all of these areas are especially needed to gain a better understanding of the terrain of recovery over time.

Interventions

Reviews and meta-analyses of the effects of psychosocial interventions in cancer survivors point to where future research endeavors should be targeted. First, intervention studies must be methodologically rigorous: There must be adequate power to detect differences; participants must be randomized to conditions; outcomes of psychosocial interventions should be chosen a priori; and researchers must find ways to improve recruitment and retention rates and to use intent-to-treat analyses to reduce attrition bias. Second, it is likely that not all cancer survivors are in need of, or will benefit from, psychosocial intervention. Routine screening for distress or the specific outcome of interest to discern who may potentially benefit from an appropriately targeted and tailored intervention will likely result in more consistent positive intervention effects. Third, the correlation between ongoing physical problems and emotional distress suggests the need for interventions to simultaneously target both physical and psychosocial symptoms (Ronson & Body, 2002). Fourth, future work should also identify how risk factors for poor outcomes interact with each other and how their respective weights can be translated into effective rehabilitation interventions. Fifth, more comprehensive interventions with both educational and counseling components are needed, because one alone is likely not enough (Andersen et al., 2004; Kornblith & Ligibel, 2003). Such interventions should also be tailored to the appropriate people. Sixth, the optimal timing of intervention in the course of survivorship is not known (Ross et al., 2002) and should be identified. Seventh, future research on psychosocial interventions with cancer survivors should attend to treatment costs and mediating–moderating processes to enable informed decisions about allocation of health care resources and widely available efficient interventions (Owen, Klapow, Hicken, & Tucker, 2001). Eighth, future studies should further test novel interventions that have shown promise to improve psychosocial and biological outcomes in cancer survivors, including physical activity interventions and online support groups. Ninth, there is a need to examine the interventions that are already widely in use in clinical settings but have never been evaluated for evidence of effectiveness. Finally, attention in all of these efforts must be paid to including in research designs strategies to evaluate the appropriateness and effectiveness of the interventions being delivered in improving outcomes for our diverse population of survivors. This includes not only those from ethnoculturally and socio-economically diverse backgrounds but also cancer survivors who are young, those who are older, those from geographically diverse areas, and those living with the effects of the full spectrum of cancers (i.e., not just breast cancer survivors).

REFERENCES

Al-Ghazal, S. K., Fallowfield, L., & Blamey, R. W. (2000). Comparison of psychological aspects and patient satisfaction following breast conserving surgery, simple mastectomy, and breast reconstruction. *European Journal of Cancer, 36,* 1938–1943.

American Psychiatric Association. (2000). *Diagnostic and statistical manual of mental disorders* (4th ed., text rev.). Washington, DC: Author.

Andersen, B. L. (2002). Biobehavioral outcomes following psychological interventions for cancer patients. *Journal of Consulting and Clinical Psychology, 70,* 590–610.

Andersen, B. L., Farrar, W. B., Golden-Kreutz, D. M., Glaser, R., Emery, C. F., Crespin, T. R., et al. (2004). Psychological, behavioral, and immune changes after a psychological intervention: A clinical trial. *Journal of Clinical Oncology, 22,* 3570–3580.

Ashing-Giwa, K. T., Padilla, G., Tejero, J., Kraemer, J., Wright, K., Coscarelli, A., et al. (2004). Understanding the breast cancer experience of women: A qualitative study of African American, Asian American, Latina and Caucasian cancer survivors. *Psycho-Oncology, 13,* 408–428.

Bouknight, R. R., Bradley, C. J., & Luo, Z. (2006). Correlates of return to work for breast cancer survivors. *Journal of Clinical Oncology, 24*, 345–353.

Bowman, K. F., Deimling, G. T., Smerglia, V., Sage, P., & Kahana, B. (2003). Appraisal of the cancer experience by older long-term survivors. *Psycho-Oncology, 12*, 226–238.

Bradley, C. J., & Bednarek, H. L. (2002). Employment patterns of long-term cancer survivors. *Psycho-Oncology, 11*, 188–198.

Bradley, C. J., Bednarek, H. L., & Neumark, D. (2002a). Breast cancer and women's labor supply. *Health Services Research, 37*, 1309–1328.

Bradley, C. J., Bednarek, H. L., & Neumark, D. (2002b). Breast cancer survival, work, and earnings. *Journal of Health Economics, 21*, 757–779.

Bradley, C. J., Neumark, D., Bednarek, H. L., & Schenk, M. (2005). Short-term effects of breast cancer on labor market attachment: Results from a longitudinal study. *Journal of Health Economics, 24*, 137–160.

Chirikos, T. N., Russell-Jacobs, A., & Jacobsen, P. B. (2002). Functional impairment and the economic consequences of female breast cancer. *Women's Health, 36*, 1–20.

Chlebowski, R. T., Aiello, E., & McTiernan, A. (2002). Weight loss in breast cancer patient management. *Journal of Clinical Oncology, 20*, 1128–1143.

Chow, E., Tsao, M. N., & Harth, T. (2004). Does psychosocial intervention improve survival in cancer? A meta-analysis. *Palliative Medicine, 18*, 25–31.

Cimprich, B., Janz, N. K., Northouse, L., Wren, P. A., Given, B., & Given, C. W. (2005). Taking charge: A self-management program for women following breast cancer treatment. *Psycho-Oncology, 14*, 704–717.

Cordova, M. J., & Andrykowski, M. A. (2003). Responses to cancer diagnosis and treatment: Posttraumatic stress and posttraumatic growth. *Seminars in Clinical Neuropsychiatry, 8*, 286–296.

Culver, J. L., Arena, P. L., Antoni, M. H., & Carver, C. S. (2002). Coping and distress among women under treatment for early stage breast cancer: Comparing African Americans, Hispanics, and non-Hispanic Whites. *Psycho-Oncology, 11*, 495–504.

Fisch, M. (2004). Treatment of depression in cancer. *Journal of the National Cancer Institute Monographs, 32*, 105–111.

Ganz, P. A., Desmond, K. A., Belin, T. R., Meyerowitz, B. E., & Rowland, J. H. (1999). Predictors of sexual health in women after a breast cancer diagnosis. *Journal of Clinical Oncology, 17*, 2371–2380.

Ganz, P. A., Desmond, K. A., Leedham, B., Rowland, J. H., Meyerowitz, B. E., & Belin, T. R. (2002). Quality of life in long-term, disease-free survivors of breast cancer: A follow-up study. *Journal of the National Cancer Institute, 94*, 39–49.

Giedzinska, A. S., Meyerowitz, B. E., Ganz, P. A., & Rowland, J. H. (2004). Health-related quality of life in a multiethnic sample of breast cancer survivors. *Annals of Behavioral Medicine, 28*, 39–51.

Goodwin, P. J. (2004). Support groups in breast cancer: When a negative result is positive. *Journal of Clinical Oncology, 22*, 4244–4246.

Grande, G. E., Myers, L. B., & Sutton, S. R. (2005). How do patients who participate in cancer support groups differ from those who do not? *Psycho-Oncology, 15*,
321–334.

Graves, K. D. (2003). Social cognitive theory and cancer patients' quality of life: A
meta-analysis of psychosocial intervention components. *Health Psychology, 22*,
210–219.

Grossman, G. (1972). On the concept of health capital and the demand for health.
Journal of Political Economy, 80, 223–255.

Gurevich, M., Devins, G. M., & Rodin, G. M. (2002). Stress response syndromes and
cancer: Conceptual and assessment issues. *Psychosomatics, 43*, 259–281.

Hamilton, A. B. (1999). Psychological aspects of ovarian cancer. *Cancer Investigation, 17*, 335–341.

Hewitt, M., Greenfield, S., & Stovall, E. (Eds.). (2005). *From cancer patient to cancer
survivor: Lost in transition.* Washington, DC: National Academies Press.

Hewitt, M., & Rowland, J. H. (2002). Mental health service use among adult cancer
survivors: Analyses of the National Health Interview Survey. *Journal of Clinical
Oncology, 20*, 4581–4590.

Hewitt, M., Weiner, S. L., & Simone, J. V. (Eds.). (2003). *Childhood cancer survivorship: Improving care and quality of life.* Washington, DC: National Academies Press.

Holzner, B., Kemmler, G., Kopp, M., Moschen, R., Schweigkofler, H., Dunser, M.,
et al. (2001). Quality of life in breast cancer patients—Not enough attention for
long-term survivors? *Psychosomatics, 42*, 117–123.

Kangas, M., Henry, J. L., & Bryant, R. A. (2002). Posttraumatic stress disorder following cancer: A conceptual and empirical review. *Clinical Psychology Review,
22*, 499–524.

Kattlove, H., & Winn, R. J. (2003). Ongoing care of patients after primary treatment
for their cancer. *CA: A Cancer Journal for Clinicians, 53*, 172–196.

Kneier, A. W. (2003). Coping with melanoma—Ten strategies that promote psychological adjustment. *The Surgical Clinics of North America, 83*, 417–430.

Knobf, M. K., Mullen, J. C., Xistris, D., & Moritz, D. A. (1983). Weight gain in
women with breast cancer receiving adjuvant chemotherapy. *Oncology Nursing
Forum, 10*, 28–33.

Kornblith, A. B. (1998). Psychosocial adaptation of cancer survivors. In J. C. Holland (Ed.), *Psycho-oncology* (pp. 223–254). New York: Oxford University Press.

Kornblith, A. B., Herndon, J. E., II, Weiss, R. B., Zhang, C., Zuckerman, E. L.,
Rosenberg, S., et al. (2003). Long-term adjustment of survivors of early-stage
breast carcinoma, 20 years after adjuvant chemotherapy. *Cancer, 98*, 679–689.

Kornblith, A. B., Herndon, J. E., II, Zuckerman, E., Cella, D. F., Cherin, E., Wolchok,
S., et al. (1998). Comparison of psychosocial adaptation of advanced stage
Hodgkin's disease and acute leukemia survivors: Cancer and Leukemia Group B.
Annals of Oncology, 9, 297–306.

Kornblith, A. B., Hollis, D. R., Zuckerman, E., Lyss, A. P., Canellos, G. P., Cooper,
M. R., et al. (1993). Effect of megestrol acetate on quality of life in a dose-response

trial in women with advanced breast cancer: The Cancer and Leukemia Group B. *Journal of Clinical Oncology, 11*, 2081–2089.

Kornblith, A. B., & Ligibel, J. (2003). Psychosocial and sexual functioning of survivors of breast cancer. *Seminars in Oncology, 30*, 799–813.

Lieberman, M. A., Golant, M., Giese-Davis, J., Winzlenberg, A., Benjamin, H., Humphreys, K., et al. (2003). Electronic support groups for breast carcinoma: A clinical trial of effectiveness. *Cancer, 97*, 920–925.

Lipscomb, J., Donaldson, M. S., & Hiatt, R. A. (2004). Cancer outcomes research and the arenas of application. *Journal of the National Cancer Institute Monographs, 33*, 1–7.

Main, D. S., Nowels, C. T., Cavender, T. A., Etschmaier, M., & Steiner, J. F. (2005). A qualitative study of work and work return in cancer survivors. *Psycho-Oncology, 14*, 992–1004.

Manne, S. L., Girasek, D., & Ambrosino, J. (1994). An evaluation of the impact of a cosmetics class on breast cancer patients. *Journal of Psychosocial Oncology, 12*, 83–99.

Massie, M. J. (2004). Prevalence of depression in patients with cancer. *Journal of the National Cancer Institute Monographs, 32*, 57–71.

Maunsell, E., Brisson, C., Dubois, L., Lauzier, S., & Fraser, A. (1999). Work problems after breast cancer: An exploratory qualitative study. *Psycho-Oncology, 8*, 467–473.

Meyer, T. J., & Mark, M. M. (1995). Effects of psychosocial interventions with adult cancer patients: A meta-analysis of randomized experiments. *Health Psychology, 14*, 101–108.

Mishel, M. H., Germino, B. B., Gil, K. M., Belyea, M., Laney, I. C., Stewart, J., et al. (2005). Benefits from an uncertainty management intervention for African-American and Caucasian older long-term breast cancer survivors. *Psycho-Oncology, 14*, 962–978.

Moyer, A. (1997). Psychosocial outcomes of breast-conserving surgery versus mastectomy: A meta-analytic review. *Health Psychology, 16*, 284–298.

Nano, M. T., Gill, P. G., Kollias, J., Bochner, M. A., Malycha, P., & Winefield, H. R. (2005). Psychological impact and cosmetic outcome of surgical breast cancer strategies. *ANZ Journal of Surgery, 75*, 940–947.

Neel, M. L. (2000). Posttraumatic stress symptomatology and cancer. *International Journal of Emergency Mental Health, 2*, 85–94.

Newell, S. A., Sanson-Fisher, R. W., & Savolainen, N. J. (2002). Systematic review of psychological therapies for cancer patients: Overview and recommendations for future research. *Journal of the National Cancer Institute, 94*, 558–584.

Nicholas, D. R. (2000). Men, masculinity, and cancer: Risk-factor behaviors, early detection, and psychosocial adaptation. *Journal of American College Health, 49*, 27–33.

Nissen, M. J., Swenson, K. K., Ritz, L. J., Farrell, J. B., Sladek, M. L., & Lally, R. M. (2001). Quality of life after breast carcinoma surgery: A comparison of three surgical procedures. *Cancer, 91*, 1238–1246.

Owen, J. E., Klapow, J. C., Hicken, B., & Tucker, D. C. (2001). Psychosocial interventions for cancer: Review and analysis using a three-tiered outcomes model. *Psycho-Oncology, 10,* 218–230.

Pinto, B. M., Clark, M. M., Maruyama, N. C., & Feder, S. I. (2003). Psychological and fitness changes associated with exercise participation among women with breast cancer. *Psycho-Oncology, 12,* 118–126.

Pinto, B. M., & Trunzo, J. J. (2004). Body esteem and mood among sedentary and active breast cancer survivors. *Mayo Clinic Proceedings, 79,* 181–186.

President's Cancer Panel. (2004). *Living beyond cancer: Finding a new balance.* Bethesda, MD: National Cancer Institute.

Rehse, B., & Pukrop, R. (2003). Effects of psychosocial interventions on quality of life in adult cancer patients: Meta analysis of 37 published controlled outcome studies. *Patient Education and Counseling, 50,* 179–186.

Ronson, A., & Body, J. J. (2002). Psychosocial rehabilitation of cancer patients after curative therapy. *Supportive Care in Cancer, 10,* 281–291.

Ross, L., Boesen, E. H., Dalton, S. O., & Johansen, C. (2002). Mind and cancer: Does psychosocial intervention improve survival and psychological well-being? *European Journal of Cancer, 38,* 1447–1457.

Roth, R. S., Lowery, J. C., Davis, J., & Wilkins, E. G. (2005). Quality of life and affective distress in women seeking immediate versus delayed breast reconstruction after mastectomy for breast cancer. *Plastic and Reconstructive Surgery, 116,* 993–1002, 1003–1005.

Rowland, J. H. (1994). Psycho-oncology and breast cancer: A paradigm for research and intervention. *Breast Cancer Research and Treatment, 31,* 315–324.

Rowland, J. H., Desmond, K. A., Meyerowitz, B. E., Belin, T. R., Wyatt, G. E., & Ganz, P. A. (2000). Role of breast reconstructive surgery in physical and emotional outcomes among breast cancer survivors. *Journal of the National Cancer Institute, 92,* 1422–1429.

Rowland, J. H., & Massie, M. J. (2004). Issues in breast cancer survivorship. In J. R. Harris, M. E. Lippman, M. Morrow, & C. K. Osborne (Eds.), *Breast diseases* (3rd ed., pp. 1419–1452). Philadelphia: Lippincott Williams & Wilkins.

Satariano, W. A., & DeLorenze, G. N. (1996). The likelihood of returning to work after breast cancer. *Public Health Reports, 111,* 236–241.

Schmitt, A., Singer, S., & Schwarz, R. (2003). Evaluation of posttraumatic psychological problems in cancer patients. *Onkologie, 26,* 66–70.

Shapiro, S. L., Lopez, A. M., Schwartz, G. E., Bootzin, R., Figueredo, A. J., Braden, C. J., & Kurker, S. F. (2001). Quality of life and breast cancer: Relationship to psychosocial variables. *Journal of Clinical Psychology, 57,* 501–519.

Sheard, T., & Maguire, P. (1999). The effect of psychological interventions on anxiety and depression in cancer patients: Results of two meta-analyses. *British Journal of Cancer, 80,* 1770–1780.

Shell, J. A., & Miller, M. E. (1999). The cancer amputee and sexuality. *Orthopaedic Nursing, 18,* 53–57, 62–64.

Short, P. F., Vasey, J. J., & Tunceli, K. (2005). Employment pathways in a large cohort of adult cancer survivors. *Cancer, 103,* 1292–1301.

Smedslund, G., & Ringdal, G. I. (2004). Meta-analysis of the effects of psychosocial interventions on survival time in cancer patients. *Journal of Psychosomatic Research, 57,* 123–131, 133–135.

Smith, M. Y., Redd, W. H., Peyser, C., & Vogl, D. (1999). Post-traumatic stress disorder in cancer: A review. *Psycho-Oncology, 8,* 521–537.

Sneeuw, K. C., Aaronson, N. K., Yarnold, J. R., Broderick, M., Regan, J., Ross, G., & Goddard, A. (1992). Cosmetic and functional outcomes of breast conserving treatment for early stage breast cancer: Part 2. Relationship with psychosocial functioning. *Radiotherapy Oncology, 25,* 160–166.

Spelten, E. R., Sprangers, M. A., & Verbeek, J. H. (2002). Factors reported to influence the return to work of cancer survivors: A literature review. *Psycho-Oncology, 11,* 124–131.

Spencer, S. M., Carver, C. S., & Price, A. A. (1998). Psychological and social factors in adaptation. In J. C. Holland (Ed.), *Psycho-oncology* (pp. 211–222). New York: Oxford University Press.

Spencer, S. M., Lehman, J. M., Wynings, C., Arena, P., Carver, C. S., Antoni, M. H., et al. (1999). Concerns about breast cancer and relations to psychosocial well-being in a multiethnic sample of early-stage patients. *Health Psychology, 18,* 159–168.

Stanton, A. L., Ganz, P. A., Kwan, L., Meyerowitz, B. E., Bower, J. E., Krupnick, J. L., et al. (2005). Outcomes from the Moving Beyond Cancer psychoeducational, randomized, controlled trial with breast cancer patients. *Journal of Clinical Oncology, 23,* 6009–6018.

Stead, M. L. (2003). Sexual dysfunction after treatment for gynaecologic and breast malignancies. *Current Opinions in Obstetrics & Gynecology, 15,* 57–61.

Steiner, J. F., Cavender, T. A., Main, D. S., & Bradley, C. J. (2004). Assessing the impact of cancer on work outcomes: What are the research needs? *Cancer, 101,* 1703–1711.

Tomich, P. L., & Helgeson, V. S. (2004). Is finding something good in the bad always good? Benefit finding among women with breast cancer. *Health Psychology, 23,* 16–23.

Weisman, A. D., & Worden, J. W. (1976). The existential plight in cancer: Significance of the first 100 days. *International Journal of Psychiatry in Medicine, 7,* 1–15.

Wortman, C. B. (2004). Posttraumatic growth: Progress and problems. *Psychological Inquiry, 15,* 81–90.

Yabroff, K. R., Lawrence, W. F., Clauser, S., Davis, W. W., & Brown, M. L. (2004). Burden of illness in cancer survivors: Findings from a population-based national sample. *Journal of the National Cancer Institute, 96,* 1322–1330.

24

PHYSICAL LATE EFFECTS OF CANCER: IMPLICATIONS FOR CARE

JACQUELINE CASILLAS AND PATRICIA GANZ

The progress made in cancer survivorship epidemiology is a success story for the 21st century. The overall 5-year survival rate is estimated to be greater than 60% for the 1.3 million adults diagnosed with cancer each year in the United States (Centers for Disease Control and Prevention, 2004). The 5-year survival rate for pediatric malignancies is estimated to be greater than 75% for the 14,000 children diagnosed with cancer each year in the United States (Jemal et al., 2005; see also National Cancer Institute [NCI], n.d.b). Data from the National Cancer Institute (n.d.c) estimate that there are 10.8 million cancer survivors in the United States today, which represents 3.4% of the population. These estimated numbers of cancer survivors continue to grow when using the NCI (n.d.a) definition of *cancer survivor:* "An individual is considered a cancer survivor from the time of diagnosis, through the balance of his or her life. Family members, friends, and caregivers are also impacted by the survivorship experience and are therefore included in this definition." There are also important differences in the types of malignancies diagnosed during childhood versus adulthood and thereby types of cancer survivors. Childhood survivors (estimated at 300,000 people) are most likely to have been diagnosed with leukemia, brain tumors, or lymphoma, whereas adults are more likely to have been diagnosed with prostate, breast, colorectal, or lung cancers. Despite these differences in cancer types between adult and pediatric survivors, much can be learned from the pediatric cancer survivorship literature due to the high enrollment rates of pediatric cancer patients onto clinical trials. We will therefore use insights gained from the pediatric cancer survivorship literature to discuss the medical complications of cure and highlight data on adult survivors, when available.

There can be long-term toxicity experienced by cancer survivors from the various multimodal treatments of surgery, chemotherapy, and radiation therapy received. It is, therefore, important to understand four key concepts when discussing the medical late effects of cancer and its treatment. First, a *late effect* is an outcome that occurs greater than 5 years from time of diagnosis of cancer, as a result of the previous cancer treatment and may be physical, psychological, or social in nature. Second, a *chronic effect* is an outcome that occurs as a result of cancer treatment, either during or after treatment, and persists for longer than 3 months after the time of initial presentation and can persist into the survivorship period. Many of these late effects and chronic effects are medical in nature and are due to the lasting influence of treatment agents. However, they have the potential to have profound effects on psychosocial functioning and quality of life. Thus, the third important concept is that cancer survivors require long-term follow-up care that should be risk based, longitudinal so as to provide continuity, and multidisciplinary in approach (Oeffinger & Hudson, 2004). Finally, survivors require a treatment summary to help focus their counseling for late effects and thereby individualize and optimize their cancer survivorship care.

MEDICAL LATE EFFECTS OF CANCER TREATMENT

Despite the advances for 5-year survival rates for cancer patients, there continues to be a high risk for the development of medical late effects years after completion of cancer treatment. Virtually every organ system is at risk for the complications of cancer treatment, which include cardiac toxicity, pulmonary dysfunction, endocrine disorders, and even second malignant neoplasms.

Cardiovascular Late Effects

Cardiovascular disease has been observed, particularly in the acute lymphoblastic leukemia (ALL) childhood cancer survivor population and in survivors of Hodgkin's disease (HD). In ALL, the increased risk for cardiovascular disease has been attributed in part to late effects of obesity, dyslipidemia, and insulin resistance or diabetes mellitus (Oeffinger et al., 2001, 2003; Reilly et al., 2001; Sklar et al., 2001). The mechanisms responsible for the obesity and subsequent comorbidities, in turn, are not completely understood but possibly include damage to the pituitary for those survivors who were exposed to cranial irradiation leading to secondary growth hormone (GH) deficiency and leptin receptor (i.e., a type of receptor that helps regulate hunger) insensitivity (Brennan et al., 1999; Carroll et al., 1998). Cardiovascular disease can result in ischemic heart disease at younger ages than is typically observed in the general population and has been observed at higher frequencies in the HD survivor population (Yung & Linch, 2003). The major contributing factor for heart disease in HD survivors is related to mantle radiation, particularly if the dose received was in excess of 30 gray (Gy; Hancock, Tucker, & Hoppe, 1993). A *gray* is the standard definition of describing the absorption of one joule of radiation energy by one kilogram of body weight.

The anthracycline class of chemotherapy (e.g., doxorubicin) is widely used in the treatment of adult and pediatric malignancies and is responsible for an established dose-related side effect of cardiomyopathy resulting in congestive heart failure (Lipshultz et al., 1991; Steinherz, Steinherz, Tan, Heller, & Murphy, 1991). The risk factors for cardiomyopathy include high cumulative total doses, older age (> 65 years), and concomitant exposure to other classes of chemotherapy (e.g., cyclophosphamide) or chest or cardiac radiation therapy (Meister & Meadows, 1993; Swain, Whaley, & Ewer, 2003; Von Hoff et al., 1979). Radiation also has unique toxicity to the heart and can result in pericarditis, pericardial thickening, valvular heart disease, and increased risk for coronary artery disease and acute myocardial infarction (Adams, Hardenbergh, Constine, & Lipshultz, 2003). A survivor may be asymptomatic for many years despite having various cardiac abnormalities and may not present with congestive heart failure until there is significant cardiac stress, such as during pregnancy. Thus, it is important for survivors to have annual follow-up examinations to assess for cardiotoxicity through a careful history and physical, as well as cardiac-focused intermittent diagnostic testing.

Obesity

As previously discussed, obesity is an important concern in the childhood cancer survivor population, particularly for ALL survivors who were exposed to cranial irradiation with damage to the hypothalamic pituitary axis and subsequent GH deficiency (Link et al., 2004; Oeffinger et al., 2003). In the adult cancer survivor population, obesity is prevalent in the breast cancer population and has been associated with the use of chemotherapy and the onset of menopause (Goodwin et al., 1999; Rock & Demark-Wahnefried, 2002). Specifically for younger breast cancer survivors (< 50 years of age), obesity has been found to be associated with premorbid obesity and decreased current physical activity (Herman, Ganz, Petersen, & Greendale, 2005). Future research, therefore, should focus on interventions designed to improve physical activity and weight reduction for cancer survivors to improve their long-term health outcomes.

Musculoskeletal Late Effects

Bone tumors that involve the extremities may require amputation for complete surgical resection of a malignancy, resulting in both cosmetic deformities and functional abnormalities (Marina, 1997). Survivors of cancer with an amputation completed during childhood or adolescence can have unique functional problems because this is a period in which there is rapid bone growth. Bony overgrowths that can occur at the distal end of the surgical stump may cause problems for prosthesis use and require repeated operations for correction of the problem (Nagarajan, Neglia, Clohisy, & Robison, 2002). Patients can also experience chronic pain in the surgical stump or in the lower extremity after amputation, which is referred to as *phantom limb pain* (Krane & Heller, 1995). For breast cancer survivors, musculoskeletal late effects as a result of mastectomy or lumpectomy include arm edema and impairment of upper limb functioning and activities of daily living (Erickson, Pearson, Ganz, Adams, & Kahn, 2001; Gosselink et al., 2003).

Radiation given at an early age for treatment of cancer can result in musculoskeletal abnormalities. In general, the larger the dose of radiation and the younger the age at time of treatment, the greater is the risk for musculoskeletal late effects (Marina, 1997; Probert & Parker, 1975). Late effects caused by radiation usually relate to the site of treatment. For example, radiation to the spine and growing bones can result in scoliosis, short stature, and leg length discrepancy (Rate, Butler, Robertson, & D'Angio, 1991). These effects of radiation therapy on the musculoskeletal system are most marked for those receiving treatment during puberty, because this is a period of rapid bone growth. Radiation therapy can also result in soft tissue loss, causing cosmetic deformities.

Osteopenia and osteoporosis occur more frequently in the cancer survivor population than the general population. Osteopenia and osteoporosis can result in musculoskeletal pain, abnormal gait, bone fractures, spinal abnormalities, and growth failure (Haddy, Mosher, & Reaman, 2001). The etiology for osteopenia most likely represents a multifactorial process that includes exposure to corticosteroids, methotrexate chemotherapy, cranial irradiation, and physical inactivity (Halton et al., 1996; Leiper, 1998; A. M. Schwartz & Leonidas, 1984; Stanisavljevic & Babcock, 1977; Warner, Evans, Webb, Bell, & Gregory, 1999). Wright, Galea, and Barr (2003) completed a study in survivors of childhood ALL in which they looked at self-perceptions of physical activity and found that the survivors have poorer self-perceptions of their ability to exercise and are less inclined to participate in exercise. This may explain, in part, the increased risk for osteopenia and osteoporosis in this population of survivors (Wright et al., 2003). Given that other contributing factors associated with osteoporosis in the general population include physical inactivity, low calcium intake, smoking, and excessive alcohol intake, practitioners caring for cancer survivors should counsel them on the importance of a healthy diet high in calcium, regular physical activity, and avoidance of smoking and frequent alcohol consumption to decrease the risk for osteopenia and osteoporosis.

Finally, treatment with prednisone and/or dexamethasone as part of chemotherapeutic regimens can also result in avascular necrosis of the femoral head and require hip replacement. Avascular necrosis typically presents with complaints of hip pain, and a limp and can occur several years after the completion of chemotherapy.

Endocrine Late Effects

Central nervous system (CNS) radiation can cause pituitary dysfunction, resulting in deficiency of various hormones, including GH, thyroid-stimulating hormone (TSH), luteinizing hormone (LH), follicle-stimulating hormone (FSH), gonadotropin-releasing hormone (GnRH), and corticotropin-releasing hormone (CRH). GH secretion is the most vulnerable to the effects of ionizing radiation to the pituitary gland and can occur at doses as low as 18 cGy. GH deficiency is a problem that particularly impacts the childhood cancer survivor, because childhood is the period during which people achieve their maximum adult height.

Infertility may result from chemotherapy and is age dependent in the childhood cancer survivor population. For men, the alkylating class of chemotherapeutic agents (e.g., cyclophosphamide, procarbazine) can result in male infertility due to azoospermia (Hobbie, Ginsberg, Ogle, Carlson, & Meadows, 2005). For women, exposure to alkylating chemotherapeutic agents and radiation can result in secondary amenorrhea or premature menopause. The risk for premature ovarian failure varies for female patients treated between 0 and 13 years of age when compared with those treated when 14 years and older (Gleeson & Shalet, 2001). Byrne et al. (1992) found that female patients treated before age 14 with chemotherapy and/or radiation therapy were not at an increased risk for premature ovarian failure. However, those between 13 and 19 years of age were 2 times as likely to reach menopause in the 3rd decade of life (Byrne et al., 1992). For female childhood cancer survivors, it is therefore important to take a careful pubertal history, menstrual and pregnancy history, and measurement of hormonal status with estradiol, FSH, and LH levels if there is a suggestive history, such as amenorrhea or irregular menses (CureSearch Children's Oncology Group, n.d.).

Adult female survivors exposed to chemotherapy are also at risk for premature menopause and amenorrhea. Increased risk for menopause does not, however, seem be related to exposure to tamoxifen therapy (Goodwin et al., 1999). The risk for premature menopause accelerates in women exposed at or around age 40 but can occur in women in their 30s. Experiencing a transition to premature menopause during treatment can lower quality of life for younger breast cancer survivors (Ganz, Greendale, Petersen, Kahn, & Bower, 2003). In addition, the vasomotor symptoms of menopause, such as hot flashes, sweats, and nighttime awakening, can be more severe in women who experience premature menopause compared with those who develop it as a natural process of aging. Finally, premature menopause and amenorrhea, in turn, place breast cancer survivors at risk for accelerated osteoporosis secondary to estrogen deficiency.

Damage to the gonadal tissue and the consequences of possible infertility have been well documented in the medical literature for those who have had abdominal irradiation because of HD, Wilms' tumor or for testicular leukemia (Bramswig et al., 1990; Nicolson & Byrne, 1993; C. L. Schwartz, 1990). Sexual dysfunction can also occur in cancer survivors and has been associated with changes in reproductive hormone levels and surgical therapies, particularly for men who undergo surgery for prostate cancer (Schover et al., 2004). Despite all of these risks, fertility and other gonadal toxicities are still not consistently discussed at the time of diagnosis and treatment (Canada & Schover, 2005; Schover, Brey, Lichtin, Lipshultz, & Jeha, 2002). Awareness of this problem is increasing, and patient-oriented resources are available (Fertile Hope: http://www.fertilehope.org; see also Schover, 1997).

Thyroid disease has been observed, particularly in the HD survivor population as a result of mantle radiation. Radiation therapy to the neck, including that for head and neck cancers and to the supraclavicular area for breast cancer, can result in hypothyroidism, which may be clinical or subclinical (i.e., only detected by blood tests in which there is an elevation in TSH with a normal thyroxin level). The greatest risk for hypothyroidism occurs within the first 5 years of completion of therapy but can occur as late as 20 years after therapy. Hyperthyroidism is a less common long-term side effect of radiation to the thyroid but also has been reported (Sklar et al., 2000).

Infectious Late Effects

Prior to 1988, surgical staging (including splenectomy) was performed in persons with HD to determine the extent of their malignancy, because radiographic imaging techniques were less sophisticated at that time. Asplenia places HD survivors at risk for serious bacterial infections, which can be life threatening (Marina, 1997). An asplenic survivor must be educated on the need to seek medical attention immediately if he or she has a fever so that antibiotics can be initiated promptly.

Cancer survivors transfused with blood products prior to July 1992 are at risk for infectious hepatitis, including hepatitis C. The natural history of infection with hepatitis C virus in this population is not yet completely understood. There are survivors of childhood ALL who are seropositive for hepatitis C but have not yet progressed to liver failure over a median of 14 years, yet there are other survivors who have chronic liver disease and fibrosis (Centers for Disease Control and Prevention, 1998; Cesaro et al., 1997; Oeffinger, Eshelman, Tomlinson, Tolle, & Schneider, 2000).

Pulmonary Late Effects

Chemotherapeutic agents, such as bleomycin and carmustine, can cause pulmonary fibrosis, resulting in impaired gas exchange. Pulmonary toxicity has been reported to occur up to 17 years postexposure to pulmonary toxic chemotherapy and may be asymptomatic for several years (Driscoll et al., 1990). Radiation therapy to the lungs can cause radiation pneumonitis, paramediastinal fibrosis, and pulmonary function abnormalities (Mertens et al., 2002). Other risk factors for developing pulmonary disease include prior pulmonary disease and older age (Meister & Meadows, 1993).

Genitourinary Late Effects

Two alkylating chemotherapeutic agents, cyclophosphamide and ifosfamide, can result in hemorrhagic cystitis during cancer treatment months to years after completion of therapy (Levine & Richie, 1989). The risk for this late effect is higher if there is also radiation exposure to the bladder. Pelvic irradiation can result in bladder fibrosis, leading to decreased bladder capacity, urinary frequency, and recurrent urinary tract infections. Pelvic irradiation can also result in scarring of the renal blood vessels with secondary hypertension (C. L. Schwartz, 1995). Surgical staging using retroperitoneal lymph node dissection can be associated with male infertility because of autonomic nervous system dysfunction, resulting in retrograde ejaculation (Heyn et al., 1992; Marina, 1997).

Neurologic Late Effects

CNS radiation therapy can result in multiple late effects including radiation necrosis; cerebrovascular accidents; and mineralizing microangiopathy, in which there is calcium deposition in the walls of the CNS blood vessels (Conomy & Kellermeyer, 1975; Marina, 1997). The radiotherapy doses used for brain tumors are usually higher in amount than for other malignancies and are therefore more often associated with neurological late effects (Anderson et al., 2001).

Chemotherapy, systemic or intrathecal, can result in neurological late effects. One such example is leukoencephalopathy, which most often occurs with the chemotherapeutic agent methotrexate in combination with cranial irradiation. Peripheral neuropathy, which can manifest as foot drop or jaw pain, can result from treatment with vinca alkaloids (i.e., vincristine and vinblastine) or cisplatin (Hansen, Helweg-Larsen, & Trojaborg, 1989). It is usually reversible once the chemotherapeutic agent is discontinued but has been observed to occur as a late effect in some pediatric cancer survivor populations. Cisplatin or other platinum chemotherapeutic agents can result in high-frequency hearing loss and thus may require consultation with an otolaryngologist for hearing aid placement (Blakley et al., 2002).

CNS radiation therapy can result in neurocognitive dysfunction in pediatric cancer survivors, with age at time of therapy being an important risk factor. Specifically, if a pediatric cancer patient has had brain irradiation before 3 years of age, the risk is very high for severe intellectual impairment. The risk for intellectual compromise from radiation therapy still exists for those who have been irradiated before 7 to 8 years of age (Duffner & Cohen, 1991). Pediatric cancer survivors who have received radiation therapy at high doses for the treatment of brain tumors can have neurocognitive deficits in memory, attention, and academic achievement (Johnson et al., 1994; Roman & Sperduto, 1995).

For adult cancer survivors, there has been recent interest in cognitive dysfunction in adults treated with chemotherapy, particularly in the breast cancer population who received adjuvant chemotherapy (Castellon et al., 2004; Rugo & Ahles, 2003; Tannock, Ahles, Ganz, & Van Dam, 2004). The mechanisms that lead to neurocognitive dysfunction are not completely understood but may include a direct toxic effect to the CNS and other indirect effects, such as anemia or a reduction in estrogen concentrations associated with chemotherapy-induced menopause (Ahles, 2004). Most studies, however, have been cross-sectional in design limiting causal inference. This is an area of increased investigation because of the widespread use of chemotherapy and hormonal therapy in breast cancer patients.

Gastrointestinal Late Effects

The chemotherapeutic agents methotrexate and 6-mercaptopurine carry the long-term risk for developing hepatic toxicity, including fibrosis and cirrhosis (Perry, 1982). Patients who develop the late effect of liver disease as a result of exposure to hepatotoxic chemotherapeutic agents may be asymptomatic for several years. Thus, liver function tests should be included in the annual laboratory evaluation of cancer survivors who have been exposed to these agents (DeLaat & Lampkin, 1992).

Survivors who have had abdominal surgery are at risk for adhesions, which can result in bowel obstruction. Counseling should be given to those survivors with a history of abdominal surgery, to seek prompt medical evaluation if they have symptoms of abdominal pain and vomiting.

Second Malignant Neoplasms

The long-term follow-up of survivors of HD has resulted in a greater understanding of the risk for secondary cancer linked to treatment exposure because of the well-documented risk for breast cancer in young female survivors of HD following chest radiation therapy (Neglia et al., 2001; Travis et al., 2003). Leukemia is another type of second malignant neoplasm that is observed in cancer survivors and is associated with exposure to alkylating agents and epipodophyllotoxins (e.g., etoposide; Curtis et al., 1992). The prognosis is unfortunately very poor for patients with a secondary leukemia and is often associated with chromosomal abnormalities of the tumor cells. Secondary solid tumors, such as soft tissue sarcomas (in particular, osteosarcoma), can occur in the field of previous exposure to radiotherapy and have been reported with exposure to the alkylating chemotherapeutic agents (Tucker et al., 1987). Radiation exposure to the thyroid is associated with an increased incidence of thyroid nodules, which can be benign or malignant, although the majority have been reported to be malignant (Sklar et al., 2000). Radiation therapy, particularly total body irradiation for bone marrow transplant recipients or cranial irradiation for treatment of brain tumors, can also result in an increased risk for skin malignancies, including basal cell carcinomas (Stavrou et al., 2001). Exposure to cyclophosphamide carries a long-term risk for bladder malignancy but is not associated with a previous history of hemorrhagic cystitis (Pedersen-Bjergaard et al., 1988). Finally, hormone therapy with tamoxifen for breast cancer treatment is associated with an increased risk for endometrial cancer, particularly if treatment with this adjuvant drug extends beyond 5 years (Swerdlow & Jones, 2005).

Other Miscellaneous Late Effects: Ophthalmologic and Dental

Cataracts can occur with exposure to corticosteroid chemotherapeutic agents, such as prednisone or dexamethasone. Cataracts have also been reported following bone marrow transplantation because of the exposure to total body irradiation (Benyunes et al., 1995; Liesner, Leiper, Hann, & Chessells, 1994; van Kempen-Harteveld, Belkacemi, Kal, Labopin, & Frassoni, 2002). In addition, radiation to the head and neck can result in dry mouth secondary to salivary gland dysfunction, poor tooth enamel, poor root formation, and increased risk for periodontal disease (i.e., plaque and gingivitis; Maguire et al., 1987).

CHRONIC EFFECTS OF CANCER TREATMENT

In addition to the late effects of treatment, which occur more than 5 years from time of diagnosis of cancer as a result of the previous cancer treatment, chronic effects may develop during cancer treatment and persist into the survivorship period. These chronic conditions must be recognized by practitioners who care for survivors because they will require continuing medical care throughout survivorship follow-up and can impact quality of life.

Lymphedema

One of the more common examples of a chronic effect of cancer treatment includes lymphedema in breast cancer survivors as a result of their primary surgical treatment. Although there are various lymphedema treatments for women who are affected by the excess of arm extracellular fluid volume because of impaired lymphatic drainage, women who have this chronic effect of cancer treatment still report poorer quality of life; fatigue; and psychological distress, including loss of confidence in their body (Ridner, 2005). The more widespread use of sentinel lymph node biopsy, which may eliminate axillary dissection, holds promise for reducing this chronic effect of cancer treatment (Salmon, Marcolet, Vieira, & Languille, 2005).

Chronic Pain

Another chronic effect of cancer treatment includes neuropathy, which can be a result of previous chemotherapy, surgery, or radiation. Neuropathy can result in chronic pain, as well as functional impairment requiring ongoing comprehensive rehabilitation that extends into the survivorship portion of care (Cheville, 2005). Survivors who are at risk for neuropathy or chronic pain include those who were exposed to (a) chemotherapeutic agents such as vincristine, taxanes, and the alkylating agent cisplatin; (b) surgical treatment for testicular cancer and breast cancer; and (c) mantle radiation resulting in cervical neuropathy (Fossa, 2004; Johansson, Svensson, & Denekamp, 2000; McFarlane, Clein, Cole, Cowley, & Illidge, 2002; Verstappen et al., 2005).

FOLLOW-UP ACTIVITIES AND SURVEILLANCE

Another essential component of the long-term care of the cancer survivor is counseling on health-protective practices, including cancer prevention practices, aimed at minimizing the risk for future morbidity and mortality. It should be noted that there are no evidence-based guidelines on specific cancer screening practices or surveillance available for the adult cancer survivor population, although the American Society of Clinical Oncology is in the process of developing some recommendations. Currently, general recommendations for cancer prevention that are used for the adult population at large, therefore, should also be communicated to the cancer survivor (Agency for Healthcare Research and Quality, n.d.). For those individuals who have a strong family history of cancer and/or have a rare hereditary susceptibility gene, such as BRCA1 and BRCA2 or HNPCC, then screening for other associated cancers in the family syndrome may be indicated. Screening for second malignant neoplasms for those cancer survivors who are at risk should be conducted through the annual history, physical, and laboratory evaluations. For pediatric cancer survivors, the Children's Oncology Group has developed risk-based, exposure-related clinical practice guidelines for screening and management of late effects, including recommendations for health-protective counseling (Landier et al., 2004; see also CureSearch Children's Oncology Group, n.d.).

CONCLUSION

There is a growing population of over 10 million cancer survivors in the United States today as a result of early detection of some cancers and improved multimodal treatment regimens. Many cures, however, are not without cost. Cancer survivors are at risk for a myriad of physical late effects as a result of their previous chemotherapy, radiation, and/or surgery. Researchers are now challenged with the need to provide high-quality follow-up care aimed at screening and early diagnosis of the physical late effects in an attempt to decrease future morbidity and mortality. However, many unanswered questions remain about the physical late effects of treatment and possible behavioral solutions that may decrease the risks for survivors. This calls for future research to provide better evidence to guide the care of childhood and adult cancer survivors and, specifically, research on the following:

- evaluation of the effects that specific cancer treatments have on the health outcomes of older cancer survivors (those who are >65) and the influence of age-related comorbidities on the risk for late effects;
- determination of the behavioral factors associated with adoption of healthy lifestyles (e.g., good dietary habits, regular physical activity) for survivors and the effect this has on this risk for developing physical late effects; and
- continued prospective cohort studies to better characterize high-risk groups of survivors, as well as defining cancer control interventions that can result in risk reduction for late effects.

The challenge will be to develop a system for high-quality care for cancer survivors, with only a limited body of knowledge of the late physical effects of treatment.

REFERENCES

Adams, M. J., Hardenbergh, P. H., Constine, L. S., & Lipshultz, S. E. (2003). Radiation-associated cardiovascular disease. *Critical Reviews in Oncology/Hematology, 45,* 55–75.

Agency for Healthcare Research and Quality. (n.d.). U.S. Preventive Services Task Force (USPSTF). Retrieved February 21, 2008, from http://www.ahrq.gov/clinic/uspstfix.htm

Ahles, T. A. (2004). Do systemic cancer treatments affect cognitive function? *The Lancet Oncology, 5,* 270–271.

Anderson, D. M., Rennie, K. M., Ziegler, R. S., Neglia, J. P., Robison, L. R., & Gurney, J. G. (2001). Medical and neurocognitive late effects among survivors of childhood central nervous system tumors. *Cancer, 92,* 2709–2719.

Benyunes, M. C., Sullivan, K. M., Deeg, H. J., Mori, M., Meyer, W., Fisher, L., et al. (1995). Cataracts after bone marrow transplantation: Long-term follow-up of adults treated with fractionated total body irradiation. *International Journal of Radiation Oncology, Biology, Physics, 32,* 661–670.

Blakley, B. W., Cohen, J. I., Doolittle, N. D., Muldoon, L. L., Campbell, K. C., Dickey, D. T., & Neuwelt, E. A. (2002). Strategies for prevention of toxicity caused by platinum-based chemotherapy: Review and summary of the annual meeting of the Blood–Brain Barrier Disruption Program, Gleneden Beach, Oregon, March 10, 2001. *Laryngoscope, 112,* 1997–2001.

Bramswig, J. H., Heimes, U., Heiermann, E., Schlegel, W., Nieschlag, E., & Schellong, G. (1990). The effects of different cumulative doses of chemotherapy on testicular function. Results in 75 patients treated for Hodgkin's disease during childhood or adolescence. *Cancer, 65,* 1298–1302.

Brennan, B. M., Rahim, A., Blum, W. F., Adams, J. A., Eden, O. B., & Shalet, S. M. (1999). Hyperleptinaemia in young adults following cranial irradiation in childhood: Growth hormone deficiency or leptin insensitivity? *Clinical Endocrinology, 50,* 163–169.

Byrne, J., Fears, T. R., Gail, M. H., Pee, D., Connelly, R. R., Austin, D. F., et al. (1992). Early menopause in long-term survivors of cancer during adolescence. *American Journal of Obstetrics and Gynecology, 166,* 788–793.

Canada, A. L., & Schover, L. R. (2005). Research promoting better patient education on reproductive health after cancer. *Journal of the National Cancer Institute Monographs, 34,* 98–100.

Carroll, P. V., Christ, E. R., Bengtsson, B. A., Carlsson, L., Christiansen, J. S., Clemmons, D., et al. (1998). Growth hormone deficiency in adulthood and the effects of growth hormone replacement: A review. *The Journal of Clinical Endocrinology and Metabolism, 83,* 382–395.

Castellon, S. A., Ganz, P. A., Bower, J. E., Petersen, L., Abraham, L., & Greendale, G. A. (2004). Neurocognitive performance in breast cancer survivors exposed to adjuvant chemotherapy and tamoxifen. *The Journal of Clinical and Experimental Neuropsychology, 26,* 955–969.

Centers for Disease Control and Prevention. (1998). Recommendations for prevention and control of hepatitis C virus (HCV) infection and HCV-related chronic disease. *Morbidity and Mortality Weekly Report, 47,* 1–39.

Centers for Disease Control and Prevention. (2004). Cancer survivorship: United States, 1971–2001. *Morbidity and Mortality Weekly Report, 53,* 526–529.

Cesaro, S., Petris, M. G., Rossetti, F., Cusinato, R., Pipan, C., Guido, M., et al. (1997). Chronic hepatitis C virus infection after treatment for pediatric malignancy. *Blood, 90,* 1315–1320.

Cheville, A. L. (2005). Cancer rehabilitation. *Seminars in Oncology, 32,* 219–224.

Conomy, J. P., & Kellermeyer, R. W. (1975). Delayed cerebrovascular consequences of therapeutic radiation: A clinicopathologic study of a stroke associated with radiation-related carotid arteriopathy. *Cancer, 36,* 1702–1708.

CureSearch Children's Oncology Group. (n.d.). Long-term follow-up guidelines for survivors of childhood, adolescent, and young adult cancers. Retrieved February 21, 2008, from http://www.survivorshipguidelines.org

Curtis, R. E., Boice, J. D., Jr., Stovall, M., Bernstein, L., Greenberg, R. S., Flannery, J. T., et al. (1992). Risk of leukemia after chemotherapy and radiation treatment for breast cancer. *New England Journal of Medicine, 326,* 1745–1751.

DeLaat, C. A., & Lampkin, B. C. (1992). Long-term survivors of childhood cancer: Evaluation and identification of sequelae of treatment. *CA: A Cancer Journal for Clinicians, 42,* 263–282.

Driscoll, B. R., Hasleton, P. S., Taylor, P. M., Poulter, L. W., Gattamaneni, H. R., & Woodcock, A. A. (1990). Active lung fibrosis up to 17 years after chemotherapy with carmustine (BCNU) in childhood. *New England Journal of Medicine, 323,* 378–382.

Duffner, P. K., & Cohen, M. E. (1991). Long-term consequences of CNS treatment for childhood cancer: II. Clinical consequences. *Pediatric Neurology, 7,* 237–242.

Erickson, V. S., Pearson, M. L., Ganz, P. A., Adams, J., & Kahn, K. L. (2001). Arm edema in breast cancer patients. *Journal of the National Cancer Institute, 93,* 96–111.

Fossa, S. D. (2004). Long-term sequelae after cancer therapy—Survivorship after treatment for testicular cancer. *Acta Oncologica, 43,* 134–141.

Ganz, P. A., Greendale, G. A., Petersen, L., Kahn, B., & Bower, J. E. (2003). Breast cancer in younger women: Reproductive and late health effects of treatment. *Journal of Clinical Oncology, 21,* 4184–4193.

Gleeson, H. K., & Shalet, S. M. (2001). Endocrine complications of neoplastic diseases in children and adolescents. *Current Opinion in Pediatrics, 13,* 346–351.

Goodwin, P. J., Ennis, M., Pritchard, K. I., McCready, D., Koo, J., Sidlofsky, S., et al. (1999). Adjuvant treatment and onset of menopause predict weight gain after breast cancer diagnosis. *Journal of Clinical Oncology, 17,* 120–129.

Gosselink, R., Rouffaer, L., Vanhelden, P., Piot, W., Troosters, T., & Christiaens, M. R. (2003). Recovery of upper limb function after axillary dissection. *Journal of Surgical Oncology, 83,* 204–211.

Haddy, T. B., Mosher, R. B., & Reaman, G. H. (2001). Osteoporosis in survivors of acute lymphoblastic leukemia. *The Oncologist, 6,* 278–285.

Halton, J. M., Atkinson, S. A., Fraher, L., Webber, C., Gill, G. J., Dawson, S., Barr, R. D. (1996). Altered mineral metabolism and bone mass in children during treatment for acute lymphoblastic leukemia. *Journal of Bone and Mineral Research, 11,* 1774–1783.

Hancock, S. L., Tucker, M. A., & Hoppe, R. T. (1993). Factors affecting late mortality from heart disease after treatment of Hodgkin's disease. *Journal of the American Medical Association, 270,* 1949–1955.

Hansen, S. W., Helweg-Larsen, S., & Trojaborg, W. (1989). Long-term neurotoxicity in patients treated with cisplatin, vinblastine, and bleomycin for metastatic germ cell cancer. *Journal of Clinical Oncology, 7,* 1457–1461.

Herman, D. R., Ganz, P. A., Petersen, L., & Greendale, G. A. (2005). Obesity and cardiovascular risk factors in younger breast cancer survivors: The cancer and menopause study (CAMS). *Breast Cancer Research and Treatment, 93,* 13–23.

Heyn, R., Raney, R. B., Jr., Hays, D. M., Tefft, M., Gehan, E., Webber, B., & Maurer, H. M. (1992). Late effects of therapy in patients with paratesticular rhabdomyosarcoma: Intergroup Rhabdomyosarcoma Study Committee. *Journal of Clinical Oncology, 10,* 614–623.

Hobbie, W. L., Ginsberg, J. P., Ogle, S. K., Carlson, C. A., & Meadows, A. T. (2005). Fertility in males treated for Hodgkin's disease with COPP/ABV hybrid. *Pediatric Blood Cancer, 44,* 193–196.

Jemal, A., Murray, T., Ward, E., Samuels, A., Tiwari, R. C., Ghafoor, A., et al. (2005). Cancer statistics, 2005. *CA: A Cancer Journal for Clinicians, 55,* 10–30.

Johansson, S., Svensson, H., & Denekamp, J. (2000). Timescale of evolution of late radiation injury after postoperative radiotherapy of breast cancer patients. *International Journal of Radiation Oncology, Biology, Physics, 48,* 745–750.

Johnson, D. L., McCabe, M. A., Nicholson, H. S., Joseph, A. L., Getson, P. R., Byrne, J., et al. (1994). Quality of long-term survival in young children with medulloblastoma. *Journal of Neurosurgery, 80,* 1004–1010.

Krane, E. J., & Heller, L. B. (1995). The prevalence of phantom sensation and pain in pediatric amputees. *Journal of Pain Symptom Management, 10,* 21–29.

Landier, W., Bhatia, S., Eshelman, D. A., Forte, K. J., Sweeney, T., Hester, A. L., et al. (2004). Development of risk-based guidelines for pediatric cancer survivors: The Children's Oncology Group long-term follow-up guidelines from the Children's Oncology Group Late Effects Committee and Nursing Discipline. *Journal of Clinical Oncology, 22,* 4979–4990.

Leiper, A. D. (1998). Osteoporosis in survivors of childhood malignancy. *European Journal of Cancer, 34,* 770–772.

Levine, L. A., & Richie, J. P. (1989). Urological complications of cyclophosphamide. *Journal of Urology, 141,* 1063–1069.

Liesner, R. J., Leiper, A. D., Hann, I. M., & Chessells, J. M. (1994). Late effects of intensive treatment for acute myeloid leukemia and myelodysplasia in childhood. *Journal of Clinical Oncology, 12,* 916–924.

Link, K., Moell, C., Garwicz, S., Cavallin-Stahl, E., Bjork, J., Thilen, U., et al. (2004). Growth hormone deficiency predicts cardiovascular risk in young adults treated for acute lymphoblastic leukemia in childhood. *The Journal of Clinical Endocrinology and Metabolism, 89,* 5003–5012.

Lipshultz, S. E., Colan, S. D., Gelber, R. D., Perez-Atayde, A. R., Sallan, S. E., & Sanders, S. P. (1991). Late cardiac effects of doxorubicin therapy for acute lymphoblastic leukemia in childhood. *New England Journal of Medicine, 324,* 808–815.

Maguire, A., Craft, A. W., Evans, R. G., Amineddine, H., Kernahan, J., Macleod, R. I., et al. (1987). The long-term effects of treatment on the dental condition of children surviving malignant disease. *Cancer, 60,* 2570–2575.

Marina, N. (1997). Long-term survivors of childhood cancer: The medical consequences of cure. *Pediatric Clinics of North America, 44,* 1021–1042.

McFarlane, V. J., Clein, G. P., Cole, J., Cowley, N., & Illidge, T. M. (2002). Cervical neuropathy following mantle radiotherapy. *Clinical Oncology, 14,* 468–471.

Meister, L. A., & Meadows, A. T. (1993). Late effects of childhood cancer therapy. *Current Problems in Pediatrics, 23,* 102–131.

Mertens, A. C., Yasui, Y., Liu, Y., Stovall, M., Hutchinson, R., Ginsberg, J., et al. (2002). Pulmonary complications in survivors of childhood and adolescent cancer: A report from the Childhood Cancer Survivor Study. *Cancer, 95,* 2431–2441.

Nagarajan, R., Neglia, J. P., Clohisy, D. R., & Robison, L. L. (2002). Limb salvage and amputation in survivors of pediatric lower-extremity bone tumors: What are the long-term implications? *Journal of Clinical Oncology, 20,* 4493–4501.

National Cancer Institute (n.d.a). *About cancer survivorship research: Survivorship definitions.* Retrieved April 11, 2008, from http://dccps.nci.nih.gov/ocs/definitions.html

National Cancer Institute. (n.d.b). *Age-adjusted SEER incidence and U.S. death rates and 5-year relative survival rates* (Table I-4). Retrieved April 11, 2008, from http://seer.cancer.gov/csr/1975_2004/results_merged/topic_survival.pdf

National Cancer Institute. (n.d.c). *Estimated U.S. cancer prevalence.* Retrieved April 11, 2008, from http://dccps.nci.nih.gov/ocs/prevalence/prevalence.html#survivor

Neglia, J. P., Friedman, D. L., Yasui, Y., Mertens, A. C., Hammond, S., Stovall, M., et al. (2001). Second malignant neoplasms in five-year survivors of childhood cancer: Childhood Cancer Survivor Study. *Journal of the National Cancer Institute, 93,* 618–629.

Nicolson, H. S., & Byrne, J. (1993). Fertility and pregnancy after treatment for cancer during childhood and adolescence. *Cancer, 17*(Suppl.), 3392–3399.

Oeffinger, K. C., Buchanan, G. R., Eshelman, D. A., Denke, M. A., Andrews, T. C., Germak, J. A., et al. (2001). Cardiovascular risk factors in young adult survivors of childhood acute lymphoblastic leukemia. *Journal of Pediatric Hematology and Oncology, 23*, 424–430.

Oeffinger, K. C., Eshelman, D. A., Tomlinson, G. E., Tolle, M., & Schneider, G. W. (2000). Providing primary care for long-term survivors of childhood acute lymphoblastic leukemia. *Journal of Family Practice, 49*, 1133–1146.

Oeffinger, K. C., & Hudson, M. M. (2004). Long-term complications following childhood and adolescent cancer: Foundations for providing risk-based health care for survivors. *CA: A Cancer Journal for Clinicians, 54*, 208–236.

Oeffinger, K. C., Mertens, A. C., Sklar, C. A., Yasui, Y., Fears, T., Stovall, M., et al. (2003). Obesity in adult survivors of childhood acute lymphoblastic leukemia: A report from the Childhood Cancer Survivor Study. *Journal of Clinical Oncology, 21*, 1359–1365.

Pedersen-Bjergaard, J., Ersboll, J., Hansen, V. L., Sorensen, B. L., Christoffersen, K., Hou-Jensen, K., et al. (1988). Carcinoma of the urinary bladder after treatment with cyclophosphamide for non-Hodgkin's lymphoma. *New England Journal of Medicine, 318*, 1028–1032.

Perry, M. C. (1982). Hepatotoxicity of chemotherapeutic agents. *Seminars in Oncology, 9*, 65–74.

Probert, J. C., & Parker, B. R. (1975). The effects of radiation therapy on bone growth. *Radiology, 114*, 155–162.

Rate, W. R., Butler, M. S., Robertson, W. W., Jr., & D'Angio, G. J. (1991). Late orthopedic effects in children with Wilms' tumor treated with abdominal irradiation. *Medical and Pediatric Oncology, 19*, 265–268.

Reilly, J. J., Kelly, A., Ness, P., Dorosty, A. R., Wallace, W. H., Gibson, B. E., et al. (2001). Premature adiposity rebound in children treated for acute lymphoblastic leukemia. *The Journal of Clinical Endocrinology and Metabolism, 86*, 2775–2778.

Ridner, S. H. (2005). Quality of life and a symptom cluster associated with breast cancer treatment-related lymphedema. *Supportive Care in Cancer, 13*, 904–911.

Rock, C. L., & Demark-Wahnefried, W. (2002). Nutrition and survival after the diagnosis of breast cancer: A review of the evidence. *Journal of Clinical Oncology, 20*, 3302–3316.

Roman, D. D., & Sperduto, P. W. (1995). Neuropsychological effects of cranial radiation: Current knowledge and future directions. *International Journal of Radiation Oncology, Biology, Physics, 31*, 983–998.

Rugo, H. S., & Ahles, T. (2003). The impact of adjuvant therapy for breast cancer on cognitive function: Current evidence and directions for research. *Seminars in Oncology, 30*, 749–762.

Salmon, R. J., Marcolet, A., Vieira, M., & Languille, O. (2005). Sentinel node biopsy or limited oriented axillary dissection (LOAD) in early breast cancer. *European Journal of Surgical Oncology, 31,* 949–953.

Schover, L. R. (1997). *Sexuality and fertility after cancer.* Hoboken, NJ: Wiley.

Schover, L. R., Brey, K., Lichtin, A., Lipshultz, L. I., & Jeha, S. (2002). Oncologists' attitudes and practices regarding banking sperm before cancer treatment. *Journal of Clinical Oncology, 20,* 1890–1897.

Schover, L. R., Fouladi, R. T., Warneke, C. L., Neese, L., Klein, E. A., Zippe, C., & Kupelian, P. A. (2004). Seeking help for erectile dysfunction after treatment for prostate cancer. *Archives of Sexual Behavior, 33,* 443–454.

Schwartz, A. M., & Leonidas, J. C. (1984). Methotrexate osteopathy. *Skeletal Radiology, 11,* 13–16.

Schwartz, C. L. (1990). Creating life on the plateau: Reproductive potential in survivors of childhood Hodgkin's disease. *International Journal of Radiation Oncology, Biology, Physics, 19,* 1099–1100.

Schwartz, C. L. (1995). Complications of treatment: Late effects of treatment in long-term survivors of cancer. *Cancer Treatment Reviews, 21,* 355–366.

Sklar, C. A., Mertens, A. C., Walter, A., Mitchell, D., Nesbit, M. E., O'Leary, M., et al. (2001). Changes in body mass index and prevalence of overweight in survivors of childhood acute lymphoblastic leukemia: Role of cranial irradiation. *Medical and Pediatric Oncology, 35,* 91–95.

Sklar, C. A., Whitton, J., Mertens, A., Stovall, M., Green, D., Marina, N., et al. (2000). Abnormalities of the thyroid in survivors of Hodgkin's disease: Data from the childhood cancer survivor study. *The Journal of Clinical Endocrinology and Metabolism, 85,* 3227–3232.

Stanisavljevic, S., & Babcock, A. L. (1977). Fractures in children treated with methotrexate for leukemia. *Clinical Orthopaedics and Related Research, 125,* 139–144.

Stavrou, T., Bromley, C. M., Nicholson, H. S., Byrne, J., Packer, R. J., Goldstein, A. M., & Reaman, G. H. (2001). Prognostic factors and secondary malignancies in childhood medulloblastoma. *Journal of Pediatric Hematology and Oncology, 23,* 431–436.

Steinherz, L. J., Steinherz, P. G., Tan, C. T., Heller, G., & Murphy, M. L. (1991). Cardiac toxicity 4 to 20 years after completing anthracycline therapy. *Journal of the American Medical Association, 266,* 1672–1677.

Swain, S. M., Whaley, F. S., & Ewer, M. S. (2003). Congestive heart failure in patients treated with doxorubicin: A retrospective analysis of three trials. *Cancer, 97,* 2869–2879.

Swerdlow, A. J., & Jones, M. E. (2005). Tamoxifen treatment for breast cancer and risk of endometrial cancer: A case-control study. *Journal of the National Cancer Institute, 97,* 375–384.

Tannock, I. F., Ahles, T. A., Ganz, P. A., & Van Dam, F. S. (2004). Cognitive impairment associated with chemotherapy for cancer: Report of a workshop. *Journal of Clinical Oncology, 22,* 2233–2239.

Travis, L. B., Hill, D. A., Dores, G. M., Gospodarowicz, M., van Leeuwen, F. E., Holowaty, E., et al. (2003). Breast cancer following radiotherapy and chemotherapy among young women with Hodgkin's disease. *Journal of the American Medical Association, 290*, 465–475.

Tucker, M. A., D'Angio, G. J., Boice, J. D., Jr., Strong, L. C., Li, F. P., Stovall, M., et al. (1987). Bone sarcomas linked to radiotherapy and chemotherapy in children. *New England Journal of Medicine, 317*, 588–593.

van Kempen-Harteveld, M. L., Belkacemi, Y., Kal, H. B., Labopin, M., & Frassoni, F. (2002). Dose–effect relationship for cataract induction after single-dose total body irradiation and bone marrow transplantation for acute leukemia. *International Journal of Radiation Oncology, Biology, Physics, 52*, 1367–1374.

Verstappen, C. C., Koeppen, S., Heimans, J. J., Huijgens, P. C., Scheulen, M. E., Strumberg, D., et al. (2005). Dose-related vincristine-induced peripheral neuropathy with unexpected off-therapy worsening. *Neurology, 64*, 1076–1077.

Von Hoff, D. D., Layard, M. W., Basa, P., Davis, H. L., Jr., Von Hoff, A. L., Rozencweig, M., & Muggia, F. M. (1979). Risk factors for doxorubicin-induced congestive heart failure. *Annals of Internal Medicine, 91*, 710–717.

Warner, J. T., Evans, W. D., Webb, D. K., Bell, W., & Gregory, J. W. (1999). Relative osteopenia after treatment for acute lymphoblastic leukemia. *Pediatric Research, 45*(4, Pt. 1), 544–551.

Wright, M. J., Galea, V., & Barr, R. D. (2003). Self-perceptions of physical activity in survivors of acute lymphoblastic leukemia in childhood. *Pediatric Exercise Science, 15*, 191–201.

Yung, L., & Linch, D. (2003). Hodgkin's lymphoma. *Lancet, 361*, 943–951.

25

PSYCHOSOCIAL AND BEHAVIORAL ISSUES IN CANCER SURVIVAL IN PEDIATRIC POPULATIONS

ANNE E. KAZAK, MELISSA A. ALDERFER, AND ALYSSA M. RODRIGUEZ

It is hardly surprising that the experience of childhood cancer has long-lasting psychological effects for both patient and family. Indeed, with improvements in survival rates for childhood cancer and the emerging evidence for late effects of treatment (Friedman & Meadows, 2002), increasing appreciation for the long-term psychological impact of childhood cancer and its treatment is imperative. Psychological late effects may be thought of as "the influence of cancer, treatment, and survivorship on survivors' and their family members' feelings, thoughts, behaviors, and relationships" (Rourke & Kazak, 2005, p. 137). This contextual view of psychological late effects emphasizes a range of potential outcomes across systems. In this chapter, we review the empirical literature from 1994 through 2004 on psychological effects of childhood cancer survival. In doing so, we balance an appreciation of the risks associated with survivorship with the resiliency that characterizes survivors and their families.

CHILDHOOD CANCER SURVIVORS

Research on the impact of childhood cancer has revealed that aside from the physiological side effects, cancer affects functioning across several areas, including the child's and adolescent's cognitive, emotional and social functioning. Despite some impairment in functioning, childhood cancer survivors also exhibit resiliency and may indeed experience overall positive adjustment, similar to their healthy peers.

Neurocognitive Effects

Among the earliest and most widely recognized late effects of childhood cancer were neuropsychological deficits. Cancers and treatments involving the central nervous system have consistently been associated with significant neurocognitive effects that can be documented with magnetic resonance imaging, computerized tomography scans, and neuropsychological testing (Mulhern et al., 2001; see also detailed reviews of this literature in Armstrong & Mulhern, 1999; Challinor, Miaskowsky, Moore, Slaughter, & Franch, 2000).

Evidence suggests impairments in cognitive functioning (Palmer et al., 2001; Ris, Packer, Goldwein, Jones-Wallace, & Boyett, 2001) and deficits in memory (Boon, Murdoch, & Jordan, 1994; Copeland, Moore, Francis, Jaffe, & Culbert, 1996; Jordan, Murdoch, Buttsworth, & Hudson-Tennent, 1995), metacognition (Kleinman & Waber, 1994; Waber, Isquith, Kahn, & Romero, 1994), visual–spatial/motor skills (Espy et al., 2001; Johnson et al., 1994), and processing speed (Langer et al., 2002; Schatz, Kramer, Ablin, & Matthay, 2000) for children surviving brain tumors and cranial radiation therapy (CRT) and intrathecal chemotherapy treatment for acute lymphoblastic leukemia (ALL). These children acquire new information and skills at lower rates than healthy peers (Palmer et al., 2001) and, ultimately, have poorer academic achievement (Espy et al., 2001; Hill et al., 1998). CRT, specifically, has been linked to significant impairment in attentional filtering, focusing, and shifting (Lockwood, Bell, & Colegrove, 1999; Rodgers, Horrocks, Britton, & Kernahan, 1999). Working memory and information processing skills are also impeded (Anderson, Smilbert, Ekert, & Godber, 1994; Johnson et al., 1994; Schatz et al., 2000).

The use of bone marrow transplantation (BMT) and stem cell transplantation (SCT) for children with leukemia and solid tumors increased from 1994 to 2004. Although this form of treatment often results in long-term disease-free survival, pre-BMT conditioning regimens involving total body irradiation (TBI) and chemotherapy can be neurotoxic. In general, BMT survivors (with or without TBI) have demonstrated stability in cognitive functioning 1 to 3 years posttransplant (Phipps, Dunavant, Srivastava, Bownam, & Mulhern, 2000; Simms, Kazak, Golomb, Goldwein, & Bunin, 2002). Despite this stability, research has indicated that a subset of these children is at higher risk for long-term cognitive difficulties, primarily those younger than age 3 at time of transplantation (Kramer, Crittenden, DeSantes, & Cowan, 1997; Phipps et al., 2000).

The specific pattern of neurocognitive deficits seen in childhood cancer survivors depends in part on age at diagnosis, type of cancer, type of cancer treatment, and tumor site (Langer et al., 2002; Palmer et al., 2001; Ris et al., 2001). In general, children diagnosed before age 7 exhibit the greatest subsequent difficulty (Langer et al., 2002; Lockwood et al., 1999; Mulhern et al., 2001; Syndikus, Tait, Ashley, & Jannoun, 1994). Further, children undergoing treatment for brain tumors tend to exhibit more neurocognitive impairments than children diagnosed and treated for leukemia. Finally, the effects of cancer and cancer treatment on neurocognitive functioning are often delayed, with most deficits not being evident until 1 or more years posttreatment (Langer et al., 2002; Mulhern et al., 2001).

Psychological Functioning

In an earlier review, Kazak (1994) summarized research on childhood cancer survivors, noting their overall competence and normative levels of psychological distress, with only a subset of survivors experiencing difficulties. Generally, this conclusion summarizes research conducted from 1994 to 2004 and can be viewed with relative confidence as still valid. However, limitations of the research (e.g., lack of comparison groups, small sample sizes, lack of ethnic diversity, heterogeneity of cancer diagnoses, broad age ranges) restrict generalizability and prevent a refined appreciation of the risks and resiliencies of survivors.

As a group, childhood and adolescent cancer survivors are as well adjusted as healthy control participants, non-ill siblings, and standardized norms (Elkin, Phipps, Mulhern, & Fairclough, 1997; Mackie, Hill, Kondryn, & McNally, 2000; Maggiolini et al., 2000; Martinson & Bossert, 1994; Ross et al., 2003). They report positive mental states, including positive self-images, and low levels of emotional distress, sometimes even less distress than healthy comparison groups (Phipps & Srivastava, 1997). Overall rates of depression and anxiety in these survivors are typically within normal limits (Radcliffe, Bennett, Kazak, Foley, & Phillips, 1996; T. Sloper, Larcombe, & Charleston, 1994; Zebrack et al., 2002).

Viewing childhood cancer as a traumatic experience has led to investigation of posttraumatic stress disorder (PTSD; in the *Diagnostic and Statistical Manual of Mental Disorders; 4th ed.* [DSM–IV]; American Psychiatric Association, 1994) and posttraumatic stress symptoms (PTSS) in childhood cancer survivors. Rates of PTSD for child and adolescent survivors are generally low (5%–12%) and roughly comparable to rates in healthy same-age peers (Butler, Rizzi, & Handwerger, 1996; Erickson & Steiner, 2001; Kazak et al., 2001). However, survivors endorse significant levels of PTSS, particularly reexperiencing and arousal (Kazak et al., 2001; Kazak, Alderfer, Rourke, et al., 2004).

The absence of anxiety and depression in child and adolescent survivors of cancer has led to speculation that childhood cancer survivors may adopt a repressive adaptive style (Phipps, Steele, Hall, & Leigh, 2001). Indeed, parents tend to observe more symptoms in their children than their children self-report (Noll et al., 1997). Furthermore, evidence is emerging that childhood cancer survivors are vulnerable to psychosocial difficulties during the transition to early adulthood. Adult survivors of childhood cancer report more negative moods, tension, and depression than their siblings (Zeltzer et al., 1997) and have shown increased suicidal symptoms and global psychological distress (Glover et al., 2003; Recklitis, O'Leary, & Diller, 2003). Finally, PTSD has been found to be higher in young adult samples than in adolescent samples, with about 20% of young adult survivors meeting PTSD criteria (Hobbie et al., 2000).

Social Functioning

Remarkably, most long-term survivors experience minimal difficulty readjusting to their social environments after treatment and have been found to exhibit social skills that are equivalent to those of healthy peers (Bessell, 2001; Garstein, Noll, & Vannatta, 2000; Newby, Brown, Pawletko, Gold, & Whitt, 2000; Noll et al., 1997). However, for survivors whose diagnoses or treatment impacted neurocognitive functioning, evidence suggests that difficulties in social competence and peer interactions may exist. Child and adolescent brain tumor survivors have greater levels of social isolation, report fewer best friends (Rieter-Purtill & Noll, 2003; Vannatta, Gartstein, Short, & Noll, 1998), and participate in fewer peer activities than other children. They also show increased social isolation and reduced social competence, on the basis of maternal, teacher, peer, and self-report (Fossen, Abrahamsen, & Storm-Mathisen, 1998; Radcliffe et al., 1996; Sawyer et al., 1995; Syndikus et al., 1994). Adolescent ALL survivors exposed to cranial radiation have also been shown to be socially isolated and shy or anxious (Noll, Bukowski, Davies, Koontz, & Kulkarni, 1993).

FAMILY-BASED PSYCHOLOGICAL LATE EFFECTS

Research on family-level effects has examined the psychological impact of cancer on parents, siblings, and family functioning. Similar to the literature on survivors, most of this research reveals overall resiliency, with concerns for a subgroup. It is interesting that family members may be at greater risk for adjustment difficulties than survivors.

Parents

The majority of studies reveal that in the 1st year after diagnosis, parents experience elevated levels of anxiety and depression. For parents of patients 6 months postdiagnosis, Hoekstra-Weebers, Heuvel, Jaspers, Kamps, and Klip (1998) reported elevated levels of anxiety and depression, estimating that 50% of mothers and 40% of fathers are clinically distressed. By 12 months postdiagnosis some reports revealed elevated distress (Hoekstra-Weebers et al., 1998), whereas others report normative levels (e.g., see Sawyer, Antoniou, Toogood, & Rice, 1997; Sawyer, Streiner, Antoniou, Toogood, & Rice, 1998). By 20 to 24 months postdiagnosis, rates of anxiety and depression are within normal limits, with approximately 10% of parents falling within clinical ranges (Dahlquist, Czyzewski, & Jones, 1996; Sawyer et al., 1997, 1998).

In the longest term study to date, parents of survivors 10 years posttreatment reported psychiatric symptomatology and psychological adjustment within normal ranges (Kupst et al., 1995). Parents of children at least 5 years posttreatment were within normal ranges on anxiety and depression, with 10% falling in the clinical range for distress (Kazak, Christakis, Alderfer, & Coiro, 1994). Similar results have been reported for parents of children 1 to 5 years posttreatment (Grootenhuis & Last, 1997) and parents of children 1 to 10 years post-BMT (Sormanti, Dungan, & Reiker, 1994).

A traumatic stress model has been helpful in understanding psychological reactions of parents of children with cancer. In field trials for the *DSM–IV*, 25% of mothers of childhood cancer survivors qualified for a current diagnosis of PTSD, compared with none of the mothers of healthy children (Pelcovitz et al., 1996). Furthermore, 54% of mothers of cancer survivors qualified for a lifetime diagnosis of PTSD, whereas only 4% of the control group did. Since then, research using diagnostic interviews has revealed more modest rates of PTSD in parents, ranging from 6% to 14% (Kazak et al., 2001; Kazak, Alderfer, Rourke, et al., 2004; Manne, DuHamel, Gallelli, Sorgen, & Redd, 1998). The percentage of parents meeting clinical cutoffs on self-report measures extends the upper end of this range, falling between 12% and 25% (Brown, Madan-Swain, & Lambert, 2003; Manne et al., 1998; Manne, DuHamel, & Redd, 2000). The largest study to date (Kazak et al., 2001) reported rates of current PTSD determined by clinical interviews to be between 11% and 14% in mothers and around 10% in fathers, with lifetime rates (i.e., PTSD at any time since cancer) of 30% for mothers and 12% for fathers.

Researchers have also attended to subclinical levels of PTSS. The earliest reports found that 40% of mothers and 33% of fathers fell into the severe range for PTSS (Stuber, Christakis, Houskamp, & Kazak, 1996). More recent reports with larger samples have been remarkably consistent, with 37% to 44% of mothers and approximately 35% of fathers falling in this range (Kazak et al., 1997; Kazak, Alderfer, Rourke, et al., 2004); these percentages are elevated, compared with parents of healthy children.

Siblings

Several studies reveal that siblings of children with cancer experience emotional and behavioral disruptions. In the largest study to date, the Sibling Adaptation to Childhood Cancer Collaborative Study (SACCCS; Barbarin et al., 1995; Sahler et al., 1994; Sargent et al., 1995), parents retrospectively reported a threefold increase in behavior problems and nearly a doubling of the incidence of emotional difficulties for siblings. Difficulties prior to cancer were consistent with norms, but adjustment after the cancer was significantly poorer than that of a nationally derived comparison group of children (Sahler et al., 1994). Of the siblings who had no problems prior to the cancer, about half experienced a problem afterward (Barbarin et al., 1995). Cohen, Friedrich, Jaworski, Copeland, and Pendergrass (1994) found more clinically significant internalizing and externalizing problems among siblings of children with cancer compared with a normative sample. Additionally, P. Sloper and While (1996) found that nearly 25% of their sample fell in the borderline to clinical range for emotional and behavioral problems on the Child Behavior Checklist (Achenbach, 1991). Some studies, however, have not replicated these results, finding that siblings of children with cancer are no different from community control participants (e.g., see Madan-Swain, Sexson, Brown, & Ragab, 1993; Van Dongen-Melman, DeGroot, Hahlen, & Verhulst, 1995). These studies, however, had smaller sample sizes than those finding significant results.

Posttraumatic stress among siblings of children with cancer is a new area of investigation. Packman et al. (1997) measured posttraumatic stress in a sample of siblings of children who had survived BMT, and approximately one third fell in the moderate to severe range for PTSS. Alderfer, Labay, and Kazak (2003) reported on PTSS in siblings of childhood cancer survivors and, similarly, found that 32% had PTSS in the moderate to severe range, exceeding rates in a comparison sample. In addition to finding difficulties, some studies have revealed positive outcomes for siblings, including valuing life more, enhanced maturity and independence, and greater compassion (Barbarin et al., 1995; Havermans & Eiser, 1994; Sargent et al., 1995).

Most sibling research includes broad age ranges and does not investigate differences as a function of current age or age at diagnosis. One of the few exceptions is the SACCCS, in which 4- to 11-year-old brothers and 12- to 17-year-old sisters had higher levels of distress than control participants. Adolescent siblings may be more likely than younger children to perceive positive benefits (Sargent et al., 1995). Alderfer et al. (2003) found that female siblings and those ages 6 and older at diagnosis were more likely to report PTSS, although P. Sloper and While (1996) found no differences in adjustment as a function of these variables.

Family Functioning

In studies of families ranging from 1 to 5 years posttreatment, family functioning, communication, satisfaction, adaptability, and cohesion were consistent with norms and/or no different from comparison families (Cohen et al., 1994; Kazak et al., 1994, 1997; Noll et al., 1995). However, a significantly larger portion of these families scored in the enmeshed range (21%) when contrasted with comparison families (14%; Cohen et al., 1994). Even within the first 2 years following diagnosis, marital adjustment and family functioning tends to be similar to norms, with a subset of families (< 25%) experiencing difficulties (Dahlquist, Czyzewski, & Jones, 1996; Streisand, Kazak, & Tercyak, 2003). Families within this time period who were off treatment, however, did report better functioning than those who were still on treatment (Streisand et al., 2003).

INTERVENTIONS FOR CHILDHOOD CANCER SURVIVORS AND THEIR FAMILIES

With a substantive body of research documenting psychological late effects for survivors and their families, the question of intervention approaches becomes increasingly pertinent. This emerging work can be organized across neurocognitive, individual psychological, and parent and family intervention targets.

Neurocognitive Interventions

The consensus regarding the presence of neurocognitive late effects provides a fruitful opportunity for intervention (Butler & Copeland, 2002). In general, most work has focused on collaborative relationships with schools and advocacy for the educational needs and concerns of survivors. In terms of systematic intervention to improve neurocognitive difficulties, a 20-session course of cognitive remediation is currently being evaluated in a multisite randomized clinical trial (Butler, 2003). Pharmacologically, methylphenidate has also been investigated as a potential treatment for attentional difficulties (Thompson et al., 2001). Additional studies will be necessary to further address the advantages and concerns associated with stimulant treatment (Butler & Mulhern, 2005).

Interventions for the Childhood Cancer Survivor

The data indicating difficulties in social functioning for some survivors suggests that targeted interventions are needed to improve social skills and interpersonal relationships (Barakat et al., 2003); however, most interventions addressing social concerns of survivors have focused on school reentry (Prevatt, Heffer, & Lowe, 2000). Although critically important, these interventions tend to be limited in scope and focused on teachers and classmates, without necessarily providing the focused intervention necessary to help survivors meet the social demands of school and the increased social sophistication necessary for the long term as they enter adolescence and young adulthood.

Health-related problems that can develop secondary to cancer and its treatment provide other opportunities for psychological intervention and are pertinent as survivors enter adulthood. For example, in a randomized clinical trial of a brief (< 1 hour) educational intervention, delivered by telephone, to reduce tobacco use, adolescent survivors who received the intervention showed increased knowledge of smoking risks, reported more perceived vulnerability, and indicated less intent to smoke cigarettes than control participants (Tyc et al., 2003).

Interventions for the Family

Interventions for parents should be specific to their psychological symptoms and timed appropriately. For example, problem-solving therapy has been shown to be effective in reducing negative affectivity and increasing problem-solving skills for mothers of children in treatment (Sahler et al., 2002). Evidence also indicates that stress reduction techniques help mothers of patients undergoing BMT (Streisand, Rodrigue, Houck, Graham-Pole, & Berlant, 2000). Empirically evaluated intervention programs for siblings are rare but are important, given their levels of adjustment difficulties. Two pilot studies of group interventions for siblings using small, nonrandom samples have offered preliminary evidence for the importance of further work in this area (Barrera, Chung, Greenberg, & Fleming, 2002; Dolgin, Somer, Zaidel, & Zaizov, 1997).

PTSS have emerged as a feasible target for intervention across multiple family members. The Surviving Cancer Competently Intervention Program (SCCIP; Kazak et al., 1999) integrates cognitive behavior therapy and family therapy in a four-session, 1-day program involving groups of families of adolescent cancer survivors. The results of a randomized clinical trial of 150 families indicate that those randomized to the SCCIP arm showed significant reductions in PTSS, particularly for survivors and fathers (Kazak, Alderfer, Streisand, et al., 2004). Interventions based on the SCCIP model have also been developed for young adult survivors (Rourke, Hobbie, Schwartz, & Kazak, 2007) and for caregivers of children at the time of diagnosis (Kazak et al., 2005).

DIRECTIONS FOR FUTURE RESEARCH

The growing literature on psychological issues in childhood cancer survival has largely confirmed and expanded the earlier work in this field. In general, survivors of childhood cancer do well psychologically. As a group, they have demonstrated remarkable resilience, given their history of serious illness in childhood. This resilience is likely multidetermined, with genetic, biological, family, and social factors contributing. However, the very treatments that increase survival have also resulted in significant sequelae that warrant additional research over the next decade, particularly focused on prevention and intervention for the subset of survivors experiencing psychological difficulties.

It is essential to move outside of deficit-oriented treatment models and to build on competency-based approaches. These approaches may be integrated into more general recommendations for cancer survivorship. For example, routine screening for psychological late effects common to survivors (e.g., neurocognitive issues, posttraumatic stress) could be part of every follow-up visit. Educational interventions during the follow-up visit are also important, especially given the significant gaps that young adults have demonstrated regarding knowledge of their medical history and vulnerability (Kadan-Lottick et al., 2002). Informal interventions include giving survivors information regarding their medical late effects while minimizing the anxiety that such education may provoke (Hudson et al., 2003), as well as providing anticipatory guidance about normative psychosocial symptoms (e.g., anxiety and worry about medical late effects, distress when reminded of cancer and late effects). More formal educational interventions can include standardized methods of educating survivors about medical and psychosocial risks (e.g., see Eiser, Hill, & Blacklay, 2000) or more targeted behavioral efforts to modify health risk behaviors (e.g., see Emmons et al., 2003; Hudson et al., 2002).

Cancer in childhood impacts the entire family, and some of the most compelling work on psychological aspects of survival focuses on the family, including not only parents but also siblings. Consistent evidence shows that although most families cope and adjust well to cancer survivorship, a subgroup of patients and their families continues to experience psychological distress. Interventions that incorporate other members of the family system and that target specific malleable outcomes are being developed and provide promise for accentuating the competence of childhood cancer survivors and their families while ameliorating the understandable distress associated with cancer and its treatment in both the short and the long term.

In thinking broadly about childhood cancer survivors, researchers should further consider the timing of intervention. The few prospective studies in this area support the consistency in psychological adjustment over time, showing, for example, that families with more adaptive coping during treatment had better long-term adjustment (Kupst et al., 1995) and that parental distress during treatment was predictive of PTSS subsequently (Best, Streisand, Catania, & Kazak, 2002). These data support the early identification of families at risk for ongoing psychological difficulties and the potential for preventive interventions to reduce the likelihood of ongoing difficulties for at-risk patients and families (Kazak et al., 2003).

A serious limitation to most of the research in this field is that it is overwhelmingly based on Caucasian samples, providing little information on the relevance of findings for ethnic minority families. To begin to address this concern, components of the problem must be defined more clearly (e.g., barriers to participation in studies, institutional characteristics such as composition of patients attending survivorship programs, perceived importance and acceptability of interventions by individuals of ethnic minority background, associations between socioeconomic status and race). Greater consideration must be given to existing interventions in terms of their cultural sensitivity and applicability to ethnic minority participants. Finally, for cancer survivors and their families generally, the delivery of care in the community and in schools, as well as using innovative formats, is vital and may enhance participation more broadly for all survivors and their families.

REFERENCES

Achenbach, T. M. (1991). *Integrative guide to the 1991 CBCL/4-18, YSR, and TRF profiles*. Burlington: University of Vermont, Department of Psychology.

Alderfer, M., Labay, L., & Kazak, A. (2003). Brief report: Does posttraumatic stress apply to siblings of childhood cancer survivors? *Journal of Pediatric Psychology, 28*, 281–286.

American Psychiatric Association. (1994). *Diagnostic and statistical manual of mental disorders* (4th ed.). Washington, DC: Author.

Anderson, V., Smilbert, E., Ekert, H., & Godber, T. (1994). Intellectual, educational, and behavioural sequelae after cranial irradiation and chemotherapy. *Archives of Diseases in Childhood, 70*, 476–483.

Armstrong, F. D., & Mulhern, R. (1999). Acute leukemia and brain tumors. In R. Brown (Ed.), *Cognitive aspects of chronic illness in children* (pp. 47–77). New York: Guilford Press.

Barakat, L., Hetzke, J., Foley, B., Carey, M., Gyato, K., & Phillips, P. (2003). Evaluation of a social skills training group intervention with children treated for brain tumors: A pilot study. *Journal of Pediatric Psychology, 28*, 299–307.

Barbarin, O., Sargent, J., Sahler, O., Carpenter, P., Copeland, D., Dolgin, M., et al. (1995). Sibling adaptation to childhood cancer collaborative study: Parental views of pre- and postdiagnosis adjustment of siblings of children with cancer. *Journal of Psychosocial Oncology, 13*, 1–20.

Barrera, M., Chung, J. Y., Greenberg, M., & Fleming, C. (2002). Preliminary investigation of a group intervention for siblings of pediatric cancer patients. *Children's Health Care, 31*, 131–142.

Bessell, A. G. (2001). Children surviving cancer: Psychosocial adjustment, quality of life, and school experiences. *Exceptional Children, 67*, 345–359.

Best, M., Streisand, R., Catania, L., & Kazak, A. (2002). Parental distress during pediatric leukemia and parental posttraumatic stress symptoms after treatment ends. *Journal of Pediatric Psychology, 26,* 299–307.

Boon, D., Murdoch, B. E., & Jordan, F. M. (1994). Performance on creative narrative tasks of children treated for acute lymphocytic leukaemia. *Aphasiology, 8,* 549–568.

Brown, R., Madan-Swain, A., & Lambert, R. (2003). Posttraumatic stress symptoms in adolescent survivors of childhood cancer and their mothers. *Journal of Traumatic Stress, 16,* 309–318.

Butler, R. (2003, November). *Neurocognitive deficits and their remediation in pediatric oncology.* Paper presented at the Children's Oncology Group meeting, Dallas, TX.

Butler, R., & Copeland, D. (2002). Attentional processes and their remediation in children treated for cancer: A literature review and the development of a therapeutic approach. *Journal of the International Neuropsychological Society, 8,* 115–124.

Butler, R., & Mulhern, R. (2005). Neurocognitive interventions for children and adolescents surviving cancer. *Journal of Pediatric Psychology, 30,* 65–78.

Butler, R., Rizzi, L., & Handwerger, B. (1996). Brief report: The assessment of posttraumatic stress disorder in pediatric cancer patients and survivors. *Journal of Pediatric Psychology, 21,* 499–504.

Challinor, J., Miaskowsky, C., Moore, I., Slaughter, R., & Franch, L. (2000). Review of research studies that evaluated the impact of treatment for childhood cancers on neurocognition and behavioral and social competence: Nursing implications. *Journal of the Society of Pediatric Nurses, 5,* 57–74.

Cohen, D. S., Friedrich, W. N., Jaworski, T. M., Copeland, D., & Pendergrass, T. (1994). Pediatric cancer: Predicting sibling adjustment. *Journal of Clinical Psychology, 50,* 303–319.

Copeland, D. R., Moore, B. D., Francis, D. J., Jaffe, N., & Culbert, S. J. (1996). Neuropsychological effects of chemotherapy on children with cancer: A longitudinal study. *Journal of Clinical Oncology, 14,* 2826–2835.

Dahlquist, L. M., Czyzewski, D. I., & Jones, C. L. (1996). Parents of children with cancer: A longitudinal study of emotional distress, coping style, and marital adjustment two and twenty months after diagnosis. *Journal of Pediatric Psychology, 21,* 541–554.

Dolgin, M. J., Somer, E., Zaidel, N., & Zaizov, R. (1997). A structured group intervention for siblings of children with cancer. *Journal of Child and Adolescent Group Therapy, 7,* 3–18.

Eiser, C., Hill, J. J., & Blacklay, A. (2000). Surviving cancer: What does it mean for you? An evaluation of a clinic based intervention for survivors of childhood cancer. *Psycho-Oncology, 9,* 214–220.

Elkin, T. D., Phipps, S., Mulhern, R. K., & Fairclough, D. (1997). Psychological functioning of adolescent and young adult survivors of pediatric malignancy. *Medical and Pediatric Oncology, 29,* 582–588.

Emmons, K. M., Butterfied, R. M., Puleo, E., Park, E. R., Mertens, A., Gritz, E. R., et al. (2003). Smoking among participants in the Childhood Cancer Survivors cohort: The Partnership for Health Study. *Journal of Clinical Oncology, 21,* 189–196.

Erickson, S., & Steiner, H. (2001). Trauma and personality correlates in long term pediatric cancer survivors. *Child Psychiatry and Human Development, 31,* 195–213.

Espy, K. A., Moore, I. M., Kaufmann, P. M., Kramer, J. H., Matthay, K., & Hutter, J. J. (2001). Chemotherapeutic CNS prophylaxis and neuropsychologic change in children with acute lymphoblastic leukemia: A prospective study. *Journal of Pediatric Psychology, 26,* 1–9.

Fossen, A., Abrahamsen, T. G., & Storm-Mathisen, I. (1998). Psychological outcome in children treated for brain tumor. *Pediatric Hematology and Oncology, 15,* 479–488.

Friedman, D., & Meadows, A. (2002). Late effects of childhood cancer therapy. *Pediatric Clinics of North America, 49,* 1083–1106.

Garstein, M. A., Noll, R. B., & Vannatta, K. (2000). Childhood aggression and chronic illness: Possible protective mechanisms. *Journal of Applied Developmental Psychology, 21,* 315–333.

Glover, D. A., Byrne, J., Mills, J. L., Robison, L. L., Nicholson, H. S., Meadows, A., & Zeltzer, L. K. (2003). Impact of CNS treatment on mood in adult survivors of childhood leukemia: A report from the Children's Cancer Group. *Journal of Clinical Oncology, 21,* 4395–4401.

Grootenhuis, M. A., & Last, B. F. (1997). Predictors of parental emotional adjustment to childhood cancer. *Psycho-Oncology, 6,* 115–128.

Havermans, T., & Eiser, C. (1994). Siblings of a child with cancer. *Child: Care, Health, and Development, 20,* 323–337.

Hill, J. M., Kornblith, A. B., Jones, D., Freeman, A., Holland, J. F., Glicksman, A. S., et al. (1998). A comparative study of the long-term psychological functioning of childhood acute lymphoblastic leukemia survivors treated by intrathecal methotrexate with or without cranial radiation. *Medical and Pediatric Oncology, 28,* 387–400.

Hobbie, W., Stuber, M., Meeske, K., Wissler, K., Rourke, M., Ruccione, K., et al. (2000). Symptoms of posttraumatic stress in young adult survivors of childhood cancer. *Journal of Clinical Oncology, 18,* 4060–4066.

Hoekstra-Weebers, J., Heuvel, F., Jaspers, J., Kamps, W., & Klip, E. (1998). Brief report: An intervention program for parents of pediatric cancer patients. A randomized clinical trial. *Journal of Pediatric Psychology, 23,* 207–214.

Hudson, M. M., Mertens, A. C., Yasui, Y., Hobbie, W., Chen, H., Gurney, J. G., et al. (2003). Health status of adult long-term survivors of childhood cancer: A report from the Childhood Cancer Survivor Study. *Journal of the American Medical Association, 290,* 1583–1592.

Hudson, M. M., Tyc, V. L., Srivastava, D. K., Gattuso, J., Quargnenti, A., Crom, D. B., & Hinds, P. (2002). Multi-component behavioral intervention to promote health protective behaviors in childhood cancer survivors: The Protect Study. *Medical and Pediatric Oncology, 39,* 2–11.

Johnson, D. L., McCabe, M. A., Nicholson, H. S., Joseph, A., Getson, P. R., Byrne, J., et al. (1994). Quality of long-term survival in young children with medulloblastoma. *Journal of Neurosurgery, 80,* 1004–1010.

Jordan, F. M., Murdoch, B. E., Buttsworth, D. L., & Hudson-Tennent, L. J. (1995). Speech and language performance of brain-injured children. *Aphasiology, 9,* 23–32.

Kadan-Lottick, N. S., Robison, L., Gurney, J. G., Neglia, J. P., Yasui, Y., Hayashi, R., et al. (2002). Childhood cancer survivors' knowledge about their past diagnosis and treatment: Childhood Cancer Survivor Study. *Journal of the American Medical Association, 287,* 1832–1839.

Kazak, A. (1994). Implications of survival: Pediatric oncology patients and their families. In D. J. Bearison & R. K. Mulhern (Eds.), *Pediatric psychooncology: Psychological perspectives on children with cancer* (pp. 171–192). New York: Oxford University Press.

Kazak, A., Alderfer, M., Rourke, M., Simms, S., Streisand, R., & Grossman, J. (2004). Posttraumatic stress symptoms (PTSS) and posttraumatic stress disorder (PTSD) in families of adolescent childhood cancer survivors. *Journal of Pediatric Psychology, 29,* 211–219.

Kazak, A., Alderfer, M., Streisand, R., Simms, S., Rourke, M., Barakat, L., et al. (2004). Treatment of posttraumatic stress symptoms in adolescent survivors of childhood cancer and their families: A randomized clinical trial. *Journal of Family Psychology, 18,* 493–504.

Kazak, A., Barakat, L., Alderfer, M., Rourke, M., Meeske, K., Gallagher, P., et al. (2001). Posttraumatic stress in survivors of childhood cancer and mothers: Development and validation of the Impact of Traumatic Stressors Interview Schedule (ITSIS). *Journal of Clinical Psychology in Medical Settings, 8,* 307–323.

Kazak, A., Barakat, L., Meeske, K., Christakis, D., Meadows, A., Casey, R., et al. (1997). Posttraumatic stress, family functioning, and social support in survivors of childhood leukemia and their mothers and fathers. *Journal of Consulting and Clinical Psychology, 65,* 120–129.

Kazak, A., Cant, M. C., Jensen, M., McSherry, M., Rourke, M., Hwang, W. T., et al. (2003). Identifying psychosocial risk indicative of subsequent resource utilization in families of newly diagnosed pediatric oncology patients. *Journal of Clinical Oncology, 21,* 3220–3225.

Kazak, A., Christakis, D., Alderfer, M. A., & Coiro, M. (1994). Young adolescent cancer survivors and their parents: Adjustment, learning problems, and gender. *Journal of Family Psychology, 8,* 74–84.

Kazak, A., Simms, A., Alderfer, M., Rourke, M., Crump, T., McClure, K., et al. (2005). Feasibility and preliminary outcomes from a pilot study of a brief psychological intervention for families of children newly diagnosed with cancer. *Journal of Pediatric Psychology, 30,* 644–655.

Kazak, A., Simms, S., Barakat, L., Hobbie, W., Foley, B., Golomb, V., & Best, M. (1999). Surviving Cancer Competently Intervention Program (SCCIP): A cognitive–behavioral and family therapy intervention for adolescent survivors of childhood cancer and their families. *Family Process, 38,* 175–191.

Kleinman, S. N., & Waber, D. P. (1994). Prose memory strategies of children treated for leukemia: A story grammar analysis of the Anna Thompson passage. *Neuropsychology, 8,* 464–470.

Kramer, J. H., Crittenden, M. R., DeSantes, K., & Cowan, M. J. (1997). Cognitive and adaptive behavior 1 to 3 years following bone marrow transplantation. *Bone Marrow Transplantation, 19*, 607–613.

Kupst, M. J., Natta, M., Richardson, C., Schulman, J., Lavigne, J., & Das, L. (1995). Family coping with pediatric leukemia: Ten years after treatment. *Journal of Pediatric Psychology, 20*, 601–617.

Langer, T., Martus, P., Ottensmeier, H., Hertzberg, H., Beck, J. D., & Meier, W. (2002). CNS late-effects after ALL therapy in childhood: III. Neuropsychological performance in long-term survivors of childhood ALL: Impairments of concentration, attention, and memory. *Medical Pediatric Oncology, 38*, 320–328.

Lockwood, K. A., Bell, T. S., & Colegrove, R. W. (1999). Long-term effects of cranial radiation therapy on attention functioning in survivors of childhood leukemia. *Journal of Pediatric Psychology, 24*, 55–56.

Mackie, E., Hill, J., Kondryn, H., & McNally, R. (2000). Adult psychosocial outcomes in long-term survivors of acute lymphoblastic leukaemia and Wilms' tumour: A controlled study. *Lancet, 355*, 1310–1314.

Madan-Swain, A., Sexson, S. B., Brown, R. T., & Ragab, A. (1993). Family adaptation and coping among siblings of cancer patients, their brothers and sisters, and nonclinical controls. *American Journal of Family Therapy, 21*, 60–70.

Maggiolini, A., Grassi, R., Adamoli, L., Corbetta, A., Charmet, G. P., Provantini, K., et al. (2000). Self-image of adolescent survivors of long-term childhood leukemia. *Journal of Pediatric Hematology/Oncology, 22*, 417–421.

Manne, S., DuHamel, K., Gallelli, K., Sorgen, K., & Redd, W. (1998). Posttraumatic stress disorder among mothers of pediatric cancer survivors: Diagnosis, comorbidity, and utility of the PTSD Checklists as a screening instrument. *Journal of Pediatric Psychology, 23*, 357–366.

Manne, S., DuHamel, K., & Redd, W. H. (2000). Association of psychological vulnerability factors to posttraumatic stress symptomatology in mothers of pediatric cancer survivors. *Psycho-Oncology, 9*, 372–384.

Martinson, L. M., & Bossert, E. (1994). The psychological status of children with cancer. *Journal of Child and Adolescent Psychiatric Nursing, 7*, 16–23.

Mulhern, R. K., Palmer, S. L., Reddick, W. E., Glass, J. O., Kun, L. E., Taylor, J., et al. (2001). Risks of young age for selected neurocognitive deficits in medulloblastoma are associated with white matter loss. *Journal of Clinical Oncology, 19*, 472–479.

Newby, W. L., Brown, R., Pawletko, T. M., Gold, S. H., & Whitt, J. K. (2000). Social skills and psychological adjustment of child and adolescent cancer survivors. *Psycho-Oncology, 9*, 113–126.

Noll, R. B., Bukowski, W., Davies, W., Koontz, K., & Kulkarni, R. (1993). Adjustment in the peer system of children with cancer: A two-year follow-up study. *Journal of Pediatric Psychology, 18*, 351–364.

Noll, R. B., Gartstein, M. A., Hawkins, A., Vannatta, K., Davies, W. H., & Bukowski, W. M. (1995). Comparing parental distress for families with children who have cancer and matched comparison families without children with cancer. *Family Systems Medicine, 13,* 11–27.

Noll, R. B., MacLean, W. E., Whitt, J. K., Kaleita, T. A., Stehbens, J. A., Waskerwitz, M. J., et al. (1997). Behavioral adjustment and social functioning of long-term survivors of childhood leukemia: Parent and teacher reports. *Journal of Pediatric Psychology, 22,* 827–841.

Packman, W. L., Crittenden, M. R., Schaeffer, E., Bongar, B., Rieger Fischer, J. B., & Cowan, M. J. (1997). Psychosocial consequences of bone marrow transplantation in donor and nondonor siblings. *Developmental and Behavioral Pediatrics, 18,* 244–253.

Palmer, S. L., Goloubeva, O., Reddick, W. E., Glass, J. O., Gajjar, A., Kun, L., et al. (2001). Patterns of intellectual development among survivors of pediatric medulloblastoma: A longitudinal analysis. *Journal of Clinical Oncology, 19,* 2302–2308.

Pelcovitz, D., Goldenberg, B., Kaplan, S., Weinblatt, M., Mandel, F., Meyers, B., & Vinciguerra, V. (1996). Posttraumatic stress disorder in mothers of pediatric cancer survivors. *Psychosomatics, 37,* 116–126.

Phipps, S., Dunavant, M., Srivastava, D. K., Bownam, L., & Mulhern, R. (2000). Cognitive and academic functioning in survivors of pediatric bone marrow transplantation. *Journal of Clinical Oncology, 18,* 1004–1011.

Phipps, S., & Srivastava, D. K. (1997). Repressive adaptation in children with cancer. *Health Psychology, 16,* 521–528.

Phipps, S., Steele, R. G., Hall, K., & Leigh, L. (2001). Repressive adaptation in children with cancer: A replication and extension. *Health Psychology, 20,* 445–451.

Prevatt, F., Heffer, R., & Lowe, P. (2000). A review of school reintegration programs for children with cancer. *Journal of School Psychology, 38,* 447–467.

Radcliffe, J., Bennett, D., Kazak, A., Foley, B., & Phillips, P. C. (1996). Adjustment in childhood brain tumor survival: Child, mother, and teacher report. *Journal of Pediatric Psychology, 21,* 529–539.

Recklitis, C., O'Leary, T., & Diller, L. (2003). Utility of routine psychological screening in the childhood cancer survivor clinic. *Journal of Clinical Oncology, 21,* 787–792.

Rieter-Purtill, J., & Noll, R. (2003). Peer relationships of children with chronic illness. In M. Roberts (Ed.), *Handbook of pediatric psychology* (3rd ed., pp. 176–197). New York: Guilford Press.

Ris, D., Packer, R., Goldwein, J., Jones-Wallace, D., & Boyett, J. M. (2001). Intellectual outcome after reduced-dose radiation therapy plus adjuvant chemotherapy for medullablastoma: A Children's Cancer Group study. *Journal of Clinical Oncology, 19,* 3470–3476.

Rodgers, J., Horrocks, J., Britton, P. G., & Kernahan, J. (1999). Attentional ability among survivors of leukaemia. *Archives of Disorders in Children, 80,* 318–323.

Ross, L., Johansen, C., Dalton, S. O., Mellemkjaer, L., Thomassen, L. H., Mortensen, P. B., & Olsen, J. H. (2003). Psychiatric hospitalizations among survivors of cancer in childhood or adolescence. *The New England Journal of Medicine, 349,* 650–657.

Rourke, M., Hobbie, W., Schwartz, L., & Kazak, A. (2007). Posttraumatic stress disorder (PTSD) in young adult survivors of childhood cancer. *Pediatric Blood and Cancer, 49,* 177–182.

Rourke, M., & Kazak, A. (2005). Psychological aspects of long-term survivorship. In C. Schwartz, W. Hobbie, L. Constine, & K. Ruccione (Eds.), *Survivors of childhood cancer* (pp. 137–149). Heidelberg, Germany: Springer-Verlag.

Sahler, O. J., Roghmann, K., Carpenter, P., Mulhern, R., Dolgin, M., Sargent, J., et al. (1994). Sibling Adaptation to Childhood Cancer Collaborative Study: Prevalence of sibling distress and definition of adaptation levels. *Developmental and Behavioral Pediatrics, 15,* 353–366.

Sahler, O. J., Varni, J., Fairclough, D., Butler, R., Dolgin, M., Phipps, S., et al. (2002). Problem-solving skills training for mothers of children with newly diagnosed cancer: A randomized trial. *Developmental and Behavioral Pediatrics, 23,* 77–86.

Sargent, J. R., Sahler, O. J., Roghmann, K. J., Mulhern, R. K., Barbarin, O., Carpenter, P. J., et al. (1995). Sibling Adaptation to Childhood Cancer Collaborative Study: Siblings' perceptions of the cancer experience. *Journal of Pediatric Psychology, 20,* 151–164.

Sawyer, M. G., Antoniou, G., Nguyen, A.-M. T., Toogood, I., Rice, M., & Baghurst, P. (1995). A prospective study of the psychological adjustment of children with cancer. *American Journal of Pediatric Hematology/Oncology, 17,* 39–45.

Sawyer, M. G., Antoniou, G., Toogood, I., & Rice, M. (1997). Childhood cancer: A two-year prospective study of the psychological adjustment of children and parents. *Journal of the American Academy of Child and Adolescent Psychiatry, 36,* 1736–1743.

Sawyer, M. G., Streiner, D. L., Antoniou, G., Toogood, I., & Rice, M. (1998). Influence of parental and family adjustment on the later psychological adjustment of children treated for cancer. *Journal of the American Academy of Child and Adolescent Psychiatry, 37,* 815–822.

Schatz, J., Kramer, J. H., Ablin, A., & Matthay, K. K. (2000). Processing speed, working memory, and IQ: A developmental model of cognitive deficits following cranial radiation therapy. *Neuropsychology, 14,* 189–200.

Simms, S., Kazak, A., Golomb, V., Goldwein, J., & Bunin, N. (2002). Cognitive, behavioral, and social outcome in survivors of childhood stem cell transplantation. *Journal of Pediatric Hematology/Oncology, 24,* 115–119.

Sloper, P., & While, D. (1996). Risk factors in the adjustment of siblings of children with cancer. *Journal of Child Psychology and Psychiatry and Allied Disciplines, 37,* 597–607.

Sloper, T., Larcombe, I. J., & Charleston, A. (1994). Psychosocial adjustment of five-year survivors of childhood cancer. *Journal of Cancer Education, 9,* 163–169.

Sormanti, M., Dungan, S., & Reiker, P. P. (1994). Pediatric bone marrow transplantation: Psychosocial issues for parents after a child's hospitalization. *Journal of Psychosocial Oncology, 12,* 23–42.

Streisand, R., Kazak, A., & Tercyak, K. P. (2003). Pediatric-specific parenting stress and family functioning in parents of children treated for cancer. *Children's Health Care, 32*, 245–256.

Streisand, R., Rodrigue, J., Houck, C., Graham-Pole, J., & Berlant, N. (2000). Brief report: Parents of children undergoing bone marrow transplantation. Documenting stress and piloting a psychological intervention program. *Journal of Pediatric Psychology, 25*, 331–337.

Stuber, M., Christakis, D., Houskamp, B., & Kazak, A. (1996). Posttrauma symptoms in childhood leukemia survivors and their parents. *Psychosomatics, 37*, 254–261.

Syndikus, I., Tait, D., Ashley, S., & Jannoun, L. (1994). Long-term follow-up of young children with brain tumors after radiation. *International Journal of Radiation Oncology Biology and Physics, 30*, 781–787.

Thompson, S., Leigh, L. Christensen, R., Xiong, X., Kun, L., Heideman, R., et al. (2001). Immediate neurocognitive effects of methylphenidate on learning-impaired survivors of childhood cancer. *Journal of Clinical Oncology, 19*, 1802–1808.

Tyc, V., Rai, S., Lensing, S., Klosky, J., Stewart, D., & Gattuso, J. (2003). An intervention to reduce intentions to use tobacco among pediatric cancer survivors. *Journal of Clinical Oncology, 21*, 1366–1372.

Van Dongen-Melman, J. E. W. M., DeGroot, A., Hahlen, K., & Verhulst, F. C. (1995). Siblings of childhood cancer survivors: How does this "forgotten" group of children adjust after cessation of successful cancer treatment? *European Journal of Cancer, 31*, 2277–2283.

Vannatta, K., Gartstein, M. A., Short, A., & Noll, R. B. (1998). A controlled study of peer relationships of children surviving brain tumors: Teacher, peer, and self-ratings. *Journal of Pediatric Psychology, 23*, 279–287.

Waber, D. P., Isquith, P. K., Kahn, C. M., & Romero, I. (1994). Metacognitive factors in the visuospatial skills of long-term survivors of acute lymphoblastic leukemia: An experimental approach to the Rey–Osterrieth Complex Figure Test. *Developmental Neuropsychology, 10*, 349–367.

Zebrack, B., Zeltzer, L., Whitton, J., Mertens, A., Odom, L., Berkow, R., & Robison, L. (2002). Psychological outcomes in long-term survivors of childhood leukemia, Hodgkin's disease, and non-Hodgkin's lymphoma: A report from the Childhood Cancer Survivor Study. *Pediatrics, 110*, 42–52.

Zeltzer, L. K., Chen, E., Weiss, R., Guo, M. D., Robison, L. L., Meadows, A. T., et al. (1997). Comparison of psychological outcome in adult survivors of childhood acute lymphoblastic leukemia versus sibling controls: A Cooperative Children's Cancer Group and National Institutes of Health study. *Journal of Clinical Oncology, 15*, 547–556.

26

LONG-TERM EFFECTS OF CANCER ON FAMILIES OF ADULT CANCER SURVIVORS

LAUREL L. NORTHOUSE, SUZANNE MELLON, JANET HARDEN, AND ANN SCHAFENACKER

With the increasing survival rates of cancer, greater attention is being given to the posttreatment phase of survivorship. This is a period in which patients and families need to adapt to the changes brought on by the cancer, to manage the lingering effects of the illness or treatments, and to learn how to live with an illness that may recur (Walker, 1997). Although more research has been conducted on the experience of adult cancer survivors during the posttreatment phase (Dorval, Maunsell, Deschenes, Brisson, & Masse, 1998; Ganz et al., 2002), less research has examined the experience of their family members. Because family members are the primary source of support to the cancer survivor (Morse & Fife, 1998), researchers and clinicians need to have a greater understanding of family members' longer term adjustment so that family members can maintain their own well-being as they care for the cancer survivor.

The purpose of this chapter is to examine published research on the experience of families of cancer survivors after completing treatment. *Family* is broadly defined as the significant others who are the primary source of support to the cancer survivor. Specifically, we (a) describe quality-of-life issues for family members during cancer survivorship, (b) identify families at greater risk for long-term adjustment problems, (c) identify interventions that have been used with survivors and their family members during survivorship, and (d) conclude with recommendations for future research.

QUALITY-OF-LIFE ISSUES OF FAMILIES IN LONGER TERM SURVIVORSHIP

A number of theoretical frameworks have been used to examine the family's quality of life during survivorship. One of the more commonly used frameworks is family stress theory (H. I. McCubbin, Thompson, & McCubbin, 1996; M. A. McCubbin & McCubbin, 1991). This theory contends that the family is a social system, that stress in one member has a reverberating effect on other family members, and that a buildup of stress can exceed the family's resources and hinder family adaptation. Stress-coping theory has also been used to guide studies with cancer survivors and their family members (Lazarus & Folkman, 1984). This theory examines how individuals appraise and cope with situations, including the stress of illness. Other frameworks or models, such as problem-solving models (Nezu, Nezu, Friedman, Faddis, & Houts, 1999), interpersonal therapy models (Donnelly et al., 2000; Klerman, Weissman, Rounsaville, & Chevron, 1984), and quality-of-life frameworks (Ferrell et al., 1996), have guided research in this area. For the purposes of this review, we used a quality-of-life framework. *Quality of life* is viewed as a multidimensional concept that includes emotional, social, physical, and spiritual well-being (Ferrell et al., 1996). Research studies in each of these four areas were examined that pertained to families of cancer survivors during the posttreatment phase.

Emotional Well-Being

Several studies examined the amount of emotional distress or the number of adjustment problems reported by family members in the posttreatment period. The consensus of these studies is that both patients' and family members' adjustment problems persist over time, even though the patient is no longer receiving treatment (Ell, Nishimoto, Mantell, & Hamovitch, 1988; Hagedoorn, Buunk, Kuijer, Wobbes, & Sanderman, 2000; Northouse, Templin, Mood, & Oberst, 1998; Oberst & Scott, 1988).

Although problems are still evident 12 to 18 months posttreatment (Northouse, 1989), it is unclear how long family members' problems continue, given the limited number of longitudinal studies with extended assessment times (i.e., beyond 1 year). However, family members' adjustment problems appear to gradually decrease over time (Hoskins, 1995). Cancer survivors and their family members reported that the cancer had no lasting or long-term negative effect on their family's quality of life when interviewed approximately 3 years postdiagnosis (Gritz, Wellisch, Siau, & Wang, 1990; Mellon, 2002). It is evident from most studies that family members' levels of adjustment are significantly related to the adjustment of the survivors (Baider & Kaplan De-Nour, 1988; Baider, Perez, & De-Nour, 1989; Gritz et al., 1990). Not only are family members' responses to cancer interdependent, but some research indicates that how well the family caregiver adjusts has a significant effect on the survivor's adjustment 1 year following diagnosis (Northouse, Mood, Templin, Mellon, & George, 2000).

Learning to deal with uncertainty is one of the major concerns reported by family members in the posttreatment phase (Hilton, 1993; Oberst & James, 1985). Husbands of women in one study reported that they were frustrated by their inability to predict what would happen in the future (Zahlis & Shands, 1991). In another study, both cancer survivors and their partners reported moderate fear of the cancer recurring (Walker, 1997). In some studies, family members have reported more fear than survivors themselves (Matthews, 2003; Mellon, Kershaw, Northouse, & Freeman-Gibb, 2007). Mellon and Northouse (2001) found that the degree of fear of recurrence reported by family members was a strong predictor of the family's quality of life: The higher the family member's fear of recurrence, the lower the family's quality of life during the extended period of survivorship.

Social Well-Being

Social well-being is another component of quality of life that is affected during cancer survivorship. Within the area of social well-being, most of the research has focused on the effect of cancer on the marital relationship (Lewis & Hammond, 1992; Lichtman, Taylor, & Wood, 1988). The good news is that most dyads report moderately high marital satisfaction during the posttreatment period. Studies of patients and/or dyads approximately 1 to 2 years after the diagnosis of cancer indicate that their marital scores on standardized measures are within the normal range and are similar to couples not dealing with cancer (Ganz, Rowland, Desmond, Meyerowitz, & Wyatt, 1998; Lichtman et al., 1988; Northouse, Templin, & Mood, 2001).

Little evidence indicates that divorce or separation occurs as a result of cancer. To the contrary, dyads who were approximately 2 years postdiagnosis reported positive effects over time (Gritz et al., 1990; Lewis & Hammond, 1992). Researchers have reported that most dyads tried to turn their cancer experience from adversity to advantage. The few dyads in which divorce or separation occurred reported that they had preexisting marital problems prior to the onset of cancer (Gritz et al., 1990). However, despite these generally positive findings, the marital relationship is not immune from stress. For example, dyads in which the survivor was depressed reported that the quality of the marital relationship suffered (Lewis & Hammond, 1992). Likewise, higher depression in the partner was also related to lower marital satisfaction during the posttreatment phase (Lewis, Woods, Hough, & Bensley, 1989).

There are areas of strain in relationships in which one person is diagnosed with cancer. In one study, 66% of the couples wanted to resolve tension in their relationship due to the cancer (Shands, Lewis, Sinsheimer, & Cochrane, 2006). One of the most frequently reported areas of strain is the extent to which patients and spouses are able to communicate openly about the cancer. Approximately one third of the breast cancer patients in one study expressed dismay over their husbands' failure to talk about cancer-related issues (Lichtman et al., 1988). Typically, the patient wanted more opportunities to express her fears freely, whereas her significant other thought that talking about these fears would hamper her adjustment and possibly even lead to a recurrence. Hilton (1994) found various communication patterns among couples dealing with cancer. In some dyads, both partners wanted to openly discuss the illness, whereas in other dyads, neither partner wanted to discuss the illness. Some couples wanted some disclosure, but not a lot, and in some couples, the partners differed in their preferences. The most beneficial pattern of communication was what was identified as "open, but selective": Partners talked about cancer together, but limited the number of negative interactions they had.

In general, more open communication has been associated with less distress in patients and their family members and with better role functioning in the family (Edwards & Clarke, 2004; Germino, Fife, & Funk, 1995; Pistrang & Barker, 1995; Vess, Moreland, & Schwebel, 1985). Some researchers have reported that the extent to which dyads discuss illness-related issues tends to decrease over time (Hilton, 1994). Once the treatment and symptoms subsided, couples reported that their communication turns to other issues. Similarly, long-term survivors and their family members reported that they tried not to talk too much or think too much about the cancer. They tried to minimize the effect of the cancer by not dwelling on it or by not letting it take control over their lives (Mellon, 2002). In two studies, dyads in the extended posttreatment period reported few illness-related communication problems with their partners (Gritz et al., 1990; Rees & Bath, 2000).

Sexuality and fertility are also social issues evident in the posttreatment phase. Sexuality issues are broader in scope and can be an issue for dyads of varying ages, whereas fertility issues are more often raised among younger dyads. Although both sexuality and fertility are relational areas that affect both members of the dyad, they have been examined almost entirely from the perspective of the survivor, and most often with long-term breast cancer survivors (Ganz et al., 1996). Although sexual problems are often attributed to the cancer survivor, some research suggests that sexual difficulties are influenced by both members of the dyad. In one study with long-term survivors of prostate cancer, 66% of the survivors reported that their partners had at least one sexual concern that interfered with their sexual relationship (Schover, Fouladi, et al., 2002). These included concerns such as wives' low sexual drive (42%), vaginal dryness (13%), or other health problems wives had that interfered with their sexual functioning (10%). The sexual relationship appears to be an area of couples' social well-being that continues to be affected in the posttreatment phase and warrants further research with both survivors and their partners (Neese, Schover, Klein, Zippe, & Kupelian, 2003).

A final issue about social well-being that emerges from the posttreatment research literature is the effect of the illness on family members' work, family, and social roles. Early in the course of illness, dyads need to change work schedules, alter household responsibilities, and balance multiple roles to accommodate the demands of illness and treatment (Zahlis & Shands, 1991). However, in the posttreatment phase, if the cancer has not recurred, dyads report less household disruption, less role strain, and less role conflict (Vess et al., 1985). Furthermore, following treatment completion, illness-related demands decrease (Lewis & Hammond, 1992), physical caregiving responsibilities decrease (McCorkle et al., 1993), disruptions in their day-to-day schedule decrease (Nijboer et al., 2000), and caregivers have less burden (Blood, Simpson, Dineen, Kauffman, & Raimondi, 1994).

Physical Well-Being

Although the impact of cancer on the physical well-being of the cancer survivor has been studied extensively in recent years, very few data are available on the physical well-being of family members during the posttreatment period. From the limited research, it is not clear whether family members have few physical effects or whether the physical effects on the family members have been overlooked in view of the very obvious physical problems reported by the patients diagnosed with the cancer.

One of the few studies of fatigue among family caregivers of cancer patients ($N = 248$) indicated that 45% of the caregivers reported mild fatigue; 25%, moderate fatigue; and 28%, severe fatigue in their caregiving role (Jensen & Given, 1993). The mean duration of caregiving was 23.6 months. No relationship was found between caregivers' age or employment status and the level of fatigue. However, caregivers who provided more hours of daily caregiving and who perceived a greater impact of the caregiving on their day-to-day schedule had more fatigue.

Although there is a lack of research on family members' physical well-being, reports indicate that approximately half of family members have chronic health problems of their own (Hilton, 1993). There are no data about the extent to which these comorbid conditions are exacerbated by the stress of the patient's cancer, nor is there information on how family members manage their own health problems when they are the primary caregiver to a spouse or relative. However, reports suggest that the patient's cancer serves as a wake-up call to other family members to start taking better care of their health (Mellon, 2002). Overall, there is insufficient research to make any definitive statements about the effects of cancer on family members' physical well-being in the posttreatment period of illness.

Spiritual Well-Being

For the purposes of this review, *spiritual well-being* refers to the way in which people make sense of their lives and find meaning and purpose in the midst of life's challenges, such as cancer (Brady, Peterman, Fitchett, Mo, & Cella, 1999). In a study of long-term survivors, Mellon (2002) found that both survivors and family members attempted to reframe the illness as something positive. For example, they were glad the cancer was diagnosed early, treated effectively, and now behind them. They also described their reliance on their spiritual faith and their increased appreciation of everyday life. Germino et al. (1995) assessed patients' and family members' level of meaning and found no difference in their scores. Both held fairly positive perspectives about the meaning of cancer in their lives. Furthermore, when they associated the cancer experience with more positive meaning, their emotional response and adjustment to the illness was better (Germino et al., 1995; Morse & Fife, 1998).

A common finding in the research literature is that cancer survivors shift their priorities to find the "right" components in their lives following a cancer diagnosis (Gall & Cornblat, 2002). Family members also shift their priorities or reevaluate them after the cancer experience (Germino et al., 1995; Hilton, 1993). Some dyads decide to carry out planned trips or to try to enjoy life more (Germino et al., 1995). In other studies, families discussed the fragility of life and their decreased emphasis on material things (Hilton, 1993). Overall, the research literature suggests that spiritual well-being is an important aspect of quality of life that is initially evident in the diagnostic phase but continues to have relevance for survivors and family members in the posttreatment phase of cancer.

Families at Risk

Although research studies on cancer survivors and their families generally show that most families do well and regain a new normalcy, there are indications that some families struggle with adjustment throughout the entire cancer trajectory and show signs of being at risk. A developing body of research indicates certain signals of distress for family members at risk, including persistent emotional distress, depression, or anxiety (Lewis et al., 1989; Northouse et al., 2002; Oberst & James, 1985); greater demands of illness (Lewis et al., 1989); concurrent stress in addition to the cancer (Ell et al., 1988;

Oberst & James, 1985); role problems and strain (Vess et al., 1985); hopelessness and uncertainty (Northouse, Laten, & Reddy, 1995; Zahlis & Shands, 1993); family communication problems (Hilton, 1994); and inadequate social support (Ell et al., 1988; Hoskins et al., 1996; Northouse et al., 2000). In addition, the developmental phase of the family can also place some families at risk for poorer adjustment (Harden, Northouse, & Mood, 2006; Rowland, 1990).

Persistent Emotional Distress

Several studies found that emotional distress, depression, or anxiety that persists over time are possible markers for a family at risk (Ell et al., 1988; Northouse et al., 1998). This pattern of ongoing distress for family members has been supported in other studies as well (Baider & Kaplan De-Nour, 1988; Northouse, 1989).

Illness Demands

Higher physical and psychological demands of illness have been correlated with the emotional distress or depression reported by family members. In a longitudinal study of mothers diagnosed with nonmetastatic breast cancer, their spouses, their school-age children, and adolescents, Lewis and colleagues (Lewis, Hammond, & Woods, 1993; Lewis et al., 1989) reported that the greater the demands imposed by the illness, the higher the depression levels of the husbands. Although higher functioning families did fairly well after the cancer, other families continued to cope with the additional burden of cancer in their usual methods, and their family functioning did not improve. These families came into the posttreatment phase functioning at a lower level and continued to do so over the 8 months. The researchers suggested that evidence of burnout from handling the cancer was present for these families at risk.

Concurrent Stressors

Other concurrent stressors may also place families at risk. Families must cope with competing demands of family life, including other illnesses, work demands, and financial concerns. Together, these stressors impose additional pressures on an already taxed family system. Hilton (1993) reported that while dealing with cancer, families often put other issues on hold, which further contributes to the pileup of stressors they face. Ell et al. (1988) reported that psychologically vulnerable family members (identified at the beginning of the illness) have greater stress unrelated to the cancer. Those family members who experienced declining mental health over time also reported increased concurrent stressors. Caregiver illnesses can take an additional toll on family members. Northouse et al. (2002) reported that family caregivers' own physical symptoms influenced their view of caregiving: The more symptom distress the family members experienced themselves, the more negative their evaluation of both caregiving and their own mental health.

Role Problems

Problems with role adjustment within the family signal another risk marker. Ell et al. (1988) found that family members with many role demands reported poorer psychological functioning. Vess et al. (1985), in a follow-up study of cancer patients and family members 5 months after diagnosis, found that families who had assumed too many role responsibilities had lower family cohesion and that families who could expand role functions internally experienced less conflict and role strain. There is some indication that the role problems a family has at the beginning of the illness may be predictive of later problems. Northouse et al. (2000) found that the number of role problems that spouses reported early in the illness directly affected their role adjustment and survivors' adjustments 1 year later.

Hopelessness and Uncertainty

In a study of recurrent breast cancer patients and their family members, investigators found that uncertainty and hopelessness reported by family members influenced their ability to carry out their roles (Northouse, Dorris, & Charron-Moore, 1995). Those family members who had higher levels of hopelessness reported more difficulty adjusting to the illness, suggesting risk susceptibility. In a large study of recurrent breast cancer patients and family members ($N = 189$ dyads), researchers found that family members reported significantly more uncertainty about the illness than did patients (Northouse et al., 2002). Additionally, when family members expressed more uncertainty, hopelessness, and a more negative appraisal of the cancer, it exerted a negative effect on their overall quality of life.

Family Communication Problems

Poor communication patterns within families can also be an additional signal of a family at risk. Several studies (Chekryn, 1984; Hilton, 1993, 1994; Lewis & Deal, 1995) indicated that there is a great deal of variety in how families talk about the cancer and its effect on their lives. What seems to be critical is the level of congruence between family members in their communication patterns. Hilton (1994) identified one communication pattern that signaled a possible family at risk. In this pattern, major discrepancies in the communication between patients and family members were found; in addition, conflict, insensitivity, lack of sharing, and uncaring behaviors were dominant. The high level of incongruence and low satisfaction with their family communication signaled possible risk for adjustment problems.

Inadequate Support

Inadequate social support from others may also identify a potential family member at risk (Eton, Lepore, & Helgeson, 2005). Northouse et al. (2000) found that spouses of colon cancer patients reported less support from other people than did patients themselves. Female spouses in particular noted the lowest levels of support. Oberst and James (1985) reported that family members expressed lack of support from multiple sources following the patient's postsurgical discharge and throughout the first 6 months, a finding also reported by Lethborg, Kissane, and Burns (2003). Hoskins et al. (1996) emphasized that marital support affects the emotional and physical adjustment of spouses of breast cancer patients over time. If husbands did not perceive support from the marital relationship, they experienced more worry and other negative emotions. Other research also substantiates the importance of social support and that lack of support contributes to lower levels of adjustment or poorer quality of life for family members dealing with a cancer illness (Ell et al., 1988; Northouse et al., 2002).

Developmental Phase of the Family

Because the needs and stressors of people change across the life span, the time at which cancer occurs and the treatments associated with it may interfere with the developmental tasks of families and put them at risk. Cancer during young adulthood creates worry about infertility associated with cancer treatments (Schover, Brey, Lipshultz, & Jeha, 2002) and problems with role strain due to multiple demands associated with raising young children, work outside the home, and household chores (Nijboer et al., 2000). Cancer during middle adulthood can interfere with retirement plans, create financial strains, and result in sexual dysfunction associated with treatment side effects (Harden et al., 2006). Cancer during older adulthood places strain on families because of the increased number of comorbid conditions both survivors and older caregivers face in addition to the cancer. The timing of cancer can affect the psychosocial issues that develop during the posttreatment phase of illness and the risk status of survivors and their family members (Cimprich, Ronis, & Martinez-Ramos, 2002; Kim, Kashy, & Evans, 2007; Rowland, 1990).

It is clear that there are several markers or signals of high-risk status for families coping with cancer. Evidence suggests that dealing with a major illness, such as cancer, can precipitate significant psychological distress in families and interfere with normal developmental processes. Furthermore, research indicates that families who come into the cancer experience with risk markers continue to exhibit ongoing symptoms of psychological vulnerability throughout the cancer survivorship trajectory.

STRATEGIES TO IMPROVE FAMILY COPING IN THE POSTTREATMENT PHASE

There is very little evidence-based research supporting proven coping methods for family members of cancer patients who have completed primary treatment. Research on coping has concentrated on the diagnosis through initial treatment phases (Mishel et al., 2002), with a few studies addressing the advanced stage (Kershaw, Northouse, Kritpracha, Schafenacker, & Mood, 2004; Manne, Pape, Taylor, & Dougherty, 1999; McMillan et al., 2006; Northouse, Kershaw, Mood, & Schafenacker, 2005). In addition, studies on coping have focused on the patient's responses to treatment-related concerns, both physical and psychological, and seldom on concerns of the significant others—spouses, family members, and other caregivers (Carver et al., 1993; Edgar, Rosberger, & Nowlis, 1993; Heim, Augustiny, Schaffner, & Valach, 1993).

Only a few randomized clinical trials testing family-based interventions have been conducted with patients and family members using longitudinal assessments that extend 6 to 12 months after active cancer treatment was begun. Interventions have been offered to family members only in some studies and to both patients and family members jointly in other studies. Examples of each of these types of family-based studies are briefly reviewed in the next subsection.

Intervention Studies With Family Members Only

Three studies typify interventions offered to family members only. First, Blanchard, Toseland, and McCallion (1996) and Toseland, Blanchard, and McCallion (1995) designed a six-session counseling intervention to help spouses cope with the stress of caring for partners with cancer. The program, Coping With Cancer, focused on problem solving, coping skills, and social support. No significant differences were found between spouses in the intervention versus control group on psychosocial outcomes; however, the intervention had differential effect on more distressed spouses. Spouses reporting more burden and poorer marital satisfaction who participated in the intervention had significantly better physical and social functioning at postintervention follow-up than distressed spouses in the control group (Toseland et al., 1995). It is interesting that patients whose spouses participated in the intervention group were significantly less depressed at 6 months follow-up than patients whose spouses did not receive the intervention, suggesting a ripple of intervention effects to patients even though they were not a part of the intervention.

In another study with family members only, Bultz, Speca, Brasher, Geggie, and Page (2000) examined the effects of a group intervention for partners of early-stage breast cancer patients. Partners randomized to the intervention participated in six weekly psychoeducational group meetings that lasted 1.5 to 2 hours. Results indicated that partners who participated in the group sessions had less mood disturbance than control participants in follow-up assessments at 3 months. In addition, patients of partners who attended the intervention sessions reported less mood disturbance ($p = .10$) and greater confident support ($p = .06$) than patients of partners in the control group. Patients reported descriptively that the intervention helped their partners be better caregivers (86%), helped their communication with one another (57%), and improved their marital relationship (43%).

Manne, Babb, Pinover, Horwitz, and Ebbert (2004) conducted an intervention with wives of men with prostate cancer. They examined the effects of a 6-week psychoeducational group intervention on wives' distress levels, coping, personal growth, and marital communication, compared with a control group. No differences were found in wives' levels of distress at 1-month follow-up, but wives who participated in the intervention reported greater use of adaptive coping and more positive growth associated with their husbands' prostate cancer.

Interventions Offered to Patients and Family Members Jointly

Some studies have offered interventions jointly to patients and one of their family members, generally the spouse. Kuijer, Buunk, DeJong, Ybema, and Sanderman (2004) offered an intervention to cancer survivors and their partners that addressed relationship equity, or the give and take, that goes on within couples confronted with serious illness. Couples who received the intervention participated in five cognitive behavior sessions that addressed relationship equity. Couples who received the intervention reported greater marital satisfaction and less bother with feelings of overinvestment or underinvestment than couples in the control group. Furthermore, patients who participated in the intervention reported less emotional distress than patients who participated in the control group.

Northouse et al. (2007) offered a family-based intervention to prostate cancer patients and their spouses or partners. Couples in the intervention group received five sessions that addressed family involvement, optimism, coping effectiveness, uncertainty reduction, and symptom management. Patients who received the family-based intervention reported less uncertainty and better communication with their spouses than did patients in the control group. Spouses who participated in the intervention reported higher quality of life, more self-efficacy, better communication, less negative appraisal of caregiving, less uncertainty, and less hopelessness than did spouses in the control group, with some intervention effects sustained to 8 and 12 months.

Jepson, McCorkle, Adler, Nuamah, and Lusk (1999) and McCorkle et al. (2000) used a longitudinal, randomized trial to test the effects of a home care intervention, Standardized Nursing Intervention Protocol, with older cancer patients just following postsurgical discharge and their family caregivers. In general, there were no significant differences in the psychosocial status of caregivers who received the intervention and those in standard care. However, patients with late-stage cancer who participated in the home care intervention group had a significantly longer survival time than patients in the control group (McCorkle et al., 2000).

The preceding six family-based studies suggest that there are positive outcomes associated with family-based interventions, whether they are offered to family members only or to family dyads jointly, a finding also reported by Martire, Lustig, Schulz, Miller, and Helgeson (2004) in their meta-analysis of family interventions in chronic illness. Although the number of family-based intervention studies in cancer is small, there appears to be a tendency to target the intervention to family members only when the goal is to reduce family caregiver distress and to target the intervention to family dyads jointly when the goal is to deal with relationship issues (e.g., equity) or to provide education and support to both members of the dyad. Some of the preceding studies indicate that family-based interventions may be more effective when offered to family members who are more distressed than others (Toseland et al., 1995). Prior research also suggests that interventions targeted to family members only may result in positive outcomes for patients, even though they are not a part of the intervention. Thus, it is important to measure both family member and patient outcomes in family-based studies (Martire et al., 2004). Because of the communication problems that have been reported in dyads dealing with cancer, some investigators have suggested that interventions offered to family dyads jointly may be more effective than interventions offered to family members only (Toseland et al., 1995). Finally, some investigators have suggested that it is important to assess a range of outcomes, rather than just emotional distress, in family-based research, because outcomes such as effective coping and the ability to find benefit in an illness are also important outcomes for families facing cancer (Manne et al., 2004).

DIRECTIONS FOR FUTURE RESEARCH

On the basis of this review of prior studies, it is evident that more research is needed on the experiences of patients and their family members during the posttreatment phase of cancer. The following is a list of recommended areas for future research.

1. In spite of the fairly universal reports about the prevalence of fear of cancer recurrence among cancer survivors and their family members, few studies have examined factors associated with heightened fear of recurrence. More research on ways to help survivors and family members manage fear of recurrence is needed.

2. More research in the area of sexuality during the posttreatment phase is also needed. The research should include both the survivors and their partners because they may differ in their views of their sexual relationship, their motivations for seeking help, and their preferences for treatments to address sexual problems (Neese et al., 2003).

3. More research is needed on the caregivers' physical well-being and how it may be affected as a result of the caregiving role. Schulz and Beach (1999) found an increased mortality rate among caregivers of cardiovascular patients who experienced strain in their caregiving role. The extent to which strain impairs the health and longevity of the caregivers of cancer patients deserves further study. Studies are also needed to explore interventions that may improve the mental and physical well-being of caregivers.

4. Little research with cancer survivors and their caregivers uses a diverse sample (Gotay & Muraoka, 1998), yet there are some indications that health disparities may exist. Maly, Leake, and Silliman (2003) found that Latina breast cancer patients received less informational support from their physicians than Caucasian patients. Because caregiver samples have been primarily Caucasian, more diversity in caregiver samples to determine how racial or ethnic characteristics affect the caregiver's role is needed.

5. A more balanced view of the positive and negative effects of cancer on patients and their family caregivers during the posttreatment phase of illness is needed. Too often, investigators have examined the negative aspects of illness without considering the benefits that may result, such as positive life changes (Kim, Schulz, & Carver, 2007), or "posttraumatic growth," as it has been called by some researchers (Weiss, 2004).

6. Finally, well-designed family-based randomized clinical trials with patients and their family caregivers are needed. Even though considerable descriptive evidence indicates that cancer creates emotional distress in patients and their key family members, intervention studies with partners have lagged far behind

the descriptive research (Cochrane & Lewis, 2005). More research is needed to test the efficacy of various strategies for reducing stress, enhancing coping, and increasing dyadic communication during the posttreatment phase of cancer.

In summary, this chapter reviewed the existing family-based research on experiences of family caregivers of cancer survivors during the posttreatment phase of cancer. From the research, it is apparent that survivors and their family members have ongoing needs that extend into the posttreatment phase. More research should be conducted to better understand the experiences of survivors and their family members, as well as to test strategies that will assist them in managing the ongoing effects of cancer.

REFERENCES

Baider, L., & Kaplan De-Nour, A. (1988). Adjustment to cancer: Who is the patient—The husband or the wife? *Israel Journal of Medical Sciences, 24,* 631–636.

Baider, L., Perez, T., & De-Nour, A. K. (1989). Gender and adjustment to chronic disease: A study of couples with colon cancer. *General Hospital Psychiatry, 11,* 1–8.

Blanchard, C., Toseland, R., & McCallion, P. (1996). The effects of a problem-solving intervention with spouses of cancer patients. *Journal of Psychosocial Oncology, 14,* 1–21.

Blood, G. W., Simpson, K. C., Dineen, M., Kauffman, S. M., & Raimondi, S. C. (1994). Spouses of individuals with laryngeal cancer: Caregiver strain and burden. *Journal of Communication Disorders, 27,* 19–35.

Brady, M. J., Peterman, A. H., Fitchett, G., Mo, M., & Cella, D. (1999). A case for including spirituality in quality of life measurement in oncology. *Psycho-Oncology, 8,* 417–428.

Bultz, B. D., Speca, M., Brasher, P. M., Geggie, P. H., & Page, S. A. (2000). A randomized controlled trial of a brief psychoeducational support group for partners of early stage breast cancer patients. *Psycho-Oncology, 9,* 303–313.

Carver, C. S., Pozo, C., Harris, S. D., Noriega, V., Scheier, M. F., Robinson, D. S., et al. (1993). How coping mediates the effect of optimism on distress: A study of women with early stage breast cancer. *Journal of Personality and Social Psychology, 65,* 375–390.

Chekryn, J. (1984). Cancer recurrence: Personal meaning, communication, and marital adjustment. *Cancer Nursing, 7,* 491–498.

Cimprich, B., Ronis, D. L., & Martinez-Ramos, G. (2002). Age at diagnosis and quality of life in breast cancer survivors. *Cancer Practice, 10,* 85–93.

Cochrane, B., & Lewis, F. M. (2005). The partner's adjustment to breast cancer: A critical analysis of intervention studies. *Health Psychology, 24,* 327–332.

Donnelly, J. M., Kornblith, A. B., Fleishman, S., Zuckerman, E., Raptis, G., Hudis, C. A., et al. (2000). A pilot study of interpersonal psychotherapy by telephone with cancer patients and their partners. *Psycho-Oncology, 9,* 44–56.

Dorval, M., Maunsell, E., Deschenes, L., Brisson, J., & Masse, B. (1998). Long-term quality of life after breast cancer: Comparison of 8-year survivors with population controls. *Journal of Clinical Oncology, 16,* 487–494.

Edgar, L., Rosberger, Z., & Nowlis, D. (1993). Coping with cancer during the first year after diagnosis. *Cancer, 69,* 817–828.

Edwards, B., & Clarke, V. (2004). The psychological impact of a cancer diagnosis on families: The influence of family functioning and patients' illness characteristics on depression and anxiety. *Psycho-Oncology, 13,* 562–576.

Ell, K., Nishimoto, R., Mantell, J., & Hamovitch, M. (1988). Longitudinal analysis of psychological adaptation among family members of patients with cancer. *Journal of Psychosomatic Research, 32,* 429–438.

Eton, D. T., Lepore, S. J., & Helgeson, V. S. (2005). Psychological distress in spouses of men treated for early-stage prostate carcinoma. *Cancer, 103,* 2412–2418.

Ferrell, B. R., Grant, M., Funk, B., Garcia, N., Otis-Green, S., & Schaffner, M. L. (1996). Quality of life in breast cancer. *Cancer Practice, 4,* 331–340.

Gall, T. L., & Cornblat, M. W. (2002). Breast cancer survivors give voice: A qualitative analysis of spiritual factors in long term adjustment. *Psycho-Oncology, 11,* 524–535.

Ganz, P. A., Coscarelli, A., Fred, C., Kahn, B., Polinsky, M. L., & Petersen, L. (1996). Breast cancer survivors: Psychosocial concerns and quality of life. *Breast Cancer Research and Treatment, 38,* 183–199.

Ganz, P. A., Desmond, K. A., Leedham, B., Rowland, J. H., Meyerowitz, B. E., & Belin, T. R. (2002). Quality of life in long-term, disease-free survivors of breast cancer: A follow-up study. *Journal of the National Cancer Institute, 94,* 39–49.

Ganz, P. A., Rowland, J. H., Desmond, K., Meyerowitz, B. E., & Wyatt, G. E. (1998). Life after breast cancer: Understanding women's health-related quality of life and sexual functioning. *Journal of Clinical Oncology, 16,* 501–514.

Germino, B. B., Fife, B. L., & Funk, S. G. (1995). Cancer and the partner relationship: What is its meaning? *Seminars in Oncology Nursing, 11,* 43–50.

Gotay, C., & Muraoka, M. (1998). Quality of life in long-term survivors of adult-onset cancers. *Journal of the National Cancer Institute, 90,* 656–667.

Gritz, E. R., Wellisch, D. K., Siau, J., & Wang, H. J. (1990). Long-term effects of testicular cancer on marital relationships. *Psychosomatics, 31,* 301–312.

Hagedoorn, M., Buunk, B. P., Kuijer, R. G., Wobbes, T., & Sanderman, R. (2000). Couples dealing with cancer: Role and gender differences regarding psychological distress and quality of life. *Psycho-Oncology, 9,* 232–242.

Harden, J., Northouse, L. L., & Mood, D. (2006). Qualitative analysis of couples' experience with prostate cancer by age cohort. *Cancer Nursing, 29,* 367–377.

Heim, E., Augustiny, K. F., Schaffner, L., & Valach, L. (1993). Coping with breast cancer over time and situation. *Journal of Psychosomatic Research, 37,* 523–542.

Hilton, B. A. (1993). Issues, problems, and challenges for families coping with breast cancer. *Seminars in Oncology Nursing, 9*, 88–100.

Hilton, B. A. (1994). Family communication patterns in coping with early breast cancer. *Western Journal of Nursing Research, 16*, 366–388.

Hoskins, C. N. (1995). Adjustment to breast cancer in couples. *Psychological Reports, 77*, 435–454.

Hoskins, C. N., Baker, S., Budin, W., Ekstrom, D., Maislin, G., Sherman, D., et al. (1996). Adjustment among husbands of women with breast cancer. *Journal of Psychosocial Oncology, 14*, 41–69.

Jensen, S., & Given, B. (1993). Fatigue affecting family caregivers of cancer patients. *Supportive Care Cancer, 1*, 321–325.

Jepson, C., McCorkle, R., Adler, D., Nuamah, I., & Lusk, E. (1999). Effects of home care on caregivers' psychosocial status. *Image: The Journal of Nursing Scholarship, 31*, 115–120.

Kershaw, T., Northouse, L., Kritpracha, C., Schafenacker, A., & Mood, D. (2004). Coping strategies and quality of life in women with advanced breast cancer and their family caregivers. *Psychology and Health, 19*, 149–156.

Kim, Y., Kashy, D. A., & Evans, T. V. (2007). Age and attachment style impact stress and depressive symptoms among caregivers: A prospective investigation. *Journal of Cancer Survivorship, 1*, 35–43.

Kim, Y., Schulz, R., & Carver, C. S. (2007). Benefit finding in the cancer experience. *Psychosomatic Medicine, 69*, 283–291.

Klerman, G. L., Weissman, M. M., Rounsaville, B. J., & Chevron, E. S. (1984). *Interpersonal psychotherapy of depression*. New York: Basic Books.

Kuijer, R. G., Buunk, B. P., DeJong, G. M., Ybema, J. F., & Sanderman, R. (2004). Effects of a brief intervention program for patients with cancer and their partners on feelings of inequity, relationship quality and psychological distress. *Psycho-Oncology, 13*, 321–334.

Lazarus, R. S., & Folkman, S. (Eds.). (1984). *Stress, appraisal, and coping*. New York: Springer Publishing Company.

Lethborg, C. E., Kissane, D., & Burns, W. I. (2003). "It's not the easy part": The experience of significant others of women with early stage breast cancer at treatment completion. *Social Work in Health Care, 37*, 63–85.

Lewis, F. M., & Deal, L. W. (1995). Balancing our lives: A study of the married couple's experience with breast cancer recurrence. *Oncology Nursing Forum, 22*, 943–953.

Lewis, F. M., & Hammond, M. A. (1992). Psychosocial adjustment of the family to breast cancer: A longitudinal analysis. *Journal of the American Medical Women's Association, 47*, 194–200.

Lewis, F. M., Hammond, M. A., & Woods, N. F. (1993). The family's functioning with newly diagnosed breast cancer in the mother: The development of an explanatory model. *Journal of Behavioral Medicine, 16*, 351–370.

Lewis, F. M., Woods, N. F., Hough, E. E., & Bensley, L. S. (1989). The family's functioning with chronic illness in the mother: The spouse's perspective. *Social Science & Medicine, 29*, 1261–1269.

Lichtman, R. R., Taylor, S. E., & Wood, J. V. (1988). Social support and marital adjustment after breast cancer. *Journal of Psychosocial Oncology, 5*, 47–74.

Maly, R. C., Leake, B., & Silliman, R. A. (2003). Health care disparity in older patients with breast carcinoma. *Cancer, 97*, 1517–1527.

Manne, S., Babb, J., Pinover, W., Horwitz, E., & Ebbert, J. (2004). Psychoeducational group intervention for wives of men with prostate cancer. *Psycho-Oncology, 13*, 37–46.

Manne, S. L., Pape, S. J., Taylor, K. L., & Dougherty, J. (1999). Spouse support, coping, and mood among individuals with cancer. *Annals of Behavioral Medicine, 21*, 111–121.

Martire, L. M., Lustig, A. P., Schulz, R., Miller, G. E., & Helgeson, V. S. (2004). Is it beneficial to involve a family member? A meta-analysis of psychosocial interventions for chronic illness. *Health Psychology, 23*, 599–611.

Matthews, B. A. (2003). Role and gender differences in cancer-related distress: A comparison of survivor and caregiver self-reports. *Oncology Nursing Forum, 30*, 493–499.

McCorkle, R., Strumpf, N. E., Nuamah, I. F., Adler, D. C., Cooley, M. E., Jepson, C., et al. (2000). A specialized home care intervention improves survival among older post-surgical cancer patients. *Journal of the American Geriatrics Society, 48*, 1707–1713.

McCorkle, R., Yost, L., Jepson, C., Malone, D., Baird, S., & Lusk, E. (1993). A cancer experience: Relationship of patient psychosocial responses to caregiver burden over time. *Psycho-Oncology, 2*, 21–32.

McCubbin, H. I., Thompson, A. I., & McCubbin, M. A. (1996). FHI: Family Hardiness Index. In H. I. McCubbin & A. I. Thompson (Eds.), *Family assessment: Resiliency, coping, and adaptation* (pp. 124–130). Madison: University of Wisconsin Press.

McCubbin, M. A., & McCubbin, H. I. (1991). Family stress theory and assessment: The resiliency model of family stress, adjustment, and adaptation. In H. I. McCubbin & A. I. Thompson (Eds.), *Family assessment inventories for research and practice* (pp. 3–22). Madison: University of Wisconsin Press.

McMillan, S. C., Small, B. J., Weitzner, M., Schonwetter, R., Tittle, M., Moody, L., & Haley, W. E. (2006). Impact of coping skills intervention with family caregivers of hospice patients with cancer. *Cancer, 106*, 214–222.

Mellon, S. (2002). Comparisons between cancer survivors and family members on meaning of the illness and family quality of life. *Oncology Nursing Forum, 29*, 1117–1125.

Mellon, S., Kershaw, T. S., Northouse, L. L., & Freeman-Gibb, L. (2007). A family-based model to predict fear of recurrence for cancer survivors and their caregivers. *Psycho-Oncology, 16*, 214–223.

Mellon, S., & Northouse, L. L. (2001). Family survivorship and quality of life following a cancer diagnosis. *Research in Nursing & Health, 24,* 446–459.

Mishel, M. H., Belyea, M., Germino, B. B., Stewart, J. L., Bailey, D. E., Jr., Robertson, C., & Mohler, J. (2002). Helping patients with localized prostate carcinoma manage uncertainty and treatment side effects: Nurse-delivered psychoeducational intervention over the telephone. *Cancer, 94,* 1854–1866.

Morse, S. R., & Fife, B. (1998). Coping with a partner's cancer: Adjustment at four stages of the illness trajectory. *Oncology Nursing Forum, 25,* 751–760.

Neese, L., Schover, L., Klein, E., Zippe, C., & Kupelian, P. A. (2003). Finding help for sexual problems after prostate cancer treatment: A phone survey of men's and women's perspectives. *Psycho-Oncology, 12,* 463–473.

Nezu, A. M., Nezu, C. M., Friedman, S. H., Faddis, S., & Houts, P. S. (1999). *Helping cancer patients cope: A problem-solving approach.* Washington, DC: American Psychological Association.

Nijboer, C., Triemstra, M., Tempelaar, R., Mulder, M., Sanderman, R., & van den Bos, G. A. (2000). Patterns of caregiver experiences among partners of cancer patients. *The Gerontologist, 40,* 738–746.

Northouse, L. L. (1989). A longitudinal study of the adjustment of patients and husbands to breast cancer. *Oncology Nursing Forum, 16,* 511–520.

Northouse, L. L., Dorris, G., & Charron-Moore, C. (1995). Factors affecting couples' adjustment to recurrent breast cancer. *Social Science & Medicine, 41,* 69–76.

Northouse, L. L., Kershaw, T., Mood, D., & Schafenacker, A. (2005). Effects of a family intervention on the quality of life of women with recurrent breast cancer and their family caregivers. *Psycho-Oncology, 14,* 478–491.

Northouse, L. L., Laten, D., & Reddy, P. (1995). Adjustment of women and their husbands to recurrent breast cancer. *Research in Nursing & Health, 18,* 515–524.

Northouse, L. L., Mood, D., Kershaw, T., Schafenacker, A., Mellon, S., Walker, J., et al. (2002). Quality of life of women with recurrent breast cancer and their family members. *Journal of Clinical Oncology, 20,* 4050–4064.

Northouse, L. L., Mood, D. W., Schafenacker, A., Montie, J. E., Sandler, H. M., Forman, J. D., et al. (2007). Randomized clinical trial of a family intervention for prostate cancer patients and their spouses. *Cancer, 110,* 2809–2818.

Northouse, L. L., Mood, D., Templin, T., Mellon, S., & George, T. (2000). Couples' patterns of adjustment to colon cancer. *Social Science & Medicine, 50,* 271–284.

Northouse, L. L., Templin, T., & Mood, D. (2001). Couples' adjustment to breast disease during the first year following diagnosis. *Journal of Behavioral Medicine, 24,* 115–136.

Northouse, L. L., Templin, T., Mood, D., & Oberst, M. (1998). Couples' adjustment to breast cancer and benign breast disease: A longitudinal analysis. *Psycho-Oncology, 7,* 37–48.

Oberst, M. T., & James, R. H. (1985). Going home: Patient and spouse adjustment following cancer surgery. *Topics in Clinical Nursing, 7,* 46–57.

Oberst, M. T., & Scott, D. W. (1988). Postdischarge distress in surgically treated cancer patients and their spouses. *Research in Nursing & Health, 11,* 223–233.

Pistrang, N., & Barker, C. (1995). The partner relationship in psychological response to breast cancer. *Social Science & Medicine, 40,* 789–797.

Rees, C. E., & Bath, P. A. (2000). Exploring the information flow: Partners of women with breast cancer, patients, and healthcare professionals. *Oncology Nursing Forum, 27,* 1267–1275.

Rowland, J. (Ed.). (1990). *Developmental states and adaptation: Adult model.* New York: Oxford University Press.

Schover, L. R., Brey, K., Lipshultz, L. I., & Jeha, S. (2002). Knowledge and experiences regarding cancer, infertility, and sperm banking in younger male survivors. *Journal of Clinical Oncology, 20,* 1880–1889.

Schover, L. R., Fouladi, R. T., Warneke, C. L., Neese, L., Klein, E. A., Zippe, C., & Kupelian, P. A. (2002). Defining sexual outcomes after treatment for localized prostate carcinoma. *Cancer, 95,* 1773–1785.

Schulz, R., & Beach, S. R. (1999). Caregiving as a risk factor for mortality: The caregiver health effects study. *Journal of the American Medical Association, 282,* 2215–2219.

Shands, M. E., Lewis, F. M., Sinsheimer, J., & Cochrane, B. B. (2006). Core concerns of couples living with early stage breast cancer. *Psycho-Oncology, 15,* 1055–1064.

Toseland, R. W., Blanchard, C. G., & McCallion, P. (1995). A problem solving intervention for caregivers of cancer patients. *Social Science & Medicine, 40,* 517–528.

Vess, J. D., Moreland, J. R., & Schwebel, A. I. (1985). A follow-up study of role functioning and the psychological environment of families of cancer patients. *Journal of Psychosocial Oncology, 3,* 1–13.

Walker, L. B. (1997). Adjustments of husbands and wives to breast cancer. *Cancer Practice, 5,* 92–98.

Weiss, T. (2004). Correlates of posttraumatic growth in husbands of breast cancer survivors. *Psycho-Oncology, 13,* 260–268.

Zahlis, E. H., & Shands, M. E. (1991). Breast cancer demands of the illness on the patient's partner. *Journal of Psychosocial Oncology, 9,* 75–93.

Zahlis, E. H., & Shands, M. E. (1993). The impact of breast cancer on the partner 18 months after diagnosis. *Seminars in Oncology Nursing, 9,* 83–97.

27

HEALTH PROMOTION AND DISEASE PREVENTION IN ADULT CANCER SURVIVORS

WENDY DEMARK-WAHNEFRIED AND NOREEN M. AZIZ

Cancer survivors are at increased risk for several conditions (i.e., progressive or recurrent disease, second primaries, obesity, diabetes, cardiovascular disease, osteoporosis, and depression), all of which may negatively influence functional status and overall health (see chap. 24, this volume). The number of known cancer-related sequelae and late effects continues to expand as the population of long-term cancer survivors grows and increasing effort is placed into more vigilant monitoring, recognizing that adverse outcomes may be more prevalent and health issues more complex among medically underserved or ethnoculturally diverse populations (Deimling, Schaefer, Kahana, Bowman, & Reardon, 2006). A variety of behavioral interventions may mitigate elevated risk for many of these late effects (Aziz, 2002; Aziz & Rowland, 2003). However, given that cancer survivorship is a fairly recent phenomenon and one that is just now receiving some of the attention it deserves, few studies have quantified longer term outcomes of lifestyle change specifically within this population (Chlebowski, 2003). Therefore, according to the 2006 American Cancer Society's *Nutrition and Physical Activity During and After Cancer Treatment: An American Cancer Society Guide for Informed Choices*, although no consensus exists to support "convincing evidence of benefit" as it relates to either disease-free or overall survival, current data do provide support for probable or possible benefit for several health behaviors, such as striving for a healthy weight, eating more fruits and vegetables (F&V) and less saturated fat, and increasing physical activity (Doyle et al., 2006). Furthermore, recent reviews of the role of exercise among cancer survivors consistently demonstrate higher levels in physical and functional well-being (e.g., functional capacity, muscular strength, body composition, fatigue) and psychological or emotional well-being (e.g., personality functioning, mood states, self-esteem, quality of life; Agency for Healthcare Research and Quality, 2004).

LIFESTYLE PRACTICES AMONG CANCER SURVIVORS

Although a substantial number of studies have reported that cancer survivors spontaneously make lifestyle changes in hopes of achieving improved health (Blanchard, Baker, et al., 2003; Blanchard, Denniston, et al., 2003; Demark-Wahnefried, Peterson, McBride, Lipkus, & Clipp, 2000; Diller et al., 2002; Earle, Burstein, Winer, & Weeks, 2003; Gritz, Nisenbaum, Elashoff, & Holmes, 1991; Gritz, Schacherer, Koehly, Nielsen, & Abemayor, 1999; Maskarinec, Murphy, Shumay, & Kakai, 2001; Maunsell, Drolet, Brisson, Robert, & Deschenes, 2002; Ostroff et al., 1995; Patterson et al., 2003; Pinto, Maruyama, et al., 2002; Pinto, Trunzo, Reiss, & Shiu, 2002; Salminen et al., 2002; Satia et al., 2004; Tangney, Young, Murtaugh, Cobleigh, & Oleske, 2002; Wayne et al., 2004), more recent population-based reports suggest that these changes may not be as prevalent or as durable as previously thought (Bellizzi, Rowland, Jeffery, & McNeel, 2005; Coups & Ostroff, 2005). Although the practice of some healthful behaviors, such as screening (Diller et al., 2002), appears to be increased among the survivor population, it is questionable whether rates are high enough to offset the additional risk.

Tobacco Use Among Cancer Survivors

At time of diagnosis, the incidence of smoking among those with cancer varies tremendously, approaching 100% among those with tobacco-related cancers of the lung, esophagus, and so on (Aziz & Rowland, 2003) and rates of approximately 8% among men and women diagnosed with non-tobacco-related cancers, such as carcinoma of the prostate or breast (Demark-Wahnefried et al., 2000). Quit rates also vary depending on the strength of association between the behavior and the disease, with quit rates among individuals with lung, head, or neck cancers ranging between 46% and 96% (with 40% "permanent cessation" at 2-year follow-up) and rates of 4% noted among women with breast cancer (Blanchard, Denniston, et al., 2003; Gritz et al., 1991; Salminen et al., 2002). Likewise, alcohol abstinence ranges from 47%

to 59% in those with head and neck cancers (for which the association between drinking and cancer is strong) and between 8% and 16% in breast and lung cancer survivors (for which the strength of association is either weaker and/or newly established; Allison, 2001; Salminen et al., 2002).

Physical Activity Among Cancer Survivors

The cross-sectional study by Demark-Wahnefried et al. (2000) suggests that 58% of breast and prostate cancer survivors "routinely exercise." However, it must be borne in mind that this study was conducted at a time when the physical activity guidelines were 20 minutes per day, three times per week. Given more recent guidelines that endorse greater standards for frequency and duration, it is doubtful whether a majority of cancer survivors would be classified as "active." In addition, although some studies report increasing levels of physical activity among survivors (Bellizzi et al., 2005; Pinto, Trunzo, et al., 2002), other studies suggest that these effects are mixed, with some subjects reporting more exercise and others reporting less (Blanchard, Denniston, et al., 2003; Salminen et al., 2002).

Dietary Intakes of Cancer Survivors

Consumption of a healthier diet after diagnosis is reported by 30% to 52% of survivors, with a majority indicating reduced intakes of meat and increased consumption of F&Vs (Maunsell et al., 2002; Salminen et al., 2002). Study findings by Tangney et al. (2002) suggest that breast cancer survivors consume diets of higher quality compared with the general population, with other studies showing that 45% to 69% of survivors consume diets with less than 30% of energy from fat and 25% to 42% consume at least five servings of F&Vs per day (Demark-Wahnefried et al., 2000; Pinto, Maruyama, et al., 2002). Findings of Wayne et al. (2004) provided evidence that some of these changes (i.e., increased F&V consumption) may be durable, whereas others (i.e., dietary fat restriction) may be subject to recidivism, thereby paralleling the findings of Gritz et al. (1991) with regard to smoking cessation. In addition, despite improved dietary intakes, the majority of successfully treated cancer survivors remain overweight or obese (Pinto, Maruyama, et al., 2002) and experience significant and continued weight gain over time (Wayne et al., 2004).

FACTORS INFLUENCING LIFESTYLE CHANGE AMONG CANCER SURVIVORS

Although some cancer survivors may initiate positive behavioral changes, others—especially men and those who are less educated, who are over age 65, or who live in urban areas—may be less likely to undertake healthful changes in behavior (Allison, 2001; Blanchard, Baker, et al., 2003; Demark-Wahnefried et al., 2000; Maunsell et al., 2002) or may be less likely to maintain them (Gritz et al., 1999). These high-risk individuals may require specific interventions to assist them with the adoption of healthful behaviors. Although a positive impact of physicians' recommendations on favorably altering lifestyle practices is observed, only about 20% of physicians do so (Blanchard, Baker, et al., 2003; Demark-Wahnefried et al., 2000); this is clearly an underused partnership in health promotion among cancer survivors. Indeed, a recent trial ($N = 450$) conducted by Jones, Courneya, Fairey, and Mackey (2004) provides strong evidence of the impact of a physician's recommendation, because breast cancer patients randomized to an arm receiving an oncologist's recommendation to exercise reported a mean increase of 3.4 metabolic equivalent task hours per week, as compared with those not receiving a similar message ($p = .011$).

BEHAVIORAL INTERVENTIONS AMONG CANCER SURVIVORS

To date, reports exist on well over 24 behavioral interventions that have used randomized controlled designs in areas of exercise (e.g., aerobic, solely; strength-training, with or without aerobics), diet (e.g., dietary fat restriction, increased F&Vs, energy restriction), multiple behavior (i.e., diet and exercise), smoking cessation, and skin protection and reduced sun exposure (Chlebowski et al., 2006; Daley et al., 2007; Demark-Wahnefried, Aziz, Rowland, & Pinto, 2005; Demark-Wahnefried et al., 2006, 2007; Nikander et al., 2007; Ohira, Schmitz, Ahmed, & Yee, 2006; Pierce et al., 2007; Pinto, Frierson, Rabin, Trunzo, & Marcus, 2005; Thorsen et al., 2005).

Roughly one third of studies among cancer survivors report any theoretical basis. Of the studies that report a reliance on behavioral theory, social-cognitive theory, the transtheoretical model, and the theory of planned behavior are evenly represented (Ajzen, 1991; Bandura, 1977; Prochaska & DiClemente, 1983).

Seventy percent of studies have relied on self-reported outcomes (e.g., change in dietary intake, quality of life) and an equal proportion have relied on physiologic measures (e.g., weight loss, walk tests) or both (e.g., quit rates with nicotine confirmation). Favorable outcomes have been reported in an overwhelming majority of studies (approximately 96%), although adequate control for confounding factors and appropriate analyses to account for attrition and adherence have not always been performed. The bias inherent with the publication of positive findings, as opposed to negative findings, also may have contributed to the high degree of reported success.

Of note, two large, well-controlled, multisite, theory-based behavioral intervention trials have recently produced results as to whether modifications in diet affect disease-free and/or overall survival (endpoints with obvious import). Findings of the Women's Intervention Nutrition Study found a reduced rate of recurrence among postmenopausal breast cancer patients who adhered to a low-fat diet (< 15% of energy from fat) compared with patients randomized to an attention control (i.e., a well-balanced diet); reductions in risk were particularly strong among women with estrogen receptor negative disease, although losses of weight may have confounded findings (Chlebowski et al., 2006). In contrast, the Women's Healthy Eating and Living Study (i.e., a trial that tested the effect of daily intakes of five vegetable servings, 16 ounces of vegetable juice, three fruit servings, 15% to 20% energy from fat, and 30 g dietary fiber in 3,088 pre- and postmenopausal breast cancer patients) found no reduction in recurrence among women randomized to the experimental arm (Pierce et al., 2007).

FUTURE DIRECTIONS

As the number of cancer survivors continues to grow and more attention is placed on health promotion and disease prevention in this high-risk population, the sophistication of behavioral interventions, the sample representation, and the import of findings should improve. Well-controlled, theory-based interventions are likely to become the norm, rather than the exception. There is a clear need, however, to develop innovative programs that can effectively accomplish the following: (a) promote behavior change in content areas that are most likely to contribute to the overall health and well-being of cancer survivors; (b) provide delivery at a point in time most likely to ensure uptake; (c) combine or sequence messages to facilitate change in multiple arenas; (d) use delivery channels and formats that are well understood, well accepted, and convenient; (e) provide guidance to overcome common barriers; and (f) target cancer populations that are currently underserved and/or most in need, that is, those with underrepresented cancers, minorities, older people, and long-term survivors (Aziz & Rowland, 2003; Stull, Snyder, & Demark-Wahnefried, 2007). Through an iterative and rigorous process of development and testing, some of the problems indigenous to current studies, that is, high rates of attrition and the accrual of samples that tend to be exclusively White and well-heeled, may be lessened as innovative and cost-effective programs become a reality.

REFERENCES

Agency for Healthcare Research and Quality. (2004). *Effectiveness of behavioral interventions to modify physical activity behaviors in general populations and cancer patients and survivors* (AHRQ Publication No. 04-E027-2). Rockville, MD: U.S. Department of Health and Human Services.

Ajzen, I. (1991). The theory of planned behavior. *Organizational Behavior and Human Decision Processes, 50,* 179–211.

Allison, P. (2001). Factors associated with smoking and alcohol consumption following treatment for head and neck cancer. *Oral Oncology, 37,* 513–520.

Aziz, N. (2002). Cancer survivorship research: Challenge and opportunity. *Journal of Nutrition, 32*(Suppl.), 3494–3503.

Aziz, N., & Rowland, J. (2003). Trends and advances in cancer survivorship research: Challenge and opportunity. *Seminars in Radiation Oncology, 13,* 248–266.

Bandura, A. (1977). *Social learning theory.* Englewood Cliffs, NJ: Prentice Hall.

Bellizzi, K. M., Rowland, J. H., Jeffery, D. D., & McNeel, T. (2005). Health behaviors of cancer survivors: Examining opportunities for cancer control intervention. *Journal of Clinical Oncology, 23,* 8884–8893.

Blanchard, C. M., Baker, F., Denniston, M. M., Courneya, K. S., Hann, D. M., Gesme, D. H., et al. (2003). Is absolute amount or change in exercise more associated with quality of life in adult cancer survivors? *Preventive Medicine, 37,* 389–395.

Blanchard, C. M., Denniston, M., Baker, F., Ainsworth, S., Courneya, K., Hann, D., et al. (2003). Do adults change their lifestyle behaviors after a cancer diagnosis? *American Journal of Health Behavior, 27,* 246–256.

Chlebowski, R. T. (2003). The American Cancer Society guide for nutrition and physical activity for cancer survivors: A call to action for clinical investigators. *CA: A Cancer Journal for Clinicians, 53,* 266–267.

Chlebowski, R. T., Blackburn, G. L., Thomson, C. A., Nixon, D. W., Shapiro, A., Hoy, M. K., et al. (2006). Dietary fat reduction and breast cancer outcome: Interim efficacy results from the Women's Intervention Nutrition Study. *Journal of the National Cancer Institute, 98,* 1767–1776.

Coups, E. J., & Ostroff, J. S. (2005). A population-based estimate of the prevalence of behavioral risk factors among adult cancer survivors and noncancer controls. *Preventive Medicine, 40,* 702–711.

Daley, A. J., Crank, H., Saxton, J. M., Mutrie, N., Coleman, R., & Roalfe, A. (2007). Randomized trial of exercise therapy in women treated for breast cancer. *Journal of Clinical Oncology, 25,* 1713–1721.

Deimling, G. T., Schaefer, M. L., Kahana, B., Bowman, K. F., & Reardon, J. (2006). Racial differences in the health of older adult long-term cancer survivors. *Psychosocial Oncology, 15,* 306–320.

Demark-Wahnefried, W., Aziz, N. M., Rowland, J. H., & Pinto, B. M. (2005). Riding the crest of the teachable moment: Promoting long-term health after the diagnosis of cancer. *Journal of Clinical Oncology, 23,* 5814–5830.

Demark-Wahnefried, W., Clipp, E. C., Lipkus, I. M., Lobach, D., Snyder, D. C., Sloane, R., et al. (2007). Main outcomes of the FRESH START trial: A sequentially tailored, diet and exercise mailed print intervention among breast and prostate cancer survivors. *Journal of Clinical Oncology, 25,* 2709–2718.

Demark-Wahnefried, W., Clipp, E. C., Morey, M., Pieper, C., Sloane, R., Snyder, D. C., & Cohen, H. J. (2006). Lifestyle intervention development study to improve physical function in older adults with cancer: Outcomes from Project LEAD. *Journal of Clinical Oncology, 24,* 3465–3473.

Demark-Wahnefried, W., Peterson, B., McBride, C., Lipkus, I., & Clipp, E. (2000). Current health behaviors and readiness to pursue life-style changes among men and women diagnosed with early stage prostate and breast carcinomas. *Cancer, 88,* 674–684.

Diller, L., Medeiros Nancarrow, C., Shaffer, K., Matulonis, U., Mauch, P., Neuberg, D., et al. (2002). Breast cancer screening in women previously treated for Hodgkin's disease: A prospective cohort study. *Journal of Clinical Oncology, 20,* 2085–2091.

Doyle, C., Kushi, L. H., Byers, T., Courneya, K. S., Demark-Wahnefried, W., Grant, B., et al. (2006). Nutrition and physical activity during and after cancer treatment: An American Cancer Society guide for informed choices. *CA: A Cancer Journal for Clinicians, 56,* 323–353.

Earle, C., Burstein, H., Winer, E., & Weeks, J. (2003). Quality of non-breast cancer health maintenance among elderly breast cancer survivors. *Journal of Clinical Oncology, 21,* 1447–1451.

Gritz, E., Nisenbaum, R., Elashoff, R., & Holmes, E. (1991). Smoking behavior following diagnosis in patients with Stage I non-small cell lung cancer. *Cancer Causes & Control, 2,* 105–112.

Gritz, E., Schacherer, C., Koehly, L., Nielsen, I., & Abemayor, E. (1999). Smoking withdrawal and relapse in head and neck cancer patients. *Head & Neck, 21,* 420–427.

Jones, L. W., Courneya, K. S., Fairey, A. S., & Mackey, J. R. (2004). Effects of an oncologist's recommendation to exercise on self-reported exercise behavior in newly diagnosed breast cancer survivors: A single-blind, randomized controlled trial. *Annals of Behavioral Medicine, 28,* 105–113.

Maskarinec, G., Murphy, S., Shumay, D., & Kakai, H. (2001). Dietary changes among cancer survivors. *European Journal of Cancer Care, 10,* 12–20.

Maunsell, E., Drolet, M., Brisson, J., Robert, J., & Deschenes, L. (2002). Dietary change after breast cancer: Extent, predictors, and relation with psychological distress. *Journal of Clinical Oncology, 20,* 1017–1025.

Nikander, R., Sievanen, H., Ojala, K., Oivanen, T., Kellokumpu-Lehtinen, P. L., & Saarto, T. (2007). Effect of a vigorous aerobic regimen on physical performance in breast cancer patients—A randomized controlled pilot trial. *Acta Oncologica, 46,* 181–186.

Ohira, T., Schmitz, K. H., Ahmed, R. L., & Yee, D. (2006). Effects of weight training on quality of life in recent breast cancer survivors: The Weight Training for Breast Cancer Survivors (WTBS) study. *Cancer, 106,* 2076–2083.

Ostroff, J. S., Jacobsen, P. B., Moadel, A. B., Spiro, R. H., Shah, J. P., Strong, E. W., et al. (1995). Prevalence and predictors of continued tobacco use after treatment of patients with head and neck cancer. *Cancer, 75,* 569–576.

Patterson, R. E., Neuhouser, M. L., Hedderson, M. M., Schwartz, S. M., Standish, L. J., & Bowen, D. J. (2003). Changes in diet, physical activity, and supplement use among adults diagnosed with cancer. *Journal of the American Dietetic Association*, *103*, 323–328.

Pierce, J. P., Natarajan, L., Caan, B. J., Parker, B. A., Greenberg, E. R., Flatt, S. W., et al. (2007). Influence of a diet very high in vegetables, fruit, and fiber and low in fat on prognosis following treatment for breast cancer: The Women's Healthy Eating and Living (WHEL) randomized trial. *Journal of the American Medical Association*, *298*, 289–298.

Pinto, B. M., Frierson, G. M., Rabin, C., Trunzo, J. J., & Marcus, B. H. (2005). Home-based physical activity intervention for breast cancer patients. *Journal of Clinical Oncology*, *23*, 3577–3587.

Pinto, B. M., Maruyama, N., Clark M., Cruess, D., Park, E., & Roberts, M. (2002). Motivation to modify lifestyle risk behaviors in women treated for breast cancer. *Mayo Clinic Proceedings*, *77*, 122–129.

Pinto, B. M., Trunzo, J., Reiss, P., & Shiu, S. (2002). Exercise participation after diagnosis of breast cancer: Trends and effects on mood and quality of life. *Psycho-Oncology*, *11*, 389–400.

Prochaska, J. O., & DiClemente, C. C. (1983). Stages and processes of self-change of smoking: Toward an integrative model of change. *Journal of Consultation Clinical Psychology*, *51*, 390–395.

Salminen, E., Heikkila, S., Poussa, T., Lagstrom, H., Saario, R., & Salminen, S. (2002). Female patients tend to alter their diet following the diagnosis of rheumatoid arthritis and breast cancer. *Preventive Medicine*, *34*, 529–535.

Satia, J. A., Campbell, M. K., Galanko, J. A., James, A., Carr, C., & Sandler, R. S. (2004). Longitudinal changes in lifestyle behaviors and health status in colon cancer survivors. *Cancer Epidemiology, Biomarkers & Prevention*, *13*, 1022–1031.

Stull, V. B., Snyder, D. C., & Demark-Wahnefried, W. (2007). Lifestyle interventions in cancer survivors: Designing programs that meet the needs of this vulnerable and growing population. *Journal of Nutrition*, *137*(Suppl.), 243–248.

Tangney, C., Young, J., Murtaugh, M., Cobleigh, M., & Oleske, D. (2002). Self-reported dietary habits, overall dietary quality and symptomatology of breast cancer survivors: A cross-sectional examination. *Breast Cancer Research and Treatment*, *71*, 113–123.

Thorsen, L., Skovlund, E., Stromme, S. B., Hornslien, K., Dahl, A. A., & Fossa, S. D. (2005). Effectiveness of physical activity on cardiorespiratory fitness and health-related quality of life in young and middle-aged cancer patients shortly after chemotherapy. *Journal of Clinical Oncology*, *23*, 2378–2388.

Wayne, S. J., Lopez, S. T., Butler, L. M., Baumgartner, K. B., Baumgartner, R. N., & Ballard-Barbash, R. (2004). Changes in dietary intake after diagnosis of breast cancer. *Journal of the American Dietetic Association*, *104*, 1561–1568.

VII

FUTURE DIRECTIONS IN BEHAVIORAL SCIENCE AND CANCER

FUTURE DIRECTIONS
IN BEHAVIORAL SCIENCE
AND CANCER

Part VII discusses the emerging clinical and research directions in the field of behavioral science and cancer. In chapter 28, Stefanek and McDonald review evidence for the role of psychological variables in the development and progression of cancer, as well as evidence relating to the biological mechanisms that may mediate a link between psychological variables and cancer. Chapter 29, by White and Dignan, reviews the approaches, theoretical frameworks, and available tools for integrating research findings into evidence-based medicine and public health practice and documents the availability of proven and promising methods to bridge the gap from research to practice. In chapter 30, McBride defines and reviews progress in achieving transdisciplinary collaboration in cancer control research and illustrates the need for transdisciplinary approaches to accelerate progress in reducing cancer incidence and mortality. Finally, chapter 31, by Strecher, addresses the potential of the Internet as a communication medium in cancer control and documents the dramatic growth in Internet use over the past decade. It also reviews the evidence base for the effectiveness of various forms of Internet-based health interventions.

28

BRAIN, BEHAVIOR, AND IMMUNITY IN CANCER

MICHAEL STEFANEK AND PAIGE GREEN MCDONALD

In this chapter, we report on the evidence for psychological variables as they relate to the development and progression of cancer. We begin by examining potential biological mechanisms that may mediate the link between psychological variables and disease. We next examine the clinical evidence that such variables relate to cancer development, progression, and survival. Finally, we address future directions in these complex research areas involving the interplay of biology and psychology.

PSYCHOLOGICAL FACTORS AND CANCER: BIOLOGICAL MECHANISMS

S. Cohen and Herbert (1996) succinctly defined *psychoneuroimmunology* as "the study of the interrelations between the central nervous system and the immune system" (p. 114). The psychoneuroimmunological paradigm postulates that the immune system, through neural and endocrine processes, mediates an association between psychological factors and disease. Because it is clearly beyond the scope of this chapter to review the comprehensive literature that has amassed on psychosocial factors and the immune system, see S. Cohen and Herbert (1996); Glaser and Kiecolt-Glaser (2005); Kiecolt-Glaser and Glaser (1991); and Kiecolt-Glaser, McGuire, Robles, and Glaser (2002) for reviews.

The Cancer Immunoediting Concept

Dunn, Bruce, Ikeda, Old, and Schreiber (2002) suggested that the ability of cancer cells to evade the extrinsic tumor suppressor function of the immune system is a result of a cancer immunoediting process. They conceptualized three phases in this process: elimination, equilibrium, and escape. The elimination phase incorporates adaptive and innate functions of the immune system in an attempt to eradicate the developing tumor. If a tumor cell evades the elimination phase, then host and tumor cell enter an active equilibrium phase in which the fight for survival results in cells that become increasingly resistant to the immune system. This phase yields continually unstable and mutating cells that eventually form tumors with lower immunogenicity. The equilibrium phase can be conceptualized as the latent period between initial carcinogenic exposure and clinical detection of the tumor. During the escape phase, tumor cells are allowed to proliferate within their microenvironment because of an established resistance to immune detection and elimination. We use the cancer immunoediting concept and recent advances in the conceptualization of the tumor microenvironment as springboards for discussing the association between psychosocial factors, cancer, and cellular immune function.

Psychosocial Factors, Cancer, and Immunity

Divergent lines of research have established that psychological factors can alter the number and functionality of cellular and humoral immunity (Maier, Watkins, & Fleshner, 1994). What remains less substantiated is whether psychologically induced changes in immunity are of the type and magnitude to influence tumor induction, growth, and metastases (S. Cohen & Rabin, 1998; Maier et al., 1994). A critical perspective to maintain is cancer as a heterogeneous group of diseases diverse in etiology, tumor microenvironments, disease course, susceptibility profiles, and immunoregulatory characteristics. Psychosocial factors may vary in level of influence with respect to cancer type and phase of tumor growth and will have differential impacts on immunity and consequently different outcomes (Maier et al., 1994). Furthermore, the effect of psychosocial factors, such as stress, depends on host characteristics, the nature of the stressor, and the immune parameters of interest (Moynihan, 2003).

The relationship between psychosocial factors and cancer has yet to be well defined or established. Although far from unequivocal, promising work has recently highlighted the potential role of chronic depression in cancer etiology and progression (Everson et al., 1996; Penninx et al., 1998; Spiegel & Giese-Davis, 2003). Depression, like cancer, should be considered a heterogenous syndrome (Kendler et al., 1996). Depression can be conceptualized as a chronic and maladaptive stress response that triggers the hypothalamic–pituitary–adrenal (HPA) axis and the sympathetic nervous system (SNS; Irwin, 1999; Maier & Watkins, 2000). The hypothalamus secretes corticotropin-releasing hormone (CRH) upon stressor stimulation. CRH causes the anterior pituitary gland to release adrenocorticotropic hormone. This hormone acts on the adrenal cortex and stimulates production and secretion of the stress hormone cortisol into peripheral blood. Cortisol is thought to be the key hormone underlying stress-mediated immune alterations in humans (Moynihan, 2003). Cells of the immune system express receptors for cortisol and other hormones. Furthermore, the SNS innervates organs of the immune system and immune cells contain receptors for the catecholamines norepinephrine (NE) and epinephrine (EPI; Madden, 2003; Maier et al., 1994). Catecholamines alter immune cell proliferation, cytokine and antibody production, lytic activity, and migration (Madden, 2003). Madden (2003) noted that SNS can either enhance or suppress the immune system, according to the characteristics of sympathetic activation (e.g., magnitude, timing) and individual differences. It is within this theoretical framework that we discuss physiological mechanisms linking depression and cancer via neuroimmune processes.

Depression and Cancer: Plausible Mechanism

As noted by Croyle (1998), the mechanisms linking depression with cancer etiology have not been clearly defined. Several pathways are plausible, ranging from the indirect effects of health behaviors (e.g., alcohol and tobacco use, physical activity, diet) to more direct biological mechanisms mediated by bidirectional interactions between the central nervous system, immune system, and endocrine system (see Exhibit 28.1). Penninx et al. (1998) offered the following explanations for a positive association between chronic depression and cancer risk among an elderly population: (a) confounding (e.g., shared genetic predisposition between depression and cancer or common alterations in neuroimmune pathways that result in immunosuppression), (b) differential cancer risk due to smoking behavior, (c) use of antidepressants, and (d) indirect influence of health behaviors associated with an increase in cancer risk. Furthermore, Penninx et al. proposed that cortisol-related dysregulation of the HPA axis may account for their findings. Indeed, chronically elevated cortisol levels are observed in depressed populations and cancer patients (Smith, 1991). Sustained release of cortisol results in immunosuppression of T-lymphocytes and natural killer (NK) cytotoxicity (Maier et al., 1994; McEwen, 1998). Shi et al. (2003) suggested that a reduction in lymphocyte number is associated with increased cancer incidence and

Lifestyle and behavior

Dysregulation of the hypothalamic–pituitary–adrenal axis
Modulation of natural killer cell number and function
Suppression of melatonin
Disruption of neuroendocrine and immune circadian rhythms
Suppression of cell-mediated immunity
Dysregulation of proinflammatory cytokines
Chronic cellular immune activation
DNA repair
Apoptosis
Angiogenesis

tumor growth. Corresponding to the immune surveillance hypothesis, Kiecolt-Glaser and Glaser (1999a, 1999b) and Spiegel and Sephton (2001) noted that psychosocial factors, such as stress, can indirectly affect carcinogenesis by suppressing the functionality of NK cells. Increasing stress levels were found to compromise NK cell lysis and cytokine response, and the proliferative response of peripheral blood lymphocytes in women surgically treated for invasive breast cancer (Andersen et al., 1998). Classic studies by Levy et al. (Levy et al., 1990; Levy, Herberman, Lippman, D'Angelo, & Lee, 1991) revealed higher NK activity in Stage I and II breast cancer patients who reported perceptions of high social support or among those actively seeking social support. Furthermore, lower NK activity has been shown to predict disease recurrence in breast cancer (Levy et al., 1991).

Several immunological models have been proposed that explore the relationship between stress, depression, and cancer progression (Holden, Pakula, & Mooney, 1998; Murr et al., 2000). Holden et al. (1998) proposed a model based on the dysregulation of inflammatory cytokines. On the basis of their synthesis of the literature, depression is associated with elevated IFN-γ, IL-1β, IL-6, β-endorphin, and soluble IL-2 receptor, down-regulated IL-2, and reduced NK activity. They hypothesize that tumor progression is facilitated through reduced NK activity due to elevated β-endorphin and an inhibition of major histocompatibility Class I molecule expression as a result of elevated TNF-α. Murr et al. (2000) asserted that depression in cancer is a result of chronic cellular immune stimulation associated with aggressive tumor types. Aggressive tumors are thought to cause sustained and elevated neopterin concentrations. This sustained immune activation results in low plasma tryptophan and serotonin concentrations. The resulting neurotransmitter imbalance increases susceptibility to mood disturbances and depression.

Stress and depression may directly affect carcinogenesis through non-neuroimmune-mediated mechanisms like DNA repair, apoptosis, and angiogenesis (Forlenza & Baum, 2000; Kiecolt-Glaser & Glaser, 1999a; Lutgendorf et al., 2003). It is likely that the influence of psychosocial factors on DNA repair is mediated by stressor and host characteristics. Conflicting findings of increases in lymphocyte-mediated DNA repair have been noted during acute stress situations (e.g., examination) with young healthy samples (L. Cohen, Marshall, Cheng, Agarwal, & Wei, 2000; Forlenza & Baum, 2000; Forlenza, Latimer, & Baum, 2000). Acute psychological stress was found to decrease lymphocyte apoptosis or immune cell death (Tomei, Kiecolt-Glaser, Kennedy, & Glaser, 1990).

Angiogenesis is the formation of new blood vessels and a critical process for the establishment of tumor growth and metastasis. Vascular endothelial growth factor (VEGF) is a potent promoter of angiogenesis and is associated with metastatic disease and poor survival in ovarian cancer (Lutgendorf et al., 2002). Although significant findings were not noted for depression, patients with ovarian cancer who reported greater helplessness or worthlessness and higher levels of distress had higher levels of VEGF (Lutgendorf et al., 2002). Furthermore, the neurotransmitters NE, EPI, and isoproterenol can directly enhance VEGF production in vitro in ovarian cancer cell lines (Lutgendorf et al., 2003). This suggests a plausible biobehavioral pathway by which stress and other psychosocial factors can influence tumor growth and disease progression (for a recent review of biobehavioral pathways, see Antoni et al., 2006).

Other mechanisms that might mediate the pathway between psychological factors and cancer have been proposed. Sephton and Spiegel (2003) proposed several indirect and direct pathways by which circadian disruption may mediate the influence of psychosocial factors on tumor growth and cancer survival. Melatonin suppression also might mediate psychosocial effects on cancer incidence (Davis, Mirick, & Stevens, 2001; Schernhammer et al., 2001). These mechanisms need research attention.

PSYCHOSOCIAL VARIABLES AND CANCER DEVELOPMENT

A host of studies have examined cancer etiology as influenced directly by psychosocial factors, including personality style (Lillberg, Verkasalo, Kaprio, Helenius, & Koskenvuo, 2002), coping style (Chen et al., 1995), life events (Geyer, 1993), stress (Roberts, Newcomb, Trentham-Dietz, & Storer, 1996), depression (Penninx et al., 1998), and hopelessness (Everson et al., 1996). In sum, the work on the role of psychosocial variables and cancer development is long on quantity and short on quality. A number of methodological concerns have been noted by Butow et al. (2000); Dalton, Boesen, Ross, Schapiro, and Johansen (2002); and Fox (1978), among others. A disproportionate number of studies have focused on breast cancer (Lillberg et al., 2001, 2003; Lillberg, Verkasalo, Kaprio, Helenius, & Koskenvuo, 2002; Lillberg, Verkasalo, Kaprio, Teppo, et al., 2002; Price et al., 2001) or all cancer sites (Dalton, Boesen, et al., 2002; Dalton, Mellemkjaer, Olsen, Mortensen, & Johansen, 2002; Penninx et al., 1998; Schapiro et al., 2000, 2001; Schapiro, Nielsen, Jorgensen, Boesen, & Johansen, 2002). No clear rationale for this selection on the basis of biological factors such as tumor growth, specific risk factors across cancer sites, genetic risk, and so on, is provided. Many earlier studies did not use multivariate analyses to estimate the independent effect of psychosocial factors on cancer risk. As noted previously, many studies have a small sample size, thus limiting power. Personality factors tested were often disparate across studies, so that few have been adequately tested, with little replication. In many cases, lifestyle factors have not been examined. This is of potential importance, because personality may impact lifestyle (i.e., healthy and unhealthy behaviors), thus mediating increased cancer risk. Recent work linking chronic depression or multiple acute episodes of depression to cancer development is intriguing (Penninx et al., 1998). Much of the work finding no link between depression and cancer risk has involved either psychiatric diagnoses or single measures of depression (Dalton, Boesen, et al., 2002; Dalton, Mellemkjaer, et al., 2002).

PSYCHOSOCIAL VARIABLES AND CANCER PROGRESSION

The role of psychosocial variables on cancer progression has also been a topic of intense debate over the past several decades, even before Spiegel, Bloom, Kraemer, and Gottheil's (1989) article assessing the role of group psychological intervention among women with metastatic breast cancer. The results of studies investigating these variables and their link to cancer progression have been quite inconsistent, with methodological critiques provided by several investigators (Cella & Holland, 1988; Edelman, Lemon, Bell, & Kidman, 1999; Fox, 1983, 1995).

As previously discussed, there is suggestive evidence that chronic depression may be linked to cancer incidence, although this connection is far from confirmed. Among diagnosed cancer patients, reports of depressed mood are clearly quite common (Derogatis et al., 1983; Stefanek, Derogatis, & Shaw, 1987) and roughly comparable to rates among patients with other medical diagnoses (Evans et al., 1999). An intriguing question related to cancer and depression is whether depression not only impacts the quality of life of a significant number of cancer patients but also affects medical outcome. The data linking depression to cancer progression are somewhat mixed, complicated by the impact of disease progression on mood and findings of certain cancer treatments creating sickness behavior, including mood changes, fatigue, and cachexia, all considered classic signs of depressive disorder.

Spiegel and Giese-Davis (2003) reviewed the literature examining the link between depression and cancer progression or survival, and they noted a positive association in 15 of 24 published studies. Restricting our discussion to findings from 1998 to 2003, several major studies indeed found such a link (Brown, Levy, Rosberger, & Edgar, 2003; Herrmann et al., 1998; Loberiza et al., 2002; Stommel, Given, & Given, 2002; Watson, Haviland, Greer, Davidson, & Bliss, 1999). Recent research (Brown et al., 2003; Teno et al., 2000; Tross et al., 1996) holds promise for better methodology and some intriguing findings. We refer readers to (a) Uchino, Cacioppo, and Kiecolt-Glaser (1996) and Uchino, Uno, and Holt-Lunstad (1999), for excellent reviews of the role of social support, physiological processes, and health; (b) House, Landis, and Umberson (1988), for their landmark work on social relationships and health; (c) Reifman (1995), for reviews of work related to social relationships, recovery from illness, and survival, including breast cancer; and (d) Geyer (1996) and Maunsell, Brisson, and Deschenes (1995), for work specifically related to cancer. The findings, as they apply to cancer, are somewhat mixed but worthy of continuing investigation.

In addition to social support, psychosocial variables, such as stressful life experiences (Graham, Ramirez, Love, Richards, & Burgess, 2002), coping styles (Faller, Bulzebruck, Drings, & Lang, 1999), fighting spirit (Greer, 1983), hopelessness (Stern, Dhanda, & Hazuda, 2001), and emotional repression (Giraldi, Rodani, Cartei, & Grassi, 1997), among many others, have been examined for their role in cancer progression or mortality. None of these psychosocial factors has a strong enough body of work in terms of solid methodology and replication to warrant confidence as major players in cancer survival.

The body of work examining depression and cancer progression is intriguing, albeit results have been mixed. Perhaps the most promising area worthy of replication studies involves the role of chronic depression and/or repeated acute depressed states and cancer progression. This area is promising because of findings that note decreased survival with higher levels of depression and also because of the quite plausible, testable psychophysiological mechanisms linking depression and cancer progression noted earlier in this chapter.

PSYCHOLOGICAL INTERVENTIONS AND CANCER SURVIVAL

A handful of studies have examined the role of psychological interventions in extending survival of cancer patients (Coyne, Stefanek, & Palmer, 2007). Roughly half of the studies listed have shown increased survival of patients receiving intervention versus those randomized to a control group. The host of differences and methodological problems across studies may help explain the disparate results. Some interventions involved individual therapy sessions (Kuchler et al., 1999; Linn, Linn, & Harris, 1982), whereas others used a group therapy format (Goodwin et al., 2001; Spiegel et al., 1989, 2007). The number of sessions of therapeutic contact varied greatly across studies, ranging from weekly group sessions for 1 year or more (Spiegel et al., 1989, 2007) to three individual contacts over a 4-week period (McCorkle et al., 2000). Cancer sites included metastatic breast cancer (Spiegel et al., 1989, 2007), malignant melanoma (Fawzy et al., 1993), gastrointestinal cancers (Kuchler et al., 1999), or multiple sites and stages within individual studies (Ilnyckyj, 1994; McCorkle et al., 2000). Finally, the content of the interventions differed greatly, from supportive–expressive group therapy (Goodwin et al., 2001; Spiegel et al., 1989, 2007), to cognitive behavior therapy (Cunningham et al., 1998, 2000; Edelman et al., 1999), to more unstructured psychotherapy (Kuchler et al., 1999).

Spiegel (2002) examined shared elements among those studies demonstrating improved survival across these trials, noting that each had an educational component, were homogeneous for disease stage and type, had supportive environments, and used as one component of the intervention some degree of coping skills and stress management teaching. Moreover, those studies showing survival benefit from intervention were also those in which intervention resulted in psychological benefit. However, these elements do not cleanly separate studies showing effect from those not favoring a psychological intervention. In the studies by Fawzy et al. (1993), Goodwin et al. (2001), and Linn et al. (1982), patients assigned to the intervention group showed psychological improvements without concomitant survival advantage.

In addition, both Goodwin et al. (2001) and Spiegel et al.(1989, 2007) enrolled only women with metastatic breast cancer, used quite structured supportive–expressive therapy interventions, and involved comparable exposure to the intervention (i.e., weekly group sessions over a 1-year period). However, although Spiegel's (1989) intervention group showed a doubling of survival versus control group participants, no survival difference between groups was found in the Goodwin et al. (2001) nor Spiegel et al. (2007) study, clearly challenging the long-standing findings of increased survival found in the original Spiegel (1989) study.

Finally, when this body of research work is reviewed or summarized (Edelman et al., 1999; Spiegel, 2002), these summaries typically include interventions that are far more educational than psychological in nature. For instance, the studies by Richardson, Shelton, Krailo, and Levine (1990) and McCorkle et al. (2000) both involved primarily, if not exclusively, educational approaches involving medication compliance checks during home visits and telephone contacts by nurses over fairly restricted time periods. These interventions did not exclude the provision of some degree of patient support, but including these in formal analyses of psychological interventions defines the term *psychological* quite loosely.

In sum, the data do not support the hypothesis that psychological interventions significantly impact the survival time of cancer patients. Examining studies both supporting and not supporting an intervention impact on disease, one can clearly see that unknown selection biases, methodological concerns, and/or poor reporting of the trials presents a challenge to interpretation and clearly dampens enthusiasm for intervention effects on survival. For an excellent systematic critical review of these studies individually and collectively, see Coyne et al. (2007).

FUTURE DIRECTIONS

It is tempting to dismiss the role of psychosocial variables in the etiology of cancer, given its long, complex, and rather unproductive history. However, research in a given area should not be abandoned prematurely because it has been a victim of methodological weaknesses. The data linking depression to cancer when examined beyond a single measurement are of interest, as is the related area of hopelessness and stressful life events. It would be comforting to hope that researchers have at last reached a level of scientific maturity that allows them to listen to the now decades-old lessons of Fox (1978). Perhaps researchers can now carefully consider the biology and complexity of the many diseases called "cancer," attend to the critical issues of validity and reliability in measurement efforts, adjust for all known risk factors, and consider very important tumor growth characteristics when assessing the role of psychosocial factors related to cancer development. Perhaps it is not now too much to ask of researchers in this field to clearly articulate the model forming the basis of their research; develop distinct hypotheses to be tested; test these hypotheses with sufficient power to detect significant differences; and consider stress or life events measures, such as the Life Events and Difficulties Scale, which move beyond simple checklist instruments. Critically, researchers need to carefully consider their selection of personality measures and attempt to integrate clearly related psychosocial concepts. Finally, this is a research area requiring skills represented by the disciplines of epidemiology, psychology, oncology, biostatistics, and other specialties linked to cancer control. To definitively address whether and how psychosocial variables play a role in cancer development, studies taking advantage of the contributions of these disciplines are sorely needed.

Much of the work intended to examine the impact of psychosocial factors on cancer progression presents considerable challenges. It is based on knowledge of sociodemographic, disease, and treatment variables that may affect disease course and vary across cancer sites, solid grounding in psychometrics and instrument selection, significant analytical skills, and a conceptual understanding of the psychosocial variables often selected as potential links to increased survival. These criteria are rarely covered adequately in any given study. Despite the energy invested in, and history of, this field, it has borne surprisingly little fruit.

The most promising areas in this body of research to date include the role of chronic and/or multiple acute episodes of depression and the role of social support. Both of these areas also present with thoughtful, testable hypotheses related to potential mechanisms of cancer progression. Selection of specific cancer sites, with clear attention to biomarkers of progression, should be considered. In addition, consideration should be given to cancers in the early stage of disease, before the biology of the disease becomes overwhelming, likely negating any impact that psychosocial factors may provide. Consistent measures of depression and social support need to be used across investigations to avoid comparing apples and oranges. Initiating studies with sufficient sample size for subgroup analyses is a necessary step to specify the distinct role of psychosocial variables.

It may be time to put the research testing the impact of psychological interventions on cancer survival to bed unless researchers learn much more about the role of psychological variables on cancer progression and test interventions specifically focused on such variables. If and as work on the role of such variables proves fruitful, several critical changes in the conduct of intervention trials need to be incorporated. First, sufficient sample size is required to avoid the possibility that a positive or negative effect could be observed on the basis of a few atypical patients. Goodwin et al. (2001) accomplished this with her sample of 235 participants providing 99% power to detect a 25% improvement in survival. Most of the other studies had a small sample size, which is problematic for at least two reasons. First, as Fox (1995) noted, the "security of conclusions in cases of significance with small N is fragile" (p. 258). Second, as Piantadosi (1990) noted, trials with low power are more likely to yield false positive results than those with high power. Moreover, imbalances in strong prognostic factors do not have to be statistically significant to cause spurious "treatment" effects.

Other considerations for further research in the area include more attention to measuring potential mechanisms for a survival effect, ranging from health behaviors to measures of the immune and endocrine systems. Careful selection of tumor types is warranted, perhaps focusing on those that are hormonally sensitive, such as breast cancer, or those that are potentially immunogenic, such as melanoma. The number of potentially predictive markers and confounds by cancer type is quite impressive and needs to be carefully controlled for during patient selection and group assignment. Again, this is particularly critical in small trials, because there is no guarantee that even a randomized clinical trial will not be affected by important chance imbalances. Targeting early-stage cancers may be more reasonable, because the natural course of more advanced stages of disease might dwarf the impact of psychological intervention.

Finally, researchers need to drastically improve the quality of reporting trials in this area. Recent work in the medical literature to improve the reporting of clinical trials has resulted in the CONSORT (i.e., Consolidated Standards of Reporting Trials) statement (Moher, Schulz, & Altman, 2001), a checklist that ensures not only improved quality of the reporting of trials but also may improve the design of such trials. Clearly, a systematic approach to the reporting of trials to ensure complete transparency from authors to consumers in the design, conduct, analysis, and interpretation of results is needed.

CONCLUSION

This chapter provided a review of evidence for psychosocial variables as they relate to the development and progression of cancer, potential mechanisms, and some thoughts on future directions in this research arena. In closing, we advocate that the suggestions outlined here be considered as ways to advance what has been a controversial area in behavioral oncology.

Biobehavioral models of psychosocial variables and disease course in cancer are clearly needed. The model by Andersen, Kiecolt-Glaser, and Glaser (1994) is one that is well developed and includes psychosocial, behavioral, and biological components, specifying the pathways by which disease may be affected. Although still undergoing testing and potentially further refinement, it nicely maps out hypotheses related to disease course and has potential applications to the area of cancer etiology as well. This model can be extended to include work related to circadian rhythm and cancer progression (Sephton & Spiegel, 2003) or can incorporate work related to stress and DNA damage, repair, or apoptosis, if and as this field develops. Related to this is the need for future research focusing on theory-driven constructs (Tross et al., 1996), rather than general psychological symptoms, and the need to untangle many potentially overlapping psychological states (e.g., hopelessness, depression, psychological distress) as links to cancer etiology or survival.

The biobehavioral models used must relate directly to the alterations in cell physiology that dictate malignant growth: (a) decreased reliance on stimulation from their normal tissue microenvironment to move to an active proliferative state, (b) insensitivity to antigrowth signals, (c) evasion of programmed cell death (i.e., apoptosis), (d) limitless replicative potential, (e) sustained angiogenesis, and (f) tissue invasion and metastasis (Hanahan & Weinberg, 2000). That is, models constructed to explain disease outcome as a function of psychological variables must describe how such variables may impact any of these hallmarks of cancer.

The issue of individual differences has not been extensively explored in this area of research. Researchers do not yet know what the key domains of individual differences are that may have physiological relevance. The role of each individual's genetic and experiential background may well be critical, as well as affective reactions to life events that may trigger different physiological responses. Precious little research has examined the role of socioeconomic status, education, or other variables related to health disparities in the studies examined in this review. Segerstrom (2003) has done some initial work in this area, noting models of individual differences related to immune system changes that may be of relevance. Finally, in a classic article, Kosslyn et al. (2002) argued that biological systems are particularly prone to variation and that such individual variations, rather than being considered "noise," are likely important in their own right. They further noted that group and individual findings mutually inform each other, helping to elucidate the complex relations between biology and psychology.

Finally, it should be noted that there are upper limits to human longevity (Carnes, Olshansky, Gavrilov, Gavrilova, & Grahn, 1999; Olshansky, Carnes, & Cassel, 1990), influenced by both nature and nurture. Although this chapter focused on disease endpoints, quality of life and the presence of psychological distress are very worthy clinical endpoints. The goal of decreasing psychological distress independent of its role in cancer etiology or progression is an important one indeed.

REFERENCES

Andersen, B. L., Farrar, W. B., Golden-Kreutz, D., Kutz, L. A., MacCallum, R., Courtney, M. E., et al. (1998). Stress and immune responses after surgical treatment for regional breast cancer. *Journal of the National Cancer Institute, 90,* 30–36.

Andersen, B. L., Kiecolt-Glaser, J. K., & Glaser, R. (1994). A biobehavioral model of cancer stress and disease course. *American Psychologist, 49,* 389–404.

Antoni, M., Lutgendorf, S. K., Cole, S. W., Dhabhar, F. S., Sephton, S. E., McDonald, P. G., et al. (2006). The influence of bio-behavioral factors on tumor biology: Pathways and mechanisms. *Nature Reviews: Cancer, 6,* 240–248.

Brown, K. W., Levy, A. R., Rosberger, Z., & Edgar, L. (2003). Psychological distress and cancer survival: A follow-up 10 years after diagnosis. *Psychosomatic Medicine, 65,* 636–643.

Butow, P. N., Hiller, J. E., Price, M. A., Thackway, S. V., Kricker, A., & Tennant, C. C. (2000). Epidemiological evidence for a relationship between life events, coping style, and personality factors in the development of breast cancer. *Journal of Psychosomatic Research, 49,* 169–181.

Carnes, B. A., Olshansky, S. J., Gavrilov, L., Gavrilova, N., & Grahn, D. (1999). Human longevity: Nature vs. nurture—Fact or fiction. *Perspectives in Biology and Medicine, 42,* 422–441.

Cella, D. F., & Holland, J. D. (1988). Methodological considerations in studying the stress–illness connection in women with breast cancer. In C. L. Cooper (Ed.), *Stress and breast cancer* (pp. 197–214). Chichester, England: Wiley.

Chen, C. C., David, A. S., Nunnerley, H., Michell, M., Dawson, J. L., Berry, H., et al. (1995, December 9). Adverse life events and breast cancer: Case-control study. *BMJ, 311,* 1527–1530.

Cohen, L., Marshall, G. D., Jr., Cheng, L., Agarwal, S. K., & Wei, Q. (2000). DNA repair capacity in healthy medical students during and after exam stress. *Journal of Behavioral Medicine, 23,* 531–544.

Cohen, S., & Herbert, T. B. (1996). Health psychology: Psychological factors and physical disease from the perspective of human psychoneuroimmunology. *Annual Review of Psychology, 47,* 113–142.

Cohen, S., & Rabin, B. S. (1998). Psychologic stress, immunity, and cancer. *Journal of the National Cancer Institute, 90,* 3–4.

Coyne J. C., Stefanek, M., & Palmer, S. C. (2007). Psychotherapy and survival in cancer: The conflict between hope and evidence. *Psychological Bulletin, 133,* 367–394.

Croyle, R. T. (1998). Depression as a risk factor for cancer: Renewing a debate on the psychobiology of disease. *Journal of the National Cancer Institute, 90,* 1856–1857.

Cunningham, A. J., Edmonds, C. V., Jenkins, G. P., Pollack, H., Lockwood, G. A., & Warr, D. (1998). A randomized controlled trial of the effects of group psychological therapy on survival in women with metastatic breast cancer. *Psycho-Oncology, 7,* 508–517.

Cunningham, A. J., Edmonds, C. V., Phillips, C., Soots, K. I., Hedley, D., & Lockwood, G. A. (2000). A prospective, longitudinal study of the relationship of psychological work to duration of survival in patients with metastatic cancer. *Psycho-Oncology, 9,* 323–339.

Dalton, S. O., Boesen, E. H., Ross, L., Schapiro, I. R., & Johansen, C. (2002). Mind and cancer: Do psychological factors cause cancer? *European Journal of Cancer, 38,* 1313–1323.

Dalton, S. O., Mellemkjaer, L., Olsen, J. H., Mortensen, P. B., & Johansen, C. (2002). Depression and cancer risk: A register-based study of patients hospitalized with affective disorders, Denmark, 1969–1993. *American Journal of Epidemiology, 155,* 1088–1095.

Davis, S., Mirick, D. K., & Stevens, R. G. (2001). Night shift work, light at night, and risk of breast cancer. *Journal of the National Cancer Institute, 93,* 1557–1562.

Derogatis, L. R., Morrow, G. R., Fetting, J., Penman, D., Piasetsky, S., Schmale, A. M., et al. (1983). The prevalence of psychiatric disorders among cancer patients. *Journal of the American Medical Association, 249,* 751–757.

Dunn, G. P., Bruce, A. T., Ikeda, H., Old, L. J., & Schreiber, R. D. (2002). Cancer immunoediting: From immunosurveillance to tumor escape. *Nature Immunology, 3,* 991–998.

Edelman, S., Lemon, J., Bell, D. R., & Kidman, A. D. (1999). Effects of group CBT on the survival time of patients with metastatic breast cancer. *Psycho-Oncology, 8*, 474–481.

Evans, D. L., Staab, J. P., Petitto, J. M., Morrison, M. F., Szuba, M. P., Ward, H. E., et al. (1999). Depression in the medical setting: Biopsychological interactions and treatment considerations. *Journal of Clinical Psychiatry, 60*(Suppl. 4), 40–55.

Everson, S. A., Goldberg, D. E., Kaplan, G. A., Cohen, R. D., Pukkala, E., Tuomilehto, J., & Salonen, J. T. (1996). Hopelessness and risk of mortality and incidence of myocardial infarction and cancer. *Psychosomatic Medicine, 58*, 113–121.

Faller, H., Bulzebruck, H., Drings, P., & Lang, H. (1999). Coping, distress, and survival among patients with lung cancer. *Archives of General Psychiatry, 56*, 756–762.

Fawzy, F. I., Fawzy, N. W., Hyun, C. S., Elashoff, R., Guthrie, D., Fahey, J. L., & Morton, D. L. (1993). Malignant melanoma: Effects of an early structured psychiatric intervention, coping, and affective state on recurrence and survival 6 years later. *Archives of General Psychiatry, 50*, 681–689.

Forlenza, M. J., & Baum, A. (2000). Psychosocial influences on cancer progression: Alternative cellular and molecular mechanisms. *Current Opinion in Psychiatry, 13*, 639–645.

Forlenza, M. J., Latimer, J. J., & Baum, A. (2000). The effects of stress on DNA repair capacity. *Psychology & Health, 15*, 881–891.

Fox, B. H. (1978). Premorbid psychological factors as related to cancer incidence. *Journal of Behavioral Medicine, 1*, 45–133.

Fox, B. H. (1983). Current theory of psychogenic effects on cancer incidence and prognosis. *Journal of Psychosocial Oncology, 1*, 17–31.

Fox, B. H. (1995). Some problems and some solutions in research on psychotherapeutic intervention in cancer. *Supportive Care in Cancer, 3*, 257–263.

Geyer, S. (1993). Life events, chronic difficulties, and vulnerability factors preceding breast cancer. *Social Science & Medicine, 37*, 1545–1555.

Geyer, S. (1996). Social factors in the development and course of cancer. *Cancer Journal, 9*, 8–12.

Giraldi, T., Rodani, M. G., Cartei, G., & Grassi, L. (1997). Psychosocial factors and breast cancer: A 6-year Italian follow-up study. *Psychotherapy and Psychosomatics, 66*, 229–236.

Glaser, R., & Kiecolt-Glaser, J. K. (2005). Stress-induced immune dysfunction: Implications for health. *Nature Reviews: Immunology, 5*, 243–251.

Goodwin, P. J., Leszcz, M., Ennis, M., Koopmans, J., Vincent, L., Guther, H., et al. (2001). The effect of group psychosocial support on survival in metastatic breast cancer. *New England Journal of Medicine, 345*, 1719–1726.

Graham, J., Ramirez, A., Love, S., Richards, M., & Burgess, C. (2002, June 15). Stressful life experiences and risk of relapse of breast cancer: Observational cohort study. *BMJ, 324*, 1420.

Greer, S. (1983). Cancer and the mind: Maudsley Bequest Lecture delivered before the Royal College of Psychiatrists, February 1983. *British Journal of Psychiatry, 143,* 535–543.

Hanahan, D., & Weinberg, R. A. (2000). The hallmarks of cancer. *Cell, 100,* 57–70.

Herrmann, C., Brand-Driehorst, S., Kaminsky, B., Leibing, E., Staats, H., & Ruger, U. (1998). Diagnostic groups and depressed mood as predictors of 22-month mortality in medical inpatients. *Psychosomatic Medicine, 60,* 570–577.

Holden, R. J., Pakula, I. S., & Mooney, P. A. (1998). An immunological model connecting the pathogenesis of stress, depression, and carcinoma. *Medical Hypotheses, 51,* 309–314.

House, J. S., Landis, K. R., & Umberson, D. (1988, July 29). Social relationships and health. *Science, 241,* 540–545.

Ilnyckyj, A. (1994). A randomized controlled trial of psychotherapeutic intervention in cancer patients. *Annals of the Royal College of Physicians and Surgeons of Canada, 27,* 93–96.

Irwin, M. (1999). Immune correlates of depression. *Advances in Experimental Medicine and Biology, 461,* 1–24.

Kendler, K. S., Eaves, L. J., Walters, E. E., Neale, M. C., Heath, A. C., & Kessler, R. C. (1996). The identification and validation of distinct depressive syndromes in a population-based sample of female twins. *Archives of General Psychiatry, 53,* 391–399.

Kiecolt-Glaser, J. K., & Glaser, R. (1991). Stress and immune function in humans. In R. Ader, D. L. Felten, & N. Cohen (Eds.), *Psychoneuroimmunology* (2nd ed., pp. 849–867). San Diego, CA: Academic Press.

Kiecolt-Glaser, J. K., & Glaser, R. (1999a). Psychoneuroimmunology and cancer: Fact or fiction? *European Journal of Cancer, 35,* 1603–1607.

Kiecolt-Glaser, J. K., & Glaser, R. (1999b). Psychoneuroimmunology and immunotoxicology: Implications for carcinogenesis. *Psychosomatic Medicine, 61,* 271–272.

Kiecolt-Glaser, J. K., McGuire, L., Robles, T. F., & Glaser, R. (2002). Emotions, morbidity, and mortality: New perspectives from psychoneuroimmunology. *Annual Review of Psychology, 53,* 83–107.

Kosslyn, S. M., Cacioppo, J. T., Davidson, R. J., Hugdahl, K., Lovallo, W. R., Spiegel, D., & Rose, R. (2002). Bridging psychology and biology: The analysis of individuals in groups. *American Psychologist, 57,* 341–351.

Kuchler, T., Henne-Bruns, D., Rappat, S., Graul, J., Holst, K., Williams, J. I., & Wood-Dauphinee, S. (1999). Impact of psychotherapeutic support on gastrointestinal cancer patients undergoing surgery: Survival results of a trial. *Hepatogastroenterology, 46,* 322–335.

Levy, S. M., Herberman, R. B., Lee, J., Whiteside, T., Kirkwood, J., & McFeeley, S. (1990). Estrogen receptor concentration and social factors as predictors of natural killer cell activity in early-stage breast cancer patients: Confirmation of a model. *Natural Immunity and Cell Growth Regulation, 9,* 313–324.

Levy, S. M., Herberman, R. B., Lippman, M., D'Angelo, T., & Lee, J. (1991). Immunological and psychosocial predictors of disease recurrence in patients with early-stage breast cancer. *Behavioral Medicine, 17,* 67–75.

Lillberg, K., Verkasalo, P. K., Kaprio, J., Helenius, H., & Koskenvuo, M. (2002). Personality characteristics and the risk of breast cancer: A prospective cohort study. *International Journal of Cancer, 100,* 361–366.

Lillberg, K., Verkasalo, P. K., Kaprio, J., Teppo, L., Helenius, H., & Koskenvuo, M. (2001). Stress of daily activities and risk of breast cancer: A prospective cohort study in Finland. *International Journal of Cancer, 94,* 888–893.

Lillberg, K., Verkasalo, P. K., Kaprio, J., Teppo, L., Helenius, H., & Koskenvuo, M. (2002). A prospective study of life satisfaction, neuroticism, and breast cancer risk (Finland). *Cancer Causes and Control, 13,* 191–198.

Lillberg, K., Verkasalo, P. K., Kaprio, J., Teppo, L., Helenius, H., & Koskenvuo, M. (2003). Stressful life events and risk of breast cancer in 10,808 women: A cohort study. *American Journal of Epidemiology, 157,* 415–423.

Linn, M. W., Linn, B. S., & Harris, R. (1982). Effects of counseling for late stage cancer patients. *Cancer, 49,* 1048–1055.

Loberiza, F. R., Jr., Rizzo, J. D., Bredeson, C. N., Antin, J. H., Horowitz, M. M., Weeks, J. C., & Lee, S. J. (2002). Association of depressive syndrome and early deaths among patients after stem-cell transplantation for malignant diseases. *Journal of Clinical Oncology, 20,* 2118–2126.

Lutgendorf, S. K., Cole, S., Costanzo, E., Bradley, S., Coffin, J., Jabbari, S., et al. (2003). Stress-related mediators stimulate vascular endothelial growth factor secretion by two ovarian cancer cell lines. *Clinical Cancer Research, 9,* 4514–4521.

Lutgendorf, S. K., Johnsen, E. L., Cooper, B., Anderson, B., Sorosky, J. I., Buller, R. E., & Sood, A. K. (2002). Vascular endothelial growth factor and social support in patients with ovarian carcinoma. *Cancer, 95,* 808–815.

Madden, K. S. (2003). Catecholamines, sympathetic innervation, and immunity. *Brain, Behavior, and Immunity, 17*(Suppl. 1), 5–10.

Maier, S. F., & Watkins, L. R. (2000). The immune system as a sensory system: Implications for psychology. *Current Directions in Psychological Science, 9,* 98–102.

Maier, S. F., Watkins, L. R., & Fleshner, M. (1994). Psychoneuroimmunology: The interface between behavior, brain, and immunity. *American Psychologist, 49,* 1004–1017.

Maunsell, E., Brisson, J., & Deschenes, L. (1995). Social support and survival among women with breast cancer. *Cancer, 76,* 631–637.

McCorkle, R., Strumpf, N. E., Nuamah, I. F., Adler, D. C., Cooley, M. E., Jepson, C., et al. (2000). A specialized home care intervention improves survival among older post-surgical cancer patients. *Journal of the American Geriatric Society, 48,* 1707–1713.

McEwen, B. S. (1998). Protective and damaging effects of stress mediators. *New England Journal of Medicine, 338,* 171–179.

Moher, D., Schulz, K. F., & Altman, D. G. (2001). The CONSORT statement: Revised recommendations for improving the quality of reports of parallel-group randomized trials. *Annals of Internal Medicine, 134*, 657–662.

Moynihan, J. A. (2003). Mechanisms of stress-induced modulation of immunity. *Brain, Behavior, and Immunity, 17*(Suppl. 1), 11–16.

Murr, C., Widner, B., Sperner-Unterweger, B., Ledochowski, M., Schubert, C., & Fuchs, D. (2000). Immune reaction links disease progression in cancer patients with depression. *Medical Hypotheses, 55*, 137–140.

Olshansky, S. J., Carnes, B. A., & Cassel, C. (1990, November 20). In search of Methuselah: Estimating the upper limits to human longevity. *Science, 250*, 634–640.

Penninx, B. W., Guralnik, J. M., Pahor, M., Ferrucci, L., Cerhan, J. R., Wallace, R. B., & Havlik, R. J. (1998). Chronically depressed mood and cancer risk in older persons. *Journal of the National Cancer Institute, 90*, 1888–1893.

Piantadosi, S. (1990). Hazards of small clinical trials. *Journal of Clinical Oncology, 8*, 1–3.

Price, M. A., Tennant, C. C., Butow, P. N., Smith, R. C., Kennedy, S. J., Kossoff, M. B., & Dunn, S. M. (2001). The role of psychosocial factors in the development of breast carcinoma: Part II. Life event stressors, social support, defense style, and emotional control and their interactions. *Cancer, 91*, 686–697.

Reifman, A. (1995). Social relationships, recovery from illness, and survival—A literature review. *Annals of Behavioral Medicine, 17*, 124–131.

Richardson, J. L., Shelton, D. R., Krailo, M., & Levine, A. M. (1990). The effect of compliance with treatment on survival among patients with hematologic malignancies. *Journal of Clinical Oncology, 8*, 356–364.

Roberts, F. D., Newcomb, P. A., Trentham-Dietz, A., & Storer, B. E. (1996). Self-reported stress and risk of breast cancer. *Cancer, 77*, 1089–1093.

Schapiro, I. R., Johansen, C., Ross-Petersen, L., Saelan, H., Garde, K., & Olsen, J. H. (2000). Personality and risk of cancer. *Psycho-Oncology, 9*, 25.

Schapiro, I. R., Nielsen, L. F., Jorgensen, T., Boesen, E. H., & Johansen, C. (2002). Psychic vulnerability and the associated risk for cancer. *Cancer, 94*, 3299–3306.

Schapiro, I. R., Ross-Petersen, L., Saelan, H., Garde, K., Olsen, J. H., & Johansen, C. (2001). Extroversion and neuroticism and the associated risk of cancer: A Danish cohort study. *American Journal of Epidemiology, 153*, 757–763.

Schernhammer, E. S., Laden, F., Speizer, F. E., Willett, W. C., Hunter, D. J., Kawachi, I., & Colditz, G. A. (2001). Rotating night shifts and risk of breast cancer in women participating in the Nurses' Health Study. *Journal of the National Cancer Institute, 93*, 1563–1568.

Segerstrom, S. C. (2003). Individual differences, immunity, and cancer: Lessons from personality psychology. *Brain, Behavior, and Immunity, 17*(Suppl. 1), 92–97.

Sephton, S., & Spiegel, D. (2003). Circadian disruption in cancer: A neuroendocrine–immune pathway from stress to disease? *Brain, Behavior, and Immunity, 17*, 321–328.

Shi, Y., Devadas, S., Greeneltch, K. M., Yin, D., Allan Mufson, R., & Zhou, J. N. (2003). Stressed to death: Implication of lymphocyte apoptosis for psychoneuro-immunology. *Brain, Behavior, and Immunity, 17*(Suppl. 1), 18–26.

Smith, R. S. (1991). The macrophage theory of depression. *Medical Hypotheses, 35,* 298–306.

Spiegel, D. (2002). Effects of psychotherapy on cancer survival. *Nature Reviews: Cancer, 2,* 383–389.

Spiegel, D., Bloom, J. R., Kraemer, H. C., & Gottheil, E. (1989). Effect of psychosocial treatment on survival of patients with metastatic breast cancer. *Lancet, 2,* 888–891.

Spiegel, D., Butler, L. D., Giese-Davis, J., Koopman, C., Miller, E., DiMicelli, S., et al. (2007). Effects of supportive–expressive group therapy on survival of patients with metastatic breast cancer. *Cancer, 110,* 1130–1138.

Spiegel, D., & Giese-Davis, J. (2003). Depression and cancer: Mechanisms and disease progression. *Biological Psychiatry, 54,* 269–282.

Spiegel, D., & Sephton, S. E. (2001). Psychoneuroimmune and endocrine pathways in cancer: Effects of stress and support. *Seminars in Clinical Neuropsychiatry, 6,* 252–265.

Stefanek, M. E., Derogatis, L. P., & Shaw, A. (1987). Psychological distress among oncology outpatients. Prevalence and severity as measured with the Brief Symptom Inventory. *Psychosomatics, 28,* 530–532, 537–539.

Stern, S. L., Dhanda, R., & Hazuda, H. P. (2001). Hopelessness predicts mortality in older Mexican and European Americans. *Psychosomatic Medicine, 63,* 344–351.

Stommel, M., Given, B. A., & Given, C. W. (2002). Depression and functional status as predictors of death among cancer patients. *Cancer, 94,* 2719–2727.

Teno, J. M., Harrell, F. E., Jr., Knaus, W., Phillips, R. S., Wu, A. W., Connors, A., Jr., et al. (2000). Prediction of survival for older hospitalized patients: The HELP survival model. Hospitalized Elderly Longitudinal Project. *Journal of the American Geriatric Society, 48*(Suppl. 5), 16–24.

Tomei, L. D., Kiecolt-Glaser, J. K., Kennedy, S., & Glaser, R. (1990). Psychological stress and phorbol ester inhibition of radiation-induced apoptosis in human peripheral blood leukocytes. *Psychiatry Research, 33,* 59–71.

Tross, S., Herndon, J., II, Korzun, A., Kornblith, A. B., Cella, D. F., Holland, J. F., et al. (1996). Psychological symptoms and disease-free and overall survival in women with Stage II breast cancer. *Journal of the National Cancer Institute, 88,* 661–667.

Uchino, B. N., Cacioppo, J. T., & Kiecolt-Glaser, J. K. (1996). The relationship between social support and physiological processes: A review with emphasis on underlying mechanisms and implications for health. *Psychological Bulletin, 119,* 488–531.

Uchino, B. N., Uno, D., & Holt-Lunstad, J. (1999). Social support, physiological processes, and health. *Current Directions in Psychological Science, 8,* 145–148.

Watson, M., Haviland, J. S., Greer, S., Davidson, J., & Bliss, J. M. (1999). Influence of psychological response on survival in breast cancer: A population-based cohort study. *Lancet, 354,* 1331–1336.

29

TRANSLATION OF RESEARCH INTO PUBLIC HEALTH PRACTICE

CAROL R. WHITE AND MARK DIGNAN

Although scientific advances have been made in the continuum of cancer control, from prevention to end-of-life care, the impact of these advances on the U.S. population has been limited because of delays in translating evidence-based findings into widespread practice. Translation of research findings to practice is important for several reasons, but two primary reasons are to ensure all populations benefit from scientific discoveries and to reduce cancer health disparities. The National Cancer Institute (NCI) describes cancer health disparities as

> differences in the incidence, prevalence, mortality, and burden of cancer and related adverse health conditions that exist among specific population groups in the United States. These population groups may be characterized by gender, age, ethnicity, education, income, social class, disability, geographic location, or sexual orientation. (2004a, ¶ 1)

The unequal burden of cancer among minority and medically underserved populations is well documented (Institute of Medicine [IOM], 1999, 2003). In its report *Unequal Treatment: Confronting Racial and Ethnic Disparities in Health Care*, the IOM (2003) assessed the extent of racial and ethnic differences in health care that are not otherwise attributable to access-related factors or

517

clinical needs, preferences, and appropriateness of intervention. They concluded that a number of sources contribute to health disparities but that some evidence suggests that health systems–level factors (e.g., financing, structure of care, cultural or linguistic barriers), patient-level factors (e.g., patient preferences, refusal of treatment, poor adherence, biological differences), and discrimination in clinical encounters (e.g., providers might be biased against minorities, feel greater clinical uncertainty when interacting with minority patients, or hold certain beliefs [i.e., stereotypes] about the behavior or health of minorities) may be associated with disparities. Specific recommendations for reducing disparities included increasing awareness about disparities among the general public, health care providers, insurance companies, and policymakers and promoting evidence-based guidelines to ensure equity and quality of care.

Recognizing the gap between research translation and practice, the NCI hosted a conference in 2002, "Designing for Dissemination," to begin identifying strategies for overcoming dissemination barriers and increasing the adoption of evidence-based interventions (NCI, 2005). As shown in Figure 29.1, increasing the adoption, reach and impact of evidenced-based cancer interventions will require synergy between scientific push, delivery capacity, and market pull and demand (NCI, 2005). Traditionally, NCI has focused more

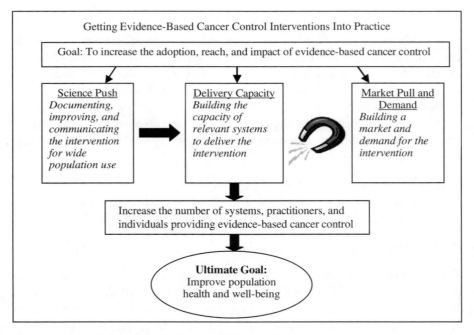

Figure 29.1. Bridging the gap: A synergistic model.

on efficacy research than on efforts to demonstrate effectiveness. Over time, the NCI has increasingly recognized the need to support efforts to enhance delivery of, and create a market or demand for, evidence-based cancer interventions. For example, NCI's strategic plan for 2006 indicated that they plan to increase allocation of resources to work with other agencies in the U.S. Department of Health and Human Services (USDHHS) to implement recommendations from the Trans-USDHHS Cancer Health Disparities Progress Review Group (CHD PRG; NCI, n.d.). In its report *Making Cancer Health Disparities History* (USDHHS, 2005), the CHD PRG developed a Call to Action consisting of 14 priority recommendations, which if implemented, could allow the USDHHS to achieve its goal of reducing cancer health disparities and progress from scientific discovery, to the development of evidence-based interventions, to the delivery of those interventions more rapidly.

Bridging the gap between research and practice requires increasing the ability to effectively communicate information about interventions and practices that research has shown to be effective—in other words, to increase the rate and success of diffusion of innovations. One factor that may be contributing to the research–practice gap is an assumption related to the logical progression of research designs—for example, the best interventions for dissemination are those that have proven successful in efficacy studies, followed by effectiveness studies, and then dissemination projects (Glasgow, Lichtenstein, & Marcus, 2003). Glasgow et al. (2003) suggested that underlying differences between efficacy and effectiveness trials exist and may account for why successful interventions identified in efficacy trials may not work exactly the same ways in real-world settings. Efficacy studies are highly controlled and conducted under very specific conditions (e.g., narrowly defined, homogeneous population; strict enrollment criteria; randomized design; strict adherence to study protocol; typically one type of setting), whereas effectiveness studies are conducted under less controlled conditions (e.g., broadly defined, heterogeneous population; adaptable enrollment criteria; more often a cross-sectional or quasi-experimental design; adaptable adherence to study protocol; more than one type of setting). As a result of these methodological differences, the characteristics of a successful intervention in an efficacy study might be quite different than those in an effectiveness study. The differences in these characteristics may explain why an efficacious intervention produces different findings in real-life settings.

This chapter focuses on the challenge of translating research to practice. Conceptually, there are three questions that need to be considered in the process of translation: Which interventions are worth implementing in the population of interest? What are the steps for implementation? and What is the overall impact of the intervention in the population of interest? This chapter provides an overview of (a) concepts of evidence-based medicine (EBM) and evidence-based public health (EBPH; the integration of best research evidence with clinical and public health practice, respectively), and implementation challenges; (b) theoretical frameworks for the dissemination, diffusion, and adoption of effective interventions; (c) tools for enhancing the practice of EBM and public health; (d) examples of current research initiatives; and (d) future research opportunities.

EVIDENCE-BASED MEDICINE AND EVIDENCE-BASED PUBLIC HEALTH

The increasing emphasis on EBM and EBPH is the result of public demands for accountability and competing demands on limited resources. Changes in health care financing, public-to-private shifts in responsibilities for the delivery of preventive services, and the increasing involvement of nontraditional partnerships are additional influences moving both medical care and public health practice toward an evidence-based approach (Baker et al., 1994). Both EBM and EBPH provide broad frameworks for a diversity of health care audiences who are responsible for decisions on strategies, policies, and programs that are most relevant, effective, and cost-effective for their communities or enrolled populations. Table 29.1 provides an overview of EBM and EBPH and illustrates the similarities and differences between the two conceptual frameworks (Brownson, Gurney, & Land, 1999; Forrest & Miller, 2002; Sackett, Straus, Richardson, Rosenberg, & Haynes, 2000).

Implementation of Evidence-Based Public Health

Recommended steps for EBPH include (a) developing an initial statement of the issue, (b) searching the scientific literature and evaluating the information, (c) quantifying the issue (i.e., identifying existing data sources), (d) developing and prioritizing program options, (e) developing an action plan and implementing interventions, and (e) evaluating the program or policy (Brownson, Baker, Leet, & Gillespie, 2003). Among these steps, finding relevant evidence in the literature, knowing what constitutes evidence, and critically appraising this evidence for its validity and usefulness (i.e., public health applicability) are especially critical. It is important to acknowledge that the challenges to understanding the scientific literature include the diversity of terminology used to describe the process of research translation to practice, varied definitions used by authors for the same terms, such as *dissemination, diffusion, knowledge transfer, uptake* or *utilization, adoption*, and *implementation*, and differences in outcome measures. Scientific evidence is usually thought of as being the result of well-designed and well-controlled research studies. Results from systematic reviews and meta-analyses are con-

TABLE 29.1
Comparison of Evidence-Based Medicine and Evidence-Based Public Health

Criterion	Evidence-based medicine	Evidence-based public health
Definition	Integration of best research evidence with clinical expertise and patient values.	Development, implementation, and evaluation of public health programs and policies through application of scientific reasoning.
Steps required	1. Convert information needs into clinical questions; 2. Review scientific literature and find best evidence; 3. Appraise relevant evidence for its validity and usefulness; 4. Apply results of appraisal in clinical practice; and 5. Evaluate the process and individual performance.	1. Develop an issue statement; 2. Review the scientific literature, and evaluate relevant information; 3. Quantify the issue (identify additional data sources); 4. Develop program or policy options; 5. Develop an action plan for program or policy; and 6. Evaluate the program or policy.
Volume of evidence	More studies reported in the literature.	Fewer studies reported in the literature.
Quality of studies	Medical studies more often rely on randomized controlled trials.	Studies often rely on other designs (e.g., cross-sectional, quasi-experimental).
Time period for observing an effect	Time period from medical treatment to outcome may be shorter.	Time period from intervention to outcome may be longer.
Professional education	Single academic credential for clinicians.	Single academic credential not available for public health practitioners.

sidered the highest level of evidence. These are followed by, in hierarchical order, evidence obtained from (a) at least one randomized controlled trial; (b) well-designed controlled trials without randomization; (c) well-designed cohort or case control analytic studies; (d) multiple time series; and (e) opinions of respected authorities on the basis of clinical experience, descriptive studies, and case reports or reports of expert committees (R. P. Harris et al., 2001).

A number of methods or systems are available for rating study quality and strength of evidence (Agency for Healthcare Research and Quality

[AHRQ], 2002). For grading the strength of evidence, important elements include quality (i.e., the aggregate of quality ratings for individual studies, predicated on the extent to which bias was minimized), quantity (i.e., magnitude of effect, numbers of studies, and sample size and power), and consistency (i.e., for any given topic, the extent to which similar findings are reported using similar and different study designs; AHRQ, 2002).

Potential Barriers to Evidence-Based Public Health

It is important to note that there are potential barriers to implementing EBPH, including lack of leadership in setting a clear agenda for EBPH; lack of a long-term view for program implementation and evaluation; external pressures that negatively impact the process toward an evidence-based approach; inadequate training in varied public health disciplines; lack of time to gather information, analyze data, and review the literature for evidence; lack of a comprehensive list, with up-to-date information on the effectiveness of programs and policies; and lack of data on the effectiveness of certain public health interventions or data for special populations (Brownson et al., 1999). Despite these barriers, translating evidence-based research into practice is still a promising approach for improving the current gap between research and practice.

THEORETICAL FRAMEWORKS

Several theoretical frameworks and models of behavioral change have been developed to explain the processes involved in developing health-related changes in knowledge, attitudes, and behaviors, but few have focused on how changes spread through populations. The health belief model is perhaps the most well-known framework designed to explain health-related changes (Hochbaum, 1958; Janz, Champion, & Strecher, 2002; Rosenstock, 1960). One of the most well-recognized theories that speaks to the process of translation is diffusion of innovations theory (Green & McAlister, 1984; Rogers, 1995). *Diffusion of innovation* is a process by which new ideas are communicated through certain channels over time among the members of a social system (Rogers, 1995). Diffusion of innovations theory predicts how and why individuals and organizations adopt or reject innovations. Adoption of innovations (e.g., new cancer prevention and control protocols) occurs through a process that begins with initial awareness of the need for a new approach, knowledge, and skills needed for implementation. The process of diffusion begins with creation of favorable attitudes toward an innovation. This often occurs through recognition of the attributes of the innovation, such as its relative advantage (i.e., benefits) over the status quo; compatibility with values, beliefs, needs; and simplicity. Observability of the innovation and its outcomes is an important part of initiation of diffusion.

In contrast to situations in which an individual contemplates adoption of an innovation, the process is more complex with organizations. This is because the process of diffusion for organizations is different from that for individuals (Parcel et al., 1995). Attitudes of gatekeepers and other stakeholders must be considered in encouraging adoption by an organization. In addition, the size and complexity of the organization, perceived advantage of adoption to the organization, availability of resources needed to support the innovation, and external forces such as financial and legal considerations are important factors that influence adoption of innovation by organizations. Once a decision to adopt an innovation is made, the next phase is implementation, which is often more difficult than the decision to adopt an innovation (McCormick & Tompkins, 1998). As a result, for implementation to be successful, a combination of effective strategies to promote change and champions to advocate for organizational change is needed.

DISSEMINATION, ADOPTION, AND EVALUATION OF EVIDENCE-BASED CANCER CONTROL INTERVENTION

When reviewing the literature related to cancer prevention and control, one should consider three questions: What types of diffusion and dissemination strategies are most effective? Are these strategies consistent across the cancer control continuum? and What are the outcomes of these diffusion and dissemination strategies? The AHRQ (2003) conducted a systematic review of primary studies evaluating strategies for disseminating cancer control interventions in five topic areas including smoking cessation, healthy diet, mammography, cervical cancer screening, and control of cancer pain. In general, the types of strategies used in these studies included train-the-trainer approaches, educational facilitators, media, and peer educators. Resulting from their review were topic-specific findings, as well as the following key findings that were generalizable across all topic areas: (a) Outcomes assessed in these studies varied considerably from process to behavioral measures; (b) terminology varied for terms related to *diffusion, dissemination,* and *implementation;* (c) passive approaches (i.e., diffusion), such as mailings, were generally ineffective; (d) active approaches (i.e., dissemination), such as train-the-trainer, were more likely to be effective; (e) the majority of evidence for strategies to disseminate cancer control interventions were identified in provider-directed interventions; and (f) several studies were primarily descriptive versus evaluative, raising the question, What are the most appropriate study designs for dissemination research?

ADOPTION OF EVIDENCE-BASED INTERVENTIONS

To bridge the research–practice gap successfully, an increase in the adoption, reach, and impact of evidence-based cancer control efforts is needed. Several tools are available to both clinical and public health practitioners who are interested in learning about evidence-based interventions—what they are and how they can be implemented. This section provides a brief overview of some of these tools.

The number of health care systems and providers providing evidence-based interventions could be enhanced through the effective dissemination of guidelines developed by an evidence-based approach, for example, the *Guide to Community Preventive Services* (see http://www.thecommunity guide.org) and the *Guide to Clinical Preventive Services* (see http://www.ahrq. gov/clinic/prevenix.htm). The *Guide to Community Preventive Services* provides public health practitioners and decision makers with recommendations regarding population-based interventions to promote community health and prevent disease (Truman et al., 2000). The *Guide to Clinical Preventive Services* provides recommendations for conditions that cause a large disease burden and that have a potentially effective preventive service (R. P. Harris et al., 2001). Preventive measures include screening tests, counseling, immunizations, and preventive medications.

The Cochrane Collaboration (see http://www.cochrane.org) is an international organization that is dedicated to producing and disseminating systematic reviews of health care interventions. These reviews, known as *Cochrane Reviews,* explore the evidence for and against the effectiveness of interventions and are designed to facilitate decision making by individuals, healthcare professionals, and policymakers.

Cancer Control PLANET (i.e., Plan, Link, Act, Network With Evidence-Based Tools) is a Web portal developed by the NCI, in partnership with the American Cancer Society, the Centers for Disease Control and Prevention (CDC), and the Substance Abuse and Mental Health Services Administration (NCI, 2004b). This portal is designed to help health educators, program staff, researchers, and cancer control planners bridge the gap from research discovery to program delivery and increase the adoption of evidenced-based approaches across the cancer control continuum. Research-Tested Intervention Programs (NCI, 2004c), developed as part of the Cancer Control PLANET, provides up-to-date and scientifically valid information about cancer prevention and control. This database consists of actual evidence-based programs and products that individuals can adapt for their own use.

Put Prevention Into Practice is a national program sponsored by the AHRQ (2004b). The program develops resources for clinicians, patients, and office staff to increase the delivery of preventive services (recommended in the *Guide to Clinical Preventive Services*) in the primary care setting.

Evaluation of Interventions

Once effective interventions are adopted, it is equally important to determine their overall public health impact. Recognizing the need to evaluate public health interventions more comprehensively than traditional methods, Glasgow and colleagues (Glasgow, 2003; Glasgow, Vogt, & Boles, 1999) have developed a new framework called RE-AIM (i.e., reach, effectiveness, adoption, implementation, and maintenance) that can be used to structure the assessment of the overall impact of a public health intervention. Building on the work of Abrams et al. (1996), who defined an intervention's impact (I) as the percentage of population receiving the intervention (R) multiplied by its efficacy (E) ($I = R \times E$), they added three additional factors (i.e., adoption, implementation, and maintenance) that account for the setting in which the intervention is adopted. Each of the factors is represented on a 0 to 1 scale (or 0%–100%). The product of the five factors is the public health impact score (i.e., population-based effect).

The RE-AIM model may be useful in balancing both internal and external validity in the planning, design, and evaluation of health behavior promotion interventions. For example, Dzewaltowski, Estabrooks, and Glasgow (2004) applied the RE-AIM model to the physical activity literature, noting that key individual and level-setting factors that moderate the impact of interventions were not often reported. They suggested that without such knowledge, the available evidence demonstrating efficacy of physical activity interventions implemented under controlled conditions may not be generalizable or sustainable when these interventions are then implemented under the conditions of practice. In a review of community-based behavioral interventions (i.e., promoting good nutrition, physical activity, or smoking cessation and prevention), Dzewaltowski, Estabrooks, Klesges, Bull, and Glasgow (2004) used the RE-AIM model to evaluate the number of studies reporting on the five factors of the model. Few studies reported on the representativeness of samples and settings and whether individuals and programs maintained the interventions. Glasgow et al. (2003) applied the RE-AIM model to differentiate key characteristics between efficacy and effectiveness studies. Public health benefits might be enhanced if all dimensions of the RE-AIM model were addressed when selecting interventions for translation.

RESEARCH INITIATIVES

The challenge of translating research findings to public health practice has prompted new research initiatives to identify best strategies for dissemination and diffusion. One example of a new initiative is the Cancer Prevention and Control Research Network (CPCRN), a network of academic, public health, and community partnerships across the United States (J. R. Harris et al., 2005), funded by the CDC and the NCI. The CPCRN conducts community-based research and is committed to accelerating the continuum of research discovery to dissemination to adoption of evidence-based interventions for cancer prevention and control, thus narrowing the gap between research translation and practice (see http://www.cpcrn.org/about.html).

A second example is an initiative called Racial and Ethnic Approaches to Community Health (REACH) 2010 (CDC, 2004). REACH 2010 is supported by the CDC in collaboration with other key partners within the USDHHS, including the Office of the Secretary, National Institutes of Health, Health Resources and Services Administration, the Administration on Aging, and the AHRQ. This initiative was developed to support Healthy People 2010 (see http://www.healthypeople.gov)—the nation's health promotion and disease prevention initiative. The goal of REACH 2010 is to eliminate disparities in health status experienced by racial and ethnic minority populations in six priority areas, including infant mortality, breast and cervical cancer screening, cardiovascular diseases, diabetes, HIV infections and AIDS, and child and adult immunizations. The racial and ethnic groups targeted by REACH 2010 are African Americans, American Indians, Alaska Natives, Asian Americans, Hispanic Americans, and Pacific Islanders. REACH 2010 supports community coalitions in designing, implementing, and evaluating community-driven and science-based interventions with the goal of replicating their successes in other communities. Such an approach could be effective in eliminating health disparities.

A third example is the establishment and ongoing support of primary care practice-based research networks (PBRNs) by the AHRQ (2004a). A PBRN is a group of ambulatory practices devoted principally to the primary care of patients, affiliated with each other (and often with an academic or professional organization). These networks have emerged as a promising approach to the scientific study of primary care, by investigating questions related to community-based practice. The PBRNs often use the experience and insight of practicing clinicians to identify and frame research questions. By linking these questions with rigorous research methods, the PBRNs can produce research findings that are immediately relevant to the clinician, more easily assimilated into everyday practice, and have the potential to improve the overall practice of primary care.

As experience with efforts to translate and disseminate cancer prevention and control research grows, the compendium of evidence-based practices and interventions available to practitioners and researchers will also grow. Research is needed to better understand (AHRQ, 2003) (a) how theoretical models of behavioral change can inform dissemination efforts, (b) what outcomes are important in dissemination research, (c) how the inconsistent use of terminology in the literature should be addressed (e.g., establishing criteria for reporting dissemination research), (d) the cost-effectiveness of different cancer control interventions and strategies to disseminate them, (e) the role of existing and new technologies in dissemination (e.g., the Internet), and (f) the characteristics of health care providers and individuals that contribute to increasing or decreasing the success of dissemination approaches. The *Guide to Community Preventive Services* is a valuable tool for researchers, as it highlights critical areas for future research on the basis of the gaps in knowledge that are revealed through the rigorous review process (Briss, Brownson, Fielding, & Zaza, 2004). Publications generated by the Cancer Prevention and Control Research Network (Bowen, Campbell, & Emmons, in press) are helping to carve out new directions for improving public health practice by using evidence-based programs and policies that have been tested, found efficacious, and then disseminated into the real world.

REFERENCES

Abrams, D. B., Orleans, C. T., Niaura, R. S., Goldstein, M. G., Prochaska, J. O., & Velicer, W. (1996). Integrating individual and public health perspectives for treatment of tobacco dependence under managed health care: A combined stepped-care and matching model. *Annals of Behavioral Medicine, 18,* 290–304.

Agency for Healthcare Research and Quality. (2002). *Systems to rate the strength of scientific evidence* (AHRQ Publication No. 02-E016). Retrieved February 28, 2008, from http//www.ahrq.gov/clinic/strevinv.htm

Agency for Healthcare Research and Quality. (2003). *Diffusion and dissemination of evidence-based cancer control interventions* (AHRQ Publication No. 03-E032). Retrieved February 28, 2008, from http://www.ahrq.gov/clinic/epcsums/canconsum.htm

Agency for Healthcare Research and Quality. (2004a). *Primary care practice–based research networks.* Retrieved February 28, 2008, from http://www.ahrq.gov/research/pbrnfact.htm

Agency for Healthcare Research and Quality. (2004b). *Put prevention into practice.* Retrieved February 28, 2008, from http://www.ahrq.gov/clinic/ppipix.htm

Baker, E. L., Melton, R. J., Stange, P. V., Fields, M. L., Koplan, J. P., Guerra, F. A., & Satcher, D. (1994). Health reform and the health of the public: Forging community health partnerships. *Journal of the American Medical Association, 272,* 1276–1282.

Bowen, S., Campbell, M., & Emmons, R. (in press). Advancing dissemination research in cancer control: I. Definitions, models, and research questions. *Cancer Causes and Control.*

Briss, P. A., Brownson, R. C., Fielding, J. E., & Zaza, S. (2004). Developing and using the *Guide to Community Preventive Services:* Lessons learned about evidence-based public health. *Annual Review of Public Health, 25,* 281–302.

Brownson, R. C., Baker, E. A., Leet, T. L., & Gillespie, K. N. (2003). *Evidence-based public health*. New York: Oxford University Press.

Brownson, R. C., Gurney, J. G., & Land, G. H. (1999). Evidence-based decision making in public health. *Journal of Public Health Management and Practice, 5,* 86–97.

Centers for Disease Control and Prevention. (2004). *REACH 2010*. Retrieved February 28, 2008, from http://www.cdc.gov/reach2010

Dzewaltowski, D. A., Estabrooks, P. A., & Glasgow, R. E. (2004). The future of physical activity behavior change research: What is needed to improve translation of research into health promotion practice? *Exercise and Sport Sciences Review, 32,* 57–63.

Dzewaltowski, D. A., Estabrooks, P. A., Klesges, L. M., Bull, S., & Glasgow, R. E. (2004). Behavior change intervention research in community settings: How generalizable are the results? *Health Promotion International, 19,* 235–245.

Forrest, J. L., & Miller, S. A. (2002). Evidence-based decision making in action: I. Finding the best clinical evidence. *Journal of Contemporary Dental Practice, 3,* 10–26.

Glasgow, R. E. (2003). Translating research to practice: Lessons learned, areas for improvement, and future directions. *Diabetes Care, 26,* 2451–2456.

Glasgow, R. E., Lichtenstein, E., & Marcus, A. C. (2003). Why don't we see more translation of health promotion research to practice? Rethinking the efficacy-to-effectiveness transition. *American Journal of Public Health, 93,* 1261–1267.

Glasgow, R. E., Vogt, T. M., & Boles, S. M. (1999). Evaluating the public health impact of health promotion interventions: The RE-AIM framework. *American Journal of Public Health, 89,* 1322–1327.

Green, L. W., & McAlister, A. L. (1984). Macro-intervention to support health behavior: Some theoretical perspectives and practical reflections. *Health Education Quarterly, 11,* 322–339.

Harris, J. R., Brown, P. K., Coughlin, S., Fernandez, M. E., Hebert, J. R., Kerner, J., et al. (2005). The Cancer Prevention and Control Research Network. *Preventing Chronic Disease, 2,* A21. Retrieved February, 28, 2008, from http://www.cdc.gov/pcd/issues/2005/jan/04_0059.htm

Harris, R. P., Helfand, M., Woolf, S. H., Lohr, K. N., Mulrow, C. D., Teutsch, S. M., & Atkins, D. (2001). Current methods of the U.S. Preventive Services Task Force: A review of the process. *American Journal of Preventive Medicine, 20*(Suppl. 3), 21–35.

Hochbaum, G. M. (1958). *Public participation in medical screening programs: A socio-psychological study* (PHS Publication No. 572). Washington, DC: U.S. Government Printing Office.

Institute of Medicine. (1999). *The unequal burden of cancer: An assessment of NIH research and programs for ethnic minorities and the medically underserved.* Washington, DC: National Academies Press.

Institute of Medicine. (2003). *Unequal treatment: Confronting racial and ethnic disparities in health care.* Washington, DC: National Academies Press.

Janz, N. K., Champion, V. L., & Strecher, V. J. (2002). The health belief model. In K. Glantz, B. K. Rimer, & F. M. Lewis (Eds.), *Health behavior and health education: Theory, research, and practice* (3rd ed., pp. 45–66). San Francisco: Jossey-Bass.

McCormick, L., & Tompkins, N. (1998). Diffusion of CDC's guidelines to prevent tobacco use and addiction. *Journal of School Health, 68,* 43–45.

National Cancer Institute. (2004a). *Applied research program.* Retrieved February 28, 2008, from http://appliedresearch.cancer.gov/areas/disparities

National Cancer Institute. (2004b). *Research and diffusion program: Cancer Control PLANET.* Retrieved February 28, 2008, from http://cancercontrolplanet.gov

National Cancer Institute. (2004c). *Research and diffusion program: Cancer Control PLANET: Research-tested intervention programs.* Retrieved February 28, 2008, from http://cancercontrol.cancer.gov/rtips

National Cancer Institute. (n.d.). *NCI annual plans & budget proposals for previous years.* Retrieved February 28, 2008, from http://planning.cancer.gov/planning/previous.shtml

National Cancer Institute. (2005). *Research diffusion and dissemination: Designing for Dissemination Conference.* Retrieved February 28, 2008, from http://cancercontrol.cancer.gov/d4d/d4d_conf_sum_report.pdf

Parcel, G. S., O'Hara-Tompkins, N. M., Harrist, R. B., Basen-Engquist, K. M., McCormick, L. K., Gottlieb, N. H., & Eriksen, M. P. (1995). Diffusion of an effective tobacco prevention program: II. Evaluation of the adoption phase. *Health Education Research: Theory & Practice, 10,* 297–307.

Rogers, E. M. (1995). *Diffusion of innovations* (4th ed.). New York: Free Press.

Rosenstock, I. M. (1960). What research in motivation suggests for public health. *American Journal of Public Health, 50,* 295–301.

Sackett, D. L., Straus, S., Richardson, W., Rosenberg, W., & Haynes, R. B. (2000). *Evidence-based medicine: How to practice and teach EBM* (2nd ed.). London: Churchill Livingstone.

Truman, B. I., Smith-Akin, C. K., Hinman, A. R., Gebbie, K. M., Brownson, R., Novick, L. F., et al. (2000). Developing the *Guide to Community Preventive Services*—Overview and rationale: The Task Force on Community Preventive Services. *American Journal of Preventive Medicine, 18*(Suppl. 1), 18–26.

U.S. Department of Health and Human Services. (2005). *Making cancer health disparities history: Report of the Trans-HHS Cancer Health Disparities Progress Review Group.* Retrieved February 28, 2008, from http://www.hhs.gov/chdprg/pdf/chdprg.pdf

30

TRANSDISCIPLINARY SOCIAL AND BEHAVIORAL RESEARCH FOR CANCER PREVENTION

COLLEEN M. McBRIDE

Since Congress launched the War on Cancer in 1971 (i.e., National Cancer Act of 1971), research across a number of disciplines now documents the complex interplay of biological, behavioral, social, and environmental factors that contribute to cancer incidence and mortality (Balmain, Gray, & Ponder, 2003). This recognition has spurred the call for transdisciplinary (TD) research approaches (Abrams, 1999; King, Stokols, Talen, Brassington, & Killingsworth, 2002; Seeman, 2003) to achieve the ambitious goal to accelerate declines in cancer incidence and mortality in the coming decade (Byers et al., 1999). Among the most pressing challenges to achieving this goal are (a) reducing behavioral risk factors, (b) applying emerging human genome discoveries to prevention and early detection of cancer, (c) addressing widely noted inequities in cancer outcomes and research, and (d) integrating cancer prevention and early detection interventions into

This chapter was authored by an employee of the United States government as part of official duty and is considered to be in the public domain. Any views expressed herein do not necessarily represent the views of the United States government, and the author's participation in the work is not meant to serve as an official endorsement.

health care delivery systems (e.g., see Byers et al., 1999; Emmons, 2000; von Eschenbach, 2004; Weir et al., 2003).

These four challenges are ideal for illustrating the need and potential for TD collaborations. Each of the four is inherently complex in nature, influenced by factors that span multiple disciplinary boundaries and analytic levels, and has persisted despite considerable research attention. Finally, they are interconnected in ways that suggest progress toward addressing one challenge could benefit progress, in some cases synergistically, toward addressing the others.

WHAT IS MEANT BY *TRANSDISCIPLINARY COLLABORATION*?

The most widely cited definition of TD collaborative research was described by Rosenfield (1992), whose taxonomy of disciplinary integration included three levels: multidisciplinary, interdisciplinary, and TD. Multidisciplinary collaborations represent the lowest level of integration in the taxonomy and typically involve representatives of different disciplines who work "in parallel or sequentially from a disciplinary-specific base" (p. 1351) to address a common research question. Interdisciplinary collaborations are the next order of integration, in which representatives of different disciplines work jointly with the shared recognition that the research question requires the combined perspectives of multiple disciplinary perspectives. However, in these collaborations, disciplinary boundaries generally are maintained as scientists work from their own discipline's conceptual models, methods, and measures to address the question at hand. TD collaboration is the highest level of integration. The ideal for these collaborations is that researchers work jointly from a shared conceptual framework that integrates knowledge across disciplinary boundaries to generate new research methods and measures. More recently, Rosenfield and Kessel (2003) have moved away from this stepped taxonomy to describe a continuum of disciplinary integration. In this model, interdisciplinary collaborations can achieve approximations of the full integration previously argued to characterize only TD collaboration.

Concurrent with this new conceptualization of the collaboration continuum, Stokols et al. (2003) have elaborated further gradations of transdisciplinarity by considering the analytic breadth and disciplinary scope of these collaborations (see Figure 30.1). In this conceptualization, TD collaborations can be horizontally integrated—occurring across disciplines at a single level of analysis (i.e., biological or societal)—or vertically integrated—occurring across a broad scope of disciplines and levels of analysis (i.e., biological to societal). An example of horizontally integrated

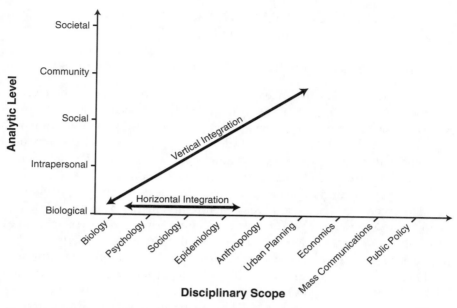

Figure 30.1. Levels of transdisciplinary collaboration.

TD research commonly described is in the area of addiction, in which collaborations occur among pharmacologists and neurologists such that these disciplinary perspectives are considered to better understand the biology of addiction (Abrams, 1999; Stokols et al., 2003). By contrast, Sallis, Linton, and Kraft's (2005) newly defined area of "active living" research represents a vertically integrated TD research in which the full breadth of analytic outcomes are considered (i.e., from biological to societal) and involves scientists with different disciplinary perspectives, from exercise physiologists to urban planners. By all accounts, vertically integrated collaborations are the most difficult to achieve yet are arguably most fruitful in their innovation potential (Stokols et al., 2003). Stokols et al. (2003) also made a distinction between TD collaboration, that is, interaction among scientists, and TD science, that is, the intellectual products (e.g., new conceptual models, measures) that can emerge from these collaborations. They suggested that TD collaborations can be judged by the quality, novelty, and scope of the scientific products and the degree of intellectual integration they embody (Stokols et al., 2003).

Irrespective of refinements in defining what constitutes TD research, behind each conceptualization is the belief that compelling and complex scientific challenges are what galvanize TD collaboration. The next section suggests four pressing challenges for cancer prevention and early detection efforts that compel TD collaboration and science.

FORCES COMPELLING TRANSDISCIPLINARY
RESEARCH INITIATIVES

Difficulty of Influencing Behavioral Risk Factors

More than half of all cancers could be prevented by reducing behavioral risk factors, such as cigarette smoking, poor diet, physical inactivity, overweight, unsafe sex practices, sun exposure, and occupational environmental toxins (Gotay, 2005). However, decades of research document the difficulty of promoting these health behaviors (Emmons, 2000). Population prevalence of physical inactivity (24%) and overweight (59%) are at historically high levels and present significant challenges for developing cost-effective population-based interventions (Behavioral Risk Factor Surveillance System, 2003). The majority of Americans (77%) report consuming fewer servings of vegetables and fruits than are recommended (Behavioral Risk Factor Surveillance System, 2003). American youth continue to take up cigarette smoking and smokeless tobacco, with an appreciable minority of adults unable to quit using tobacco despite a strong desire and earnest attempts to do so (Fiore et al., 2004). Across all cancer-related behaviors, posttreatment relapse continues to be a substantial challenge. Adherence rates to annual mammography are less than optimal (Sondik, 2000). Acceptance of colorectal cancer screening among Americans remains low, at about 40% nationally (Sondik, 2000).

Concurrent with these challenges, researchers have learned that behavioral risk factors arise from a complex interplay of physiological (e.g., genetic, metabolic, neurological), psychological (e.g., confidence, motivation, emotion), interpersonal (e.g., social support), and environmental (e.g., resource availability, social policy) reinforcements (Emmons, 2000). Thus, to be maximally effective, interventions should consider multiple analytic levels and a broad scope of disciplinary perspectives. For example, growing evidence that risk behaviors cluster suggests that common neurological factors (e.g., dopamine receptors) may play a reinforcement role in the adoption of health habits. Risk habits also may be mutually reinforcing in that poor eating habits can lead to overweight and, thus, make it more difficult to be physically active. In turn, the physical environment may simultaneously present barriers to multiple health habits such as limited options for healthy eating and physical activity and readily accessible cigarettes (Emmons, 2000). These challenges have been acknowledged in several research reports, with the call for innovative intervention approaches that consider multiple disciplinary perspectives and analytic levels that could be facilitated by TD research collaborations (e.g., see Emmons, 2000).

Applying Emerging Human Genome Discoveries

Advances in biology and molecular epidemiology have established clearly that cancer is a genetic disease (Balmain et al., 2003). A plethora of evidence suggests that genes, alone or in complex interaction with environmental exposures (including lifestyle) are integral in initiating and promoting the multistep carcinogenesis process. Moreover, researchers increasingly suggest that the effects of environmental exposures (e.g., sun exposure, cigarette smoking, pollution) on cancer development may differ among individuals with genetic polymorphisms (i.e., variants) that augment susceptibility (Lerman & Shields, 2004).

These advances bring growing appreciation that cancer prevention and screening recommendations are not one size fits all and herald the coming of personalized medicine in which DNA variations can be used to customize these recommendations (e.g., see Subramanian, Adams, Venter, & Broder, 2001). Identification of several cancer susceptibility genes for breast, ovarian (BRCA1 and BRCA2), and colorectal (MLH1/2, familial adenomatous polyposis) cancers that confer significant lifetime risk (50%–80%) for carriers of these mutations is just the beginning of what is predicted to be rapid development of additional genetic susceptibility testing (Subramanian et al., 2001). Contributing to this is the recent completion of the sequence of the human genome and evolving laboratory technology that will speed discovery of susceptibility genes, understanding of the function of their protein products (i.e., proteomics), and the genetics of complex traits and diseases (Subramanian et al., 2001).

Customizing cancer prevention and screening recommendations on the basis of genomic risk profile and providing related risk feedback introduces a host of fascinating and challenging research questions that conceivably could cross all levels of analysis (i.e., biological to societal) and should be informed by the perspectives of scientists who represent multiple disciplines (Lerman & Shields, 2004). Indeed, the quest for and discovery of genetic markers of susceptibility, damage, and early-stage disease provides a natural bridge for TD collaborations among clinicians, bench scientists, social scientists, and behavioral scientists (Vainio & Husgafvel-Pursiainen, 1996).

CANCER CONTROL RESEARCH QUESTIONS FOR TRANSDISCIPLINARY RESEARCH COLLABORATIONS

This section describes two examples of important challenge areas to illustrate their interrelationships, and the horizontally- and vertically-integrated TD research that could accelerate progress toward achieving national goals for cancer prevention and control.

Tobacco Use: A Complex Biopsychosocial Phenomenon

Over the past decade, a number of scientists have presented comprehensive and compelling reviews of the multiple factors that influence tobacco use (e.g., see Abrams, 1999). Briefly, these reviews juxtapose smokers' strong desire to quit against the backdrop of low population quit rates, high relapse rates, and disproportionately high smoking rates among those with mental health comorbidities (e.g., alcoholism, schizophrenia, attention-deficit/hyperactivity disorder; Dierker, Avenevoli, Merikangas, Flaherty, & Stolar, 2001; Tercyak, Lerman, & Audrain, 2002), to suggest that nicotine dependence has strong physical and psychological underpinnings. They describe the clustering of tobacco use in families, to suggest the likely conjoint contributions of heredity and social–environmental influences on tobacco use (Shenassa et al., 2003). Moreover, they describe dramatic declines in tobacco use observed in states with progressive tobacco control policies to demonstrate the power of social and policy influences on tobacco use (e.g., see Gilpin, Emery, White, & Pierce, 2003).

In the late 1990s, these observations prompted several retreats, conferences, and advisory groups to consider what was needed to advance tobacco research in promoting adult cessation and preventing adolescent initiation (Morgan et al., 2003). The groups' consensus was that Transdisciplinary Tobacco Use Research Centers (TTURCs) could engender TD collaborations to study tobacco use within a broad biopsychosocial context. Issues for particular emphasis for TTURCs included research to understand trajectories of tobacco use in adolescence, development of treatments for tobacco dependence tailored to individual genetic and psychosocial profiles, and dissemination of tobacco control programs at social and organizational levels. Seven TTURCs were funded in 1999, through a request for applications jointly sponsored by the National Cancer Institute and the National Institute for Drug Abuse, with the Robert Wood Johnson Foundation providing supplemental support to centers for communication and policy research.

Each TTURC was organized around a theme, and investigators were charged to involve investigators from the basic sciences, bearing in mind translational applications of the research for clinical and public health settings. In addition, the collaborators were expected to devise a common conceptual framework that would enable tobacco use to be considered across multiple levels of analysis and disciplinary perspectives. TTURC themes ranged from "Genes, Environment and Tobacco Use Across Cultures" to "Building the Evidence Base for Tobacco Control Policies" (see http://cancer control.cancer.gov/tcrb/tturc).

Recent publications have yielded new insights into the interplay of genetics and nicotine dependence derived from vertically integrated TD collaborations among behavioral and molecular geneticists. The TD science emerging from these collaborations implicate genes involved in dopaminergic pathways (Lerman et al., 2003, 2004), drug metabolism (Miksys, Lerman, Shields, Mash, & Tyndale, 2003), and behavioral characteristics such as hostility (Fallon, Keator, Mbogori, Turner, & Potkin, 2004) as significant factors in nicotine dependence. These contributions suggest new directions for developing more effective therapies and selecting optimal pharmacologic interventions for smokers.

Physical Inactivity: Developing Effective Microlevel and Macrolevel Interventions

As with tobacco use, physical activity patterns too are influenced by biological, psychological, social, and environmental factors (e.g., see King et al., 2002). However, to date, physical activity interventions have been based largely on social-cognitive models that target an individual's subjective experience of interpersonal and microenvironmental factors (e.g., immediate conditions within one's home or workplace) and how they impinge on that individual's choice to be active (King et al., 2002). A number of these interventions have been evaluated in randomized trials, with inconsistent outcomes (e.g., see Marcus et al., 1998; Pinto et al., 2002).

TD collaborations that involve disciplinary expertise in the structured physical environment (e.g., environmental psychology, city planning) have been suggested to stimulate new paradigms and interventions that can produce sustainable increases in physical activity. Consideration of the physical environment has led to the development of new measures, such as environmental friendliness toward physical activity (e.g., whether communities are structured to facilitate walking rather than traffic flow; see Saelens, Sallis, & Frank, 2003). In this way, TD research that melds structural–environmental perspectives with cognitive and behavioral perspectives could suggest new intervention targets, evaluation methodologies, and primary outcomes (Saelens et al., 2003).

This TD research also must consider health disparities, as they affect many of the factors that underlie physical inactivity. For example, Boslaugh, Luke, Brownson, Naleid, and Kreuter (2004) reported that African Americans view their neighborhoods as less safe and less pleasant for physical activity than do Whites. Thus, vertically integrated TD research that crosses disciplines and simultaneously targets multiple analytic levels from individual skills building to community activation, such as community watch programs or other collaborations with police departments and local leaders, could address the challenge to reduce health disparities in cancer outcomes.

These vertically integrated TD collaborations that cross multiple levels from micro- to macroenvironmental factors will be enormously challenging. Conceptual models such as behavioral choice theory (BCT; Epstein, 1998) have been suggested to facilitate disciplinary cross talk. For example, BCT posits that the reinforcing value of an alternative, such as being physically inactive, can be considered across individual, community, and environmental levels of analysis. This and other conceptual models could provide a starting point for facilitating TD collaboration.

WHAT IS IT GOING TO TAKE TO MOVE TRANSDISCIPLINARY COLLABORATION FORWARD?

By all accounts, attaining TD collaboration in its ideal form is an extremely difficult and slow process (Seeman, 2003; Stokols, Harvey, Gress, Fuqua, & Phillips, 2005). The literature is replete with case studies that suggest the considerable barriers that occur throughout the process (e.g., see Magill-Evans, Hodge, & Darrah, 2002; Potter, 2001; Rosenfield & Kessel, 2003; Seeman, 2003; Stokols et al., 2003). In response, a number of interpersonal process models have been described that could guide the development of TD collaborations (Fong, 2003; Magill-Evans et al., 2002). Although process models can be used to suggest practical steps for developing and sustaining TD collaborations, they may not overcome the more amorphous and idiosyncratic barriers that can make TD collaborations so difficult to initiate and sustain. More recently, Stokols et al. (2003, 2005) have suggested a model for evaluating the process and scientific outputs of TD collaborative teams that lend qualitative insights into the behavioral, affective, interpersonal, and intellectual processes that facilitate and undermine TD research.

Overcoming Barriers to Transdisciplinary Collaborations

The numerous and considerable barriers to TD collaborations have been described by many (Potter, 2001; Rosenfield, 1992; Rosenfield & Kessel, 2003; Seeman, 2003; Stokols et al., 2003) and include professional specialization, cross-disciplinary communication, physical proximity, and availability of extrinsic incentives. First, professional specialization, that is, the almost uniform alignment of academic departments, national meetings, and scientific publications within single disciplines, is a significant impediment to TD collaboration. Accordingly, promotion and tenure policies give greater value to scientific accomplishments that impact a single field of study and emphasize lead authorship that may not be as readily attained in TD collaborations. Disciplinary chauvinism or disrespect (Stokols et al., 2003), fueled by differences in perceived rigor of methodological approaches of different disciplines, can also create tensions across disciplines that inhibit collaboration.

Second, communication across disciplines is inhibited by differences in vocabulary used even when describing similar measures and methods (Potter, 2001). Vocabulary plays a central role in professional specialization, enabling in-group and out-group distinctions that can be obstacles to cross-disciplinary communication (Potter, 2001). The time involved in arriving at mutual understandings of terminology can be frustrating and a strong disincentive to TD collaboration (Seeman, 2003).

Third, physical proximity can also make TD collaboration more challenging. Clinical, basic, social, and behavioral scientists are often located in different physical settings that create logistical inconveniences (e.g., parking) and impede coming together for formal and informal interactions. Reliance on more convenient alternatives, such as electronic communication, may lead to miscommunications and misunderstandings among team members who have different disciplinary perspectives or vocabularies or do not know each other well (Stokols et al., 2003).

Finally, extrinsic incentives, such as infrastructure, funding, and formalized reward systems, are lacking. The realities of careers in contemporary biomedical research mean that scientists often must secure significant proportions of their own salary through grant support. The considerable time involved in forging TD collaborations and the relatively slow evolution of the scientific products of these collaborations also can reduce the attraction of TD collaboration. Considering these sizeable barriers, it is surprising that comparatively little work has been published to guide research teams in navigating the interpersonal processes needed to build TD collaborations.

Collaborative Process Models Can Inform Transdisciplinary Collaborations

The consensus among those doing TD research (e.g., see Magill-Evans et al., 2002; Seeman, 2003; Stokols et al., 2003) is that group process factors play an instrumental and facilitative role in TD collaboration. Collaborative process models with roots in knowledge creation theory used in business settings (Fong, 2003) and professional alliance models used in academic management (Magill-Evans et al., 2002) suggest a number of strategies to facilitate communication and cooperation among individuals from a broad array of disciplines. Taken together, these models suggest that boundary crossing is a first step in TD collaboration, followed by an ongoing and iterative process of knowledge sharing, creation, and integration (Fong, 2003).

In these frameworks, "boundary crossing" is conceptualized as willingness to engage in interpersonal interactions that cross disciplines and hierarchical divisions. This willingness is often catalyzed by commitment to the solution of a compelling problem. Formalizing this commitment with a contract to collaborate (e.g., submission of a grant application), intentional pooling of existing financial resources, or an external stimulus such as an institutional initiative can increase the sustainability of these interactions (Magill-Evans et al., 2002).

The products of boundary crossing, knowledge sharing, and knowledge creation are most likely to occur when scientists and other stakeholders (e.g., community representatives, advocacy groups) respect and trust each other. Shared leadership is essential (Rosenfield, 1992), as is that each team member has an understanding of what he or she has to gain from the collaboration (Magill-Evans et al., 2002). This can be fostered through retreats or ongoing meetings in which the agenda is to promote co-teaching through group exploration of a research question with the goal to acquire a shared understanding of the different disciplinary perspectives relating to assumptions, constraints, and knowledge gaps (Fong, 2003; Magill-Evans et al., 2002; Seeman, 2003).

Knowledge sharing and identification of knowledge gaps can be used to prompt the knowledge creation necessary for innovation (Fong, 2003). This can be facilitated by ongoing group interactions that include joint problem-solving activities to identify possible new knowledge products, such as new hypotheses, integrated theoretical frameworks for analyzing important problems, novel methodological and empirical analyses of those problems, and evidence-based recommendations for public policy (Stokols et al., 2003). Once these products have been identified, knowledge integration can occur, in which the team seeks to marry the different perspectives and values of the team and their stakeholders to guide a decision-making process for prioritizing how to pursue full development of these products. These processes are iterative and may be cycled through again and again as knowledge integration raises new questions and considerations for the TD team.

Evaluating Outcomes of Transdisciplinary Collaborations

Given the substantial investment of resources to build and sustain TD collaborations, evaluation of the collaborative process and scientific outputs will be critical for their long-term sustainability. A number of challenges for developing an evaluative model for TD research have been suggested, including the impracticality of randomized trials to compare TD and non-TD collaborative teams, the tendency for evaluators to be team insiders, the lack of methodological tools to use, and uncertainty about the time frame needed for TD collaborations to generate scientific returns (Stokols et al., 2003).

Stokols et al. (2003) have developed a conceptual model to evaluate the process and scientific outputs of several of the TTURCs. Their evaluative model was derived through a series of qualitative and quantitative data collection strategies and behavioral observations conducted with TTURC investigators, staff, scientific consultants, and representatives from funding agencies. Concept mapping was used to synthesize the data across sources, and it suggested five key outcome clusters: collaboration, scientific integration, professional validation, communication, and health impacts. In turn, a logic map was developed to suggest a temporal order (i.e., immediate, intermediate, and long term), and causal pathways driving the outcomes were identified (see Figure 30.2). This logic model was used as a framework to guide

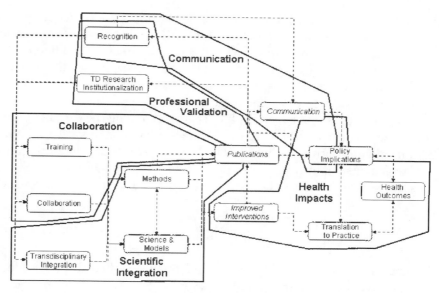

Figure 30.2. Evaluative model for evaluating the Transdisciplinary Tobacco Use Research Centers. TD = transdisciplinary. Long-term outcomes such as health impacts (e.g., improved interventions) derive from immediate collaboration and training through their effects on intermediate markers of scientific integration, including TD integration, methods, science, and model development. In turn, improved health impacts influence other long-term outcomes related to communication such as policy implications. Development of evaluative models such as this is needed to provide a framework for assessment of the value of future TD collaborations and science.

development of evaluation instruments being used to conduct a comprehensive and longitudinal evaluation of the TTURCs (see Stokols et al., 2003, for a detailed description of the methods).

Most recently, Stokols et al. (2005) described findings from the first 5 years of in vivo evaluation of these TTURCs. Their findings confirm and give new insights into the complex behavioral and affective mechanisms that can facilitate and impede efforts to achieve TD-integrated research. They confirmed that behavioral processes suggested by Fong's (2003) model (e.g., attending retreats and conferences outside one's major field, participating in working groups and brainstorming sessions) are important for increasing cross talk and for determining the extent to which participating scientists perceive that transdisciplinarity has been achieved.

In-depth prospective surveying as part of one of the TTURCs indicated that involved neuroscientists and behavioral scientists reported emotional ups and downs, periods of both great frustration and satisfaction, over their 5-year collaboration (Stokols et al., 2005). These ups and downs were more accentuated, with the lows being markedly lower, for the behavioral scientists than the neuroscientists. Neuroscientists reported consistently higher levels of satisfaction and perceptions of scientific integration than the behavioral scientists. Stokols et al. (2005) likened this to the "Mars–Venus effect" used in popular culture (Gray, 1993) to characterize gender differences in relationship orientation. This effect may reflect disciplinary differences in cultures, interpersonal needs, and tolerance for group processes that must be considered in building TD collaborations. Indeed, these differences in subjective experience, as well as geographic separation among the two disciplinary groups, led to some fragmentation, as day-to-day collaborative activities became aligned within discipline. Thus, evaluative models like this can be used to gain insight into qualitative barriers to TD collaboration, and the lessons learned can be directed to improve the next generation of TD research.

FUTURE DIRECTIONS

Several promising and large National Institutes of Health (NIH) funding initiatives have laid the groundwork for TD collaborative teams, and the next decade and new evaluative models will lead to a better understanding of their promise. However, the forecasted leveling off of NIH funding means additional strategies will be needed if TD research is to flourish.

First, development of TD training opportunities will be important to overcome barriers and foster TD research teams of the future (King et al., 2002; Seeman, 2003). These opportunities could take a variety of forms, including programs that expose trainees early in their careers to a broad array of disciplinary perspectives, as well as midcareer training opportunities that emphasize cross-disciplinary training and skills needed to lead TD teams. To this end, professional societies could partner or take the lead in sponsoring premeeting training workshops, interest groups that enable cross-disciplinary mentoring, and other mechanisms that encourage disciplinary boundary crossing.

It undoubtedly will be challenging to build programs that achieve a truly TD training milieu. This will require involvement and collaboration among a number of schools (e.g., public health, business, medicine, liberal arts), departments (e.g., biology, psychology, epidemiology), and centers (e.g., cancer, bioethics, genomics). Considerable time and resources must be committed to identifying core funding, agreeing on and establishing the curricula, and enlisting and sustaining active involvement from mentors. New programs in public health genomics ongoing or in development at the Universities of Michigan, North Carolina, and Washington represent exciting examples of a new generation of these TD training programs that might be used as models for future efforts.

Second, national scientific meetings could be organized to bring together different disciplines with the expressed purpose to learn about and foster TD collaborations (King et al., 2002). These efforts might include minimeetings that have a specialized focus on TD research. However, reluctance to attend additional meetings may be a significant impediment. Incentives to attend could be considered (e.g., low meeting costs, format options that enable more informal interactions, high profile keynote speakers, opportunities to submit talks to special journal editions). The recent conference on active living research held in 2004 (Sallis, Linton, & Kraft, 2005), and the special issue of the *American Journal of Preventive Medicine* (Sallis, Moudon, Linton, & Powell, 2005) that resulted, show that these efforts are already under way.

Third, funding initiatives sponsored by universities, cancer centers, medical centers, private foundations, and private industry could provide seed monies earmarked to TD collaborations to address pressing cancer control challenges. NIH initiatives beyond the expensive program project mechanism could also be augmented by special program announcements for investigator-initiated grants, and in so doing, could facilitate broader distribution of funding for TD collaborations. These initiatives could offer incentives that recognize the unique challenges of TD research to encourage scientists that these collaborations are worth the time investment, such as longer funding timelines or quick-turnaround options for competing renewals. Appointment of a standing study section specifically for TD research could also be an extrinsic incentive to galvanize TD collaborations.

As cancer prevention and early detection research grows increasingly more complicated, the need for TD collaborations has become more urgent. Although TD collaboration in its ideal form has the potential to accelerate research innovation in cancer control, these collaborations face considerable challenges and will require dedicated resources and visionary leaders if the full potential is to be achieved.

REFERENCES

Abrams, D. B. (1999). Transdisciplinary paradigms for tobacco prevention research. *Nicotine & Tobacco Research, 1*, 15–23.

Balmain, A., Gray, J., & Ponder, B. (2003). The genetics and genomics of cancer. *Nature Genetics, 33*, 238–244.

Behavioral Risk Factor Surveillance System. (2003). *Trends data, negative behavior circumstance.* Retrieved on April 21, 2004, from http://www.cdc.gov/brfss/Trends

Boslaugh, S. E., Luke, D. A., Brownson, R. C., Naleid, K. S., & Kreuter, M. W. (2004). Perceptions of neighborhood environment for physical activity: Is it "who you are" or "where you live"? *Journal of Urban Health, 81*, 671–681.

Byers, T., Mouchawar, J., Marks, J., Cady, B., Lins, N., Swanson, G. M., et al. (1999). The American Cancer Society challenge goals. *Cancer, 8*, 715–727.

Dierker, L. C., Avenevoli, S., Merikangas, K. R., Flaherty, B. P., & Stolar, M. (2001). Associations between psychiatric disorders and the progression of tobacco users' behaviors. *Journal of the American Academy of Child Adolescent Psychiatry, 40,* 1159–1167.

Emmons, K. M. (2000). Behavioral and social science contributions to the health of adults in the United States. In Institute of Medicine (Eds.), *Promoting health: Intervention strategies from social and behavioral research* (pp. 254–321). Washington, DC: National Academies Press.

Epstein, L. H. (1998). Integrating theoretical approaches to promote physical activity. *American Journal of Preventive Medicine, 15,* 257–265.

Fallon, J. H., Keator, D. B., Mbogori, J., Turner, J., & Potkin, S. G. (2004). Hostility differentiates the brain metabolic effects of nicotine. *Cognitive Brain Research, 18,* 142–148.

Fiore, M. C., Croyle, R. T., Curry, S. J., Cutler, C. M., Davis, R. M., Gordon, C., et al. (2004). Preventing 3 million premature deaths and helping 5 million smokers quit: A national action plan for tobacco cessation. *American Journal of Public Health, 94,* 205–210.

Fong, P. S. W. (2003). Knowledge creation in multidisciplinary project teams: An empirical study of the processes and their dynamic interrelationships. *International Journal of Project Management, 21,* 479–486.

Gilpin, E. A., Emery, S., White, M. M., & Pierce, J. P. (2003). Changes in youth smoking participation in California in the 1990s. *Cancer Causes Control, 14,* 985–993.

Gotay, C. C. (2005). Behavior and cancer prevention. *Journal of Clinical Oncology, 23,* 301–310.

Gray, J. (1993). *Men are from Mars, women are from Venus: A practical guide for improving communication and getting what you want in your relationships.* New York: HarperCollins.

King, A. C., Stokols, D., Talen, E., Brassington, G. S., & Killingsworth, R. (2002). Theoretical approaches to the promotion of physical activity: Forging a transdisciplinary paradigm. *American Journal of Preventive Medicine, 23*(Suppl. 2), 15–25.

Lerman, C., & Shields, A. E. (2004). Genetic testing for cancer susceptibility: The promise and the pitfalls. *Nature Reviews: Cancer, 4,* 235–241.

Lerman, C., Shields, P. G., Wileyto, E. P., Audrain, J., Hawk, L. H., Jr., Pinto, A., et al. (2003). Effects of dopamine transporter and receptor polymorphisms on smoking cessation in a bupropion clinical trial. *Health Psychology, 22,* 541–548.

Lerman, C., Wileyto, E. P., Patterson, F., Rukstalis, M., Audrain-McGovern, J., Restine, S., et al. (2004). The functional mu opioid receptor (OPRM1) Asn40Asp variant predicts short-term response to nicotine replacement therapy in a clinical trial. *The Pharmacogenomics Journal, 4,* 182–192.

Magill-Evans, J., Hodge, M., & Darrah, J. (2002). Establishing a transdisciplinary research team in academia. *Journal of Allied Health, 31,* 222–226.

Marcus, B. H., Bock, P. C., Pinto, B. M., Forsyth, L. H., Roberts, M. B., & Traficante, R. M. (1998). Efficacy of an individualized, motivationally tailored physical activity intervention. *Annals of Behavioral Medicine, 20,* 174–180.

Miksys, S., Lerman, C., Shields, P. G., Mash, D. C., & Tyndale, R. F. (2003). Smoking, alcoholism, and genetic polymorphisms alter CYP2B6 levels in human brain. *Neuropharmacology, 45*, 122–132.

Morgan, G. D., Kobus, K., Gerlach, K. K., Neighbors, C., Lerman, C., Abrams, D. B., & Rimer, B. K. (2003). Facilitating transdisciplinary research: The experience of the transdisciplinary tobacco use researcher centers. *Nicotine & Tobacco Research, 5*(Suppl. 1), 11–19.

National Cancer Act of 1971, Public Law 92-218, 92nd Congr., Senate 1828, December 23, 1971.

Pinto, B. M., Friedman, R., Marcus, B. H., Kelley, H., Tennstedt, S., & Gillman, M. W. (2002). Effects of a computer-based, telephone-counseling system on physical activity. *American Journal of Preventive Medicine, 23*, 113–120.

Potter, J. D. (2001). At the interfaces of epidemiology, genetics, and genomics. *Nature Reviews: Genetics, 2*, 142–147.

Rosenfield, P. L. (1992). The potential of transdisciplinary research for sustaining and extending linkages between the health and social sciences. *Social Science & Medicine, 35*, 1343–1357.

Rosenfield, P. L., & Kessel, F. (2003). Fostering interdisciplinary research: The way forward. In F. Kessel, P. L. Rosenfield, & N. Anderson (Eds.), *Expanding the boundaries of health and social science: Case studies in interdisciplinary innovation* (pp. 378–413). New York: Oxford University Press.

Saelens, B. E., Sallis, J. F., & Frank, L. D. (2003). Environmental correlates of walking and cycling: Findings from the transportation, urban design, and planning literatures. *Annals of Behavioral Medicine, 25*, 80–91.

Sallis, J. F., Linton, L., & Kraft, K. (2005). The first active living research conferences: Growth of a transdisciplinary field. *American Journal of Preventive Medicine, 28*(Suppl. 2), 93–95.

Sallis, J. F., Moudon, A. V., Linton, L. S., & Powell, K. E., (Eds.). (2005). Active living research [Special issue]. *American Journal of Preventive Medicine, 28*(Suppl. 1).

Seeman, T. E. (2003). Integrating psychosocial factors with biology. In F. Kessel, P. Rosenfield, & N. Anderson (Eds.), *Expanding the boundaries of health and social science: Case studies in interdisciplinary innovation* (pp. 206–227). New York: Oxford University Press.

Shenassa, E. D., McCaffery, J. M., Swan, G. E., Khroyan, T. V., Shakib, S., Lerman, C., et al. (2003). Intergenerational transmission of tobacco use and dependence: A transdisciplinary perspective. *Nicotine & Tobacco Research, 5*(Suppl. 1), 55–69.

Sondik, E. J. (2000). *Clinical preventive services progress review: Setting priorities for the delivery, quality, measurement, and coverage of clinical preventive services.* Retrieved April 19, 2004, from http://www.cdc.gov/nchs/about/otheract/hp2000/cps/clinprog.htm

Stokols, D., Fuqua, J., Gress, J., Harvey, R., Phillips, K., Baezconde-Garbanati, L., et al. (2003). Evaluating transdisciplinary science. *Nicotine & Tobacco Research, 5*(Suppl. 1), 21–39.

Stokols, D., Harvey, R., Gress, J., Fuqua, J., & Phillips, K. (2005). In vivo studies of trans-disciplinary scientific collaboration: Lessons learned and implications for active living research. *American Journal of Preventive Medicine, 28*(Suppl. 2), 202–213.

Subramanian, G., Adams, M. D., Venter, J. C., & Broder, S. (2001). Implications of the human genome for understanding human biology and medicine. *Journal of the American Medical Association, 286,* 2296–2307.

Tercyak, K. P., Lerman, C., & Audrain, J. (2002). Association of attention-deficit/hyperactivity disorder symptoms with levels of cigarette smoking in a community sample of adolescents. *Journal of the American Academy of Child & Adolescent Psychiatry, 41,* 799–805.

Vainio, H., & Husgafvel-Pursiainen, K. (1996). Mechanisms of carcinogenesis and molecular epidemiology. *British Journal of Hospital Medicine, 56,* 162–170.

von Eschenbach, A. C. (2004). A vision for the National Cancer Program in the United States. *Nature Reviews: Cancer, 4,* 820–828.

Weir, H. K., Thun, M. J., Hankey, B. F., Ries, L. A. G., Howe, H. L., Wingo, P. A., et al. (2003). Annual report to the nation on the status of cancer 1975–2000, featuring the use of surveillance data for cancer prevention and control. *Journal of the National Cancer Institute, 95,* 1276–1299.

31

INTERACTIVE HEALTH COMMUNICATIONS FOR CANCER PREVENTION AND CONTROL

VICTOR STRECHER

This chapter examines the current evidence for, and future of, *interactive health communications* (IHC) in cancer prevention and control. Other terms referring to similar domains include *consumer health informatics* and *eHealth*. The computer-based technologies relevant to IHC can include the Internet, mobile phones, personal digital assistants, computer-tailored print materials, interactive voice response, computer-driven kiosks, and CD-ROM, although a number of emerging technologies will also be relevant to IHC. In most cases, however, this chapter focuses on the Internet as the currently dominant instantiation of IHC. The variety of multimedia, interactivity, and connectivity formats offered by the Internet is extensive. Health-related organizations can now provide timely, interesting, and relevant cancer prevention and control programming on the Internet with the potential of reaching millions of users.

IHCs here are considered in terms of their reach and their effectiveness. Because IHCs, by definition, must interact in some manner with the user, different models of interaction are discussed. Finally, future directions for IHCs are explored, with a focus on emerging linkages to medical and bioinformatics systems.

THE REACH OF INTERACTIVE HEALTH COMMUNICATIONS

The growth of Internet access, broadband (i.e., high-speed Internet) access, amount of Internet use, and amount of Internet use for health-related reasons have all significantly increased over the past decade and appear to increase with every new survey on these subjects. Nearly all estimates of Internet access are out of date by the time they are published. It is, however, clear that the proportion of adults in the United States with Web access exceeds 75% and that the average Internet user reports spending over 12 hours per week using the Internet (Center for the Digital Future, 2005). After an early "dot-bomb" bubble washed away much of the eHealth field's initial snake-oil hype, the majority of Americans are now using IHCs. The Pew Internet and American Life Project 2006 survey of American adults with access to the Internet found that 80% of respondents (roughly 113 million adults) reported using the Web to obtain health information (Fox, 2006). In this survey, 64% of respondents reported using the Internet for a specific disease, 51% for a medical treatment or procedure, 49% for information about diet and nutrition, and 44% for information about exercise or fitness. The 2005 HINTS survey estimates that over 8.6 million smokers reported using the Internet for information about quitting smoking in the past 12 months (Health Information National Trends Survey, 2005). This compares favorably with the estimate that roughly 800,000 smokers in the United States call "quitlines" each year for cessation advice (Ossip-Klein and McIntosh, 2003). In addition to the home, Americans are also receiving eHealth programming through their health care organizations and employers.

Seekers of Web-based health information are more likely to be women, better educated, and White, and have higher incomes. A consistent finding from Web usage studies is the greater use among younger individuals, both cancer patients (Metz et al., 2003; Satterlund, McCaul, & Sandgren, 2003; Smith et al., 2003) and the general public (Fox & Fallows, 2003). Yet older patients, even those without Internet experience, readily participate in Internet-based self-management programs (Feil, Glasgow, Boles, & McKay, 2000; Gustafson et al., 1998; McTavish et al., 1995). More important is the increasing acceptability of the medium, even in populations for whom Internet access has been traditionally low.

Internet access and use continues to be exceptionally high among teens. Popular subjects among a broad socio-demographic spectrum of high school girls include disease-related information, diet and nutrition, exercise and fitness, sex, alcohol and drug abuse, mental health, medicines, and violence (Borzekowski & Rickert, 2000). The majority of girls in this survey felt it was particularly important to have access to contraceptive and nutrition information.

THE EFFECTIVENESS OF INTERACTIVE
HEALTH COMMUNICATIONS

Unfortunately, the majority of Internet-based health programming continues to focus on simple information transfer models. As Cline and Haynes (2001) stated in their appraisal of the field, "Much of the literature . . . focuses on the Internet as a high-tech conveyor in the rapid diffusion of information or health lessons. However, to do so is to ignore the very nature of the Internet" (p. 687). The Internet, and IHCs in general, can create more than a simple clearinghouse of health information (Cassel, Jackson, & Cheuvront, 1998; Neuhauser & Kreps, 2003). One starting point might be to consider the ways in which IHCs can interact with the user. Four types of interactivity, discussed in the next four sections, seem relevant: (a) user navigation, (b) collaborative filters, (c) expert systems, and (d) human-to-human interaction.

User Navigation: A Library at Your Fingertips

The most commonly used IHC strategy requires users to search for information, identifying what they consider the most relevant to their needs and interests. An appropriate metaphor to this form of navigation is "library": Similar to a library, the Internet has methods of searching for the large amount of available health information. Also like a library, however, the Internet does not automatically make available the best information or advice that an individual needs at a particular time. Studies in the educational literature have found that, when compared against fixed sequencing of instructional material, user control results in deviations from important information or methods of instruction (see Clark, 1982, for a review) and subsequent lower performance (Coldevin, Tovar, & Brauer, 1993; Gay, 1986; Ross & Morrison, 1989; Ross & Rakow, 1981; Steinberg, 1977).

Collaborative Filtering: What Others Like You Are Doing

It is common to use the actions and subsequent outcomes of similar peers to inform one's own decisions. Collaborative filtering uses software algorithms for identifying to the user the behaviors of other individuals who have similar behaviors (e.g., purchasing behavior). Collaborative filtering in the health area could match coping strategies and medical decisions of similar others. Collaborative filtering programs, however, will also face a number of challenges (Claypool, Brown, Le, & Waseda, 2001; Resnick & Varian, 1997). First, early users have very few others with whom they can compare. Predictions of what the user needs, when there are only a few users similar to them, will likely be inaccurate. Second, it may be difficult to find other users matching in more than just a few domains. Finally, individuals who do not consistently agree or disagree with anyone else (so-called gray sheep in collaborative filtering; Claypool et al., 2001) will fail to receive consistently useful information from an algorithm.

Expert Systems: When You Need a Counselor

A third interactive approach, closely approximating a counseling experience, is termed an *expert system*. Having undergone more experimental research than any other IHC system, this approach attempts to apply an expert's assessment, decision rules, and feedback strategies to software. The expert systems tested in the health behavior area typically require (a) a collection of characteristics, at an individual level, relevant to the targeted behavior change (or movement through stages of change); (b) an algorithm that uses these data to generate messages tailored to the specific needs of the user; and (c) a feedback protocol that combines these messages in a clear, vivid manner. The inferences made from the data are an attempt to reflect standards of a human expert (Negotia, 1985; Velicer, 1993). Selection of tailoring factors is based on two criteria: what is most important (i.e., predictive of behavior and behavior change) and what is most changeable (Green & Kreuter, 2000). Selection of factors on which to tailor feedback to the user is one of the most important steps in the development of an expert system.

The weight of evidence from randomized trials suggests that tailored communications for cancer prevention and control have a greater influence on relevant behavioral and decision-making outcomes than one-size-fits-all approaches (e.g., Noar, Benac, & Harris, 2007; Richards et al., 2007; Strecher, 2007), even among those with low literacy skills (Lipkus, Lyna, & Rimer, 1999; Skinner, Strecher, & Hospers, 1994). Moreover, we are beginning to understand why tailored communications have an influence. One of the key effect moderators in tailored expert systems appears to be the increased relevance of the message (Dijkstra, in press; Strecher et al., 2008).

Human-to-Human Interaction: A Channel for Social Support

Using high tech to facilitate high touch through online support groups provides patients a convenient way to give and receive informational and emotional support (Brennan & Fink, 1997; Shaw, McTavish, Hawkins, Gustafson, & Pingree, 2005). The 24-hours-per-day, 7-days-per-week accessibility to online support is considered a significant advantage to patients who, whether because of stress, pain, or the cancer treatment itself, have irregular sleeping habits. Patients report frequent use of discussion groups late at night (Shaw et al., 2005). Anonymity is a frequently cited benefit of computer-mediated groups (Shaw et al., 2005). Use of computer-mediated support services, however, has been found to be somewhat lower among underserved populations, including minority and older patients (Gustafson et al., 1998).

A review of 10 studies of online cancer support groups (Klemm et al., 2003) found significant support for improved patient coping. Many of these studies lacked controlled experimental designs, and many were conducted among small, homogeneous groups of patients, mainly White women (Klemm et al., 2003). Although the differential influence of peer-moderated versus professionally moderated groups is an important issue to online discussion group developers, published research, to the knowledge of this author, has not examined this issue (Till, 2003).

Online therapists offer another human-to-human interaction relevant to IHCs (Carlbring, Ekselius, & Andersson, 2003; Tate, Jackvony, & Wing, 2003). Online Internet interactions with therapists offer significant convenience to both the user and the therapist. Although this issue has not been examined, online therapy may offer an added degree of anonymity and therefore the possibility of more honest expression of behaviors, attitudes, and emotions. As is the case with telecounseling services, however, proactive online therapy could be difficult and expensive to scale in a high-quality manner to large populations. Hybrid models could combine expert system (e.g., identifying current ability and barriers to tailor cooking and shopping skills messages), user navigation (e.g., an information library with accurate, timely information regarding obesity and cancer), collaborative filtering (e.g., a personalized recipe book filtering on taste preferences), and human-to-human interactions (e.g., an online support group) in the same program (Gustafson et al., 1998, 1999; Smaglik et al., 1998).

In a comprehensive review of computer-generated health behavior interventions (including the Web), Revere and Dunbar (2001) concluded, "It is notable that only those studies using print and telephone devices reported a theoretical basis for their methodology" (p. 76). Doshi, Patrick, Sallis, and Calfas's (2003) review of 24 Web sites designed to promote physical activity found very low use of health behavior change theory and a lack of attention to assessment or feedback tailored to characteristics of the user. IHCs would benefit from new conceptual frameworks that integrate psychosocial and communications constructs. An important step for the IHC field would be the conceptualization and integration of interactivity as a construct in these frameworks.

FUTURE DIRECTIONS

The IHC field continues to change rapidly in terms of access to the relevant technologies, consumer attitudes toward the technologies, and the technologies themselves. These changes pose a tremendous challenge to IHC researchers in remaining timely and relevant (Cline & Haynes, 2001). IHC interventions tested in randomized trials as "black boxes" are often out of date by the time the results are published. Even if an effect is demonstrated in such trials, there are rarely mechanisms of effect that can be clearly identified to help other IHC developers. Researchers are therefore encouraged to consider innovative intervention approaches and research paradigms to identify active, inert, and possibly negative components of IHC (Abrams, Mills, & Bulger, 1999; Collins, Murphy, & Strecher, 2007; Kreps, 2003).

Identifying the Active Components and Mechanisms of Interactive Health Communications

Why do IHCs generally have a stronger effect on behavioral and decision-making outcomes than more traditional mass communication strategies? Given the large number of potentially active IHC components, innovation in experimental approaches to their evaluation is important. Multiphase optimization strategy (MOST) designs may be particularly relevant to IHC development (Collins et al., 2007; Collins, Murphy, Nair, & Strecher, 2005). These designs begin with the systematic screening of large numbers of potentially active factors, then refine and ultimately optimize interventions with the factors found to be most effective. MOST provides a principled, efficient approach to testing, using a randomized trial design, large numbers of potentially active factors that normally would be too unwieldy to test using more traditional means. Recent research has used a MOST design to efficiently identify several active components of IHCs (Strecher et al., 2008).

Since IHCs can often tailor information to specific needs and interests of the user, research examining how users differentially respond to intervention components is highly relevant to IHC development. For example, Williams-Piehota, Schneider, Pizarro, Mowad, and Salovey (2003) found that an individual's need for cognition moderated the impact of mammography screening messages and that tailoring the message to the subject's need for cognition produced a positive effect on mammography screening behavior at 6-month follow-up. Other interesting psychosocial and communication factors that could be examined in tailored communications include narrative stories, message timing, appeals to core values, normative feedback, message density and length, graphics, culture, literacy, media type, risk feedback, and many others.

Another area for IHC research relevant to cancer prevention and control is the study of risk communication for informed decision making. Eliciting patient preferences and values to provide feedback that is accurate, balanced, and easy to comprehend for individuals varying in their ability to understand risk information is an important challenge. IHCs allow risk information to be tailored to an individual's actual and perceived risk, numeracy, need for cognition, and locus of control. There is also a need to bulletproof risk perceptions from sensational or anecdotal information that has been found to unduly influence these perceptions (e.g., Ubel, Jepson, & Baron, 2001).

Integrating Consumer and Medical Informatics

Interactions between the types of IHCs discussed in this chapter and other informatics systems of clinical medicine, biology, and public health are now emerging. With organizations such as the U. S. Department of Veterans Affairs taking a lead in demonstrating the effectiveness and efficiency of electronic medical records systems (Haugh, 2003), large managed care systems, including Kaiser Permanente and Group Health Cooperative, are beginning to integrate tools to prompt and record cancer-related screening, counseling, and decision support activities (McAfee, Grossman, Dacey, & McClure, 2002). At Kaiser Permanente, links are being made between the electronic medical record, the patient health record, and consumer-focused IHCs including health risk appraisal and tailored behavior change and decision-making tools.

Online communication between clinicians and patients seems, on the face of it, to be another logical extension of the medical–consumer informatics integration. Such interactions, however, have yielded mixed results (Katz, Moyer, Cox, & Stern, 2003), with both physician and patient preferences for some types of e-mail interactions (e.g., simpler clinical issues and requests for normal lab results) over others (e.g., complex or sensitive issues such as mental health or pain management). Moreover, researchers must recognize the fundamental transitions in the structure and process of clinical practice that are likely to occur as a result of integrating online communications systems (Katz & Moyer, 2004). Although various reimbursement models are being explored, payment for online communication is only beginning to be adopted. Other significant steps toward systematic integration would be an effective triage (e.g., physician–nurse–Web site) of patient questions and complete documentation of online communication in the electronic medical record (Katz et al., 2003).

For nearly 4 decades, researchers have found that knowledge is generally unrelated to health behavior and that simple information transmission fails to change health-related behaviors. Yet, the concept of the pamphlet rack outside of the doctor's office endures, even in electronic form. Successful integration of these fields of informatics can probably yield outcomes greater than the sums of their parts, but a scientific, theoretically grounded understanding of both fields will be required to achieve success.

Integrating Consumer and Bioinformatics

The application of statistical and computational methods to understanding the human genome should yield tremendous benefits in the understanding of cancer susceptibility, responsiveness to prevention efforts, and survivorship. To date, estimates of an individual's health risk are calculated from population-based data (Beery et al., 1986). In other words, researchers currently use population-based mortality data to calculate a risk age on the basis of an individual's demographic characteristics and health habits (Beery et al., 1986; Strecher & Kreuter, 1995). Feedback from such health risk assessments can provide only averaged, usually bland, feedback regarding risk that generally has little impact on behavior change (Kreuter & Strecher, 1996; Strecher & Kreuter, 1995). Assessing an individual's risk that incorporates genotypic, environmental, and behavioral data will ultimately allow far more accurate, detailed, and personalized feedback to that individual. IHCs will play an important role in creating very personalized feedback tailored to the abilities and preferences of the individual. Once this feedback is provided, genetic information could be used in combination with behavioral, psychosocial, and environmental data to create a far more tailored intervention plan. For example, genetic and smoking history data could inform the type and dosing of pharmacotherapy for smoking cessation in combination with a tailored behavioral treatment plan (Lerman & Berrettini, 2003).

CONCLUSIONS

IHCs, particularly through the Internet, now reach the majority of the North American, European, and Australian populace. Use of IHCs for cancer prevention has been lower than use by cancer patients. This finding is not surprising and remains an important challenge with which prevention researchers are familiar. Randomized controlled trials specifically comparing different methods of reaching individuals for prevention are needed.

Users of IHCs find them palatable because of their convenience, availability, and anonymity. Computer-driven interventions, however, are clearly not for everyone. For nearly 2 decades, education researchers have examined individual differences in learning from computer-assisted instruction. This research direction should be further developed for IHCs in an effort to determine the types of individuals who benefit most and least from these interventions.

As the IHC field develops, researchers and practitioners would benefit from more careful consideration of what it means to be interactive. This chapter presented different approaches to IHC interactivity, approaches that likely will be differentially effective on the basis of an individual's health and behavioral issues, optimal (not necessarily preferred) learning style, need for cognition, ability, and many other characteristics. Unfortunately, the IHC interaction approach most commonly used, requiring the user to navigate through an electronic library of information (i.e., pamphletware), may be the least effective among individuals with low ability or prior knowledge.

Controlled trials comparing the impact of different interactivity approach, media, content, and message frequency, among other factors, by characteristics of the individual would likely improve the quality and understanding of IHCs. One of the most egregious errors of this field has been to generalize IHCs into one class of intervention. Asking "Are IHCs effective?" is like asking "Do movies entertain?" Clearly, some do and some do not. The challenge is to determine the optimal fit of IHCs to individual needs and preferences. This issue is completely consistent with the adaptive potential of IHCs.

REFERENCES

Abrams, D. B., Mills, S., & Bulger, D. (1999). Challenges and future directions for tailored communication research. *Annals of Behavioral Medicine, 21,* 299–306.

Beery, W. L., Schoenbach, V. J., Wagner, E. H., Graham, R., Karon, J. and Pezzullo, S. (1986). *Health risk appraisal: Methods and programs, with annotated bibliography* (U.S. Department of Health and Human Services Publication No. 86-3396). Washington, DC: National Center for Health Services Research and Health Care Technology.

Borzekowski, D. L., & Rickert, V. I. (2000). Urban girls, Internet use, and accessing health information. *Journal of Pediatric and Adolescent Gynecology, 13,* 94–95.

Brennan, P., & Fink, S. (1997). Health promotion, social support, and computer networks. In R. Street, W. Gold, & T. Manning (Eds.), *Health promotion and interactive technology* (pp. 157–169). Mahwah: NJ: Erlbaum.

Carlbring, P., Ekselius, L., & Andersson, G. (2003). Treatment of panic disorder via the Internet: A randomized trial of CBT vs. applied relaxation. *Journal of Behavior Therapy and Experimental Psychiatry, 34,* 129–140.

Cassel, M. M., Jackson, C., & Cheuvront, B. (1998). Health communication on the Internet: An effective channel for health behavior change? *Journal of Health Communication, 3,* 71–79.

Center for the Digital Future. 2005. *Digital future report.* Available at http://www.digitalcenter.org

Clark, R. E. (1982). Antagonism between achievement and enjoyment in ATI studies. *Educational Psychologist, 17,* 92–101.

Claypool, M ., Brown, D., Le, P., and Waseda, M. (2001). Inferring user interest. *IEEE Internet Computing, 5,* 32–39.

Cline, R. J., & Haynes, K. M. (2001). Consumer health information seeking on the Internet: The state of the art. *Health Education Research, 16,* 671–692.

Coldevin, G., Tovar, M., & Brauer, A. (1993). Influence of instructional control and learner characteristics on factual recall and procedural learning from interactive video. *Canadian Journal of Educational Communication, 22,* 113–130.

Collins, L. M., Murphy, S. A., Nair, V., & Strecher, V. (2005). A strategy for optimizing and evaluating behavioral interventions. *Annals of Behavioral Medicine, 30,* 65–73.

Collins, L. M., Murphy, S. A., & Strecher, V. (2007). The multiphase optimization strategy (MOST) and the sequential multiple assignment randomized trial (SMART): New methods for more potent eHealth interventions. *American Journal of Preventive Medicine, 32*(Suppl. 5), 112–118.

Dijkstra, A. (in press). The psychology of tailoring: Ingredients in computer-tailored persuasion. *Social and Personality Psychology.*

Doshi, A., Patrick, K., Sallis, J. F., & Calfas, K. (2003). Evaluation of physical activity Web sites for use of behavior change theories. *Annals of Behavioral Medicine, 25,* 105–111.

Feil, E. G., Glasgow, R. E., Boles, S., & McKay, H. G. (2000). Who participates in Internet-based self-management programs? A study among novice computer users in a primary care setting. *Diabetes Education, 26,* 806–811.

Fox, S. (2006, October 29). *Online health search 2006.* Available at http://www.pewinternet.org/PPF/r/190/report_display.asp

Fox, S., & Fallows, D. (2003). *Internet health resources: Health searches and email have become more commonplace, but there is room for improvement in searches and overall Internet access.* Retrieved February 28, 2008, from http://www.pewinternet.org/PPF/r/95/report_display.asp

Gay, G. (1986). Interaction of learner control and prior understanding in computer-assisted video instruction. *Journal of Educational Psychology, 78,* 225–227.

Green, L., & Kreuter, M. (2000). *Health promotion planning: An educational and environmental approach* (2nd ed.). Mountain View, CA: Mayfield.

Gustafson, D. H., Hawkins, R., Boberg, E., Pingree, S., Serlin, R., Graziano, F., & Chan, C. L.. (1999). Impact of a patient-centered, computer-based health information/support system. *American Journal of Preventive Medicine, 16,* 1–9.

Gustafson, D. H., McTavish, F., Hawkins, R., Pingree, S., Arora, N., Mendenhall, J., & Simmons, G. E. (1998). Computer support for elderly women with breast cancer. *Journal of the American Medical Association, 280,* 1305.

Haugh, R. (2003). Reinventing the VA: Civilian providers find valuable lessons in a once-maligned health care system. *Hospitals & Health Networks, 77,* 50–52.

Health information national trends survey (HINTS). (2005). Available at http://hints.cancer.gov/index.jsp

Katz, S. J., & Moyer, C. A. (2004). The emerging role of online communication between patients and their providers. *Journal of General Internal Medicine, 19,* 978–983.

Katz, S. J., Moyer, C. A., Cox, D. T., & Stern, D. T. (2003). Effect of a triage-based e-mail system on clinic resource use and patient and physician satisfaction in primary care: A randomized controlled trial. *Journal of General Internal Medicine*, *18*, 736–744.

Klemm, P., Bunnell, D., Cullen, M., Soneji, R., Gibbons, P., & Holecek, A. (2003). Online cancer support groups: A review of the research literature. *CIN: Computers, Informatics, Nursing*, *21*, 136–142.

Kreps, G. L. (2003). The impact of communication on cancer risk, incidence, morbidity, mortality, and quality of life. *Health Communication*, *15*, 163–171.

Kreuter, M. W., & Strecher, V. J. (1996). Do tailored behavior change messages enhance the effectiveness of health risk appraisal? Results from a randomized trial. *Health Education Research*, *11*, 97–105.

Lerman, C., & Berrettini, W. (2003). Elucidating the role of genetic factors in smoking behavior and nicotine dependence. *American Journal of Medical Genetics: B. Neuropsychiatric Genetics*, *118*, 48–54.

Lipkus, I. M., Lyna, P. R., & Rimer, B. K. (1999). Using tailored interventions to enhance smoking cessation among African-Americans at a community health center. *Nicotine & Tobacco Research*, *1*, 77–85.

McAfee, T., Grossman, R., Dacey, S., & McClure, J. (2002). Capturing tobacco status using an automated billing system: Steps toward a tobacco registry. *Nicotine & Tobacco Research*, *4*(Suppl. 1), 31–37.

McTavish, F. M., Gustafson, D. H., Owens, B. H., Hawkins, R. P., Pingree S., Wise, M., et al. (1995). CHESS (Comprehensive Health Enhancement Support System): An interactive computer system for women with breast cancer piloted with an underserved population. *Journal of Ambulatory Care Management*, *18*, 35–41.

Metz, J. M., Devine, P., DeNittis, A., Jones, H., Hampshire, M., Goldwein, J., & Whittington, R. (2003). A multi-institutional study of Internet utilization by radiation oncology patients. *International Journal of Radiation Oncology, Biology, Physics*, *56*, 1201–1205.

Negotia, U. N. (1985). *Expert systems and fuzzy systems*. Menlo Park, CA: Benjamin Cummings.

Neuhauser, L., & Kreps, G. L. (2003). Rethinking communication in the e-health era. *Journal of Health Psychology*, *8*, 7–22.

Noar, S. M., Benac, C. N., & Harris, M. S. (2007). Does tailoring matter? Meta-analytic review of tailored print health behavior change interventions. *Psychological Bulletin*. *133*, 673–693.

Ossip-Klein, D. J., & McIntosh, S. (2003). Quitlines in North America: Evidence base and applications. *American Journal of Medical Sciences*, *326*, 201–205.

Resnick, P., & Varian, H. R. (1997). Recommender systems. *Communications of the ACM*, *40*, 56–58.

Revere, D., & Dunbar, P. J. (2001). Review of computer-generated outpatient health behavior interventions: Clinical encounters "in absentia." *Journal of the American Medical Informatics Association*, *8*, 62–79.

Richards K. C., Enderlin, C. A., Beck, C., McSweeney, J. C., Jones, T. C., & Roberson, P. K. (2007). Tailored biobehavioral interventions: A literature review and synthesis. *Research and Theory for Nursing Practice*, *21*, 271–285.

Ross, S., & Morrison, G. (1989). In search of a happy medium in instructional technology research: Issues concerning external validity, media replications, and learner control. *Educational Technology, Research, and Development, 37*, 19–33.

Ross S., & Rakow, E. (1981). Learner control as adaptive strategies for selection of instructional support on math rules. *Educational Psychology, 73*, 745–753.

Satterlund, M. J., McCaul, K. D., & Sandgren, A. K. (2003). Information gathering over time by breast cancer patients. *Journal of Medical Internet Research, 5*, e15. doi:10.2196/jmir.5.3.e15

Shaw, B. R., McTavish, F., Hawkins, R., Gustafson, D. H., & Pingree, S. (2005). Experiences of women with breast cancer: Exchanging social support over the CHESS computer network. *Journal of Health Communication, 5*, 135–159.

Skinner, C. S., Strecher, V. J., & Hospers, H. (1994). Physicians' recommendations for mammography: Do tailored messages make a difference? *American Journal of Public Health, 84*, 43–49.

Smaglik, P., Hawkins, R. P., Pingree, S., Gustafson, D. H., Boberg, E., & Bricker, E. (1998). The quality of interactive computer use among HIV-infected individuals. *Journal of Health Communication, 3*, 53–68.

Smith, R. P., Devine, P., Jones, H., DeNittis, A., Whittington, R., & Metz, J. M. (2003). Internet use by patients with prostate cancer undergoing radiotherapy. *Urology, 62*, 273–277.

Steinberg, E. R. (1977). Review of student control in computer-assisted instruction. *Journal of Computer-Based Instruction, 3*, 84–90.

Strecher, V. J. (2007). Internet methods for delivering behavioral and health-related interventions (eHealth). *Annual Review of Clinical Psychology, 3*, 53–76.

Strecher, V. J., & Kreuter, M. W. (1995). The psychosocial and behavioral impact of health risk appraisals. In R. T. Croyle (Ed.), *Psychosocial effects of screening for disease prevention and detection* (pp. 126–143). New York: Oxford University Press.

Strecher, V. J., McClure, J. B., Alexander, G. L., Chakraborty, B., Nair, V. N., Konkel, J. M., et al. (2008). Web-based smoking cessation programs: Results of a randomized trial. *American Journal of Preventive Medicine, 34*, 373–381.

Tate, D. F., Jackvony, E. H., & Wing, R. R. (2003). Effects of Internet behavioral counseling on weight loss in adults at risk for Type 2 diabetes: A randomized trial. *Journal of the American Medical Association, 289*, 1833–1836.

Till, J. E. (2003). Evaluation of support groups for women with breast cancer: Importance of the navigator role. *Health and Quality of Life Outcomes, 1*, 16.

Ubel, P. A., Jepson, C., & Baron, J. (2001). The inclusion of patient testimonials in decision aids: Effects on treatment choices. *Medical Decision Making, 21*, 60–68.

Velicer, W. F. (1993). An expert system intervention for smoking cessation. *Addictive Behaviors, 18*, 269–290.

Williams-Piehota, P., Schneider, T. R., Pizarro, J., Mowad, L., & Salovey, P. (2003). Matching health messages to information-processing styles: Need for cognition and mammography utilization. *Health Communication, 15*, 375–392.

AUTHOR INDEX

Numbers in italics refer to listings in the references.

Aapro, M. S., 349, *354*
Aaro, L. E., *164*
Aaron, J., 328, 331, 339, *342, 376*
Aaronson, N. K., 116, 120, 121, *125,*
    128, 362, *372, 376, 430*
Aarts, H., 45, *52*
Abboud, P. A., *181*
Abell, T., *144*
Abemayor, E., 488, *493*
Ablin, A., *450*
Abraham, L., *443*
Abrahamsen, T. G., 452, *460*
Abrams, D. B., 5–6, *20,* 45, *52,* 92, 97,
    113, 169, *180, 181, 182, 186,*
    239, 246, *247, 248,* 525, *527,*
    531, 533, 536, *543, 545,* 552, *555*
Abramson, L. Y., 347, 352, 353, *354*
Absetz, P., 282, *293, 295*
Achenbach, T. M., 454, *458*
Ackerson, L., *234*
Adami, H. O., 36, 38, *39*
Adamolli, *462*
Adams, J., 110, *111,* 401, *407, 434, 443*
Adams, J. A., *442*
Adams, J. E., *387*
Adams, J. H., *388*
Adams, M., 213, *222*
Adams, M. A., *221*
Adams, M. D., 535, *546*
Adams, M. J., 433, *442*
Adams, T. B., 169, *187*
Addy, C. L., *248*
Adelbratt, S., 332, *341*
Adenis, C., *318*
Adler, D., 395, *405,* 478, *482*
Adler, D. C., 483, *514*
Adlis, S. A., 292, *300*

Advisory Committee on Cancer
    Control of the National Cancer
    Institute of Canada, The, 6, *20*
Agarwal, S. K., 503, *511*
Agency for Healthcare Research and
    Quality (AHRQ), 140, *143,* 190,
    196, *201,* 441, *442,* 488, *491,*
    521–522, *523, 524, 526, 527*
Agrawal, S., 176, *187*
Ahearn, E. M., *339*
Ahearn, S., *345*
Ahles, T., 219, 438, *446*
Ahles, T. A., 351, *354,* 438, *442, 447*
Ahmed, R. L., 490, *493, 493*
Ahmedzai, S., *125*
Ahn, C., 399, *404*
Ahnen, D. J., *277*
Ahrens, M. B., *165*
Aickin, M., 98, *202*
Aiello, E., 417, *426*
Aiken, L. S., 138, *143,* 257, *273*
Aitchison, T., 215, *221*
Ajzen, I., 44, *52, 53,* 490, *492*
Akechi, T., 350, *358*
Albanes, D., *112*
Albers, M., *128*
Albertson, P. C., *127*
Albrecht, G. L., *163*
Albrecht, T. L., 104, *111*
Albright, J., *318*
Alcalay, R., 105, *112*
Aldana, E., 351, *359*
Aldana, S. G., 239, *249*
Alderfer, M., 451, 453, 454, 456, *458,*
    461
Alexander, G. L., *558*
Alexander, S. C., *341*

559

Al-Ghazal, S. K., 417, *425*
Allan Mufson, R., *516*
Allen, C., *112, 247*
Allen, J. D., 92, *97*
Allen, R. S., *407*
Allenby, A., *375*
Allison, C. J., *101*
Allison, P., 489, 490, *492*
Almendingen, K., 291, *298*
Altman, D., 268, *276*
Altman, D. G., 62, 83, 171, *183*, 509, *515*
Alvarez, F. B., *38*
Ambrosino, J., 421, *428*
Ambrozy, D. M., *346*
American Academy of Pediatrics, Committee on Public Education, 199, *201*
American Cancer Society, 61, 66, 79, 209, *217*, 226, 227, *231*, 487
American Dietetic Association, 198, *201*
American Journal of Preventive Medicine, 543, *543*
American Psychiatric Association (APA), 171, *181*, 416, *425, 458*
Ammerman, A., 190, 191, *201*
Ammerman, A. S., *205*
Amon, A., 228, *234*
Anda, R. F., 171, *181*
Anderman, C., 63, 66, 80, 82, 137, *144*
Andersen, A., *164*
Andersen, B. L., 362, 368, 369, 371, *372*, 421, 425, *425*, 502, 509, *510*
Andersen, M. R., 272, *273*
Andersen, P. A., 214, *217, 222*
Anderson, B., *514*
Anderson, B. L., *318*, 420
Anderson, C., 244
Anderson, C. A., 142, *144, 246*
Anderson, D. M., 437, *442*
Anderson, E. D. C., *315*
Anderson, G. L., 92, *102, 112*
Anderson, J., 192, *204*
Anderson, J. E., *187*
Anderson, K. B., *112*

Anderson, M., 188, 214, *219, 301*
Anderson, N., *545*
Anderson, V., 450, *458*
Andersson, G., 551, *555*
Andersson, S. O., *36*
Andersson-Ellströöm, T., 286, *298*
Andreski, P., 176, *181*
Andrews, H., 226, *233*
Andrews, S., 395, *403*
Andrews, T. C., *446*
Andrykowski, M. A., 280, 295, 364, 366, 367, *372, 373, 376*, 416, 417, 418, 420, *426*
Angeli, N., *297*
Anliker, J., 194, *204*
Annyas, A. A., *345*
Ansell, D., *278*
Anthony, J. C., 92, *100*, 177, *183*
Antin, J. H., *514*
Anton-Culver, H., *112*
Antoni, M., 503, *510*
Antoni, M. H., *376*, 418, *426, 430*
Antoniou, G., 453, *464*
Antonucci, T., 307, *320*
Antonucci, T. C., 194, *203*
Applegate, B. W., 170, *187*
Applegate, W., *247*
Appley, M. H., *233*
Apter, A., 194, *204*
Arbeit, M. L., 195, *206*
Arber, A., 329, 330, 337, *341*
Archbold, P., 397, *407*
Ardern-Jones, A., *316*
Arena, P., *376, 430*
Arena, P. L., 418, *426*
Arkinson, J. O., *112*
Armstrong, B. K., 24, 33, 34, *37*, 215, *220*
Armstrong, C. A., *248*
Armstrong, F. D., 450, *458*
Armstrong, K., 304, 306, *313, 314, 319*
Arndt, L. A., 368, *374*
Arnold, A., *374*
Arnold, R. M., 338, *341*
Aro, A. R., 281, 282, *295, 296*
Ary, D. V., 156, *162*

Asbury, R., *357*
Ascherio, A., *37, 38*
Ashbury, F. D., 27, *39*
Ashikaga, T., *314*
Ashing-Giwa, K. T., 415, 417, *425*
Ashley, S., *321*, 451, *465*
Aspinwall, L. G., 143, *143*
Assman, S. F., 75, 76, 77, *79*
Atherton, P. J., *386*
Atkin, W., *278*, 289, 290, *299, 301*
Atkin, W. S., 290, *296*
Atkins, D., *528*
Atkins, J. N., *356*
Atkinson, C., *405*
Atkinson, S. A., *444*
Atwood, K., 35, *35, 148*
Audrain, J., 70, 80, *144*, 304, 310, *314, 317, 536, 544, 546*
Audrain-McGovern, J., 161, *162, 164, 185, 544*
Augustiny, K. F., 476, *481*
Ault, K. A., *38*
Auslander, W., *204*
Austin, D. F., *442*
Austoker, J., *281*, 282, *284*, 296, *299*
Avenevoli, S., 536, *543*
Ayala, G. X., 64, *81, 99*
Aziz, N., 487, 488, 490, 491, *492*
Aziz, N. M., *492*
Azizi, E., 214, *217*
Azzouz, F., 395, *405*

Baalbergen, A., *318*
Babb, J., *147, 315*, 396, 406, 477, *483*
Babb, J. S., *315*
Babcock, A. L., 434, *447*
Bacak, S. J., 245, *247*
Bach, J. V., 312, *314*
Bachiocco, V., 351, *354*
Bachman, J. G., *164*
Back, A. L., 337, 338, 339, 340, *341, 342, 344*
Backinger, C., 160, *162*
Bacon, C. G., 381, *386*
Baden, L. R., 226, *231*
Badger, G. J., *163*

Baer, N., *164*
Baezconde-Garbanati, L., *545*
Baghurst, P., *464*
Baider, L., 469, 473, *480*
Baildam, A., *297*
Baile, D., 336
Baile, W. D. F., *341*
Baile, W. F., *182*, 328, 329, 331, 332, 338, 339, *341, 342, 344, 345, 365, 375*
Bailey, D. E., Jr., *357, 484*
Bailey, W. C., *183*
Bailie, A. J., 137, *143*
Bain, C., *273*
Baker, A. H., 294, *296*
Baker, D. I., *250*
Baker, E. A., 245, *247*, 520, *528*
Baker, E. L., 520, *527*
Baker, F., 488, 490, *492*
Baker, L. C., 171, *182, 274*
Baker, M. W., *316*
Baker, S., *482*
Baker, T. B., 175, *186, 188*
Baker, W. L., 89, 92, *100, 102*
Bakke, A. C., 349, *355*
Balanda, K. P., 92, *100*, 211, *220*
Balch, G., 160, *163*
Balch, G. I., 68, *80*
Balcueva, E. P., *386*
Baldwin, S., *232*
Bales, C., *233*
Bales, C. B., 311, *318*
Ballard-Barbash, R., *205, 257, 274, 300, 494*
Ballard-Reisch, D. S., 336, *342*
Balmain, A., 531, 534, *543*
Balmes, J., *39*
Balshem, A., 141, *145*, 304, *317*
Bandiwala, S. I., *249*
Bandura, A., 45, *53*, 239, 246, 490, *492*
Banerjee, T. K., 358, *359*
Bankhead, C., 281, *296*
Bankhead, C. R., 283, 287, *296*
Bansal, N., *247*
Bansod, A., 174, *185*
Bantle, J. P., *54*

Barakat, L., 455, *458*, *461*

Barakat, R., *319*, *388*

Barakat, R. R., *235*

Baranowski, J., 98, 200, *201*

Baranowski, T., 92, 97, 98, *101*, 190,
    192, 195, 200, *201*, 206, 244, 246

Barbarin, O., 454, *458*, *464*

Barber, L. T., *234*

Bard, M., *372*

Barg, F., 397, 398, 400, *403*, *407*

Barker, C., 470, *485*

Barker, D. C., *80*

Barker, J., *144*

Barley, G. C., *341*

Barlow, W. E., 66, 80, 82, 137, *144*, 277

Barnwell, E., *21*

Barofsky, I., 116, *125*, *128*

Baron, J., 141, *148*, 553, *558*

Baron, J. A., 30, *35*

Baron, R. M., 77, *80*

Baronowski, J., *97*

Barr, E., *38*

Barr, R. D., 434, *444*, *448*

Barratt, A., *318*, *344*

Barrera, M., 456, *458*

Barrett, R. J., *234*

Barsevick, A., *315*

Bartee, R. T., 199, *203*

Barton, D. L., 385, *386*

Basa, P., *448*

Basch, C. E., 68, *80*

Basen-Enguist, K., 98, 229, 232, *300*,
    529

Baskin, M., *202*

Baskin, M. L., 196, *201*

Bastani, R., 67, 81, 269, 273, *273*, 277,
    287, *296*

Batenhorst, A., *128*

Bath, P. A., 470, *485*

Batterwall, A., *112*

Baty, B., 307, *315*

Baty, B. J., 312, *314*

Baum, A., 63, 80, *148*, 235, *318*, 503,
    512

Bauman, A., 239, 245, 246, 248, *250*

Bauman, K. I., 156, *162*

Baumgartner, K. B., *494*

Baumgartner, R. N., *494*

Baumiller, R. C., *318*

Baxter, J. S., *203*

Baxter, K., 286, *300*

Bayliss, M. S., *128*

Beach, B., 216, *218*

Beach, B. H., *218*

Beach, K. E., *187*

Beach, M., *35*

Beach, M. L., *165*

Beach, S. R., 479, *485*

Beacham, A., *295*

Beale, E. A., 332, *342*

Bearison, D. J., *461*

Beatty, P. C., 270, *273*

Beck, C., *557*

Beck, J. D., *462*

Beckham, J., 395, *404*

Beckman, H. B., 337, 338, 339, *342*

Becona, E., 177, *182*

Bedell, E., 331, *342*

Bedell, S. E., 331, *342*

Bedell, B. T., 215, *218*

Bednarek, H. L., 422, *426*

Beebe, T. J., 292, *300*

Beemer, F. A., 308, *316*

Beene-Harris, R. Y., 312, *314*

Beery, W. L., 554, *555*

Beeson, L., *38*

Beeson, W. L., *39*

Begg, C., 77, *80*

Behar, E. S., 68, *80*

Behavioral Risk Factor Surveillance
    System, 534, *543*

Bekkers, M. J. T. M., 367, *372*

Belch, G., *221*

Belcher, D. W., *102*

Belckers, M. J. T. M., *372*

Belin, T. R., 387, 417, *426*, *429*, *481*

Belizzi, K. M., 488, *492*

Belkacemi, Y., 439, *448*

Bell, D. R., 504, *512*

Bell, R. M., 153, *163*

Bell, R. S., *125*

Bell, S., 286, *296*

Bell, T. S., 450, *462*

Bell, W., 434, *448*

Bellg, A. J., 353, *357*

Bellizzi, K. M., 489, *492*

Belton, L., *20, 98, 202, 207*

Belyea, M., *357, 428, 484*

Benac, C. N., 550, *557*

Benedetti, F., 352, *355*

Benedict, S., *20, 98, 202, 207*

Bengtsson, B. A., *442*

Benjamin, H., *428*

Bennett, D., 451, *463*

Bennett, J. W., 63, *100*

Bennett, N. E., *80*

Bennetts, A., 286, *296*

Benowitz, N. L., 17, *20, 175, 181, 185*

Bensley, L. S., 470, *483*

Benyunes, M. C., 439, *442*

Bepler, G., *318*

Beral, V., *20*

Berenson, G. S., 195, *206*

Beresford, S., 196, *202*

Beresford, S. A., 63, *82, 92, 97, 102,*
    196, 201, 202

Berg, A. O., 255, *276*

Berger, A., 350, *355*

Bergh, J., 281, *298*

Berglund, B., 290, *298*

Bergman, B., *125*

Bergner, M., 118, *125, 126*

Bergstrom, R. L., 135, *143*

Berkow, R., *465*

Berkowitz, R., *235*

Berlant, N., 456, *465*

Berman, M. L., *234*

Bernaards, C. A., *372*

Bernard, L., *402, 403*

Bernard, L. J., *102*

Bernene, J., *249*

Bernhard, J., 394, *407*

Bernhardt, B. A., 304, *317*

Bernhardt, J. M., *98*

Bernstein, I., 118, *127*

Bernstein, L., *443*

Bernstein, M., *235*

Berrettini, W., 554, *557*

Berrino, F., *387*

Berry, C., *184*

Berry, D., *22, 320*

Berry, H., *511*

Berry-Bobovski, L., 306, *318*

Berther, P., *318*

Bertz, J., 215, *223*

Berwick, M., 210, *217*

Bessell, A. G., 452, *458*

Best, A., 5–6, *20*

Best, J. A., *98, 162, 163*

Best, M., 457, *459, 461*

Beunen, G., 246, *248*

Beveridge, H. A., 332, *343*

Bhatia, S., *444*

Bibeau, D., 45, *53*

Bickel, W. K., 176, *181*

Biemer, P., *275*

Biener, L., 92, 98, 157, *165*

Biesecker, B. B., 304, 306, 307, *314*

Biglan, A., 156, *162*

Bingler, R., *315*

Binkley, D., *101, 206*

Binstock, M. A., 228, *232*

Biradavolu, M., 134, *145*

Biran, A., *301*

Birch, L. L., 190, 199, *201, 203*

Bird, J. A., 269, *276*

Bird, S. T., 270, *277*

Birkett, N., 88, *98*

Bishop, A. J., 226, *232*

Bishop, D., 195, *206*

Bishop, M., *375, 376*

Bjordal, K., *128*

Bjork, J., *445*

Bjorner, J. B., *128*

Black, C., 156, *162, 179, 185*

Black, J. B., 245, *250*

Black, J. T., 116, *126*

Black, N., *273*

Black, W. C., 134, *149*

Blackburn, G. L., *492*

Blacker, C., *389*

Blacklay, A., 457, *459*

Blaine, T. M., *163*

Blair, S. N., 245, *247*

Blake, S. M., 244, *247*
Blakeley, B. W., 438, *442*
Blakely, T., 199, *205*
Blake-Mortimer, J., 369, *372*
Blakeny, N., *202*
Blalock, J. A., *182*
Blanchard, C., 399, *403, 408, 476, 480*
Blanchard, C. G., 332, *342, 476, 485*
Blanchard, C. M., 488, 489, *490, 492*
Blanchard, E. B., 332, *342*
Blanck, H. M., 197, *207*
Blanco, A. M., *319*
Bland, S. D., 27, *35*
Blanks, R., *300*
Blarney, R. W., 417, *425*
Blazeby, J., *128*
Blettner, M., 78, *83*
Blinson, K., *232*
Bliss, J. M., 505, *516*
Blitstein, J. L., 85, 88, 90, 91n, 94n,
     95n, 100, 101, 102
Block, S. D., 337, *344*
Blomhoff, S., 290, *301*
Blood, G. W., 471, *480*
Bloom, J. R., 350, *359, 372, 504, 516*
Blum, W. F., *442*
Bobbitt, R. A., 118, *125, 126*
Boberg, E., *556, 558*
Bobo, J. K., 176, *181*
Bochner, M. A., *428*
Bock, P. C., *544*
Bodurka, D. C., *232*
Body, J. J., 365, 415, 416, 424, *429*
Boesen, E. H., 368, *376, 419, 429, 503,
     504, 511*
Boggess, J. F., 255, *274*
Boggis, C., *297*
Boice, J. D., Jr., *443*
Boldeman, C., 210, 214, *217*
Bole, C., *358*
Bole, C. W., 348, *356*
Bolen, J. C., 25, 27, *35, 38*
Boles, S., 548, *556*
Boles, S. M., 64, *81, 525, 528*
Bolognia, J. L., 210, *217*
Bonacore, L. B., 256, *274*

Bonadona, V., 307, 308, *314, 318*
Bonfill, X., 258, 260, *266, 267, 269, 273*
Bongar, B., *463*
Bonner, J. A., *182*
Bonney, G., *317*
Bonollo, D. S., *186*
Bonomi, A., *125*
Bonomi, A. E., *125*
Bonomi, P., 45, *54, 125*
Boogaerts, A., *314*
Bookwala, J., 396, *403*
Boon, D., 450, *459*
Bootzon, R, *429*
Bor, D. H., *185*
Borawski, E. A., 216, *218*
Bordeleau, L. J., 116, *126*
Borkovec, T. D., 68, *80*
Borland, R., 210, 211, 213, 214, 216,
     217, 218, 219, 221
Borrelli, B., 177, 178, 179, *181, 185*
Borstelmann, N., 307, *320*
Borwhat, M. J., *112*
Borzekowski, D. L., 548, *555*
Bosch, F. X., 226, *232, 234, 284, 296,*
     299
Boslaugh, S. E., 537, *543*
Bosompra, K., 305, *314*
Bossert, E., 451, *462*
Bostic, D., *300*
Bostwick, J. M., 369, *373*
Bosworth, H., 395, *404*
Botkin, J. R., 304, 306, 307, 308, 309,
     314, 315, 320, 320
Bottomley, A., 363, *372*
Bottorff, J. L., 136, *144, 258, 261, 276*
Botvin, E. M., 153, *162*
Botvin, G. J., 153, 154, *162*
Bouknight, R. R., 422, *426*
Boutwell, W. B., *97*
Bovbjerg, D. H., 135, *146, 320, 349,*
     352, 357
Bove, B., *315*
Bowen, D. J., 137, 142, *144, 179, 181,*
     197, 202, 205, 305, 314, 493
Bowen, J. B., *21*
Bowen, S., 527, *527*

Bower, J. E., 364, 370, *372*, *377*, *387*, *430*, 436, *443*

Bowling, A., 118, 122, *125*

Bowman, A., 176, *181*

Bowman, D., *343*

Bowman, K. F., 415–416, *426*, 487, *492*

Bowman, L., 450, *463*

Boyce, A., 396, *404*

Boyd, J. W., *185*

Boyd, N. R., 80, *314*, *317*

Boyer, M., *342*

Boyer, M. J., 334, *342*

Boyes, A., *296*

Boyett, J. M., 450, *463*

Boyko, E. J., *102*

Braden, C. J., 363, *376*, *429*

Bradley, C. B., *249*

Bradley, C. J., 393, 401, *403*, 422, 423, *425*, *426*, *430*

Bradley, E., 395, *403*, *405*

Bradley, P., *147*, *277*

Bradley, S., *514*

Brady, M. J., 472, *480*

Braithwaite, D., 307, *314*

Bramadat, I. J., 46, *53*

Bramswig, J. H., 436, *442*

Brandberg, Y., 215, 216, *217*

Brand-Driehorst, S., *513*

Brandon, T. H., 172, 174, *186*

Branstetter, A. D., 137, *146*

Branstrom, R., 215, *217*

Brasher, P., 400, *404*

Brasher, P. M., 477, *480*

Brassington, G. S., 245, *248*, 531, *544*

Brasure, M., 192, *202*

Brauer, A., 549, *556*

Braunstein, G. D., *389*

Braverman, M. T., 92, *99*

Brawley, O., *113*

Breast and Cervical Cancer Prevention and Treatment Act, 34, *36*

Brecht, M. L., *127*

Bredson, C. N., *514*

Breen, N., *22*, 34, 40, *113*, 256, 257, *274*, *275*, *277*

Breen, N. L., 257, *274*

Breitbart, W., 395, *403*

Breitlow, K. K., *203*

Brekelmans, C. T. M., *318*

Brelje, K., *99*

Brennan, B. M., 433, *442*

Brennan, L. K., 245, *247*

Brennan, P., 550, *555*

Breslau, E. S., 271, *276*

Breslau, N., 176, *181*

Breslow, N. E., 75, 76, *81*

Brett, J., 281, 282, *296*

Brewer, N. T., 283, *296*

Brewster, W. R., 110, *112*

Brey, K., 436, *447*, 475, *485*

Bricker, E., *558*

Brinn, L. S., 213, *220*

Brinton, L. A., 226, *234*

Briss, P., 272, *273*

Briss, P. A., 269, 272, 273, *276*, *277*, *527*, *527*

Brisson, C., 422, *428*

Brisson, J., 467, *481*, 488, *493*, 505, *514*

Britton, A., 272, *273*

Britton, P. G., 450, *463*

Broder, S., 535, *546*

Broderick, M., *430*

Brodersen, J., 282, *296*, *297*

Brody, D. S., 335, *345*

Bromley, C. M., *447*

Bronstein, B. R., *222*

Brook, R. H., *127*

Brooks, R., 395, *404*

Brotto, L. A., 384, *386*

Brower, L., 305, *315*

Browman, G. P., 179, *181*

Brown, C., *388*

Brown, D., 549, *555*

Brown, D. R., *38*

Brown, H., 90, 97, *98*

Brown, K., *320*

Brown, K. L., 305, *317*

Brown, K. S., 92, *98*, *162*, *163*

Brown, K. W., 505, *510*

Brown, M., *250*

Brown, M. L., 422, *430*

Brown, P., 351, *359*

Brown, P. K., *528*

Brown, R., 452, 453, *459*, *462*

Brown, R. A., 177, *181*

Brown, R. T., 454, *462*

Brown, S. A., 177, *188*

Brown, T., *20*

Brownell, K. D., 198, *204*

Brownson, R. C., *204*, 245, *247*, *248*,
    520, 522, 527, *527*, *528*, *529*,
    537, *543*

Broz, S. L., 338, 340, *342*

Bruce, A. T., 500, *511*

Brug, H., 192, *202*

Brug, J., 192, *205*, *206*

Bruvold, W. H., 153, *162*

Bryant, R. A., 416, 420, *427*

Bryce, J., 272, *277*

Bryk, A. S., 90, *101*

Bubela, N., 351, *356*

Buchanan, G. R., *446*

Buchner, D. M., 242, *248*

Bucholtz, D. C., *205*

Buck, C., 88, *98*

Buck, E. L., 228, *234*, 258, 259, 263,
    264, 265, 266, 267, *277*

Buckman, R., *315*, 329, 332, *342*

Budin, W., *482*

Budney, A., 176, *181*

Buettner, P. G., 215, *223*

Bukach, C., *296*

Bukowski, W., 452, *462*

Bulger, D., 552, *555*

Bull, F. C., 192, *205*

Bull, S., 525, *528*

Bull, S. S., 17, *20*, 269, *274*

Buller, D. B., 92, *98*, 194, 196, *202*, 210,
    211, 212, 213, 214, 215, 216,
    217, *219*, *220*, *221*, *222*, *223*

Buller, M. K., *98*, *202*, 210, 211, 216,
    218

Buller, R. E., *514*

Bullinger, M., *125*

Bultz, B., 400, *404*

Bultz, B. D, 477, *480*

Bulzebruck, H., 505, *512*

Bundred, N., *297*

Bunin, N., 450, *464*

Bunnell, D., *557*

Burant, C., 393, *404*

Burchenal, J. H., 121, *126*

Burciaga Valdez, R., *235*

Burger, C., *318*

Burgess, C., 363, 366, *373*, 505, *512*

Burgess, C. C., *300*

Burgess, P., 366, *373*

Burgoon, M., 213, *218*

Buring, J. B., *38*

Burish, T. G., 348, 349, 350, *355*, *360*

Burke, W., 305, *314*

Burling, A. S., 176, *181*

Burling, T. A., 176, *181*

Burman, M., 283, *300*

Burnett, A. L., 381, *389*

Burnett, W., 226, *233*

Burns, D. M., 179, *184*

Burns, R., *247*

Burns, S., *298*

Burns, W. I., 475, *482*

Burstein, H., 488, *493*

Burton, D., 163, *184*

Burton, N. W., 240, *250*

Burton, R., *99*

Burton, R. C., 24, *37*

Busby-Earle, C., 136, *145*

Bush, A., *162*

Bush, N., *144*

Bushey, M. T., *315*

Bushunow, P., *358*

Busic, A. J., *218*

Buster, J. E., *389*

Butler, B. A., 45, *54*

Butler, L. M., *494*

Butler, M. S., 434, *446*

Butler, R., 451, 455, *459*, *464*

Butow, P., *318*, *343*, *515*

Butow, P. N., 328, 330, 334, 339, *344*,
    345, *346*, 503, *510*

Butterfield, R. M., *459*

Buttsworth, D. L., 450, *461*

Buunk, B. P., 468, 477, *481*, *482*

Buzaglo, J., *232*, *233*, *318*, *319*

Byers, T., 5, 20, 23, *37*, 61, 62, *80*, *234*, *493*, 531, 532, *543*
Byock, I. R., 332, *342*
Byrne, J., 435, 436, *442*, *446*, *447*, *460*
Byrom, J., 288, *297*

Caan, B. J., *494*
Caballero, B., 195, *202*
Cabana, M. D., 173, *181*
Cacioppo, J. T., 47, *54*, 505, *513*, *516*
Cady, B., *80*, *543*
Caggiula, A. R., 179, *186*
Calfas, K., 551, *556*
Calfas, K. J., *221*, 240, *250*
Calhoun, P., 395, *404*
Calingaert, B., *22*, *320*
Callas, P., 174, *185*
Callas, P. W., 176, *185*
Calle, E. E., 28, *36*
Calvert, *298*
Cameron, C. L., *376*
Cameron, J., 393, 399, *404*
Cameron, L., 44, *53*
Cameron, L. D., 138, 139, *144*, 305, *314*
Cameron, R., 5–6, *20*, 92, 98, 148, 154, *162*
Campbell, F., 77, *81*
Campbell, F. C., *442*
Campbell, M., 527, *527*
Campbell, M. K., 16, 17, *20*, *21*, *22*, 92, 98, 140, *147*, 192, 194, 196, 197, *201*, *202*, *203*, 205, 206, 207, *208*, *494*
Campbell, N. R., *99*
Campbell, R., *112*
Campo, M. C., *234*
Canada, A. L., 384, *386*, 436, *442*
Canadian Strategy for Cancer Control, 7, *20*
Canellos, G. P., 337, *345*, *427*
Canevello, A. B., 134, *146*
Cannuscio, C. C., 26, *36*
Cant, M. C., *461*
Cantor, J. C., 171, 172, *182*
Cantor, M., *218*
Caparso, N. E., *314*
Capelleri, J. C., 383, *388*

Capone, M. A., 383, *386*
Caporaso, N. F., *80*
Carbone, E., 192, *202*
Carey, M., *458*
Carey, M. P., 349, *355*, 383, *388*
Carey, T. S., 272, *274*
Carlbring, P., 551, *555*
Carli, G., 351, *354*
Carline, J. D., *346*
Carlson, C. A., 435, *444*
Carlson, C. R., 364, *373*
Carlson, M., *403*
Carlsson, L., *442*
Carmack, C., 244, *246*
Carman, N., *300*
Carmona, R. H., 313, *316*
Carnes, B. A., 510, *510*, *515*
Carney, A., 306, *314*
Carpenter, J. H., *163*
Carpenter, J. S., *295*
Carpenter, P., 458, *464*
Carpenter, P. J., *464*
Carr, A. B., 169, *183*
Carr, C., 206, *494*
Carr, J. E., 351, *359*
Carrell, D. S., 46, *53*
Carriere, K. C., *343*
Carroll, J. K., *358*
Carroll, M. D., 28, *37*, 39
Carroll, P. V., 433, *442*
Carson, S., 92, *99*
Cartei, G., 505, *512*
Carter, B. L., *182*
Carter, P., 393, *404*
Carter, W. B., 118, *125*
Caruso, L., *357*
Carver, C., 348, *360*
Carver, C. S., 353, *359*, 365, 367, *373*, *376*, 415, 418, 426, 430, 476, 479, 480, *482*
Casamitjana, M., *101*
Case, L. D., *232*
Casey, R., *461*
Casey, V., *408*
Caspersen, C. J., *247*
Cass, O. W., 292, *300*

Cassel, C., *510*, *515*
Cassel, M. M., 549, *555*
Cassidy, R. C., 104, *112*
Casson, P. R., *389*
Castellon, S. A., 438, *443*
Castells, X., *101*
Castellsague, X., *232*
Castro, C., *248*
Castro, C. M., *248*
Catalan, J., 384, *387*
Catania, L., 457, *459*
Catton, C. N., *125*
Catton, P., 340, *344*
Cavalleri, A., *387*
Cavallin-Stahl, E., *445*
Cavender, T. A., 422, 423, *428*, *430*
Cavill, N. A., 239, *248*
Cegala, D. J., 338, 340, *342*
Cella, D., 231, *235*, 472, *480*
Cella, D. F., 120, 121, *125*, *427*, 504, *511*, *516*
Cen, S., *165*
Center for the Digital Future, 548, *555*
Centers for Disease Control and Prevention, National Center for Health Statistics, 28, 32, 36, 39, 431, *443*
Centers for Disease Control and Prevention (CDC), 25, 27, 36, 168, 171, *182*, 189, *202*, 217, *218*, 238, *247*, 437, *443*, 526, *528*
Cepeda Benito, A., 178, *182*
Cerhan, J. R., *515*
Cesaro, S., 437, *443*
Chakraborty, B., *558*
Chalker, D. K., *36*
Challinor, J., 450, *459*
Chalmers, K. L., 46, *53*
Chaloupka, F., 160, *162*, *163*
Chamberlain, F., *300*
Chamberlain, J., *297*
Chamberlain, R. M., *220*
Chambers, S. L., 290, *301*
Champion, V. L., 134, *148*, *405*, 522, *528*
Chan, B. K. S., 255, *274*

Chan, C. L., *556*
Chan, E. C., 269, *276*
Chan, F. Y. S., 348, *357*
Chan, J., 399, *404*
Chan, J. M., 30, *36*
Chang, L., 213, *219*
Chang, V., *373*
Chao, A., 30, *36*
Chao, C., 140, *144*
Chapko, M. K., *102*
Charleston, A., 451, *464*
Charmer, G. P., *462*
Charron-Moore, C., 474, *484*
Chatenoud, L., *234*
Chatterjee, R., 384, *386*
Cheadle, A., *100*
Chee, E., 351, *359*
Chekryn, J., 474, *480*
Chen, A. H., *248*
Chen, C. C., 503, *511*
Chen, C. J., *233*
Chen, D., 245, *250*
Chen, E., *465*
Chen, E. H., *278*
Chen, F. L., *101*
Chen, H., *460*
Chen, M., 22, *165*
Chen, X., 242, *250*
Cheng, L., 503, *511*
Chenoy, R., *298*
Chepaitis, A. E., *188*
Cherlin, E., *403*, *427*
Chernew, M., *405*
Chesebro, B. B., *102*
Chesney, M., 230, *232*
Chesney, M. A., *102*
Chessells, J. M., 439, *445*
Chesson, H., *233*
Cheung, A., 393, *404*
Cheuvront, B., 549, *555*
Cheville, A. L., 440, *443*
Chevron, E. S., 468, *482*
Chi, D., *388*
Chiang, Y. P., 122, *127*
Chiarelli, A. M., 280, 284, *297*
Chihara, S., 395, *406*

Chilcoat, H., 176, *181*

Chirikos, T. N., 422, *426*

Chittenden, A., *319*

Chlebowski, R. T., 417, *426*, 487, 490, 491, *492*

Cho, M., *80*

Cho, Y. I., 92, *100*

Chochinov, H. M., 332, *342*

Choi, W. S., 152, *164*

Cholewinski, S., *37*

Chollette, V., 275, 289, *301*

Chompret, A., *318*

Chou, C., *165*

Chou, S. P., 176, *184*

Chow, E., 421, *426*

Chow, J., *36*

Christakis, D., *461*, *465*

Christakis, N. A., *346*, 453, *461*

Christensen, C., L., 142, *144*, 220

Christensen, D. N., 210, 383, *386*

Christensen, R, *465*

Christiaens, M. R., *444*

Christiani, D. C., 35, *39*

Christians, A., *297*

Christiansen, J. S., *442*

Christianson, A., *97*

Christie, A., 396, *404*

Christoffersen, K., *446*

Chu, P. W., *300*

Chung, J. Y., 456, *458*

Church, T. R., *299*

Chvetzoff, G., 352, *355*

Chye, R., *343*

Cimprich, B., *355*, 423, *426*, 475, *480*

Cinciripini, L. G., *182*

Cinciripini, P. M., 174, 178, *182*

Claes, E., 306, 308, 309, *314*

Clancy-Hepburn, K., 199, *202*

Clapp, E. J., *221*

Clark, E. M., 192, *205*

Clark, L. C., 31, *36*

Clark, M., *494*

Clark, M. A., 256, 257, 269, 272, *274*, *276*

Clark, M. B., *320*

Clark, M. M., 169, *180*, 369, *373*, 421, *429*

Clark, R. E, 549, *555*

Clarke, V., 470, *481*

Clarke, V. A., 135, *149*

Clarridge, B. R., *408*

Claus, E. B., *250*

Clauser, S., 422, *430*

Clay, T., *202*

Claypool, M., 549, 550, *555*

Clayton, J., 339, *343*

Clayton, J. M., 328, *346*

Cleaveland, B. L., *223*

Clegg, A., *275*

Clein, G. P., 440, *445*

Clemmons, D., *442*

Clinch, J., *405*

Cline, R. J., 549, 552, *555*

Cline-Elsen, J., 351, *355*

Clipp, E., 488, *493*

Clipp, E. C., *346*, *492*

Clohisy, D. R., 434, *445*

Clyburn, L., 393, *404*

Coates, R. C., *273*

Coates, R. J., 10, *22*, 34, *40*, 256, *277*

Cobleigh, M., 488, *494*

Cochrane, B., *480*

Cochrane, B. B., 470, *485*

Cockburn, J., 281, 282, 282, 283, 296, 297, *299*

Codori, A., 305, *315*

Cody, R., 213, 241, *247*

Cofer, M., *21*

Coffey, C., *297*

Coffin, J., *514*

Cohen, D. A., 45, 49, 53, *183*

Cohen, D. S., 454, 455, *459*

Cohen, H. J., *492*

Cohen, J. I., *442*

Cohen, L., 329, *342*, 345, 365, *375*, 503, *511*

Cohen, M. E., 438, *443*

Cohen, N., *207*

Cohen, R. D, *512*

Cohen, S., 364, 367, 368, 370, *374*, 499, 500, *511*

Coiro, M., 453, *461*

Colabianchi, N., 334, *346*

Colan, S. D., *445*

Colby, S. M., 176, *182*, *184*

Coldevin, G., 549, *556*

Colditz, G., 35, *35*, 92, 97, *148*

Colditz, G. A., 9, *20*, *23*, *26*, *30*, *35*, *36*, *37*, *38*, *39*, *40*, *41*, *204*, *222*, *515*

Cole, B. F., *221*

Cole, D. C., 352, *357*

Cole, G., 239, *247*

Cole, J., 440, *445*

Cole, S., *514*

Cole, S. W., *510*

Colegrove, R. W., 450, *462*

Coleman, E. A., 241, *247*

Coleman, K. J., 70, *80*

Coleman, R., *492*

Collet, J.-P., 370, *373*

Collins, C., 395, *408*

Collins, C. A., *376*

Collins, F. S., 303, 313, *315*, *316*

Collins, L. M., 552, *556*

Collins, M., *275*

Collins, S., 215, *219*

Collins, V., 309, *315*

Collyar, D. E., *112*

Colman, L. K., *359*

Coltman, C., *112*

Colwell, H. H., *387*

Combs, G. F., Jr., *36*

Commerce Clearing House, 198, *202*

Compas, B. E., 365, 367, 368, 369, 372, *373*, *375*

Conaway, M., *234*

Concato, J., *405*

Connell, C. J., *36*

Connelly, R. R., *442*

Conner, P., *187*

Connor-Kuntz, F. J., 238, *247*

Connors, A., Jr., *516*

Connors, M., *183*

Conomy, J. P., 437, *443*

Conrad, K. M., 155, *163*

Constantino, J. P., *112*, *125*

Constanzo, D., *249*

Constine, L. S., *358*, 433, *442*

Conway, T. L., *250*

Cook, E. D., 110, *112*

Cook, N. R., *38*

Cook, R., 258, 261, *276*

Cook, T., 177, *188*

Cook, V. A., 213, *219*

Cooke, L., *296*

Coole, D., *100*

Cooley, M. E., *514*

Coombes, C., *344*

Coon, K. A., 199, *203*

Cooper, B., *514*

Cooper, D. B., *184*

Cooper, K. D., 216, *218*

Cooper, M. R., *113*, *427*

Cooperberg, M. R., 381, *387*

Copeland, D., 454, 455, 458, *459*

Copeland, D. R., 450, *459*

Copeland, L. A., *183*

Coppola, P. R., *98*

Corbett, K. K., *55*

Corbett, M., 290, *301*

Corbetta, A., *462*

Corcoran, M., 396, *404*

Cordes, J. E., *299*

Cordova, M. J., 295, 364, 367, *373*, 416, 417, 418, 420, *426*

Coristine, M., 396, 402, *404*

Corkrey, R., *99*

Corle, D., *205*

Cornblat, M. W., 472, *481*

Cornbleet, M. A., 340, *345*

Cornelius, V., *373*

Cornfeld, M., *147*, *277*

Cornfield, J., 87, 88, 89, *98*

Cornuz, J., 172, *185*

Cortina, K. S., 194, *203*

Coscarelli, A., 425, *481*

Costa, C., 219, *221*

Costalas, J. W., 309, 312, *315*, *315*, *316*

Costanza, M. C., *163*

Costanzo, E., *514*

Cotugna, N., 199, 200, *203*

Coughlin, S., 320, *528*

Coughlin, S. S., 330, *343*

Coups, E. J., 488, *492*
Courneya, K. S., 237, *247*, 490, *492, 493*
Courtney, M. E., *510*
Covey, L. S., 177, *184, 188*
Covin, J., *221*
Cowan, M. J., 450, *462, 463*
Cowley, N., 440, *445*
Cox, C. E., 328, *345*
Cox, D. T., 553, *556*
Cox, E., 228, *235, 258, 259, 277*
Cox, J. T., 285, *301*
Cox, L. S., 179, *182*
Cox, T., 285, *297*
Coyle, D., *405*
Coyne, C., *275*
Coyne, J., *313*
Coyne, J. C., 505, 507, *511*
Craft, A. W., *445*
Craig, S., *163, 165*
Crandall, S. J., 172, *187*
Crane, L. A., 213, *218, 220, 228, 233, 271, 274*
Crank, H., *492*
Craufurd, D., 304, *315*
Crawford, M. A., 160, *163*
Creamer, M., 366, *373*
Creech, L., *219*
Creech, L. L., 216, *218*
Cremo, J., *221*
Crespin, T. R., *372, 425*
Crews, K. M., 170, *187*
Crittenden, K. S., 92, *100*
Crittenden, M. R., 450, *462, 463*
Croghan, I. T., *185*
Crom, D. B., *460*
Cronin, W. M., *112, 125, 126*
Crooks, D., 396, *404*
Cross, D., *219, 221*
Crow, R. A., *247*
Croyle, R. T., 138, *144, 145*, 171, *183*, 230, *232, 268, 275*, 304, *307, 308, 314, 315, 317, 320*, 501, *511, 544, 558*
Cruciani, G., *356*
Cruess, D., *494*
Crump, T., *461*

Crystal, S., 305, *314*
Cuddeford, L., 286, *299*
Culbert, S. J., 450, *459*
Cull, A., *125, 128, 136, 145*, 312, *315*
Cullen, J. W., 6, *20, 21, 62, 81*
Cullen, K. W., 92, *97, 98*, 200, *201*
Cullen, M., *557*
Cullen, M. R., *39*
Culley, C. A., 216, *218*
Culver, J. L., 418, *426*
Culyer, A. J., *163*
Cummings, C., 352, *359*
Cummings, K. M., 92, *98*
Cunningham, A. J., 506, *511*
Cunningham, L. L., *295*
Cunningham, L. L. C., 364, *373*
CureSearch Children's Oncology Group, 435, 441, *443*
Curfman, G. D., 226, *231*
Curry, S., 16, *23, 25, 29, 37*, 140, *147*
Curry, S. J., 5, *20, 22, 61, 63, 66, 79, 80, 82, 137, 144*, 173, *182, 183*, 257, *258, 274, 299, 544*
Curtis, J. R., *346*
Curtis, R. E., 439, *443*
Cusinato, R., *443*
Cutler, C. M., *183, 544*
Cutter, G. R., 212, *217, 218, 221, 222*
Cuzick, C. D., *320*
Cuzick, J., 285, *296, 297, 301*
Czyzewski, D. I., 453, *455, 459*

Dacey, S., 553, *557*
Daeppen, J. B., 176, *182*
Dahl, A. A., *494*
Dahlof, C. G., *128*
Dahlquist, L. M., 453, *455, 459*
Dahme, B., 349, *356, 368, 375*
Dale, L. C., 169, *183*
Daley, A. J., 490, *492*
Dalton, M. A., *165, 376*
Dalton, R. J., *386*
Dalton, S. O., 368, 419, *429, 463, 503, 504, 511*
Daly, M., 142, *145, 147*, 229, *234, 309, 319*

Daly, M. B., 45, 53, 280, 299, 309, 313, 315, 316, 319, 320
Damian, D., 339, 343
Damron, D., 194, 204
Damus, K., 288, 301
Dancel, M., 220
D'Angelo, T., 502, 514
D'Angio, G. J., 434, 446, 448
Daniel, M., 201, 204
Danko, G. P., 182
Danoff-Burg, S., 376
Dar, A. R., 188
Darke, S., 176, 182
Darrah, J., 538, 544
Das, L., 462
Daston, C., 205
Daugherty, C. K., 329, 330, 331, 335, 336, 343, 346
David, A. S., 511
David, D., 349, 352, 357
Davidann, B., 99
Davidson, J., 505, 516
Davidson, K. W., 80, 268, 274, 275
Davidson, R., 321
Davidson, R. J., 513
Davies, D. R., 304, 315
Davies, W., 452, 462
Davies, W. H., 462
Davis, A. M., 120, 125, 278
Davis, C., 328, 343
Davis, D. A., 188
Davis, H. L., Jr., 448
Davis, J., 417, 429
Davis, J. M., 343
Davis, K. C., 163
Davis, L. J., Jr., 185
Davis, M. W., 351, 359
Davis, R. B., 38
Davis, R. M., 171, 181, 183, 544
Davis, S., 503, 511
Davis, S. M., 202
Davis, T., 112
Davis, W. W., 388, 430
Dawson, D. A., 176, 184
Dawson, J. L., 511
Dawson, S., 444

Day, N. E., 23, 39, 75, 76, 80
Day, R., 116, 120, 125
De, A. K., 101
Deal, L. W., 474, 482
DeAlba, I., 231, 232
Dean, C., 281, 297
Deas, A., 218
Debanne, S. M., 216, 218
deBruin, W. B., 134, 145
Deci, E. L., 193, 194, 203, 207
Decker, T. W., 351, 355
Decker, V. B., 389
Decruyenaere, M., 314
Dee, B., 358
Deeg, H. J., 442
Degner, L. F., 335, 343
DeGraffinreid, C. R., 104, 112
DeGroot, A., 454, 465
deHaes, J. C., 120, 125, 328, 345, 359
Deimling, G. T., 415–416, 426, 487, 492
Dejong, G. M., 477, 482
DeJong, W., 20, 23, 36
Del Mar, C. B., 211, 220
DeLaat, C. A., 438, 443
Delaney, E. A., 349, 359
de Leeuw, C., 275
De Leeuw, J., 90, 97, 100
de Leon, J., 177, 182
Delgado, M., 247
Delichatsios, H. K., 100, 193, 203
Dell, J., 278
Dellavalle, R., 218
Dellinger, A., 92, 99
DeLorenze, G. N., 422–423, 429
DeLuise, T., 281, 297
DeMarco, T., 319
Demark-Wahnefried, W., 92, 98, 194, 196, 202, 433, 446, 488, 489, 490, 491, 492, 493, 494
Dement, J., 146
Demierre, M. F., 220
Deming, W., 139, 146
Demisse, S., 202
Demko, C. A., 216, 218
Demmy, T. L., 104, 112

DeMonner, S., *405*

deMoor, C., 97, 98, *345, 365, 375*

Denayer, L., *314*

Denekamp, J., 440, *444*

Deng, S., *249*

DeNittis, A., *558*

Denke, M. A., *446*

Denman, S., 211, *220*

Denniston, M., 488, *489*

Denniston, M. M., *492*

De-Nour, A. K., 469, *480*

Dent, C. W., 153, *163, 165*

DePauw, S., *127*

DePue, J. D., 173, *182*

Derogatis, L. P., 504, *516*

Derogatis, L. R., 504, *511*

Derose, K. P., 92, *99*

Desai, M., 298, *299*

DeSantes, K., 450, *462*

Deschenes, L., 467, *481*, 488, *493*, 505, *514*

Desmond, K., *469*

Desmond, K. A., 366, *372, 374, 375, 387, 417, 426, 429, 481*

Desseigne, F., *314*

Detmar, L. D. V., *376*

Detmar, S. B., 116, *125*

Detweiler, J. R., 215, *218*

Deuson, R. R., *356*

Deutsch, G., 339, *343*

Dev, P., *219*

Devadas, S., *516*

Devane-Hart, K., *101*

DeVellis, B., 20, 98, 202, 207, *220*

DeVellis, R. F., *205*

Devessa, S. S., 226, *234*

Devine, E. C., 352, *355*

Devine, P., 557, *558*

Devins, G. M., 416, *427*

DeVoe, D., 241, *249*

DeVoss, D., *405*

DeVries, H., 17, 20, 169, *183*

deWitte, L., *408*

Dey, P., 215, 284, *297*

Dhabhar, F. S., *510*

Dhanda, R., 505, *516*

Diaz, F. J., 177, *182*

Diaz, T., 153, *162*

DiBartola, L. M., 339, *343*

Dibble, S., 397, *407*

Di Blasi, Z., 352, *355*

Dickens, L. L., *183*

Dickey, D. T., *442*

DiClemente, C., *206*

DiClemente, C. C., 44, *54*, 193, 239, *249*, 490, *494*

Diefenbach, L., 175, *186*

Diefenbach, M., *320*

Diefenbach, M. A., *21*, 44, *53*, 205, 305, 311, *315, 318*

Diehr, P., 92, *99*

Diehr, P. H., *100*

Dienemann, J. A., *357*

Dierker, L. C., 536, *543*

Dietrich, A. J., 92, 212, 219, *221*

Dietz, W. H., *204*

DiGianni, L. M., 310, *315, 319*

Dignan, F. L., 337, *345*

Dignan, M., 228, *232*

Dignan, M. B., 217, *222*

Dijkstra, A., 17, 20, 170, *183*, 550, *556*

Dillard, A. J., 139, 141, *144*

Diller, L., 452, *463*, 488, *493*

DiLorenzo, T., 135, *146*

Di Marino, M. E., 174, *187*

Dimeo, F. C., 351, *355*

DiMicelli, S., *516*

Dimond, E., *316*

Dinee, S., *144*

Dineen, M., 471, *480*

Dippo, C., *275*

Ditto, P., *144*

Ditto, P. H., 138, 139, *145*

Dixon, R., 363, *374*

Dixon, S., 283, *299*

Dobbinson, S., 214, *219*

Dobkin, P., *357*

Dobkin, P. L., 349, *358*

Dodd, M., 397, *407*

Dodd, M. J., 136, *145*

Dodds, J., *202*

Dogan-Ates, A., *235*

Dohan, E., *374*
Doherty, I., 288, *300, 301*
Dolgin, M., *458, 464*
Dolgin, M. J., 456, *459*
Doll, R., *40*
Dominitz, J. A., *102*
Donaldson, G. W., 351, 352, *359*
Donaldson, M. S., 116, *127*, 421, *428*
Donnelly, J. M., 468, *481*
Donner, A., 85, 88, 89, 90, 91, 97, 98,
    100, 101
Donny, E., 179, *186*
D'Onofrio, C. N., 92, 99, 269, *276*
Donovan, K. A., 136, *144, 180–181,*
    306, *315*
Doolittle, M., *112*
Doolittle, N. D., *442*
Dores, G. M., *448*
Dorevitch, A., 215, *222*
Dorfman, L., 47, *55, 183*
Dorgan, K. A., 305, *316*
Dorosty, A. R., *446*
Dorrenbos, A., 392, 395, *407*
Dorris, G., 474, *484*
Dorsey, A., *342*
Dorval, M., 307, 308, *315, 319*, 467, *481*
Doshi, A., 551, *556*
Dougherty, J., 476, *483*
Dow, K. H., *357*
Dowda, M., *249*
Dowsett, S., 330, *342*
Doyle, C., *201*, 488, *493*
Dratt, J., 241, *249*
Drazen, J., 226, *231*
Drewnoski, A., 199, *203*
Drings, P., 505, *512*
Driscoll, B. R., 437, *443*
Drolet, M., 488, *493*
Druley, J., 393, *408*
Drysdale, S., 294, *298*
Duan, N., 9, *99*
Dube, C. E., *274*
Dubois, L., 422, *428*
Dudley, W. N., *101*, 206
Duez, N. J., *125*
Duffner, P. K., 438, *443*

Duffy, S. A., 179, *183*
Duggan, A., *221*
DuHamel, K., 453, *462*
DuHamel, K. N., 349, *355*
Dukes, K. A., 334, *345*
Dummer, G. M., 238, *247*
Dunavant, M., 450, *463*
Dunbar, P. J., 551, *557*
Duncan, C., *184*
Duncan, T., 156, *162*
Dundee, J. W., 349, *355*
Dungan, S., 453, *464*
Dunn, A. L., 244, 245, *247, 248*
Dunn, G. P., 500, *511*
Dunn, J. K., *249*
Dunn, P. D., 297, *298*
Dunn, S. M., 334, 339, *342, 346, 515*
Dunne, E. F., *233*
Dunser, M., 126, *427*
Durham, C., 316, *317*
Duteau-Buck, C., *320*
Dutson, D. S., 307, *314, 315*
Duvall, R. C., *101*
Dwyer, J. H., 92, *100, 164*
Dzewaltowski, D. A., 17, *20*, 525, *528*

Earle, C., 17, *21*, 405, 488, *493*
Earp, J. A., 205, 270, *276*
Eastwood, S., *80*
Eaton, C. A., *184*
Eaves, L. J., *513*
Ebbert, J., 396, *406*, 477, *483*
Ebbert, J. O., 169, *183*
Eberman, K. M., *185*
Ebie, N., *278*
Eccles, D., *321*
Eccleston, P., 172, *187*
Eckhardt, L., *100*, 216, *218, 219, 221*
Eckles, A., *221*
Edelman, S., 504, 506, *512*
Eden, O. B., *442*
Edgar, L., 370, *373*, 476, *481*, 505, *510*
Edmonds, C. V., *511*
Edwards, A., 136, 140, *144*
Edwards, A. G. K., 368, *373*
Edwards, B., 470, *481*

Edwards, B. K., 24, *37*
Edwards, E. K., 5, *20*
Edwards, K., 214, *222*
Edwards, R., *188, 278, 296, 301*
Eeles, R., *316*
Ehrich, B., 257, *274, 276*
Ehrsam, G., *218, 271, 274*
Eichenfield, L. F., *218, 221*
Eisenmann, J. C., 199, *203*
Eiser, C., 454, 457, *459, 460*
Ekert, H., 450, *458*
Ekselius, L., 551, *555*
Ekstrom, D., *482*
Elam, L. C., *102*
Elashoff, R., 488, *493, 512*
Elder, J. P., 64, *81, 92, 99, 100,* 206,
     219, 221, 250
Eley, J. W., 382, *387*
Elkin, T. D., 451, *459*
Elkins, G., 349, *355*
Ell, K., 468, 472, 473, 474, *475, 481*
Ell, K. O., 366, *375*
Eller, L. S., 349, 350, *355*
Ellickson, P. L., 153, 161, *163*
Ellis, P. M., 331, *343*
Ellis, S. E., 312, *314*
Ellison, R. C., *206*
Ellman, R., 284, *297*
Ellsworth, R., *218*
Elton, R. A., *315*
Elwyn, G., 136, *144*
Emerson, J., 210, *220*
Emery, C. F., *372, 425*
Emery, J., 307, *314*
Emery, S., 536, *544*
Emmons, K., 17, *21, 99, 220,* 310, *315*
Emmons, K. M., 45, 51, *52, 53,* 148,
     181, 186, 239, *247,* 257, 258,
     274, 457, *459,* 532, 534, *544*
Emmons, R., 527, *527*
Emparanza, J., 258, 260, *273*
Emrich, L. J., 92, *99*
Emster, V. L., *102*
Enderlin, C. A., *557*
Eng, E., 194, *207,* 305, *314*
Engeland, A., *164*

Engelhard, D. A., *299*
Engler, J., 92, *100*
English, D. R., 33, 34, *37,* 211, 215, 216,
     219, 220, 221
Engstrom, P. E., 45, *53,* 299
Engstrom, P. F., 141, 280, *315, 320*
Ennett, S. T., *162*
Ennis, M., *444, 512*
Enos, L. E., 75, *79*
Epping-Jordan, J. E., 363, 364, 365, 367,
     373
Epps, R. P., 172, *183*
Epstein, J. A., 153, *162*
Epstein, L. H., 70, 80, 537, *544*
Epstein, S. A., 136, *144*
Erath, S., 178, *182*
Erblich, J., 135, *146*
Erickson, P., 118, *125*
Erickson, S., 451, *460*
Erickson, V. S., 434, *443*
Eriksen, M. P., *529*
Ernst, E., 352, *355*
Ersboll, J., *446*
Ertl, G., 216, *218*
Erwin, P. C., *183*
Eshelman, D. A., 437, *444, 446, 446*
Espinel, C. F., *162*
Espy, K. A., 450, *460*
Esselsyn, C. B., *388*
Estabrooks, P., 17, *20*
Estabrooks, P. A., 525, *528*
Ethelbah, B., *202*
Eton, D. T., 475, *481*
Etschmaier, M., 422, *428*
Ettinger, D. S., *188*
Ettinger, W. H., Jr., 240, *247*
European Organization for Research and
     Treatment of Cancer, 119, *125*
Evangelista, L., *127*
Evans, D. G. R., 304, *315*
Evans, D. L., 504, *512*
Evans, G., *145*
Evans, R. B., 380, *388*
Evans, R. G., *445*
Evans, T. V., 475, *482*
Evans, W., *147*

Evans, W. D., 434, *448*
Everaerd, W., *387*
Everett, J., *318*
Evers-Kiebooms, G., *314*
Everson, S. A., 270, *275*, 501, 503, *512*
Ewer, M. S., 433, *447*
Ewings, J. A., 92, *102*
Eyler, A. A., *248*
Eyler, A. E., 172, *183*
Ezzati, M., 23, 24, 26, 28, 31, 32, *37*

Fabrigar, L. R., *148*
Facione, N. C., 136, *145*
Faddis, S., 468, *484*
Fagan, P., 160, *162*
Fagerstrom, K., 151, *163*
Fagg, J., 384, *387*
Fahey, J. L., *512*
Fainaru, M., 194, *204*
Fairclough, D., 451, *459, 464*
Fairclough, D. L., 78, 79, *81*
Fairey, A. S., 490, *493*
Fakhrabadi-Shokoohi, D., *39*
Faller, H., 505, *512*
Fallon, J. H., 536, *544*
Fallowfield, L., 331, 332, 333, 334, 337, 339, *343, 344*, 417, *425*
Fallows, D., 548, *556*
Fang, C. Y., 45, *53*, 280, 299, 309, 311, *315, 318*
Farkas, A. J., 152, *164*
Farley, T. A., 45, *53*
Farmer, A., *298*
Farmer, M., 294, *298*
Farrar, W. B., *372, 425, 510*
Farrell, D., 192, *202, 205*
Farrell, J. B., *428*
Farrelly, M. C., 158, *163, 164*
Farrenkopf, M., 92, *99*
Fasaye, G., 307, *316*
Fatone, A., *320*
Fava, J. L., 70, *83*
Fawzy, F. I., 368, 369, *372, 373, 374*, 506, *512*
Fawzy, N. W., 368, 369, *373, 374, 512*
Fears, T., *446*

Fears, T. R., *442*
Feder, S. I., 421, *429*
Feil, E. G., 548, *556*
Feldman, C. S., 351, *359*
Feldman, H. A., 89, 99, *204*
Feldman, R., 194, *204*
Feldstein, M., *372*
Felton, G., *249*
Feng, Z., 92, 97, 97, 99, 179, *181, 202*
Fenn, K., 134, *145*
Fernandez, M. E., *528*
Ferrans, C. E., 117, *126*
Ferrell, B. A., 399, *404*
Ferrell, B. R., 399, *404*, 468, *481*
Ferri, J., *344*
Ferrucci, L., *515*
Ferry, L. H., 172, 174, *183*
Ferster, D., *55*
Feskanich, D., 29, *37*
Fetscher, S., 351, *355*
Fetting, J., *511*
Feyerabend, C., *187*
Fielding, J., 527, *527*
Fields, M. L., *527*
Fife, B., 467, 472, *484*
Fife, B. L., 470, *481*
Figueiredo, M. I., 196, *203*
Figueredo, A. J., *429*
Figuero-Moseley, C., *358*
Filiberti, A., 363, *374*
Fillit, H., 395, *404*
Filsinger, S., *98*
Finch, C., 307, *316*
Fine, J. A., 210, *217*
Fink, S., 550, *555*
Finn, J. D., 70, *80*
Finnegan, J., *247*
Finnegan, J. R., *101*
Fins, J. J., 339, *343, 344*
Finucane, M., 135, *147*
Fiore, M. C., 168, 169, 170, 171, 172, 175, *183, 186, 187, 188*, 534, *544*
Fiori, K. L., 194, *203*
Fisch, M., 419, *426*
Fischoff, B., 134, 135, *144, 145, 148*
Fiset, V., *147*

Fishbein, M., 44, *52*, *53*, 257, *274*
Fisher, B., 103, *112*, 116, *125*, *126*
Fisher, J. O., *201*
Fisher, L., *442*
Fisher, P., *296*
Fitch, T. R., *356*
Fitchett, G., 472, *480*
Fitzgerald, G., *313*
Fitzgerald, J. T., *183*
Fitzpatrick, R., *298*, *407*
Flaherty, B. P., 536, *543*
Flanders, W. D., *36*
Flannery, J. T., *443*
Flatt, S. W., *494*
Flay, B., 152, *163*, *165*
Flay, B. R., 68, *81*, 152, 153, 154, 155, 160, *163*, 164
Flegal, K. M., 28, 29, *37*, *39*
Fleischman, A. R., 339, *344*
Fleisher, L., 311, *318*
Fleishman, S., *481*
Fleiss, J. L., *184*
Fleming, C., 33, *37*, 212, *219*, 456, *458*
Fleshner, M., 500, *514*
Fletcher, I., *298*
Fletcher, J., *22*
Fletcher, R., *148*
Flint, P., *217*
Flores, R., 238, 241, *247*
Flynn, B. S., *22*, 157, *163*, *165*, *314*
Flynn, P. J., *358*
Foegbe, W. H., 151, *164*
Foley, B., 451, *458*, *461*, *463*
Foley, K. L., 172, *187*
Folkman, S., 44, *53*, 230, *232*, *233*, 392, *404*, 468, *482*
Folsom, A. R., *38*
Fong, G. T., *148*
Fong, P. S. W., 538, 539, 540, 541, *544*
Forbes, C., 17, *20*, 258, 259, 266, *274*, *275*
Ford, D. E., 177, *183*
Ford, L., *113*
Ford, M. E., *113*
Ford, S., 339, *343*, *344*
Ford, V. Y., *101*

Forlenza, M. J., 503, *512*
Forman, J. D., *484*
Formenti, S. C., 366, *375*
Forrest, J. L., 520, *528*
Forrest, S., *299*
Forsberg, C., 352, *360*
Forster, J., *220*
Forster, J. L., 92, 99, 160, *163*
Forsyth, L. H., 239, *248*, *544*
Forte, K. J., *444*
Fortinsky, R., 393, *404*
Fortmann, S. P., 171, *183*
Foshee, V. A., *162*
Fossa, S. D., 440, *494*
Fossen, A., 452, *460*
Foster, C., *316*, *321*
Fotheringham, M. J., *9*, *22*, 249, 257, 276
Fouad, M., *113*
Fouladi, R. T., *182*, *388*, *447*, 471, *485*
Fowler, F. J. J., 281, *300*
Fox, B. H., 503, 504, 507, 508, *512*
Fox, B. J., 175, *186*
Fox, S., 141, *145*, 548, *556*
Fox, S. A., 92, 99
Fraher, L., *444*
France, E. K., 179, *183*
Franceschi, S., *234*
Franch, L., 450, *459*
Franche, R., 393, *404*
Francis, D. J., 450, *459*
Francis, L. A., 199, *203*
Frank, C., *218*
Frank, E., 171, *183*
Frank, J. W., 352, *357*
Frank, L. D., 537, *545*
Frank, R. G., *235*
Frankel, R. M., 337, 338, 339, *342*
Franklin, F. A., *101*, *206*
Franks, M. M., 104, *111*
Fraser, A., 422, *428*
Fraser, C., *296*
Frassoni, F., 439, *448*
Fraumeni, J., 226, *234*
Frazier, A. L., 26, *36*
Fred, C., *376*, *481*

Freda, M. C., 288, *301*

Freedman, L., *205*

Freedman, L. S., *113*

Freeman, A., *460*

Freeman, M. A., 139, *145*

Freeman-Gibb, L., 469, *483*

Freemantle, N., *188*

Freeman-Wang, T., 287, *297*

French, K., 281, *297*

French, S. A., 195, 196, 197, 198, 199, 203, *207*

Frenn, M., 241, *247*

Frets, P. G., *317*

Freudenheim, J. L., 29, *37*

Fridinger, F., 239, *247, 248*

Friebel, T., *319*

Fried, T., *405*

Friedenreich, C. M., 237, *247*

Friedlander, M., *318*

Friedman, A., 340, *344*

Friedman, D., 448, 449, *460*

Friedman, D. L., *445*

Friedman, L. C., *316*

Friedman, R., *545*

Friedman, R. H., 193, *203, 203*, 271, *274*

Friedman, S. H., 468, *484*

Friedrich, W. N., 454, *459*

Friedrichsen, M. J., 330, *343*

Frierson, G. M., 490, *494*

Fries, E. A., 196, *203*

Frink, B., 398, *405*

Frohardt, M., 139, *146*

Fry, A., 136, *145*

Fryer-Edwards, K. A., 338, *341*

Fu, Q., *205*

Fuchs, C., *37*

Fuchs, C. S., 30, *37, 41*

Fuchs, D., *515*

Fuemmeler, B. F., 190, 197, *203*

Fukkala, E., *512*

Fulkerson, J. A., 199, *207*

Fuller, A., *298*

Funk, S. G., 470, *481*

Fuqua, J., 538, *545, 546*

Future II Study Group, The, 285, *297*

Gaff, C., 309, *315, 344*

Gaffney, C., 179, *185, 221*

Gage, M., *199*

Gail, M. H., *442*

Gajjar, A., *463*

Galanko, J. A., *494*

Galanter, E., 353, *357*

Galea, V., 434, *448*

Gall, T. L., 472, *481*

Gallager, M., 351, *355*

Gallagher, A., 329, 330, 337, *341*

Gallaher, P., *165, 461*

Gallant, S. J., *375*

Gallelli, K., 453, *462*

Galper, D., *223*

Galvao, D. A., 237, *247*

Galvin, E., *407*

Gamble, M., 199, 200, *203*

Ganz, P. A., 116, 120, *125, 126, 127, 128*, 364, 366, *372, 374, 375, 376, 377*, 380, 384, 385, 387, 417, 418, 426, 429, 430, 433, 434, 436, 438, 443, 444, 447, 467, 469, 470, *481*

Gao, D. L., *101*

Gappmayer-Locker, 287, *297*

Garber, J. E., 310, *315, 319*

Garcia, N., *481*

Garde, K., *515*

Garr, D. R., 228, *234*

Garrett, J. M., *220*

Garrett, P., *250*

Garssen, B., *359*

Gartlehner, G., 272, *274*

Gartstein, M. A., 452, *465*

Garwicz, S., *445*

Gasparro, F. P., 209, *220*

Gattamaneni, H. R., *443*

Gattas, M., *318*

Gattuso, J., 460, *465*

Gattuso, J. S., *21*

Gaugler, J. E., 396, *404*

Gavrilov, L., 510, *510*

Gavrilova, N., 510, *510*

Gay, G., 549, *556*

Gebbie, K. M., *529*

Gee, L., *102*
Geggie, P., 400, *404*
Geggie, P. H., 477, *480*
Gehan, E., *444*
Geiger, A. M., 228, *232*
Gelber, R. D., 122, *126*, *445*
Geling, O., *356*
Gellar, B. M., *165*
Geller, A., 211, *221*
Geller, A. C., 92, 99, 172, *184*, 213, 214, *218*, *219*
Geller, B. M., *22*, *163*, 283, *300*
Gendrano, N. III, 383, *388*
Geno, C., *221*
Geno, C. R., 216, *218*, *223*
Gent, M., *127*
Gentle, A. F., 211, *220*
George, G., 172, *187*
George, M. A., 201, *204*
George, T., 391, *406*, 469, *484*
Georgiou, A., *355*
Gerhardt, C., *373*
Gerlach, K. K., *545*
Germak, J. A., *446*
Germino, B. B., *357*, *428*, 470, 472, *481*, *484*
Gerrard, M., *146*, 213, *221*
Getson, P. R., *444*, *460*
Geyer, S., 503, 505, *512*
Geyer, S. M., *182*
Ghaffari, A. M., *232*
Ghafoor, A., *233*, *444*
Ghosh-Dastidar, B., 153, *163*
Giambarresi, T. R., *314*
Gianola, F. J., 116, *128*
Giardiello, F. M., 309, *317*
Gibbons, F. X., *146*, 213, *221*
Gibbons, P., *557*
Gibbs, A., *297*
Gibertinin, M., 328, *345*
Gibson, B. E., *446*
Gibson, C., 395, *403*
Gibson, J. J., *221*
Gidron, Y., 353, *355*
Giedzinska, A. S., 364, 365, *374*, 417, 418, *426*

Giese, A. J., *218*
Giese-Davis, J., *373*, *428*, 501, 505, *516*
Gift, A., *405*
Giglio, M., 339, *345*
Gil, K. M., *428*
Gilchrist, L. D., 176, *181*
Giles, G. G., 24, *37*
Giles-Corti, B., 211, *219*, *221*
Gill, G. J., *444*
Gill, P., 177, *186*
Gill, P. G., *428*
Gillespie, A., 92, *100*
Gillespie, A. M., 211, *220*
Gillespie, C. C., *188*
Gillespie, D., 309, *316*
Gillespie, K. N., 520, *528*
Gilliland, F. D., *127*, 382, *387*
Gillman, M. W., *100*, *545*
Gilmore, N., 288, *297*
Gilpin, E., 171, *184*
Gilpin, E. A., 152, *164*, 536, *544*
Gilson, B. S., 118, *125*, *126*
Gilson, J. S., *126*
Ginsberg, J., *445*
Ginsberg, J. P., 435, *444*
Giovannucci, E., 26, 29, 30, 36, *37*, *386*
Giovannucci, E. L., 30, *37*, *39*, *41*
Giovino, G., 159, *183*, *184*
Giovino, G. A., *40*, *80*, *165*
Giraldi, T., 505, *512*
Girardi, F. L., 287–288, *297*
Girasek, D., 421, *428*
Girgis, A., 214, 216, *219*, *220*, 330, 332, *343*
Gitchell, J. G., 174, *187*
Gitlin, L., 396, *404*
Giulano, A. R., 226, *232*
Given, B., 391, 392, 393, 395, 396, 401, *403*, *404*, *405*, *406*, *407*, *408*, *426*, 471, *482*
Given, B. A., 336, *343*, 505, *516*
Given, C., 391, 392, 393, 395, 396, 397, *403*, *404*, *405*, *406*, *407*, *408*
Given, C. W., 336, *343*, *355*, *404*, *426*, 505, *516*
Given, G., 352, *355*

Glanz, K., 22, 45, 52, 53, 54, 67, 81, 98, 99, 102, 112, 203, 206, 213, 214, 216, 219, 220, 230, 235, 276, 306, 316, 365, 368, 374, 528
Glare, P., 343
Glasby, M., 215, 223
Glaser, R., 372, 372, 374, 405, 425, 500, 502, 503, 509, 510, 512, 513, 516
Glasgow, R. E., 17, 20, 64, 65, 65n, 81, 137, 146, 179, 183, 195, 204, 269, 271, 272, 274, 277, 519, 525, 528, 548, 556
Glass, A., 39, 271, 277
Glass, J. O., 462, 463
Glasser, B., 297
Glasser, D. B., 386
Glassman, A. H., 177, 184
Glassman, B., 16, 22, 234
Glassman, M., 364, 367, 375
Gledhill-Hoyt, J., 25, 40
Gleeson, H. K., 435, 443
Glenn, B., 269, 273, 287, 296
Glicksman, A. S., 460
Glober, G., 332, 342
Glover, D. A., 452, 460
Gnys, M., 82, 178, 187
Gochman, D. S., 148
Godar, D. E., 209, 210, 220
Godber, T., 450, 458
Goddard, A., 430
Godfrey, H., 393, 405
Godwin, A. K., 315, 319
Goel, M. S., 35, 38
Goeppiger, J., 407
Goff, B., 386
Goggin, K. J., 248
Goins, K. Y., 173, 188
Golan, M., 194, 204
Golant, M., 373, 428
Gold, K., 310, 313, 317
Gold, R., 306, 318
Gold, S. H., 452, 462
Gold, W., 555
Goldberg, D. E, 512
Goldberg, D. P., 286, 297
Goldberg, J., 199, 203

Goldenberg, B., 463
Golden-Kreutz, D. M., 372, 425, 510
Goldfarb, N., 99
Goldhirsch, A., 122, 126
Goldstein, A. M., 447
Goldstein, D., 235
Goldstein, M., 80, 169, 274
Goldstein, M. G., 171, 173, 181, 182, 183, 186, 527
Goldstein, N., 399, 405
Goldwein, J., 450, 463, 464, 557
Golomb, V., 450, 461, 464
Goloubeva, O., 463
Gomez-Caminero, A., 317
Gonzales, R., 305, 312, 321
Gonzales-Pinto, A., 177, 182
Gonzalez, L. C., 232
Gonzalez, R. E., 92, 99
Good, R. S., 383, 386
Goodday, R., 353, 355
Goodman, G. E., 39
Goodman, J., 184
Goodman, P. J., 112
Goodman, R. M., 270, 277
Goodwin, P. J., 116, 126, 370, 374, 421, 426, 433, 436, 444, 506, 508, 512
Goodyear, M. D, 127
Goold, S. D., 304, 319
Gordon, C., 183, 544
Gordon, E. J., 330, 331, 335, 336, 343
Gordon, J. R., 64, 81
Gordon, L., 182
Gore-Felton, C., 369, 372
Gorin, S. S., 170, 184
Gortmaker, S. L., 199, 204
Gospodarowicz, M., 448
Gosselink, R., 434, 444
Gotay, C., 479, 481
Gotay, C. C., 116, 121, 126, 127, 306, 316, 534, 544
Gottheil, E., 504, 516
Gottlieb, L. K., 529
Gottschalk, M., 250
Gould, S. M., 192, 204
Graber, J. E., 3, 21, 175, 185
Graboys, T. B., 331, 342

Graham, J., *373, 505, 512*
Graham, R., *555*
Graham, S., *37, 147*
Graham-Pole, J., *456, 465*
Grahn, D., *510*
Gram, I. T., *282, 297*
Grana, R., *160, 162*
Grande, G. E., *418, 427*
Graney, M., *179, 187*
Grant, B., *493*
Grant, B. F., *176, 177, 184*
Grant, K., *176, 187*
Grant, M., *399, 404, 481*
Grant-Petersson, J., *92, 98, 212, 219*
Grasse, C., *147*
Grassi, L., *505, 512*
Grassi, R., *462*
Graul, J., *513*
Graverstein, S., *405*
Graves, C., *98*
Graves, D. R., *142, 144*
Graves, K. D., *368, 369, 370, 374, 419, 427*
Gray, G., *125*
Gray, J., *531, 542, 543, 544*
Graydon, J. E., *351, 356*
Graziano, G., *556*
Greco, F. A., *349, 355*
Green, D., *447*
Green, E. D., *303, 315*
Green, L., *550, 556*
Green, L. S. G., *146*
Green, L. W., *201, 204, 522, 528*
Green, M. J., *312, 316*
Green, S. B., *113*
Green, V., *233*
Greenberg, E. R., *494*
Greenberg, J., *396, 406*
Greenberg, M., *456, 458*
Greenberg, M. D., *233*
Greenberg, R. S., *443*
Greendale, G. A., *385, 387, 433, 436, 443, 444*
Greene, K., *213, 220*
Greeneltch, K. M., *516*
Greenfield, S., *423, 427*

Greenfield, T. K., *32, 38*
Greenwald, P., *6, 21, 62, 81*
Greer, B., *386*
Greer, S., *505, 513, 516*
Greer, Y., *247*
Gregory, J. W., *434, 448*
Gregson, J., *195, 206*
Greil, R., *126*
Greimel, E. R., *287, 297*
Gress, J., *538, 545, 546*
Grieco, E. M., *104, 112*
Grieve, R., *51, 53*
Griffin, A. M., *339, 346*
Griffin, C. A., *309, 317*
Griffin, S., *194, 205*
Grimm, P., *398, 405*
Grimm, P. M., *357*
Grimshaw, J. M., *277*
Grissino, L. M., *172, 183*
Gritz, E., *488, 489, 490, 493*
Gritz, E. R., *21, 67, 81, 92, 99, 179, 183, 184, 205, 210, 212, 220, 459, 469, 470, 481*
Grizzle, J., *97*
Groenvold, M., *128*
Grootenhuis, M. A., *453, 460*
Grosfeld, F. J. M., *308, 316*
Gross, C. R., *299*
Grossfeld, G. D., *387*
Grossman, G., *422, 427*
Grossman, J., *461*
Grossman, M., *160, 162*
Grossman, R., *553, 557*
Grothaus, L. C., *63, 82, 299*
Grotmol, T., *291, 298*
Grove, J., *306, 316*
Grunberg, S. M., *348, 356*
Grunfeld, E., *393, 396, 404, 405*
Gruskin, E., *234*
Guadagnoli, E., *335, 343*
Guamaccia, C., *402, 403*
Guerra, F. A., *527*
Guerrero, E., *232*
Guevarra, J., *320*
Guido, M., *443*
Guillem, J., *275*

Gulliver, C., *185*
Gulliver, S. B., 176, 177, *182, 184*
Guo, M. D., *465*
Guralnik, J. M., *515*
Gurevich, M., 416, 420, *427*
Gurney, J. G., *442, 460, 461, 520, 528*
Gurpegui, M., 177, *182*
Gussow, J., 199, *204*
Gustafson, D. H., 548, 550, 551, *556, 556, 557, 558*
Gustavsson, G., *187*
Guther, H., *512*
Guthrie, D., *512*
Gutterman, E., 395, *404*
Guttmacher, A. E., 303, 313, *315, 316*
Guyatt, G. H., 124, *127*
Guyer, M. S., 303, *315*
Gwaltney, C. J., *182*
Gyato, K., *458*

Ha, C. N., *101*
Haaga. D. A. F., 368, *373*
Haas, A. L., 177, *184*
Haas, J. S., 270, *274*
Habbal, R., *235*
Habicht, J. P., 272, *277*
Hack, T., *342*
Hackett, J. R., 228, *232*
Haddock, K., *249*
Haddy, T. B., 434, *444*
Hadjistavropoulos, T., 393, *404*
Hadley, D. W., 304, *314, 316*
Hadley, E. C., *249*
Hadley, T., *144*
Hafertepen, A., *318*
Hafstad, A., 157, *164*
Hagedoorn, M., 468, *481*
Hagerty, K., *330*
Hagerty, R., *342*
Haggmark, C., 352, *360*
Haglind, E., 290, *298*
Hahlen, K., 454, *465*
Hahn, A., 135, *145*
Hahn, D. E., *387*
Haile, R. W., *35*
Hailey, S., 368, *373*

Haines, P., *207*
Haire-Joshu, D., 194, *205*
Haisfield, W., *357*
Hakama, M., 20, 23, *39*
Halam, J., 239, *248*
Halapy, E., *297*
Halbert, C. H., 231, *232*, 309, *316*
Haley, W., *407*
Haley, W. E., *483*
Hall, A., 339, *343*
Hall, H. I., *222*
Hall, J. R., *218*
Hall, K., 452, *463*
Hall, S., 226, *232*
Hall, S. A., 255, *274*
Hall, S. M., 169, 177, *184, 186, 209*
Hall, W., 137, *143*, 176, *182*
Haller, D., *275*
Halliday, J., 309, *315*
Hallion, M. E., 169, *187*
Hallowell, N., 313, *316*
Halton, J. M., 434, *444*
Hamilton, A. B., 415, *427*
Hamilton, A. S., *127*
Hamilton, R. D., 327, *346*
Hamilton, S. J., *112*
Hammon, S., *357*
Hammond, M. A., 469, 471, 473, *482*
Hammond, S., *112*, 239, 387, *445*
Hamovitch, M., 468, *481*
Hampshire, M., *557*
Hanahan, D., 509, *513*
Hancock, L., 92, *99*
Hancock, S. L., 433, *444*
Handwerger, B., 451, *459*
Hanjani, P., *298*
Hankey, B. F., *546*
Hankinson, S. E., *41*
Hann, I. M., 439, *445*
Hanna, D., *318, 492*
Hanna, N., *404*
Hannan, P., 199, *203*
Hannan, P. J., 89, 92, *100*
Hanrahan, P. F., 214, *220*
Hansen, M., *356*
Hansen, R. A., 272, *274*

Hansen, S. W., 438, *444*
Hansen, V. L., *446*
Hansen, W. B., *164*
Hansis-Diarte, A., *300*
Harari, G., *217*
Hardcastle, J. D., 290, *299*
Hardeman, W., 194, *205*
Harden, J., 473, 475, *481*
Hardenbergh, P. H., 433, *442*
Haris, T. M., *305*
Harkness, E., 352, *355*
Harlan, L. C., *127, 388*
Harlos, M., *342*
Harlow, L. L., 365, 366, *376*
Harper, G. R., *316*
Harrell, J., 213, *221*
Harrell, J. S., *249*
Harrington, J. M., *112*
Harrington, K. F., *101, 206*
Harris, E. L., 68, *83*
Harris, J., 393, *405*
Harris, J. R., *429, 526, 528*
Harris, M. S., *550, 557*
Harris, R., *232, 506, 514*
Harris, R. P., *521, 524, 528*
Harris, S., 64, *81*
Harris, S. D., *373, 480*
Harris, S. R., 336, *344*
Harris, T. M., 305, *316*
Harrist, R. B., *220, 529*
Hart, A., Jr., *202*
Hart, S., 362, *375*
Harth, T., 421, *426*
Hartman, K. E., 255, *274*
Hartz, D. T., *184*
Harvey, C., *112*
Harvey, E. L., *188*
Harvey, J., 364, *375*
Harvey, R., 538, *545, 546*
Hasenbring, M., 349, 356, 368, *375*
Hasin, D. S., 176, *184*
Hasleton, P. S., *443*
Hassard, T., *342*
Hatcher, M. B., 363, *374*
Hatsukami, D. K., 169, *185*
Hatziandreu, E., *183*

Hauck, W., 396, *404*
Haugh, R. 553, *556*
Haughey, B. P., *37*
Haughton, L., *202*
Hauser, J., 401, *407*
Hauser, J. M., 401, *405*
Havas, S., 194, *204*
Havermans, T., 454, *460*
Havice, M., *247*
Haviland, J. S., 505, *516*
Haviland, M. L., 158, 159, *163, 164*
Havlik, R. J., *515*
Hawk, L. H., Jr., *544*
Hawkins, A., *462*
Hawkins, R., 550, *556, 558*
Hawkins, R. P., *557, 558*
Hawley, S. T., 270, *276*
Hawton, K., 384, *387*
Hay, J. L., 283, *297*
Hayashi, R., *461*
Hayes, L., 211, *220*
Hayes Roth, B., 353, *359*
Hayman, J., 393, 395, *405*
Haynes, K. M., 549, 552, *555*
Haynes, R. B., *188, 520, 529*
Haynes, S., 121, *126*
Hays, D. M., *444*
Hays, J., 110, *112*
Hays, R. D., 118, 123, *126, 127, 128,*
    290, 300
Hazuda, H. P., 505, *516*
Health Information National Trends
    Survey, 548, *556*
Healton, C. G., *163*
Heath, A. C., *513*
Heath, C. W., Jr., *40*
Heath, G. W., *248*
Heatherton, T. F., *165*
Hebert, D., *97*
Hebert, J. R., *206, 528*
Heck, J. E., 170, *184*
Hedderson, M. M., *493*
Hedley, D., *511*
Heenan, P. J., 215, *220*
Heffer, R., 455, *463*
Heflin, L., *375*

Heideman, R., *465*
Heiermann, E., *442*
Heikkila, S., *494*
Heim, E., *481*
Heiman, J., 388
Heiman, J. R., 383, *386, 387*
Heimans, J. J., *448*
Heimendinger, J., 97, 192, *204, 206*
Heimes, U., *442*
Heiney, S., 338, *344*
Heinrich, R. L., 120, *128*
Heintz, A. P., *387*
Heisler-Mackinnon, J., *202*
Helenius, H., 503, 504, *514*
Helfand, M., 255, *274, 528*
Helft, P. R., *344*
Helgeson, V. S., 364, 365, 366, 367,
    368, 370, *374, 375,* 417, 420,
    430, 475, 478, *481, 483*
Heller, G., 433, *447*
Heller, L. B., 434, *444*
Helweg-Larsen, S., 437, *444*
Helzlsouer, K. J., 304, *317*
Henderson, B., 281, *296*
Henderson, B. E., 227, *232*
Henley, S. J., *40*
Henne-Bruns, D., *513*
Hennekens, C. H., 31, *38*
Hennessy, E. V., 139, *145*
Henning, J. M., *387*
Hennrikus, D. J., 92, *99*
Henry, J. L., 416, 420, *427*
Hensley, M., *388*
Hepworth, J., 398, *408*
Herberman, R. B., 502, *513, 514*
Herbert, T. B., 499, 500, *511*
Herman, D. R., 433, *444*
Hermann, C., 505, *513*
Hermann, R. E., *388*
Hern, H. E. J., 335, *344*
Herndon, J. E. II, *427, 516*
Herr, N., 199, *204*
Herrell, F. E., Jr., *516*
Herrero, R, *234*
Herrmann, C., 505
Hersey, J., 190, *201*

Hersey, J. C., *163*
Hertzberg, H., *462*
Heslop, S. D. M., 339, *346*
Hester, A. L., *444*
Hetzke, J., *458*
Heuvel, F., 453, *460*
Hewett, P., 292, *298*
Hewitt, M., 5, 20, 23, *37,* 61, 80, 211,
    220, 418, 423, *427*
Heydenreich, J., 214, *222*
Heyn, R., 437, *444*
Hiatt, R., 5–6, 6, *20*
Hiatt, R. A., 6, 9, *21,* 61, *81,* 116, *127,*
    234, 257, 269, *274, 276,* 421, *428*
Hickcox, M., *82,* 178, *187*
Hicken, B., 368, *375,* 425, *429*
Hickey, A. A., *202*
Hickman, S. A., *248*
Hickok, J. T., 347, 348, 349, 335051,
    354, 356, *358*
Higgins, S. T., 176, *181*
High, J. L., *113*
Hill, D., 155, 215, *222*
Hill, D. A., *448*
Hill, J., 451, *462*
Hill, J. J., 457, *459*
Hill, J. M., 450, *460*
Hill, J. O., 27, *38*
Hillenberg, B., *389*
Hiller, J. E., *510*
Hillhouse, J., 213, *222*
Hillier, V. F., 286, *297*
Hillman, A. L., 92, *99*
Hilton, B. A., 469, 470, 471, 472, 473,
    474, *482*
Hilton, J. F., *102*
Himmelstein, D. U., *185*
Hinds, P., *460*
Hinds, P. S., 16, *21*
Hines, J. M., *218*
Hinman, A. R., *529*
Hirji, K., *376*
Hirst, K., *102*
Hitsman, B., 177, 178, *181, 185*
Hla, K. M., 235, 258, 259, *277*
Hla, K. M. A., 228, *235*

Hlubocky, F. J., 329, *346*

Ho, M., *247*

Hobbie, W., 452, 456, 460, *464*

Hobbie, W. L., 435, *444*

Hoben, K., *98*

Hochbaum, G. M., 522, *528*

Hochberg, Y., 75, *81*

Hockemeyer, J. R., *146*

Hodge, M., 538, *544*

Hodson, I., *181*

Hoekstra-Weebers, J. E. H. M., *320*, 453, *460*

Hoelscher, D. M., 195, *204*

Hoelzer, K. L., *356*

Hoff, G., 290, 291, *298, 298*

Hoff, G. S., 290, *301*

Hoffman, B., 364, *374*

Hoffman, B. R., *165*

Hoffman, M., 328, 337, *344*

Hoffman, R. M., *388*

Hoffman-Goetz, L., 257, *274*

Hofman, M., *358*

Hogbin, B., 339, *344*

Hogg, A., *298*

Holcombe, C, 334, *346*

Holden, R. J., 502, *513*

Holecek, A., *557*

Holland, J., 7, *21*

Holland, J. C., 118, *127, 374*

Holland, J. D., 504, *511*

Holland, J. F., 460, *516*

Hollis, D. R., *427*

Hollis, J. F., 68, 77, *81*, 171, *186*

Hollis, S., *81*

Holm, L. E., 210, *217*

Holman, H., 240, *248*

Holmes, C., *127*

Holmes, E., 488, *493*

Holmes, M. D., *41*

Holowaty, E., *448*

Holst, K., *513*

Holt, C. L., *205*

Holt-Lunstad, J., 505, *516*

Holtom, R., 288, *300, 301*

Holtzman, D., 25, 27, 35, *38*

Holzner, B., *126*, 415, *427*

Honess, L., 192, *202*

Honess-Morreale, L., *202*

Honeycutt, C., *222*

Hood, K., *144*

Hoogerbrugge, N., *320*

Hopkins, K. D., 88, *99*

Hoppe, R. T., 433, *444*

Hopwood, P., 139, *145, 297*

Horgen, K. B., 198, *204*

Hornbrook, M. C., *249*

Horning, R. L., 211, *220*

Hornslien, K., *494*

Horowitz, E., *483*

Horrocks, J., 450, *463*

Horrowitz, M. M., *514*

Horton, R., *80*

Horwitz, E., 396, 406, 477, *483*

Hoskins, C. N., 468, 473, 475, *482*

Hoskins, W. J., *235*

Hosmer, D. W., 76, *81*

Hospers, H., 550, *558*

Houck, C., 456, *465*

Houfek, J., *320*

Hough, E. E., 470, *483*

Hou-Jensen, K., *446*

House, J. S., 505, *513*

Housemann, R. A., 245, *247*

Houskamp, B., 453, *465*

Houston, C., *204*

Houston, D. M., 294, *298*

Houts, P. S., 468, *484*

Howe, H. L., 20, 37, *546*

Howe, S., *112*

Howell, A., *145*

Howell, S. J., 384, *387*

Howells, R., 288, *298*

Howells, R. E., *298*

Howze, E. H., *248*

Hoy, M. A., *492*

Hryniuk, W. M., *127*

Hrywna, M., *377*

Hsee, C. K., 135, *146*

Hsieh, C. Y., *233*

Hsing, A. W., *233*

Hu, F. B., 27, 38, *39*

Huang, T., *165*

Hubbell, F. A., *112*, 231, *232*
Huber, H. P., 287–288, *297*
Huber, M. H., *188*
Hudis, C. A., *481*
Hudson, M., 194, *202, 208*
Hudson, M. A., *202*
Hudson, M. M., 432, *446, 457, 460*
Hudson-Tennent, L. J., 450, *461*
Hufford, D., *218*
Hufford, M., *82*
Hugdahl, K., *513*
Hughes, C., 306, 307, *316, 317, 319*
Hughes, G. M., *297*
Hughes, J. R., 174, 176, *185*
Hughes, R. G., 171, *182*
Huijgens, P. C., *448*
Hulscher, M. E., *277*
Humair, J. P., 172, *185*
Humfleet, G. L., 177, *184*
Humphrey, L. L., 255, *274*
Humphreys, K., *428*
Humphris, G., 363, *374*
Hung, L., *165*
Hunt, J. R., *112*
Hunt, M. K., 92, *100*, 196, *202, 207*
Hunt, S. M., 118, *126*
Hunter, D. J., 20, 23, 30, 36, 37, 38, *41,*
515
Hunter, S., *102*
Hurd, S., 103, 110, *113*
Hurley, K., 13, *21*, 45, *54*, 141, *146,*
229, *233*, 280, *299*, 305, *319,*
348, *357*
Hurley, L. B., *234*
Hurley, S. F., 281, *297*
Hurley. K. E., 309, *316*
Hurt, R. D., 176, *185*
Husgafvel-Pursianinen, K., 535, *546*
Husten, C., 168, *185*
Hutchinson, J., 240, *250*
Hutchinson, R., *445*
Hutter, J. J., *460*
Hwang, W. T., *461*
Hyde, R. T., *39*
Hyland, A., *98*
Hytten, K., 331, *344*
Hyun, C. S., *512*

Iacovino, V., 368, 369, *374*
Ideströöm, M., 286, 287, *298*
Ikeda, H., 500, *511*
Ilan, S., *320*
Illidge, T. M., 440, *445*
Ilnyckyj, A., 506, *513*
Inskip, P. D., *387*
Institute of Medicine, U. S., 32, 40, 257,
275, 312, *316*, 385, *387*, 517, *528*
International Agency for Research on
Cancer (IARC), 26, 27, *38*
Irvine, D., 351, *356*
Irvine, D. M., 351, *356*
Irwig, L., *296*
Irwin, M., 501, *513*
Isaacs, C., *319*
Isasi, T., *298*
Ishibe, N., *314*
Islam, N., *201*
Isnec, M. R., 99, 213, *219*
Isquith, P. K., 450, *465*
Itzen, M., *315*

Jabbari, S., *514*
Jackvony, E. H., 239, *250*
Jackson, A., *101, 206*
Jackson, C., 549, *555*
Jackson, E., 194, *202, 208*
Jackson, K., 168, *185, 388*
Jackson, T. C., *183*
Jackvony, E. H., 192, *207*, 551, *558*
Jacobs, A., *358*
Jacobs, D. R., Jr., 31, *38*
Jacobs, E. J., 36, *39*
Jacobsen, P., 395, *408*
Jacobsen, P. B., *21*, 205, 305, *317*, 351,
354, *356*, 422, *426, 493*
Jacobson, M. F., 197, 198, *204, 206*
Jacobson, P. E., 92, *102*
Jacoby, P., *219*
Jacovino, V., *374*
Jaffe, N., 450, *459*
James, A., 197, *202, 494*
James, R. H., 469, 472, 473, 475, *484*
James, A. S., *220*
Jamner, L. D., 162, *164*

Janega, J. B., 85, 91n, 95n, *102*
Jannoun, L., 451, *465*
Jansen, A. M., *232*
Jantz, C., 192, *204*
Janz, N. K., 305, *321, 426, 522, 528*
Jarvis, M. J., *188, 301*
Jasmine, M., 210, *217*
Jaspers, J., 453, *460*
Jaworski, T. M., 454, *459*
Jean-Pierre, P., *358*
Jeffery, D. D., 488, *492*
Jeffrey, R. W., 99, 198, 199, *203*
Jeha, S., 436, *447, 475, 485*
Jemal, A., 225, 226, 227, *233*, 431, *444*
Jemmott, J. B., 138, *145*
Jenkins, D., 286, *298, 299*
Jenkins, G., P., *511*
Jenkins, J., *316*
Jenkins, R., *388*
Jenkins, R. A., 350, *360*
Jenkins, R. G., 228, *234*
Jenkins, V., 333, 334, 337, *343*
Jenkins, V. A., 331, 332, *343*
Jensen, M., *461*
Jensen, S., 471, *482*
Jenson, A. B., *233*
Jepsen, C., *482*
Jepson, C., 141, *148*, 395, 400, *405*, 478, *483, 514, 553, 558*
Jepson, R., 17, *20*, 257, 258, 259, 270, *274, 275*
Jereczek-Fossa, B. A. M., 350, 351, *356*
Jernigan, D, 47, *55*
Jernigan, J. C., *113*
Jernigan, S., 213, *220*
Jiang, Y., 199, *205*
Joab, S. A., 136, *144*
Jobe, J. B., *278*
Johansen, C., 368, *376*, 419, *429, 463, 503, 504, 511, 515*
Johansson, S., 440, *444*
Johnsen, E. L., *514*
Johnson, A., *297*
Johnson, C. A., 156, *164*
Johnson, C. C., *204*
Johnson, C. L., 28, 37, *39*, 46, *53*

Johnson, D. L., 438, *444, 450, 460*
Johnson, J. L., 136, *144*, 258, 261, *276*
Johnson, K. A., 309, 310, *317*
Johnson, K. C., 179, *187*
Johnson, N., 198, *205*
Johnson, R., 398, *408*
Johnson, R. J., *146*
Johnson, T., 269, *275*
Johnson, T. P., *278*
Johnson-Hurzeler, R., 403, *405*
Johnston, J. A., *187*
Johnston, L. D., 152, *164*
Johnston, M. R., *219*
Johnston, R., 219, *221*
Jones, C. L., 453, 455, *459*
Jones, D., *460*
Jones, H., 557, *558*
Jones, J. L., 213, *220*
Jones, J. M., 287, 289, *301*, 340, 341, *344*
Jones, K., *221*
Jones, L., *97*
Jones, L. W., 490, *493*
Jones, M. E., 439, *447*
Jones, M. H., 286, *298*
Jones, P. W., *298*
Jones, Q. J., 339, *342*
Jones, R. H., *218*
Jones, T. C, *557*
Jones-Wallace, D., 450, *463*
Joorman, J., 89, *101*
Jordan, F. M., 450, *459, 461*
Jorenby, M. E., *183, 187, 188*
Jorgensen, T., 504, *515*
Joris, F., 215, *222*
Joseph, A., *460*
Joseph, A. L., *444*
Joseph, F., 226, *234*
Julesberg, K., *204*
Jung, D. L., *39*
Jung, E. G., 215, *223*
Jungner, G., 255, 256, *278*
Juraskova, I., 334, *345*

Kaasa, S., 331, *344*
Kabeto, M., *405*

Kachur, E., *188*
Kadan-Lottick, N. S., 457, *461*
Kahana, B., 416, *426*, 487, *492*
Kahler, C. W., *181*
Kahn, B., 387, 436, *443*, *481*
Kahn, C. M., 450, *465*
Kahn, E. B., 240, 241, 242, *248*
Kahn, K. L., 434, *443*
Kaizer, L., *358*
Kakai, H., 488, *493*
Kakaz, A., 449, *464*
Kal, H. B., 439, *448*
Kalbeek, W. D., *202*
Kaldor, J., *232*
Kaleita, T. A., *463*
Kalkbrenner, K. J., *315*
Kalman, D., *184*
Kalsbeek, W., *100*
Kaminsky, B., *513*
Kampert, J. B., *39*
Kamps, W., 453, *460*
Kane, I. L., *218*
Kaneda, M., 350, *358*
Kangas, M., 416, 420, *427*
Kaplan, C. P., *274*
Kaplan, G. A., 270, 275, *512*
Kaplan, R. M., 80, *125*, 234, 268, *274*, *275*
Kaplan, S., *463*
Kaplan, S. H., 334, *345*
Kaplan De-Nour, A., 469, 473, *480*
Kaprio, J., 503, 504, *514*
Karanja, N., 68, *81*
Karatoprakli, P., *317*
Karnofsky, D. A., 121, *126*
Karon, J., *555*
Kase, R. G., *314*
Kashiwagi, T., 395, *406*
Kashy, D. A., 475, *482*
Kasl, S., *403*, *405*
Kassel, J. A., 178, *187*
Kassel, J. D., *82*
Kasten, L. E., 75, *79*
Katapodi, M. C., 136, 137, *145*
Kataria, R., *404*
Katsumata, N., 350, *358*

Kattlove, H., 414, 415, *427*
Katz, M. L., 104, *112*
Katz, R. C., 213, *220*
Katz, S., *405*
Katz, S. J., *101*, 553, *556*
Kauff, N., *319*
Kauffman, S. M., 471, *480*
Kaufman, M. E., *358*
Kaufmann, P. G., 80, *274*
Kaufmann, P. M., *460*
Kaufmann, V., *185*
Kavanah, M., *112*, *126*
Kawachi, I., 35, *35*, 39, 386, *515*
Kayser, K., 364, *374*
Kazak, A., 450, 451, 453, 454, 455, 456, 457, *458*, *459*, *461*, *463*, *464*, *465*
Kazura, A., *182*
Kealey, K. A., 154, *164*
Keator, D. B., 536, *544*
Keefe, F. J., 368, *373*
Keeling, F., *145*
Kelder, S., *206*
Kellam, S. G., 92, *100*
Keller, P., 134, *145*
Kellermeyer, R. W., 437, *443*
Kelley, K., 138, *145*, 545
Kellokumpu-Lehtien, P. L., *493*
Kellum, L., *218*
Kelly, A., *446*
Kelly, B., *319*
Kelner, M., 332, 337, *346*, 346
Kelsey, K., 20, 98, 202, *207*
Kelsey, K. S., 194, *205*
Kelso, P. D., 139, *144*
Kemmler, G., 120, *126*, 427
Kenady, D. E., *373*
Kendler, K. S., 501, *513*
Kenford, S. L., *188*
Kennedy, C., 241, *249*
Kennedy, S., 503, *516*
Kennedy, S. J., *515*
Kenney, L. B., 385, *387*
Kenny, D. A., 77, *80*
Kenny, D. T., 334, *344*
Kercher, K., 393, *404*
Kernahan, J., 450, *463*

Kerner, J., 17, *21*, 226, *233*, *528*
Kershaw, T., 396, 476, 482, 483, *484*
Kershaw, T. S., 469, *483*
Kessel, F., 532, 538, *545*
Kessler, R. C., *513*
Keul, J., 351–352, *355*
Kewenter, J., 290, *298*
Keyserling, T. C., *205*
Khan, L. K., 197, *207*
Khroyan, T. V., *545*
Kicks, K., *162*
Kidd, J., 286, *299*
Kidman, A. D., 504, *512*
Kiecolt-Glaser, J. K., 372, *374*, 393, *405*,
    500, 502, 503, 505, 509, *510*,
    512, *513*, *516*
Kieffer, S. A., *315*
Kierman, G. L., *482*
Killen, J. D., 179, *188*
Killingsworth, R., 245, *248*, 531, *544*
Kim, Y., 351, *356*, 475, 479, *482*
Kimerling, R., 369, *372*
King, A. C., 62, *83*, 179, *188*, 242, 245,
    246, *248*, 531, 537, 542, *544*
King, D. K., *356*
King, T. K., 169, 179, *180*, *185*
King, T. S., *162*
Kinne, S., 45, 46
Kinney, A. Y., 312, *314*
Kinney, J. P., *219*
Kippes, M. E., 351, *359*
Kirk, J., *318*
Kirk, K. A., *101*, 206
Kirk, S. B., *376*
Kirkley, B. G., *205*
Kirkpatrick, J., *388*
Kirkwood, J., *513*
Kirsch, I., 347, 352, *356*
Kirshner, J. J., *359*
Kirtland, K. A., 245, *248*
Kish, L., *100*
Kissane, D., *375*, 475, *482*
Kitchener, H., 286, 296, *298*
Kitchens, K., *182*
Kiviniemi, M. T., 139, *147*
Klabunde, C., 274, *277*

Klabunde, C. N., 256, 257, *274*, *275*
Klapow, J. C., 368, *375*, 425, *429*
Klar, N., 85, 88, 90, 91, 97, 98, *100*, *101*
Klastersky, J., 348, *356*
Kleijnen, J., 352, *355*
Klein, E., 471, *484*
Klein, E. A., 110, *112*, 388, *447*, *485*
Klein, J. E., 339, *344*
Klein, W. M., 138, *148*
Klein, W. M. P., 134, 139, *144*, *145*,
    146, *147*
Kleinbaum, D. G., 76, 77, *81*
Kleinman, S. N., 450, *461*
Klemm, P., 551, *557*
Klerman, G. L., 468, *482*
Klesges, L. M., 17, *20*, 525, *528*
Klijn, J. G. M., *317*
Klip, E., 453, *460*
Klosky, J., *465*
Knatterud, G. L., 80, *274*
Knaus, W., *516*
Kneier, A. W., 415, *427*
Knight, R., 393, *405*
Knight, S. J., *128*
Knobf, M. K. 417, *427*
Knowles, G., 340, *345*
Kobrin, S., 289, *301*
Kobus, K., *545*
Koch, G. G., *162*
Kocha, W. I., *188*
Kodl, M., 156, *164*
Koehly, L., 488, *493*
Koenig, B. A., 335, *344*
Koepke, D., *163*
Koeppen, S., *448*
Koepsell, T. D., 88, 89, *100*
Koh, H., 211, *221*
Koh, H. K., *184*
Kohn, L. S., 134, *145*
Kollias, J., *428*
Kolonel, L. N., 30, *38*
Kondryn, H., 451, *462*
Konkel, J. M., *558*
Koo, J., *444*
Koontz, K., 452, *462*
Koopman, C., *516*

Koopmans, J., *374, 512*
Koops, H. S., *345*
Koplan, J. P., *527*
Kopp, M., *126, 427*
Koppie, T. M., *387*
Kornblith, A. B., 118, *127,* 362–363,
  363, 364, 365, *374,* 414, 415,
  416, 417, 418, 419, *425, 427,*
  428, 460, 481, 516
Korzun, A., *516*
Kosinski, M., *128*
Koskenvuo, M., 503, 504, *514*
Kosslyn, S. M., *510, 513*
Kossoff, M. B., *515*
Kottaridis, P. D., 384, *386*
Kottke, T. E., 46, *54*
Koutsky, L. A., 33, *38*
Kozachik, S., 336, *343, 355,* 392, 393,
  395, 396, 398, 399, *403, 404, 405*
Krabbendam, P. J., *345*
Kraemer, H. C., 504, *516*
Kraemer, J., *425*
Kraft, K., 533, 543, *545*
Krag, D. N., *373*
Krailo, M., 506, *515*
Kramer, B. J., 401, *405*
Kramer, J. H., 450, 460, *462, 464*
Kramish Campbell, M., 92, *100*
Krane, E. J., 434, *444*
Krasnov, C. L., *112*
Kreft, I., 90, 97, *100*
Kreiner, S., 282, *297*
Kreps, G. L., 549, 552, 557, *557*
Kresge, C. L., *389*
Kressel, S., *126*
Kretzman, J., 46, *53*
Kreuger, R. A., 68, *82*
Kreuter, M., 16, *21,* 550, *556*
Kreuter, M. W., 192, 204, 271, 275,
  311, *317,* 537, 543, *554, 557, 558*
Kricker, A., 33, *37,* 215, *220, 510*
Krishnan-Sarin, S., *164*
Kristal, A. R., 63, *82,* 102, *206*
Kristeller, J., 179, *184*
Kristjanson, L. J., *342, 343*
Kritpracha, C., 476, *482*

Kroeze, W., 192, *205*
Kronnenwetter, C., *373*
Krozely, M. G., 349, *355*
Krueger, R. A., *299*
Krumm, S., 398, *405*
Krupnick, J. L., *377, 430*
Kryscio, R. J., *101*
Kucharski, S., *316*
Kuchler, T., 506, *513*
Kudelka, A. P., 332, *342, 345*
Kuebler, P. J., *358*
Kuehn, B. M., 289, *298*
Kuijer, R. G., 468, 477, *481, 482*
Kulik, J. A., 213, *221*
Kulkarni, R., 452, *462*
Kumanyika, S. K., 68, *81*
Kumpfer, K., 244, *249*
Kun, L., 463, *465*
Kun, L. E., *462*
Kupelian, P. A., *388,* 447, 471, *484, 485*
Kupper, L. L., 76, *81*
Kupst, M. J., 453, 457, *462*
Kurker, S. F., 363, *376, 429*
Kurman, R. J., *233*
Kurtin, P. S., 121, *128*
Kurtz, J., 391, 393, 396, *405, 406*
Kurtz, M., 391, 393, 394, 395, 396, *405,*
  406
Kurtz, S. M., 337, *344*
Kushi, L. H., *493*
Kutz, L. A., *510*
Kuzel, T., *128*
Kwan, L., *377, 430*
Kwate, N. O., *320*
Kwong, C. A., *54*
Kylstra, W. A., *387*

Laara, E., 23, *39*
Labay, L., 454, *458*
Labopin, M., 439, *448*
Labrecque, M. S., 332, *342*
Lacey, L., 275, *278*
La Chance, P. A., 271, *277*
LaCroix, A. Z., *247*
Laden, F., *515*
Laforge, R. G., 70, *83*

Lally, R. M., *428*
Lambert, R., 453, *459*
Lamdan, R. M., *377*
Lammes, F. B., 328, *345*
Lampic, C., 281, 282, 284, *298*
Lampkin, B. C., 438, *443*
Lancaster, T., 179, *186*
Lancaster, W., *233*
Land, G. H., 520, *528*
Landi, N. A., *182*
Landier, W., 441, *444*
Landis, K. R., 505, *513*
Lang, H., 505, *512*
Langa, K., *405*
Langenberg, P., 194, *204*
Langer, T., 450, 451, *462*
Langmark, F., *164*
Langstrom, H., *494*
Languille, O., 440, *447*
Lansky, S. B., 122, *127*
Lanz, P. M., 161, *164*
Lanza, E., *113*, 191, *205*
Lapitsky, L., *182*
Larcombe, I. J., 451, *464*
Largent, J., *112*
Larkin, E. K, *315*
Larsen, I. K., 291, *298*
Larson, P., *234*
LaSalle, V. H., 307, *316*
Lashley, J., *98*
Lasser, K., 177, *185*
Last, B. F., 453, *460*
Laten, D., 473, *484*
Latimer, J. J., 503, *512*
Latini, D., 176, *181*
Latini, D. M., 384, *387*
Latreille, J., *358*
Laurant, M. G. H., 242, *250*
Lauzier, S., 422, *428*
la Vecchia, C., *234*
Lavigne, J., *462*
Lawrence, D., 17, *21*, 175, *185*
Lawrence, W. F., 422, *430*
Lawson, H. W., *233*
Layard, M. W., *448*
Lazarus, R., 392, *406*

Lazarus, R. S., 44, *53*, 230, *233*, 468, *482*
Lazovich, D., 216, *220*
Le, P., 549, *555*
Le, T., *300*
Leake, B., *127*, 479, *483*
Leakey, T. A., 271, *274*
Leary, M. R., 213, *220*
Lechner, L., 192, *206*
Ledochowski, M., *515*
Lee, C., 168, 213, 241, *247*
Lee, E. S., *275*
Lee, H., 25, *40*
Lee, I. M., *39*
Lee, J., 502, *513*, *514*
Lee, J. E., 25, *39*
Lee, K. A., 136, *145*
Lee, N. C., 10, *22*, 34, *40*, 256, *273*, *277*
Lee, R. E., 241, *248*, 312
Lee, S., 304, *317*
Lee, S. J., 17, *21*, 337, *344*, *514*
Lee, Y., 199, *203*
Leedham, B., 366, *375*, 387, 425, *481*
Lee-Jones, C., 363, *374*
Leenhouts, G. H., 382, *387*
Leet, T. L., 520, *528*
Legius, E., *314*
Legler, J., 260, 265n(d), 266, 269, *275*,
 382, *387*
Lehman, J. M., 376, *430*
Leibing, E., *513*
Leiblum, S., *388*
Leiblum, S. R., 383, *388*
Leigh, L., 452, *463*, *465*
Leiper, A. D., 434, 439, *445*
Leischow, S., *187*
Leitenberg, H., 368, *373*
Le Marchand, L., 306, *316*
Lemeshow, S., 76, *81*
Lemon, J., 504, *512*
Lemon, S., *316*
Lenert, L., 174, *185*
Lennon, P. A., *220*
Lensing, S., *465*
Lentz, G. M., *386*
Lentz, L., 339, *346*
Lenzi, R., 329, 332, *342*, *345*

Leonard, B., 239, *247*
Leonard, R. C., 340, *345*
Leonidas, J. C., 434, *447*
Lepore, S. J., 367, *375*, 475, *481*
Lerman, C., 80, 136, 139, 141, 142, *144*,
        145, *147*, *162*, 170, *185*, 229,
        230, *232*, *234*, 268, *275*, 286,
        298, 304, 305, 306, 307, 308,
        309, 310, 313, *314*, *316*, *318*,
        365, 368, *374*, 535, 536, *544*,
        545, *546*, 554, *557*
Lerman, Y., *217*
Leslie, E., *249*
Leszcz, M., *374*, *512*
Lethborg, C. E., 475, *482*
Letner, J. A., 336, *342*
Leveille, S. G., *247*
Levenkron, J. C., 304, *317*
Leventhal, E. A., 44, *53*, 138, *145*
Leventhal, H., 44, *53*, 138, 139, 141,
        144, *145*
Levin, B., *234*, 290, *298*
Levin, N., 306, *318*
Levine, A., *249*
Levine, A. M., 506, *515*
Levine, L. A., 437, *445*
Levine, M. N., 121, *127*
Levy, A. R., 505, *510*
Levy, M., 327, *344*
Levy, S. M., 502, *513*, *514*
Lew, R. A., 211, 213, 214, *219*, *220*, *221*
Lewis, B. A., 244, *248*
Lewis, E. M., 339, *345*
Lewis, F. M., *52*, *54*, 67, *81*, *112*, *221*,
        276, 469, 470, 471, 472, 473,
        474, 480, *480*, *482*, *483*, *485*, *528*
Lewis, J. A., 77, *81*
Lewis, K. E., 304, *319*
Lewis, R., *275*
Lewis, S., 339, *343*, *344*
Li, F. P., *448*
Li, L., 396, *406*
Li, S., *102*
Li, T., 38
Li, Y. F., 339, *342*
Liang, K. Y., 76, *81*

Liaw, K. L., 226, *233*
Lichstein, K. L., 51, *53*
Lichtenstein, E., 17, *21*, 65, 65n, 195,
        204, 271, *277*, 519, *528*
Lichtenstein, S., 135, *148*
Lichtin, A., 436, *447*
Lichtman, R. R., 469, 470, *483*
Lieberman, M. A., 418, *428*
Liesner, R. J., 439, *445*
Ligibel, J., 415, 416, 418, 419, 425, *428*
Lillberg, K., 503, 504, *514*
Lillie, S. E., 283, *296*
Limacher, M., *112*
Lin, L. S., *201*
Lin, T. H., *144*, *317*
Linch, D., 433, *448*
Linch, D. C., 384, *386*
Linder, J., *404*
Lindholm, E., 290, 291, *298*
Lindquist, C. H., 190, *201*
Linehan, J., *297*
Link, K., 433, *445*
Linn, B. S., 506, *514*
Linn, E., *125*
Linn, M. W., 506, *514*
Linnan, L. A., 45, *52*, 239, *247*
Lins, B., 80
Lins, N., *543*
Linton, L., 533, 543, *545*
Linville, L. H., *101*
Lipkus, I., 488, *493*, 550, *557*
Lipkus, I. M., 17, *21*, 134, 137, 139, 140,
        145, *146*, 169, 170, *185*, *234*,
        318, 492, *557*
Lippman, M., 502, *514*
Lippman, M. E., *429*
Lippman, S. M., *112*
Lips, C. J. M., 308
Lipscomb, J., 116, *126*, *127*, 421, *428*
Lipsey, M. W., 63, *81*
Lipshultz, L. I., 436, *447*, 475, *485*
Lipshultz, S. E., 433, *442*, *445*
Lipsitz, L. A., *249*
List, M. A., 122, *127*
Lister-Sharp, D., 294, *300*
Litrownik, A. J., 99

Littenberg, B., 283, *300*
Little, R. J. A., 75, 78, *81*
Littlejohns, P., *300*
Litwin, M. S., 121, *127*
Liu, Y., *445*
Lloyd, K., 294, *298*
Lloyd, S. R., *125*
Loader, S., 304, 306, *317*
Lobach, D., *492*
Lobb, E. A., 334, *344*
Lobb, R., *100*
Loberiza, F. R., 505, *514*
Lockett, J., *297*
Lockwood, G. A., *511*
Lockwood, K. A., 450, 451, *462*
Lodder, L. N., 308, *317*
Loescher, L. J., 210, *220*
Loewenstein, G. F., 135, 136, *146*
Loge, J. H., 331, 332, *344*
Lohman, T., *202*
Lohr, K. N., 255, 272, *274, 276, 528*
Lombard, D. N., *223*
Long, A., *145*
Long, K., *248*
Longshore, D. L., 153, *163*
Lopez, A., 23, *39*
Lopez, A. D., 23, *37, 40*
Lopez, A. M., 363, *376, 429*
Lopez, D. F., 139, *144*
Lopez, S. T., *494*
LoPiccolo, J., 383, 384, *387, 388*
Lorig, K., 240, *248*
Lorincz, A., 284, *296*
Lorincz, A. T., 226, *233*
Lorn, K., 190, *201*
Loughlin, S. E., *164*
Louie, D. H., 138, *144*
Lovallo, W. R., *513*
Lovato, C. Y., 99, 136, *144*, 214, *222, 258, 261, 276*
Lovato, L. C., 116, *127*
Love, S., *373, 505, 512*
Lovely, M., *407*
Lowe, J., 215, *223*
Lowe, J. B., 92, *100*, 211, *220*
Lowe, P., 455, *463*

Lower, T., 216, *220*
Lowery, J. C., 417, *429*
Lown, B., 331, *342*
Lu, M., *102*
Lubeck, D. P., *387*
Lucassen, A., *316*
Luck, A., 292, *298*
Ludman, E., 82, *277, 299*
Ludman, E. J., 173, *182*
Ludwig, A., *144*
Lue, T. F., *387*
Luebbert, K., 349, 350, 356, 368, *375*
Luecken, L., 365, 367, *373*
Luecken, L. J., 372, *375*
Luepker, R. V., 206, 238, *248*
Lui, K. J., *219*
Luke, D. A., 537, *543*
Lund, E., 282, *297*
Luo, Z., 422, *426*
Lurie, N., 228, *233*
Lusk, E., 99, 395, 405, 478, *482*
Lustbader, E., *145*
Lustig, A. P., 478, *483*
Lutgendorf, S. K., 503, *510, 514*
Luus, C. A. E., *146*
Luxford, K., *22*
Lyberg, L., *275*
Lyles, J. N., *349*
Lyna, P., *318*
Lyna, P. R., 17, *21*, 137, *145*, 169, *185, 234, 550, 557*
Lynch, E., *249*
Lynch, H., *316*
Lynch, H. T., 304, 308, *317, 318, 319, 320*
Lynch, J., *316, 317*
Lynch, J. F., *317*
Lynch, J. W., 270, *275*
Lynch, T. J. J., 337, *345*
Lyss, A. P., *427*
Lytle, L. A., 195, *204, 206*

Mabry, M., *188*
MacCallum, R., *510*
MacGregor, D. G., 135, *147*
Machin, D., 77, *81*

Macia, F., *101*
Mackay, J., *315*
Mackey, J. R., 490, *493*
Mackie, E., 451, *462*
MacKie, R., 212, 215, *219, 221*
MacKinnon, D. P., *164*
MacKinnon, J. G., 92, *100*
Maclean, M., 334, *342*
MacLean, W. E., *463*
MacLehos, R., 82, *277*
MacLeod, C. M., *126*
Macleod, R., 304, *315*
Madan-Swain, A., 453, 454, *459, 462*
Madden, T. J., 44, *52*
Madden, K. S., 501, *514*
Maddern, G., 292, *298*
Maddock, J., 99, *219*
Maddock, J. E., 213, 214, 215, *220, 222*
Madigan, S. D., *101*
Madill, C., *98*
Madill, D. L., *162*
Maggiolini, A., 451, *462*
Magill-Evans, J., 538, 539, 540, *544*
Maglione, M. A., *277*
Magnan, R. E., 283, *297*
Maguire, A., 439, *445*
Maguire, P., 329, 339, *344,* 362, 368,
    369, 370, *376,* 418, 419, *429*
Maher, E. R., 304, *315*
Mahler, H. I., 213, 215, *221*
Mahoney, D., *407*
Mai, V., *297*
Maia, J. A., 246, *248*
Maier, S. F., 500, 501, *514*
Main, C. J., 351, *356*
Main, D., 80, *314, 316, 317, 319*
Main, D. S., 422, 423, *428, 430*
Maislin, G., *482*
Majpruz, V., *297*
Malarkey, W. B., *405*
Malick, J., *315*
Malone, M. E., *101*
Malouf, J., 139, *146*
Maloy, J., 212, *221*
Maloy, J. A., 216, *218, 223*
Maly, R. C., 479, *483*

Malycha, P., *428*
Mancini, J., 312, *318*
Mandel, F., *463*
Mandel, J. S., *35*
Mandelblatt, J., 226, 228, *233, 235,* 258,
    278
Mandelblatt, J. S., 258, 261, 263,
    265n(i), 266, 267, *269, 275, 278*
Manetta, A., *112,* 231, *232*
Manfredi, C., 92, *100*
Mangan, C. E., *233*
Mangan, P., 228, *235,* 258, 261,
    265n(i), *278*
Manley, M. W., 172, *183*
Mann, E., *296*
Mann, S. L., 154, *164*
Manne, S., 257, *275,* 364, 367, *375,*
    396, 406, 453, *462,* 477, 478, *483*
Manne, S. L., 45, *53,* 280, *299,* 421,
    428, 476, *483*
Manning, T., *555*
Manos, M. M., *232*
Manske, S. R., 98, *162*
Manson, J. E., 27, *38, 39*
Mansson-Brahme, E., 210, *217*
Mant, D., 291, *298*
Mantell, J., *468, 481*
Mantelli, D., 139, *146*
Marani, S. K., *319*
Marceau, L., 243, *249*
Marco, C. A., *82*
Marcolet, A., 440, *447*
Marcom, P. K., *22,* 320
Marcoux, M., 238, *248*
Marcus, A., *232*
Marcus, A. C., 17, *21,* 179, *183,* 195,
    204, 228, 233, *269, 274,* 519, *528*
Marcus, B., 239, *247*
Marcus, B. H., 179, *185,* 239, 244, *248,*
    490, *494,* 537, *544, 545*
Marcus, F. M., *22*
Marcus, J., 349, *355*
Marek, P. M., 154, *164*
Margitic, S. E., 104, *112*
Margolis, K. L., 228, *233*
Margreiter, R., *126*

Marina, N., 434, 436, 437, *445, 447*
Marion, M. S., *388*
Mark, M. M., 368, 369, *375*, 418, *428*
Markman, M., *235*
Markowitz, A., *275*
Markowitz, L. E., 226, *233*
Marks, J., 80, *543*
Marks, L. B., *358*
Marks, R., 215, *222*
Marlatt, G. A., 64, *81, 181*
Marlow, L. A. V., 289, *301*
Marquart, L., 31, *38*
Marrett, L. B., 27, *39*
Marschke, P., 381, *389*
Marsh, T., *201*
Marshall, D. G., *165*
Marshall, G. D., Jr., 503, *511*
Marshall, J. R., *37, 113*
Marshall, P. A., 335, *344*
Marshall, S., *248*
Marsiglia, H. R., 350–351, *356*
Marteau, T. M., 226, *232*, 286, 288,
    299, 313, *318, 319*
Marti, B., 239, *250*
Marti, J., 258, 260, *273*
Martin, B. W., 239, *250*
Martin, D. C., *100*
Martin, D. K., 332, *346*
Martin, J. B., 351, *354*
Martin, R., 141, 142, *148*
Martin, R. C., *218*
Martinez-Cross, J., *300*
Martinez-Ramos, G., 475, *480*
Martin-Hirsch, P., 17, *20*, 258, 259, *274*
Martinson, L. M., 451, *462*
Martire, L., 393, 408, *483*
Martire, L. M., 478, *483*
Martus, P., *462*
Marucha, P. T., *405*
Maruyama, N., 488, 489, *494*
Maruyama, N. C., 237, *249*, 421, *429*
Marzo, M., 258, 260, *273*
Marzullo, D. M., 139, *145*
Mash, D. C., 536, *545*
Maskarinec, G., 488, *493*
Masny, A., 229, *234*

Masouredis, C. M., *102*
Massad, L. S., 285, *301*
Masse, B., 467, *481*
Masse, L. C., *203*
Massie, M. J., 414, 417, *428, 429*
Mathwig, J. L., 134, *146*
Matteson, S., 354, *356*
Matthay, K., *460*
Matthay, K. K., 450, *464*
Matthews, B. A., 469, *483*
Matthews, E., *144*, 160, *162*
Matthews, J., *375*
Mattick, R. P., 137, *143*
Mattox, S., *21*
Matulonis, U., *493*
Mauch, P., *493*
Mauger, D. T., *316*
Maunsell, E., 422, *428*, 467, *481*, 488,
    489, 490, 505, *514*
Maurer, H. M., *444*
Maurer, L. H., 110, *112*
Mavros, P., *356*
Maxwell, M., 368, *373*
Mayer, J. A., 92, *100*, 214, 215, 216,
    218, 219, 221, 222
Mayer, R. N., 306, *320*
Mayhew, K. P., 152, *164*
Mays, J., 92, *97*
Mazonson, P., 240, *248*
Mbogori, J., 536, *544*
McAdams, M., *234*
McAfee, T., 553, *557*
McAlister, A. L., 522, *528*
McAlpine, L., *181*
McAvay, G., *250*
McBride, C., 66, 80, 137, *144*, 488, *493*
McBride, C. M., 63, *82*, 137, *146*, 287,
    299, 310, *318*
McBride, J., 287, 289, *301*
McCabe, M. A., *444, 460*
McCaffery, J. M., *545*
McCaffery, K., 278, 290, *299*
McCaffery, K. J., 288, *299*
McCaffrey, D. F., 153, *163*
McCallion, P., 399, *403*, 408, 476, *480*,
    485

McCallum, R. C., *405*

McCarthy, D. E., 175, *183*

McCarthy, E. P., *38*

McCarty, F., *101*, *206*

McCaul, K. D., 134, 135, 136, 137, 138, 139, *143*, *144*, *146*, 283, *297*, 548, *558*

McChargue, D. E., 177, *185*, *187*

McClelland, J. W., 98, *100*

McClement, S., *342*

McClure, J., 553, *557*

McClure, J. B., 137, *146*, 173, 174, *182*, *558*

McClure, K., *461*

McCorkle, R., *355*, 395, 397, 398, *405*, *407*, 471, 478, *482*, *483*, 506, *514*

McCormack, L. A., 226, *233*

McCormick, D., *185*

McCormick, K. M., *529*

McCormick, L., 270, *277*, 523, *529*

McCoy, S. B., 135, *146*

McCready, D., *444*

McCubbin, H. I., 468, *483*

McCubbin, M. A., 468, *483*

McCulloch, C. E., 90, 97, *100*, *274*

McCullough, M. L., 36, *39*

McDaniel, J. S., 363, *375*

McDonald, P. G., *510*

McEwen, B. S., 501, *514*

McEwen, J., 118, *126*

McFarlane, V. J., 440, *445*

McFarlin, S., *373*

McFeeley, S., *513*

McGarrigle, H. H., 384, *386*

McGinnis, J. M., 151, *164*

McGinnis, K. A., *248*

McGinnis, W. L., *182*

McGivern, B., 306, *318*

McGovern, P., *101*

McGovern, P. G., 228, *233*

McGovern, P. M., 290, *299*

McGrath, P. C., *373*

McGrath, P. J., 353, *355*

McGuire, L., 500, *513*

McGuire, P., *297*

McGuire, W., 46, *53*

McHugh, P., 339, 339–340, *344*

McIlvain, H. E., 176, *181*

McIntosh, S., 173, *186*, 548, *557*

McIntyre, L., *346*

McKay, H. G., 548, *556*

McKee, M., *273*

McKenzie, T. L., *248*, *250*

McKinlay, J., 243, *249*

McKinlay, S. M., 89, 99, *248*

McKinney, M., 210, *220*

McKnight, J., 46, *53*

McLachlan, S.-A., 370, *375*

McLean, N., 194, *205*

McLeroy, K. R., 45, *53*, 270, *277*

McLerran, D., 92, 97, 98, 99, 196, *201*

McLerran, D. F., *206*

McMillan, C., 349, *355*

McMillan, S., 395, 396, *406*, *408*

McMillan, S. C., 476, *483*

McMurray, R. G., 238, *249*

McNally, R., 451, *462*

Mcneel, T., 488, *492*

McNeilly, M., *346*

McPherson, K., *273*

McQueen, A., 270, *275*

McSherry, M., *461*

McSweeney, J. C., *557*

McTavish, F., 550, *558*

McTavish, F. M., 548, *556*, *557*

McTiernan, A., 179, 417, *426*

Meade, B., 198, *205*

Meadows, A., 449, 460, *461*

Meadows, A. T., 433, 435, 437, *444*, *445*, *465*

Meares, C. J., *357*

Medeiros Nancarrow, C., *493*

Meekin, S. A., 339, *344*

Meeske, K., 460, *461*

Mehta, S. S., *387*

Meier, W., *462*

Meijer, C. J., 234, 284, *296*

Meijers-Heijboer, E. J., 308, 309, *317*, *318*

Meinert, C. L., 75, *82*

Meischke, H., *144*

Meiser, B., 307, 309, 315, *318*, *344*

Meisler, E., *388*

Meissner, H., 257, *274, 277*

Meissner, H. I., 6, 17, *21, 22,* 175, *185,* 256, 268, 270, 272, 273, *275, 276,* 289, *301*

Meister, L. A., 433, 437, *445*

Melanson, E. L., 27, *38*

Mellemkjaer, L., *463,* 504

Mellon, S., *318,* 391, *406, 407,* 469, 470, 472, *483, 484*

Melton, R. J., *527*

Melvin, C., 179

Mendelsohn, A. B., *407*

Mendenhall, J., *556*

Meneghini, E., *387*

Menke-Pluymers, M., *318*

Merajver, S. D., 304, 305, 312, *321*

Mercado, A. B., *405*

Merikangas, K. R., 536, *543*

Mermelstein, R., 80, 151, 152, 156, 160, *163, 164, 165, 186*

Meropol, N. J., *275*

Merritt, R. K., 152, *164*

Mertens, A., *447, 459,* 465

Mertens, A. C., *387,* 437, *445, 447, 460*

Messeri, P., *163*

Messier, S. P., *247*

Meston, C., *388*

Metcalfe, K., *317*

Metcalfe, K. A., 310, *318*

Metz, J. M., 548, *557, 558*

Mewborn, C. R., 44, *54*

Meyer, D. M., 82, *277*

Meyer, T. J., 368, 369, *375, 418, 428*

Meyer, W., *442*

Meyerowitz, B. E., 362, 364, 366, *372, 374, 375, 376, 377, 387,* 417, *426, 429, 430,* 469, *481*

Meyers, B., *463*

Mhurchu, N. C., 199, *205*

Micco, E., 306, *314*

Michaud, D. S., *37*

Micheli, A., 385, *387*

Michell, M., *511*

Michielutte, R., *232*

Mielke, M., *183*

Mielke, M. M., *187*

Miglioretti, D. L., 300, *315*

Mignotte, H., *314*

Mihm, M. C., Jr., *222*

Miksys, S., 536, *545*

Miles, A., 283, 290, *299*

Miller, D. R., *184, 211, 221*

Miller, D. S., *40*

Miller, E., *516*

Miller, G., 348, *360*

Miller, G. A., 353, *357*

Miller, G. E., 478, *483*

Miller, H., *315*

Miller, J. P., *249*

Miller, K., *342*

Miller, M. E., 417, *429*

Miller, N. E., 351, *357*

Miller, S. A., 520, *528*

Miller, S. M., 6, 13, *21, 22,* 45, 53, *54,* 141, *145, 146, 147,* 192, *205,* 229, 230, 232, 233, *234, 277,* 280, 298, 305, 309, 311, *315, 316, 318, 319, 320,* 329, 335, *345,* 348, *357*

Miller, W. R., 64, *82,* 193, *206*

Milliron, K. J., 304, 305, 312, *321*

Mills, J. L., *460*

Mills, M., 229, *233*

Mills, M. E., 334, *345*

Mills, S., 552, *555*

Mills, S. L., 17, *21,* 175, *185*

Milne, E., 211, 212, *219, 219, 221*

Milsom, I., 286, *298*

Minkler, M., 46, *54,* 104, *112*

Mirick, D. K., 503, *511*

Mischel, W., 229, *233, 320*

Mishel, M. H., 330, 335, *345,* 352, *357,* 419, 420, *428,* 476, *484*

Mishra, A., *388*

Mitchell, D., *447*

Mitchell, J. B., 226, *233*

Mitchell, J. L., 329, 336, *345*

Mitchell, P. D., *206*

Mittleman, M. A., *386*

Mittlemark, M. B., *247*

Mo, M., 472, *480*
Moadel, A. B., *493*
Mock, P., *296*
Mock, V., 351, *357*, 398, *405*
Moell, C., *445*
Moen, I. E., *298*
Moeykens, B. A., 46, *55*
Moher, D., 80, 268, *276*, 509, *515*
Mohler, J., *357*, *484*
Moinpour, C. M., 110, *112*, 116, *127*
Mok, T. S., 348, *357*
Mokrohisky, S. T., *218*
Molassiotis, A., 348, 349, 353, *354*, *357*
Molenberghs, G., 79, *83*
Molleman, E., 328, *345*
Moloney, T. W., 46, *55*
Monaco, J. H., *40*
Mondloch, M. V., 352, *357*
Mondul, A. M., *39*
Monson, R. R., *39*
Montano, D. E., 63, 82, 257, *276*
Montgmery, D. H., *205*
Montgomery, G. H., 135, *146*, 348, 349, 352, 353, *357*
Montgomery, S., *315*
Monti, P. M., *182*, *184*
Montie, J. F., *484*
Montori, V., *183*
Mood, D., 391, 396, 406, 407, 468, 469, 473, 476, *476*, 481, 482, *484*
Moody, L., 396, 406, *483*
Moody-Thomas, S., *112*
Mook, D. G., 138n, *147*
Mooney, P. A., 502, *513*
Moore, B. D., 450, *459*
Moore, I., 450, *459*
Moore, I. M., *460*
Moore, L. J., 335, *344*
Mor, V., *408*
Morales, L. S., 123, *126*
Moran, E., *128*
Moran-Klimi, K., *377*
Moravan, V., *297*
Moreland, J. R., 470, *485*
Morey, M., *492*
Morgan, D. L., 68, *82*

Morgan, G. D., 536, *545*
Morgan, T., *247*
Morgenstern, H., 76, *81*
Mori, M., *442*
Morita, T., 395, *406*
Moritz, D. A., 417, *427*
Morra, M., *204*
Morrill, C., 98, *202*
Morris, S. M., *222*
Morrison, G., 549, *558*
Morrison, M. F., *512*
Morrissey, S., 226, *231*
Morrow, G. R., 347, 348, 349, 350, 351, 353, 354, 356, *357*, 358, 359, *511*
Morrow, M., *429*
Morse, R. M., 185, *484*
Morse, S. R., 467, 472, *484*
Morselli, A. M., 351, *354*
Mortensen, P. B., *463*, 504, *511*
Morton, D. L., *512*
Morton, S. C., *277*
Moschen, R., *427*
Mosher, R. B., 434, *444*
Moskowitz, J. M., 92, *99*
Moss, S., *297*
Mott, J. A., 152, *164*
Mott, L. A., *165*
Mouchawar, J., 80, *543*
Moudon, A. V., 543, *545*
Mowad, L., 295, *301*, 552, *558*
Moyer, A., 375, 417, *428*
Moyer, C. A., 553, *556*
Moyer-Mileur, L., *250*
Moynihan, C., *316*
Moynihan, J. A., 500, 501, *515*
Mueller, N. H., *220*
Muggia, F. M., *448*
Mulder, M., 406, *484*
Muldoon, L. L., *442*
Mulhern, R., 450, 455, 458, 459, 463, *464*
Mulhern, R. K. 450, 451, 459, 461, *462*
Mullen, J. C., 417, *427*
Mullen, M., 45, *54*
Mullen, P., *273*
Mullens, A. B., 135, 136, *146*

Muller, M. J., 116, *125*
Mulrow, C. D., *249, 528*
Munafo, M. R., 179, *186, 296*
Muneoka, L., 213, *219*
Munoz, N., 284, *296*
Munoz, R. F., 169, 174, 177, *184, 185*
Muññoz, N., *232*
Murakami-Akatsuka, L., 214, *220*
Muraoka, M., 479, *481*
Murata, P. J., 141, *145*
Murdoch, B. E., 450, *459, 461*
Murman, D., *407, 408*
Murphy, B., 398, *408*
Murphy, D., *249*
Murphy, M. F., 179, *186*
Murphy, M. L., 433, *447*
Murphy, S., 488, *493*
Murphy, S. A., 552, *556*
Murr, C., 502, *515*
Murray, C., 23, *39*
Murray, C. J., 23, *37*
Murray, D. M., 85, 88, 89, 90, 91, 92, 94n, 95n, 96, 97, *99, 100, 101, 102, 155, 163, 165*
Murray, N., *188*
Murray, T., *233, 444*
Murtaugh, M., 488, *494*
Musa, D., 110, *111*
Musselman, D. L., 363, *375*
Must, A., *204*
Mustian, K. M., 350, 351, *356, 358*
Mutrie, N., *492*
Myers, A., *298*
Myers, L. B., 418, *427*
Myers, M. G., 177, *188*
Myers, R., *102*
Myers, R. E., 269, 273, 275, 287, *296*

Nader, P. R., 195, 206, *248*
Nadler, R., *128*
Nagarajan, R., 434, *445*
Nair, V., 552, *556*
Nair, V. N., *558*
Naleid, K. S., 537, *543*
Nanda, K., 255, *274*
Nanny, M. S., *204*

Nano, M. T., 417, *428*
Napolitano, M. A., 243, *249*
Napuli, I., 228, *234*
Narod, S., *232*, 316, 317, *318, 319*
Nash, J., 307, *315*
Natarajan, L., *494*
Nathoo, V., 285, *299*
National Cancer Act of 1971, 531, *545*
National Cancer Institute (NCI), 6, 7, 17, *21*, 46, *54*, 152, 160, *164*, 196, 226, *233*, 397, 406, 431, *445, 524, 529*
National Center for Health Statistics, 28, 32, *36, 39*
National Institutes of Health, 123, *127*
National Institutes of Health Consensus Development Panel, 226, *233*
National Institutes of Health Consensus Development Panel on Physical Activity and Cardiovascular Health, 237–238, *249*
Natta, M., *462*
Naud, P., *299*
Navarro, A. M., 228, *234*
Neale, J., *297*
Neale, J. M., *82*
Neale, M. C., *513*
Neel, M. L., 416, *428*
Neese, L., 384, 386, 388, *447*, 471, 479, *484, 485*
Neet, M. J., *248*
Neglia, J. P., 387, 434, 439, 442, *445, 461*
Negotia, U. N., 550, *557*
Negri, E., *234*
Neighbors, C., *545*
Neijt, J. P., 120, *125*
Nelson, L., *298*
Nemeroff, C. B., 363, *375*
Nesbit, M. E., *447*
Ness, P, *446*
Nestle, M., 197, *206*
Nettekoven, L., *55*
Neuberg, D., *493*
Neuhausen, S. L., *319, 319*
Neuhauser, L., 549, *557*

Neuhouser, M. L., *493*
Neumark, D., 422, *426*
Neumark-Sztainer, D., 199, *203*
Neuwelt, E. A., *442*
Neville, G., 199, *202*
Newby, W. L., 452, *462*
Newcomb, P. A., *183*, 503, *515*
Newell, J., 212, *219*
Newell, S. A., 418, 419, *428*
Newhouse, J. P., *163*
Newlands, E., *344*
Newport, D. J., 363, *375*
Newton, P., 349, *355*
Newton, R. U., 237, *247*
Nezu, A. M., 468, *484*
Nezu, C. M., 468, *484*
Ngo-Metzger, Q., 38
Nguyen, A.-M. T., *464*
Niaura, R., 169, 177, 178, *181*, 185, *186*
Niaura, R. S., *527*
Nichaman, M. Z., *205*
Nicholas, D. R., 415, *428*
Nicholson, H. S., *444*, *447*, *460*
Nicklas, T., 195, *206*
Nicklas, T. A., 195, *205*, *206*
Nicolson, H. S., 436, *446*
Nides, M. A., *187*
Niederdeppe, J., 158, 159, *163*, *164*
Nielsen, I., 488, *493*
Nielsen, I. R., 99
Nielsen, L. F., 504, *515*
Nieschlag, E., *442*
Nijboer, C., 394, 395, 396, *406*, 471, *475*, *484*
Nikander, R., 490, *493*
Niknian, M., 89, 99
Nilson, E. G., 339, *343*
Nisenbaum, R., 488, *493*
Nishimoto, R., 468, *481*
Nissen, M. J., 417, *428*
Nissman, D., 272, *274*
Nixon, D. W., *492*
Noar, S. M., 257, 276, 550, *557*
Noel, M., *343*
Nogues, C., *318*
Noland, M. P., 92, *101*

Noll, R., 452, *463*
Noll, R. B., 452, 455, 460, *462*, *463*, *465*
Nolte, S., *298*
Norat, G., 189, *207*
Norcross, J., 193, *206*
Noriega, V., *373*, *480*
Norman, G. J., 211, 212, *221*
Norman, G. R., 76, *82*, 124, *127*
North, N., 340, *345*
Northouse, L., 391, 393, 395, 396, 398, 399, 400, *406*, *407*, 425, 476, *482*
Northouse, L. L., 468, 469, 472, 473, 474, 475, 476, 477, *481*, *483*, *484*
Northover, J., *298*
Northover, J. M. A., *296*
Novelli-Fischer, U., 351, *355*
Novick, L. F., *529*
Novotny, T. E., *183*
Nowels, C. T., 422, *428*
Nowlis, D., 476, *481*
Nuamah, I., 395, 397, 398, 405, *407*, 478, *482*, *483*
Nuamah, I. F., *514*
Nuamah, R., *403*
Numberger, J. I., Jr., *182*
Nunnally, J., 118, *127*
Nunnally, J. C., 72, *82*
Nunnerly, H., *511*
Nwachokor, A., 98
Nyhof-Young, J., 340, *344*

Oakland, D., *250*
Oates, V., 194, *208*
Oberst, M., 396, *407*, 468, *484*
Oberst, M. T., 468, 469, 472, 473, 475, *485*
Obeso, J. L., *235*
Ochshorn, P., *165*
Ockene, J. K., 99, 168, 171, 172, 173, *186*, *188*
O'Connor, A. M., 140, *147*
Odom, L., *465*
O'Donnell, S., 135, *146*
Oeffinger, K. C., 432, 433, 437, *446*
Oenema, A., 192, *202*, *206*
Offit, K., 305, *317*, 388

Offord, K. P., 185
Ogden, C. L., 28, 37, 39
Ogle, S. K., 435, 444
Oh, M. S., 183
Oh, S., 366, 375
Oh, S. S., 216, 221
O'Hara-Tompkins, N. M., 529
Ohira, T., 490, 493
Ohsuga, M., 350, 358
Ojala, K., 493
Okunieff, P., 356, 358
Old, L. J., 500, 511
Oldenburg, B., 240, 250, 296
Oldenburg, F., 359
O'Leary, A., 229, 233
O'Leary, M., 447
O'Leary, T., 452, 463
Oleske, D., 488, 494
Olevera, N. E., 249
Olevitch, L., 192, 205
Olivanen, T., 493
Olkin, I., 80
Olsen, J. H., 463, 504, 515
Olsen, M. K., 78, 82
Olshansky, S. J., 510, 515
Olson, A. L., 92, 98, 212, 219, 221
Olver, I., 349, 354
O'Malley, A., 258, 261, 265n(i), 278
O'Malley, P. M., 152, 164
Omenn, G. S., 31, 39
O'Neil, J., 343
O'Neill, C., 204
O'Neill, S., 241, 249
Ong, G., 282, 284, 296, 299
Ong, L. M. L., 328, 335, 337, 345
Oosterwijk, J. C., 320
Oppedisano, G., 373
Orecchia, R., 350–351, 351, 356
O'Riordan, D. L., 219
Orleans, C., 181
Orleans, C. T., 80, 169, 184, 186, 191,
    206, 274, 317, 527
Ornstein, S. M., 228, 234
O'Rourke, D., 278
Osborne, C. K., 429
Osganian, S. K., 204, 206

Osler, M., 92, 101
Osoba, D., 123, 127, 348, 358
Osowiecki, D. M., 373
Ossip-Klein, D. J., 173, 186, 548, 557
Osterloh, I. H., 388
Ostroff, J. S., 137, 146, 488, 492, 493
Osuch, J., 405
O'Sullivan, B., 125
O'Sullivan, I., 283, 299
Oswald, D. L., 192, 205
Otis-Green, S., 481
Ottensmeier, H., 462
Otter, R., 281, 300
Owen, J. E., 368, 369, 375, 425, 429
Owen, N., 9, 19, 22, 239, 248, 249, 257,
    276
Owens, B. H., 557
Oxman, A. D., 188
Oyama, H., 350, 358

Paavonen, J., 285, 299
Packer, R., 450, 463
Packer, R. J., 447
Packman, W. L., 454, 463
Padilla, G., 127, 425
Padma-Nathan, H., 383, 388
Paffenberg, R. S., Jr., 26, 39
Page, S., 400, 404
Page, S. A., 477, 480
Pagell, F., 169, 187
Pahor, M., 515
Pakula, I. S., 502, 513
Palamara, L., 349, 355
Palmer, P., 165
Palmer, S. C., 505, 511
Palmer, S. L., 450, 451, 462, 463
Pandya, K., 357
Papandonatos, G., 178, 181, 182
Pape, S. J., 476, 483
Papenfuss, M. R., 232
Parazzini, F., 234
Parcel, G. S., 195, 204, 206, 220, 248,
    523, 529
Park, E. R., 459
Park, T. L., 366, 376
Parker, B. R., 434, 446

Parker, M. A., 290, 291, *299*
Parker, P. A., 329, 331, 332, 334, 335,
  342, 345, 365, 366, *375, 494*
Parkin, D. M., *20*
Parle, M., 328, *343*
Parra-Medina, D., 99
Parrott, R., *221, 222,* 305, *316, 342*
Partridge, F., 393, *405*
Parzuchowski, J., *112*
Pasacreta, J., 397, 398, 401, *403, 407*
Pascale, R. W., 45, *54*
Pasick, R. J., 269, 271, *276*
Paskett, E. D., 104, 107, *112, 232,* 269,
  276, 282, 299
Pasnau, R. O., 368, *374*
Passin, H., 63, 80
Pate, R. R., 241, 244, *248, 249*
Patenaude, A. F., 306, *315, 319*
Pater, J., *358*
Patrick, D. L., 97, 122, *127*
Patrick, J. H., 110, *112*
Patrick, K., 551, *556*
Patten, C. A., *182*
Patterson, F., *185, 544*
Patterson, R. E., 196, 206, 488, *493*
Pattison, P., *373*
Paty, J. A., *82,* 174, 178, *187*
Paulussen, T., 45, *52*
Pavalko, E, 393, *407*
Pawletko, T. M., 452, *462*
Paxton, A., *202*
Payne, M. E., 98, *162*
Payne, T. J., 170, 175, *186, 187*
Payne-Wilks, K., *102*
Pbert, L., 171, 172, 173, *186, 188*
Pearce, R., 214, *222*
Pearlman, D. N., 257, *276*
Pearson, J., 211, *220*
Pearson, M. L., 434, *443*
Pearson, S., 292, *298*
Pechacek, T. F., *98*
Pedersen, K., *22*
Pedersen-Bjergaard, J., 439, *446*
Pee, D., *442*
Peele, P., 110, *111*
Peersman, G., 228, *234*

Pelcovitz, D., 453, *463*
Pelkman, C. L., 98, *162*
Pemberton, M., *162*
Pendergrass, T., 454, *459*
Penman, D., *511*
Penner, L. A., 104, *111*
Penninx, B. W., 501, 503, 504, *515*
Penson, D. F., *387, 388*
Penson, R. T., 337, *345*
Pentz, M. A., 156, *164*
Pentz, R. D., *319*
Perez, C. A., *235*
Perez, J. E., 174, *185*
Perez, M. A., 363, *376*
Perez, T., 469, *480*
Perez-Ayayde, A. R., *445*
Perez-Stable, E. J., *235*
Periasamy, S., *206*
Perkins, J., *99*
Perkins, K., *185*
Perkins, K. A., 179, *186*
Perla, J., *98*
Pernet, A., 285, *301*
Perrin, E. B., *100*
Perry, C. L., 195, 205, 206, *248*
Perry, M. C., 438, *446*
Perry, N., 283, *299*
Person, S., *101, 206*
Pertschuk, M., 46, *54*
Pescatello, L. S., 244, *249*
Peshkin, B. N., *232, 316, 319*
Peterman, A. H., 472, *480*
Peters, E., 135, *147*
Peters, L., 214, *222*
Peters, N., 306, *319*
Peters, T., 286, 288, *300*
Peters, T. J., 288, *300,* 313, *319*
Petersen, G. M., 309, *317*
Petersen, L., *376,* 385, *387,* 433, 436,
  443, 444, 481
Peterson, A., 92, *99*
Peterson, A. V., 154, *164*
Peterson, B., 488, *493*
Peterson, E., 176, *181*
Peterson, G. M., *315*
Peterson, K. E., 92, 97, *204, 207*

Peterson, S. K., 258, 276, 312, *316, 319*
Peterson, T. R., 239, *249*
Petitto, J. M., *512*
Peto, J., *232*
Peto, R., *40*
Petosa, R., 239, *248*
Petraitis, J., 153, *163*
Petris, M. G., *443*
Pett, M., 244, *249*
Petticrew, M., 294, *300*
Petty, R. E., 47, *54*
Peyser, C., 416, *430*
Pezzullo, S., *555*
Philippe, K., *314*
Philipsen, P. A., 214, *222*
Phillips, C., *511*
Phillips, C. W., *278*
Phillips, K., 394, *407, 538, 545, 546*
Phillips, K. A., *274*
Phillips, K. M., 172, 174, *186*
Phillips, P., *458*
Phillips, P. C, 451, *463*
Phillips, R. S., *38, 516*
Phipps, S., 450, 451, 452, *459, 463, 464*
Piantadosi, S., 508, *515*
Piasetsky, S., *511*
Picard, C. L., 337, *345*
Pichon, L. C., *221*
Piedmonte, M. R., 92, *99*
Pieper, C., *492*
Pierce, H. I., *358*
Pierce, J. P., 152, *164, 183, 184, 490, 491, 494, 536, 544*
Pierce, S., *405*
Pignone, M., 255, *276*
Pilvikki Absetz, S., 281, *296*
Pinckney, R. G., 283, *300*
Pingitore, R., 177, *187*
Pingree, S., 550, *556, 557, 558*
Pinover, W., 396, *406, 477, 483*
Pinquart, M., 393, 394, 395, 396, *407*
Pinto, A., *544*
Pinto, B. M., 179, *185, 203, 237, 243, 249, 420, 421, 429, 488, 489, 490, 492, 494, 537, 544, 545*
Piot, W., *444*

Pipan, C., *443*
Piper, M. E., 175, 178, 179, *186*
Pirie, P. L., *163*
Pistrang, N., 470, *485*
Pizarro, J., 295, *301, 552*
Pizzaro, J., *558*
Pladevall, M., 258, 260, *273*
Plane, M. B., 228, 235, 258, 259, *277*
Plummer, M., 226, *234*
Pocock, S. J., 75, *79*
Pohlamus, B., 98, *100*
Polinsky, M. L., *376, 481*
Pollack, H., *511*
Pollard, W. E., *126*
Ponder, B., 531, *543*
Pool, C., *145*
Poole, K., 244, *249*
Porta, M., *101*
Porter, M. *296*
Porter, M. R., 363, *375*
Porterfield, T., *315*
Posluszny, D. M., 63, *80*
Posner, T., 295, *300*
Poston, W. S. C., 241, *249*
Potischman, N., 227, *234*
Potkin, S. G., 536, *544*
Potosky, A. L., 116, *127, 381, 382, 387, 388*
Potter, D. E., *248*
Potter, J. D., 538, *545*
Poulter, L. W., *443*
Poussa, T., *494*
Powe, N. R., *181*
Powell, K. E., 248, *543, 545*
Powell-Griner, E., 25, 27, 35, *38*
Powers, D., 142, *144, 179, 181*
Powers, P., *218*
Powers, P. J., *218*
Poyner, E., *388*
Pozo, C., *373, 480*
Pratt, M., 239, 245, *250*
Preacher, K. J., *405*
Prescott, R., 90, 97, *98*
President's Cancer Panel, 423, *429*
Prevatt, F., 455, *463*
Prevost, A. T., 307, *314*

Pribram, K. H., 353, *357*
Price, A. A., 365, *376*, 415, *430*
Price, M. A., 504, *510*, *515*
Prigerson, H., 395, *403*
Primo, K., *373*
Prislin, M. D., 339, *345*
Pritchard, K. I., *444*
Probert, J. C., 434, *446*
Prochaska, J., *181*, 193, *206*
Prochaska, J. J., 177, *186*, *250*
Prochaska, J. O., 16, *22*, 44, *54*, 70, 83,
    140, *147*, 239, *249*, 490, *494*, *527*
Pronin, E., 215, *218*
Prout, M. N., *184*
Provantini, K., *462*
Province, M. A., 240, *249*
Pruchno, R. A., 110, *112*
Psaty, B. M., *100*
Pueleo, E., *148*
Pukrop, R., 362, 368, *376*, 418, *429*
Puleo, E., *459*
Purtzer, M. Z., 349, *355*
Puska, P., 46, *54*
Putnam, J., 198, *206*
Putt, M., 306, *314*

Quargnenti, A., *460*
Quick, B. L., 213, *221*
Quinlan, K., *146*
Quirt, G., *374*

Raasch, B., 215, *223*
Raatz, S. K., *54*
Rabin, B. S., 500, *511*
Rabin, C., 490, *494*
Rabow, M., 401, *407*
Raczynski, J. M., *101*, 206
Radcliffe, J., 451, 452, *463*
Radcliffe, N. M., 134, *147*
Radecki, S., 339, *345*
Radford, J. A., *387*
Raffle, A. E., 295, *300*
Ragab, A., 454, *462*
Rahbar, M., *405*
Rahbar, M. H., *355*
Rahim, A., *442*

Rai, S., *465*
Raimondi, S. C., 471, *480*
Rairikar, C., *314*
Raizman, P. S., *184*
Raju, K. S., 288, *300*, *301*
Rakow, E., 549, *558*
Rakowski, W., 256, 257, 271, *274*, *275*,
    276
Ramirez, A., *373*, 505, *512*
Ramirez, A. J., 281, *300*
Ramsey, L. T., *248*
Ramsey, P. G., *346*
Ramsey, S., 272, *273*
Ramsey, S. E., *181*
Rand, C. S., *181*
Randall, M. E., *235*
Raney, R. B., Jr., *444*
Rankin, N., *22*
Ransdell, L. B., 241, 242, *249*, *250*
Ransohoff, D., *146*
Rappat, S., *513*
Raptis, G., *481*
Rate, W. R., 434, *446*
Ratner, P. A., 136, *144*, 258, 261, *276*
Raudenbush, S. W., 90, *101*
Rauscher, G. H., 270, *276*
Ravdin, P., 334, *346*
Rawl, S., *405*
Ray, R. M., *101*
Raynov, J., 348, *358*
Reaman, G. H., 434, *444*, *447*
Reardon, J., 487, *492*
Rebbeck, T. R., 308, *319*
Recklitis, C., 452, *463*
Redd, W. H., 347, 349, 350, *355*, *358*,
    373, 416, *430*, 453, *462*
Redding, C. A., 215, *222*
Reddy, P., 473, *484*
Redman, C. W., *297*
Redman, S., 328, *343*
Redmon, C. K., *112*, *126*
Redmon, J. B., 45, *54*
Redmond, G. P., *389*
Reed, D. A., 363, *375*
Rees, C. E, 470, *485*
Reesor, K., 369, *374*

Reesor, P., *374*
Reesor, S. O., 368
Reeve, J., 305, *314*
Reeves, R. S., *249*
Regan, J., *430*
Regan, K., 307, *320*
Rehse, B., 362, 368, *376*, 418, *429*
Reid, R., *233*
Reid, S., 99
Reifman, A., 505, *515*
Reiker, P. P., 453, *464*
Reilley, B., *273*
Reilly, B. M., 257, *278*
Reilly, J. J., 432, *446*
Reintgen, D. S., 328, *345*
Reis, T. J., *146*
Reise, S. P., 123, *126*
Reiss, P., *182*, 488, *494*
Reither, E. N., 29, *39*
Rejeski, W. J., 242, *247, 248*
Remington, P. L., 171, *181*
Rennard, S. I., *187*
Renner, B., 135, 139, *145, 147*
Rennie, K. M., *442*
Reno, R. R., 138, *143*, 257, *273*
Resnick, P., 549, *557*
Resnicow, K., 92, *101*, 193, 194, 196, 197, *201, 202, 203, 206*
Restine, S., *544*
Reus, V. I., 169, 177, *184*
Reutter, L., 47, *54*
Revenson, T., *148*
Revere, D., 551, *557*
Rexrode, K. M., *38*
Reyno, L., *405*
Reynolds, K. D., 92, *101*, 194, 195, *206*, 210, 212, 213, 216, *218, 221, 223*, 257, *273*
Reynosa, J. T., 178, *182*
Rhodes, L., 25, 27, 35, *38*
Ribisl, K., 161, *165*
Riboli, E., 189, *207*
Rice, M., 453, *464*
Rich, M., 255, *276*
Richards, K. C., 550, *557*
Richards, M., 373, 505, *512*

Richards, M. A., *300*
Richardson, C., *462*
Richardson, J. L., 506, *515*
Richardson, P., 288, *301*
Richardson, P. H., 288, *300*
Richardson, W., 520, *529*
Rich-Edwards, J. W., *38, 39*
Richie, J. P., 437, *445*
Richmond-Avellaneda, C., *320*
Ricker, D., 381, *389*
Rickert, V. I., 548, *555*
Ridner, S. H., 440, *446*
Riedel, B. W., 51, *53*
Rieger Fischer, J. B., *463*
Rielinger, K., 171, *186*
Ries, L. A. G., *20, 37, 40, 546*
Rietbroek, R. C., *345*
Rieter-Purtill, J., 452, *463*
Riggs, R. S., *101*
Rigotti, N. A., 25, *39, 40*, 171, 179, 180, *186, 188*
Riley, A., *388*
Rimer, B., 5–6, 9, 17, 20, 21, 141, 142, *144, 145, 147*, 273, *275*
Rimer, B. K., 10, 16, 17, *21, 22, 34, 40*, *52, 54, 61, 67, 81, 112*, 134, 137, 140, *145, 147*, 169, *185*, 228, *234*, 256, 257, 269, 271, *274, 275, 276, 277*, 282, 299, 307, *309, 319, 320, 528, 550, 557*
Rimm, E. B., *37, 38, 386*
Ringdal, G. I., 421, *430*
Ripamonti, C., 363, *374*
Ripley, J. S., 196, *203*
Ripley, K., 99
Ris, D., 450, 451, *463*
Rittenberry, L., 97
Ritter, P. L., 179, *188*
Ritter-Sterr, C., 122, *127*
Ritt-Olson, A., *165*
Ritz, L. J., *428*
Rivers, J. K., 214, *222*
Rizzi, L., 451, *459*
Rizzo, J. D., *514*
Roalfe, A., *492*
Roberson, P. K., *557*

Robert, J., 488, *493*
Robert, S. A., 29, *39*
Roberts, C. S., 328, *345*
Roberts, F. D., 503, *515*
Roberts, M., *494*
Roberts, M. B., *544*
Roberts, M. M., 281, *297*
Roberts, N. E., 137, *148*
Robertson, C., *357*
Robertson, C., *484*
Robertson, W. W., Jr., 434, *446*
Robinson, D. S., *373, 480*
Robinson, J., 213, *222*
Robinson, J. D., 215, *222*
Robinson, K., 398, *403*
Robinson, M. H. E., 290, *299*
Robinson, S., 281, *297*
Robison, L., *461, 465*
Robison, L. L., 434, *445, 460, 465*
Robison, L. R., *442*
Robles, T. F., 500, *513*
Robson, M., *319*, 380, *388*
Roche, A. M., 172, *187*
Rock, B. H., *202*
Rock, C. L., 433, *446*
Rockhill, B., 35, *39*, 171, *183*
Rodani, M. G., 505, *512*
Rodehaver, C. B., 349, *359*
Rodgers, A., 23, *37*, 199, *205*
Rodgers, J., 450, *463*
Rodgers, R. W., 44, *145*
Rodin, G. M., 416, *427*
Rodrigue, J. R., 366, *376*, 456, *465*
Rodriguez, C., 28, 30, 36, *39*
Roe, D. J., *232*
Roetzer, L., *144*
Rogers, B. L., 199, *203*
Rogers, E. M., 46, *54*, 522, *529*
Rogers, J. D., 32, *38*
Rogers, L. Q., 179, *187*
Rogers, R. W., 44, *54*, 134, *145*
Roghmann, K., *464*
Rogstad, K. E., 285, 286, *300*
Rohay, J. M., 174, *187*
Rohsenow, D. J., *182, 184*
Roijackers, J., 17, *20*, 169, *183*

Roland, C. L., *102*
Roland, M., 77, *82*
Rollnick, S., 64, *82*, 193, *206*
Roman, D. D., 438, *446*
Romberger, D. J., 176, *187*
Romero, I., 450, *465*
Ronis, D. L., 134, *147, 183*, 475, *480*
Ronson, A., 365, *376*, 415, 416, 424,
    429
Roona, M. R., *165*
Rooney, B. L., 96, *101*, 155, *165*
Roppe, B., *234*
Rosberger, Z., 370, *373*, 476, *481*, 505,
    510
Roscoe, J., 354, *356*
Roscoe, J. A., 348, 349, 351, 353, 354,
    356, 358, 359
Rosdahl, I., 216, *217*
Rose, A., 306, *319*
Rose, M. S., 110, *112*
Rose, R., *513*
Rosen, R. C., 383, *388*
Rosen, S., 198, *205*
Rosenberg, H. M., 37, *40*
Rosenberg, S., *219, 427*
Rosenberg, S. A., 116, *128*
Rosenberg, W., 520, *529*
Rosenfield, P. L., 532, 538, 540, *545*
Rosenstock, I. M., 134, *148*, 522, *529*
Rosenthal, S., *357*
Rosner, B., 37, *38*
Rosner, B. A., 30, *37, 40*
Ross, A., 425, *429*
Ross, L., 368, 369, 370, *376*, 419, *429*,
    451, *463*, 503, *511*
Ross, S., 549, *558*
Rosseel, K., *218*
Rossetti, F., *443*
Rossi, J. S., 70, *83*, 215, *222*
Rosso, S., 215, *222*
Rossouw, J. E., 103, 110, *112, 113*
Ross-Petersen, L., *515*
Roter, D., *344*
Rotger, A., *235*
Roth, E. A., *277*
Roth, J., 80, 314, *319*

Roth, R. S., 417, *429*
Rothenberger, D., *234*
Rothman, A. J., 139, 143, *147*, 215, *218*
Rothman, J., 46, *54*
Rottenstreich, Y. S., 140, *147*
Rotter, J. B., 347, 352, 353, *359*
Rouffaer, L., *444*
Rounsaville, B. J., 468, *482*
Rourke, M., 449, 451, 453, 456, 460,
        461, 464
Roussi, P., 309, *318, 319*
Rowland, J., 475, *485, 487, 488, 491,
        492*
Rowland, J. H., 364, 366, *372, 374, 375,
        387, 413, 417, 418, 426, 427,
        429, 469, 473, 481, 488, 490, 492*
Rowland, L. C., 169, *183*
Rowley, P. T., 304, *317*
Rozencweig, M., *448*
Rubin, D. B., 75, 78, *81, 82*
Rubin, P., *358*
Rubinstein, W. S., *316*
Ruccione, K., *460*
Ruckdeschel, J. C., 104, *111*, 332, *342*
Rudd, R. E., 46, *55*
Rudnick, A., 336, 337, *345*
Rue, M., 310, *315*
Ruger, U., *513*
Rugo, H. S., 438, *446*
Rukstalis, M., *185, 544*
Rumelhart, D. E., 353, *359*
Rummans, T. A., 369, *373*
Runfola, P. S., 172, *183*
Runowicz, C. D., 288, *301*
Rush, R., 136, *145*
Russ, C. R., *223*
Russell, D., *144*
Russell, I., *144*
Russell, M. A., 169, *187*
Russell, R., *181*
Russell, W. D., 240, *250*
Russell-Jacobs, A., 422, *426*
Rust, P. F., 228, *234*
Rustgi, A. K., *316*
Rustin, G., *344*
Ryan, R. M., 193, 194, *203, 207*

Saal, H. M., *318*
Saario, R., *494*
Saarto, T., *493*
Saba, L. M., *218*
Sackett, D. L., 520, *529*
Sadetzki, S., *217*
Saelan, H., *515*
Saelens, B. E., 70, 80, 245, *250*, 537,
        545
Sage, P., 416, *426*
Sahler, O., *458*
Sahler, O. J., 454, *456, 464*
Sales, A. E., 339, *342*
Sales, S. D., *181*
Sallen, S. E., *445*
Sallis, J. F., 9, 19, *21, 22, 100*, 218, 219,
        221, 239, 245, *248, 250*, 257,
        268, 276, 533, 537, 543, 545,
        551, 556
Salmeróón, J., *299*
Salminen, E., 488, 489, *494*
Salminen, S., *494*
Salmon, P., 334, *346*
Salmon, R. J., 440, *447*
Salonen, J. T., 46, *54, 512*
Salovey, P., 215, *218*, 295, *301*, 552,
        558
Saltel, P., *314*
Salz, T., 283, *296*
Samsa, G., *318*
Samsa, G. P., *146*
Samuels, A., *233, 444*
Sanderman, R., 281, 300, 394, 395, *406*,
        468, 477, *481, 482, 484*
Sanders, K., *102*
Sanders, S. P., *445*
Sanderson, C., *273*
Sandgren, A. K., 548, *558*
Sandler, H. M., *484*
Sandler, R. S., 35, *494*
Sandman, P. M., 137, *148*
Sands, C., 142, *145, 147*, 309, *319*
Sanhueza, A., 20, 98, *202*
Sanjose, S., *232*
Sanson-Fisher, R., 99, 172, *187*, 211,
        214, 216, 219, 220, 222, 330,
        332, *343*, 418, *428*

Santi, S., *163*
Sarafian, B., *125*
Saraiya, M., 209, 214, *219, 220, 222, 233*
Sarason, I. G., 154, *164*
Sargent, J., *458, 464*
Sargent, J. D., 157, *165*
Sargent, M. G., 454, *464*
Sarna, L., 120, *127*
SAS Institute, 79, *82*
Sasieni, P., *188, 301*
Sasso, B., 80
Satagopan, J., *319*
Satariano, W. A., 422, *429*
Satcher, D., *527*
Sateren, W. B., 103, 110, *113*
Saterlund, M. J., 548, *558*
Sathya, J., *181*
Satia, J. A., 488, *494*
Sauar, J., 290, *298, 301*
Saul, J., 334
Saunders, R. P., *249*
Saunders-Martin, T., 98
Saurin, J., *314*
Savolainen, N. J., 418, *428*
Sawe, U., *187*
Sawyer, M. G., 452, 453, *464*
Saxton, J. M., *492*
Scaf-Klomp, W., 281, *300*
Scanlan, J., *393, 408*
Scarborough, R., *298*
Schaalma, H., 45, *52*
Schacherer, C., 488, *493*
Schaefer, M. L., 487, *492*
Schaeffer, E., *463*
Schafenacker, A., 396, 406, 407, 476, *482, 484*
Schafer, J. L., 78, *82*
Schaffner, L., 476, *481*
Schaffner, M. L., *481*
Schag, C. A., 120, *128*
Schag, C. A. C., *364, 376*
Schapira, L., *344*
Schapiro, I. R., 503, 504, *511, 515*
Schatz, J., 450, *464*
Schatzkin, A., 103, *113, 205*

Schechtman, K., *204*
Scheier, M., 348, *360*
Scheier, M. F., 353, *359, 373, 480*
Schellong, G., *442*
Schenk, M., 422, *426*
Schenker, N., 78, *82*
Scherbring, M., *407*
Schernhammer, E. S., 503, *515*
Scheuch, E. K., 269, *276*
Scheuer, L., 308, 309, *319*
Scheulen, M. E., *448*
Schiffman, M. H., 226, *233, 234, 389, 407, 408*
Schiffman, S., *383, 389*
Schildkraut, J. M., *22, 320*
Schilling, A., *182*
Schimpff. S. C., 348, *356*
Schinka, J. A., 80
Schinke, S. P., 153, *162*
Schipper, R., *408*
Schlegel, W., *442*
Schmale, A. M., *511*
Schmidt, J., *250*
Schmidt, J. E., 366, *367, 376*
Schmitt, A., 416, *429*
Schmitz, K. H., 490, *493*
Schneider, G. W., 437, *446*
Schneider, K. A., *315, 319*
Schneider, T. R., 295, *301, 552, 558*
Schnoll, R., *318*
Schnoll, R. A., 137, *147, 268, 277, 305, 315, 365, 366, 376*
Schoenbach, V. J., *555*
Schofield, M. J., 214, *222*
Schofield, P. E., 334, *345*
Scholefield, J. H., *299*
Scholes, D., *299*
Scholefield, J. H., 290, *299*
Schonwetter, R., *483*
Schornagel, J. H., 116, *125, 376*
Schover, L., *232, 471, 484, 485*
Schover, L. R., 380, 381, 382, 383, 384, *386, 388, 436, 442, 447, 471, 475, 485*
Schreiber, R. D., 500, *511*
Schroder, K. E. E., *383, 388*
Schroeder, D. M., 137, *146*

Schubert, C., *515*

Schulenberg, J. E., 152, *164*

Schulman, J., *462*

Schulman, K., *317*

Schultz, B., *250*

Schultz, L., 176, *181*

Schulz, R.,

Schultz, W. C., *387*

Schulz, K. F., 268, *276*, 509, *515*

Schulz, R., 348, *360*, 370, *374*, 396, *402,
    403, 407*, 478, 479, 482, 483, 485

Schumacher, K., 397, *407*

Schutte, N., 139, *146*

Schwartz, A. M., 434, *447*

Schwartz, C. L., 436, 437, *447*

Schwartz, G. E., 363, *376, 429*

Schwartz, J. E., *82*

Schwartz, L., 456, *464*

Schwartz, L. M., 134, 140, *149*, 281,
    293, 295, *300*

Schwartz, M., 142, *147*, 229, *234*, 316

Schwartz, M. D., *188*, 305, 307, 308,
    309, *317, 319*

Schwartz, S. M., *493*

Schwarz, N., *275*

Schwarz, R., 416, *429*

Schwebel, A. I., 470, *485*

Schweigkofler, H., *427*

Sciamanna, C., *182, 249*

Scott, D. W., 468, *485*

Scott, M. D., *217, 222*

Scribner, R. A., 45, *53*

Searle, S. R., 90, 97, *100*

Seay, J., 304, *317*

Seay, S., *182*

Secker-Walker, R. H., *22*, 163, *165*

Secreto, G., *387*

Sedjo, R. L., *232*

Seeman, T., 242, *250*

Seeman, T. E., 531, 538, 539, 540, 542,
    545

Sees, K. L., *184*

Seger, D., *82, 277*

Segerstrom, S. C., *510, 515*

Segura, J. M., 92, *101*

Seid, M., 121, *128*

Seidel, J., *318*

Seiler, R., 239, *250*

Sejr, H. S., 92, *101*

Selhub, J., *41*

Seligman, M. E., 347, *354*

Seltman, H., 365, *374*

Seltz, M., 352, *357*

Seltzer, M., 396, *406*

Senior, V., 313, *319*

Senn, H. J., 348, *356*

Senn, K. L., *234*

Sennott-Miller, L., 98, 134, *147, 202*

Sephton, S., 509, *515, 516*

Sephton, S. E., 502, 503, *510*

Serdula, M., 197, *207*

Serlin, R., *556*

Severson, H. H., 169, *185*

Sexson, S. B., 454, *462*

Seymour, J. D., 197, *207*

Seynaeve, C., *317, 318*

SF-36 Health Survey, *128*

Shabsigh, R., *388*

Shadbolt, B., 290, *301*

Shadel, W. G., 239, *247*

Shaffer, K., *493*

Shah, J. P., *493*

Shah, K. V., 284–285, *296*

Shakib, S., *545*

Shalet, S. M., *387*, 435, *442*

Shamban, J., *219*

Shands, M. E., 469, 470, 471, 473, *485*

Shannon, C., 199, *207*

Shannon, J., 63, *82*, 92, *102*, 196, *201*

Shannon, S. E., *346*

Shapiro, A., *492*

Shapiro, S. L., 363, *376*, 418, *429*

Sharp, L. K., 120, *128*

Sharp, P., *232*

Sharpe, P. A., *248*

Shaw, A., 504, *516*

Shaw, B. R., 550, *558*

Shaw, E. G., *188*

Shaw, M. J., 292, *300*

Sheard, T., 362, 368, 369, 370, *376,*
    418, 419, *429*

Sheffer, C. E., 170, *187*

Shelby, R., *377*
Shelke, A. R., 348, *358, 359*
Shell, J. A., 417, *429*
Shelton, D. R., 506, *515*
Shelton, L. G., *22, 165*
Shenassa, E. D., 536, *545*
Shepherd, J., 228, *234*
Sherbourne, C. D., 118, *128*, 290, *301*
Sherman, D., *482*
Sherman, K., *319*
Sherman, M., *232*
Sherr, L., *297*
Sherwood, P., 392, 393, 395, 397, *405,*
    407, 408
Shi, Y., 501, *516*
Shield, R., *408*
Shields, A. E., *162*, 535, *544*
Shields, P. G., 536, *544, 545*
Shiffman, S., 71, *82*, 174, 178, *185, 187*
Shifren, J. L., 385, *389*
Shigaki, D., 99, 213, *219*
Shiloh, S., *320*
Shin, J., 399, *404*
Shinn, E., 286, *300*
Shiu, S., 488, *494*
Shoda, Y., 13, *21*, 45, *54*, 141, *146*, 229,
    233, 280, *299*, 305, *308, 319,*
    348, *357*
Shopland, D. R., 40, 46, *54*
Short, A., 452, *465*
Short, P. F., 422, *430*
Shoveller, J. A., 214, *222*
Shumay, D., 488, *493*
Siau, J., 469, *481*
Sickles, E. A., *300*
Sidlofsky, S., *444*
Siegel, B., *184*
Siegel, J. E., *377*
Siegel, M., 157, *165*
Siegel, R., *233*
Siemer, M., 89, *101*
Sienko, D. G., 171, *181*
Sievanen, H., *493*
Sigal, R. J., *38*
Siiteri, P. K., 227, *234*
Silk, K. J., *22*

Silliman, R. A., 334, *345*, 479, *483*
Silverio, R., 213, *219*
Silverman, J. D., 337, *344*
Silverman, M., 110, *111*
Silverstein, J. H., 349, 352, *357*
Siminoff, L., 136, *147*
Siminoff, L. A., 334, *346*
Simmons, G. E., *556*
Simmons-Morton, 240
Simms, A., *461*
Simms, S., *233*, 450, *461*
Simon, J. A., *389*
Simon, T. R., *165*
Simone, J. V., 423, *427*
Simons-Morton, D. G., 240, *250*
Simpson, J. M., 85, *101*, 296
Simpson, K. C., 471, *480*
Simpson, N. K., *113*
Simpson, P., 210, *217*
Singal, R., 305, *314*
Singer, A., 286, *298*
Singer, D. E., 171, *188*
Singer, E., 307, *320*
Singer, J., *148*
Singer, P. A., 332, *346*
Singer, S., 416, *429*
Sinsheimer, J., 470, *485*
Sison,, C., *344*
Sjoberg, L., 140, *147*
Sjoden, P., 216, *217*, 298
Sjoden, P. O., 281, *298*
Skinner, C. S., 16, 17, *21, 22*, 134, 140,
    146, 147, 205, 311, *320*, 550, *558*
Skinner, E. C., 364, *376*
Sklar, C. A., 432, 436, 439, 446, *447*
Skovlund, E., *494*
Slade, J., *184, 186*
Sladek, M. L., *428*
Slate, E. H., *36*
Slater, E., *318*
Slater, J. S., 92, *101*, 228, *233*
Slaughter, R., 450, *459*
Slavin, J., 31, *38*
Sleijfer, D. T., *345*
Slenker, S. E., 282, *297*
Sloan, D. A., *373*

Sloan, J. A., *182, 343, 386*
Sloane, R., *492*
Sloman, R., 351, *359*
Sloper, P., 454, *464*
Sloper, T., 451, *464*
Slovic, P., 134, 135, *147, 148*
Slygh, C., *219*
Slymen, D. J., 99, *100, 221*
Smaglik, P., 551, *558*
Small, B. J., *483*
Smedley, B. D., 190, *207, 275*
Smedslund, G., 421, *430*
Smeenk, F., 400, *408*
Smerglia, V., 415–416, *426*
Smets, E. M., 351, *359, 387*
Smigelski, C., *203*
Smilbert, E., 450, *458*
Smith, D., *298*
Smith, E., *112*
Smith, H. L., 63, *80*
Smith, J., 194, *207*
Smith, K. R., 304, 306, 307, *314, 315, 320*
Smith, M., *201*
Smith, M. Y., 416, *430*
Smith, P. O., 170, *187*
Smith, R. A., 227, *234*, 268, 273, *275, 283, 299*
Smith, R. C., *515*
Smith, R. P., 548, *558*
Smith, R. S., 501, *516*
Smith, S. S., 170, 178, *187, 188*
Smith, T. L., *182*
Smith-Akin, C. K., *529*
Smith-Bindman, R., 280, *300*
Smith-Warner, S. A., 29, *39*
Smoklowski, T. D., 156, *162*
Sneeuw, K. C., 121, *128*, 417, *430*
Sneeuw, K. C. A., 362, *376*
Snell, J. L., 228, *234*, 258, 259, 263, 264, 265, 266, *267, 277*
Snider, P. R., 366, *367, 377*
Snijders, P., *234*
Snyder, C., 116, *126, 127*, 316, *317, 318*
Snyder, D. C., 491, *492, 494*
Snyder, P., 365, *374*

Sobell, L. C., 176, *187*
Sobell, M. B., 176, *187*
Sobol, A. M., *204*
Society for Research on Nicotine and Tobacco, 171, *187*
Sodergren, K. M., 349, *359*
Soler, M., 227, *234*
Solomon, A., *217*
Solomon, C. G., *38*
Solomon, L. J., *314*
Somer, E., 456, *459*
Somerset, M., 286, *288, 300*
Somerville, M. A., *288, 297*
Somkin, C. P., 228, *234*
Sondik, E. J., 534, *545*
Soneji, R., *557*
Song, V., 213, *219*
Sonneborn, D., *274*
Sood, A. K., *514*
Soots, K. I., *511*
Sorensen, B. L., *446*
Sorensen, G., 92, 97, 98, 196, *207*, 202, *220*
Söörensen, S., 393, 394, 395, *396, 407*
Sorgen, K., 453, *462*
Sormanti, M., 364, *374*, 453, *464*
Sorosky, J. I., *514*
Sowden, A., 294, *300*
Sox, C. H., 92, 98, 212, *219*
Spangler, J. G., 172, *187*
Spanswick, C. C., 351, *356*
Speca, M., 400, 404, 477, *480*
Speer, J. J., 385, *389*
Speizer, F. E., 30, 37, 40, 222, *515*
Spelten, E. R., 422, *423, 430*
Spencer, L., 169, *187*
Spencer, S. M., 365, *376*, 415, *430*
Sperduto, P. W., 438, *446*
Sperner-Unterweger, B., 126, *515*
Spiegel, D., 350, *359*, 369, *372, 373*, 501, 502, 503, 504, 505, 506, 509, *513, 515, 516*
Spiegelman, D., 38, *39*
Spilker, B., 118, *126, 128*
Spiro, R. H., *493*
Sprangers, M. A., 121, *128*, 422, *430*

Sprangers, M. A. G., *376*
Spring, B., 177, 178, *181, 185, 187*
Sridhar, F. G., 124, *127*
Srivastava, D. K., 450, 451, *460, 463*
St. John, D. J., 309, *315*
Staab, J. P., *512*
Staats, H., *513*
Stables, G., 195, 197, *203*
Stacey, D., *147*
Stackpole, K. M., *165*
Stacy, A. W., *163, 165*
Stafford, R. S., 171, *188*
Stallings, F. L., 110, *113*
Stalmeier, P. F. M., 308, *320*
Stampfer, M. J., 26, 30, *37, 38, 39, 40, 222*
Standish, L. J., *493*
Stanford, J. L., *127, 382, 387, 388*
Stange, K. C., 216, *218*
Stange, P. V., *527*
Stanisavljevic, S., 434, *447*
Stanley, L. C., 46, *53, 55*
Stanton, A. L., 366, 367, 370, *375, 376,*
        377, 419, 430
Stanton, W. R., 92, *100*
Staples, M., 281 *297*
Staples, M. P., 24, *37*
Stapleton, J., 213, *222*
Stapleton, J. A., *187*
Starr, P., *221*
Stavrou, T., 439, *447*
Stead, L. F., 179, *183, 186*
Stead, M. L., 417, *430*
Stearns, V., 349, *355*
Stebbens, J. A., *463*
Steckler, A., 45, *53, 270, 277*
Steel, C. M., *315*
Steele, R. G., 452, *463*
Steele, S. J., *188, 301*
Stefanek, M., *144, 505, 511*
Stefanek, M. E., *504, 516*
Steger-May, K., *204, 205*
Steggles, N., 307, *314*
Stein, E., *207*
Stein, J. A., 92, 99, 141, *145*
Stein, K. D., 354, *359*
Steinberg, E. R., 549, *558*

Steiner, C., *221, 222*
Steiner, D. L., 453, *464*
Steiner, H., 451, *460*
Steiner, J. F., 422, 423, *428, 430*
Steinhauser, K. E., 332, *346*
Steinherz, L. J., 433, *447*
Steinherz, P. G., 433, *447*
Step, M. M., 136, *147*
Stepanski, B. M., *100, 214, 222*
Stephens, D., 285, *301*
Stephens, L. M., *102*
Stephens, M., 393, 395, *408*
Stephenson, M. T., 213, *221, 222*
Stephenson, R. A., *388*
Stern, D. T., 553, *556*
Stern, R. M., 348, *358*
Stern, S. L., 505, *516*
Stetner, F., *184*
Stetz, K. M., 396, *408*
Stevens, M., *219*
Stevens, R. G., 503, *511*
Stevens, V. J., 68, *81*
Stewart, A. L., 118, *128, 179, 188, 290,*
        300
Stewart, B., 68, 83, 397, *407*
Stewart, D., 393, 399, *404, 465*
Stewart, J., *428*
Stewart, J. L., *357, 484*
Stewart, S. K., 337, *344*
Stewart, S. L., 269, *276*
Stewart-Brown, S., *296*
Stewart-Williams, S., 352, *359*
Stieglitz, R. D., 351, *355*
Stinson, F. S., 176, *184*
Stitt, L. W., *188*
Stoddard, A., 92, *207*
Stoddard, A. M., *97*
Stokols, D., 45, *55, 245, 248, 531, 532,*
        533, 538, 539, 540, 541, 542,
        544, 545, 546
Stolar, M., 536, *543*
Stommel, M., 395, *405, 408, 505, 516*
Stone, A. A., 70, 71, *82, 383, 389*
Stone, C., *100*
Stone, E. G., 258, 259, 263, 264,
        265n(b), 266, 267, *277*

Stone, E. J., 205, 206, 248
Stonebridge, C., 396, 404
Stonegger, W., 239, 250
Stones, M., 393, 404
Stopfer, J., 306, 313, 314
Storer, B. E., 503, 515
Storm-Mathisen, I., 452, 460
Story, M., 199, 203, 207
Stovall, E., 423, 427
Stovall, M., 443, 445, 446, 447, 448
Strahan, E. J., 139, 148
Strainchamps, E., 364, 374
Strander, H., 352, 360
Strang, P., 332, 341
Strang, P. M., 330, 343
Strang, V., 396, 408
Straus, S., 520, 529
Stray-Pedersen, B., 164
Strecher, V. J., 134, 148, 220, 311, 312,
    317, 321, 522, 528, 550, 552,
    554, 556, 557, 558
Street, R., 555
Streiner, D. L., 76, 82, 464
Streisand, R., 455, 456, 457, 459, 461,
    465
Streke, A. V., 165
Strickman-Stein, N., 235
Stromme, S. B., 494
Stronegger, W., 250
Strong, E. W., 493
Strong, L. C., 448
Struewing, J. P., 314
Strumberg, D., 448
Strumpf, N. E., 483, 514
Stryker, J., 220
Stuba, M. P., 512
Stuber, M., 453, 460, 465
Studts, J. L., 144, 295
Stull, V. B., 491, 494
Sturm, C. M., 334, 346
Stuver, S. O., 33, 40
Stuyt, E. B., 176, 188
Subramanian, G., 535, 546
Sudman, S., 275, 278
Sufka, A. V. W., 146
Sugarbaker, P. H., 116, 125, 128

Sugerman, J., 22, 320
Sugg-Skinner, C., 205
Sugrue, D. P., 389
Sui, D., 384, 386, 388
Sullivan, K., 334, 345
Sullivan, K. M., 442
Sullivan, L. M., 334, 345
Sullivan, M. A., 177, 188
Suls, J., 141, 142, 146, 148
Suminski, R. R., 249
Summerton, J., 335, 345
Sun, P., 165
Sun, T., 99, 184, 219
Sun, Y., 307, 315
Sun, Y.-C., 138, 144
Surbone, A., 329, 346
Susser, M., 273, 277
Sussman, S., 153, 163, 165
Sutherland, L., 192, 207
Sutton, S., 278, 283, 289, 299, 300, 301,
    307, 314
Sutton, S. R., 282, 295, 418, 427
Svensson, H., 440, 444
Swain, S. M., 433, 447
Swan, G. E., 545
Swan, J., 10, 22, 34, 40, 256, 257, 274,
    277
Swanson, C. A., 234
Swanson, G. M., 543
Swanson, J. E., 54, 80
Sweeney, T., 444
Swenson, K. K., 428
Swerdlow, A. J., 439, 447
Swisher, E., 386
Syme, S. L., 190, 207, 275
Symons, M., 98, 202, 207
Syndikus, I., 451, 452, 465
Syrjala, K. L., 351, 359
Szabo, A., 396, 408
Szarewski, A., 179, 188, 287, 299, 301

Tainsky, M. A., 306, 318
Tait, D., 451, 465
Talen, E., 245, 248, 531, 544
Tan, C. T., 433, 447
Tangney, C., 488, 489, 494

Tangrea, J. A., 103, 110, *113*

Tannock, I., 352, *355*

Tannock, I. F., 438, *447*

Taplin, S., *82*

Taplin, S. H., 63, 66, 78, 80, 82, 137, 144, 257, 271, *276, 277*

Taras, H. L., 199, *207*

Taren, D., 98, *202*

Tashkin, D., *127*

Task Force on Community Preventive Services, The, 258, *277*

Tate, D., *249*

Tate, D. F., 192, 193, *207*, 223, 239, 250, *551, 558*

Tatla, R. K., *297*

Tattersall, M., *343*

Tattersall, M. H., 339, *342, 343, 344*

Tattersall, M. H. N., 328, 330, 331, 334, 339, *342, 343, 346*

Tatum, C. M., 104, *112*

Taupin, D., 290, 292, *301*

Taylor, A., 210, 220, *250, 301*

Taylor, A. M., 211, 212, 216, *218*

Taylor, J., *462*

Taylor, K. L., 370, *377*, 476, *483*

Taylor, K. M., 337, *346*

Taylor, P. M., *443*

Taylor, P. R., *112*

Taylor, S., *207*

Taylor, S. E., 469, *483*

Taylor, T., 278, 289, *301*

Teasdale, J. D., 347, *354*

Tefft, M., *444*

Tejeda, W. B., 103, 110, *113*

Tejero, J., *425*

Television Bureau of Advertising, 199, *207*

Tempelaar, R., 394, 395, *406, 484*

Templeton, E., 336, *344*

Templin, T., 391, 396, *406, 407*, 468, 469, *484*

ten Kroode, H. F. J., 308, *316*

Tennant, C. C., *510, 510, 515*

Tennstedt, S., *203, 545*

Teno, J. M., 401, *408*, 505, *516*

Teppo, L., 504, *514*

Teran, L., *165*

Tercyak, K. P., *162*, 455, 465, 536, *546*

Terrell, J. E., *183*

Tessaro, I., 20, 98, 194, *202, 207*, 307, *320*

Tessaro, I. A., 194, *207*

Teutsch, S. M., 255, *276, 528*

Thackway, S. V., *510*

Theis, B., 27, *39*

Themba, M., 47, *55*

Theobald, T., 215, *222*

Thieden, E., 214, *222*

Thiesse-Duffy, E., 138, *146*

Thiis-Evensen, E., 290, 292, 298, *301*

Thilen, U., *445*

Thomas, D. B., 92, *101*

Thomas, M., 246, *248*

Thomas, S. M., *112*

Thomas, W., *54*

Thomassen, L. H., *463*

Thompson, A. I., 468, *483*

Thompson, B., 45, 46, 55, 92, 97, 97, 98, 99, *102*, 196, *201, 203*

Thompson, H. S., 306, 307, 312, *320*

Thompson, I. M., *112*

Thompson, J., 46, 53, *55*

Thompson, N. J., 92, *102*

Thompson, S., 455, *465*

Thompson, T. L., *342*

Thomson, C. A., *492*

Thomson, S. J., *163*

Thomson O'Brien, M. A., 173, *188*

Thorndike, A. N., 171, *188*

Thorndyke, P. W., 353, *359*

Thornquist, M. D., 39, 92, *102*

Thors, C. L., 351, *356*

Thorsen, H., 282, 296, *297*

Thorsen, L., 490, *494*

Thrasher, J., 194, *208*

Thun, M. J., 28, 32, 35, 36, 37, 40, 233, *546*

Thurfjell, E., 281, *298*

Thursfield, V. J., 24, *37*

Tickle, J. J., *165*

Tieman, A., *181*

Tiffany, S. T., 67, 71, *82*

Tilanus-Linthorst, M. M. A., *318*

Till, J. E., 551, 558
Tilley, B. C., 93, 102, 275
Tinetti, M. E., 240, 250
Tinker, L., 202
Tinley, S., 317
Tinley, S. T., 309, 320
Tiro, J. A., 269, 277, 289, 301
Tittle, M., 483
Titze, S., 239, 250
Tiwari, R. C., 233, 444
Tobias, J. S., 327, 346
Tobler, N. S., 153, 154, 155, 165
Tolbert, V., 404
Tolle, M., 437, 446
Tomaino-Brunner, C., 288, 301
Tomei, L. D., 503, 516
Tomiak, A. T., 188
Tomich, P. L., 417, 420, 430
Tomlinson, G. E., 437, 446
Tompkins, N., 523, 529
Tomshine, P. A., 292, 300
Toney, K., 194, 205
Toogood, I., 453, 464
Tope, D. M., 348, 349, 350, 355, 360
Torgerson, D. J., 77, 82
Toseland, R., 399, 403, 408, 476, 480
Toseland, R. W., 476, 478, 485
Tosteson, T. D., 92, 98, 212, 219
Tosti, S., 46, 53
Tovar, M., 549, 556
Townsend, A., 393, 408
Traficante, R. M., 544
Tran, V. T., 307, 315
Trappido, E. J., 226, 235
Trauth, J. M., 113
Travis, L. B., 439, 448
Tremaine, W., 116, 123, 128
Tremblay, A., 395, 403
Trentham-Dietz, A., 503, 515
Trewin, D., 275
Trichopoulos, D., 20, 23, 36, 38
Triemstra, M., 394, 395, 406, 484
Trijsburg, R. W., 317
Trimbath, J. D., 309, 317
Trimble, E. L., 113
Tripp, M. K., 220

Trock, B., 141, 145
Troesch, L. M., 349, 359
Trojaborg, W., 438, 444
Troosters, T., 444
Tross, S., 505, 509, 516
Trost, S. G., 249
Trowonou, A., 317
Trudeau, K. J., 268, 275
Truman, B. I., 524, 529
Trumbull, R., 233
Trunzo, J., 488, 489, 494
Trunzo, J. J., 420, 429, 490, 494
Truong, P. T., 188
Tsao, M. N., 421, 426
Tseng, D. S., 228, 235, 258, 259, 266, 267, 277
Tuason, L. J., 388
Tucker, D. C., 136, 306, 315, 368, 375, 425, 429
Tucker, J. A., 180
Tucker, K. L., 199, 203
Tucker, M. A., 179, 188, 433, 439, 444, 448
Tucker, T. C., 101
Tulsky, D. S., 125
Tulsky, J. A., 338, 341, 346
Tunceli, K., 422, 430
Tuokko, H., 393, 404
Tuomilehto, J., 46, 54, 512
Turcotte, R., 125
Turk, D. C., 351, 359
Turnbull, B. W., 36
Turner, J., 16, 22, 328, 343, 536, 544
Turner, L., 152, 165
Turner, S., 212, 219
Turner-Cobb, J. M., 369, 372
Turrisi, R., 213, 222
Tversky, A., 140, 147
Twiggs, L. B., 285, 301
Twombly, R., 151, 165
Tworek, C., 80
Tyc, V., 456, 465
Tyc, V. L., 460
Tyll, L., 247
Tyndale, R. F., 536, 545
Tyrrell, M., 228, 233

U. S. Department of Health, Education, and Welfare, 167–168, *188*

U. S. Department of Health and Human Services (USDHHS), 25, 26, 27, *40*, 151, 155, 161, *165*, 171, *188*, *208*, 237, 237n, 238, 240, 240n, *250*, *529*

U. S. Food and Drug Administration, 117, *128*

Ubel, P. A., 141, *148*, 553, *558*

Uchino, B. N., 505, *516*

Uhler, R. J., 209, *222*

Ullen, H., 210, 215, *217*

Umberson, D., 505, *513*

Underwood, S. M., *112*

Unger, E. R., *233*

Unger, J. B., 154, *165*

Unger, M., *147*, *277*

Ungerleider, R. S., *113*

Unic, I., 308, *320*

Uno, D., 505, *516*

Unrod, M., 177, *188*

Unruh, H. K., *144*

Urbach, F., 209, *220*

Urban, N., 272, *273*

Vach, W., 78, *83*

Vainio, H., 535, *546*

Valach, L., 476, *481*

Valanis, B., 68, *83*

Valdimarsdottir, H. B., 305, *317*, *320*

Valenstein, M., *183*

Vanable, P. A., 383, *388*

van Berge-Henegouwen, G. P., 367, *372*

van Breukelen, G., 17, *20*, 169, *183*

Vanchieri, C., 197, *208*

Van Daal, W. A. J., 308, *320*

Van Dam, F. S., 438, *447*

van den Borne, H. W., 367, *372*

van den Bos, G., 394, 395, *406*, *484*

van den Brandt, P. A., *38*, *39*

van den Heuvel, W. J., 281, *300*

van der Bij, A. K., 242, *250*

Vander Hoorn, S., 23, *37*

van der Kamp, L. J., 281, *296*

van der Leun, J. C., 209, *220*

van der Ploeg, E., 281, *296*

van de Wiel, H. B., 281, *300*, *387*

van Dongen-Melman, J. E. W. M., 454, *465*

van Elderen, T. M., 281, *296*

Van Fleet, S., 349, 350, *360*

van Haastregt, J., *408*

Vanhelden, P., *444*

VanHoewyk, J., 307, *320*

van Kempen-Harteveld, M. L., 439, *448*

van Knippenberg, F. C., 120, *125*, 367, *372*

van Leeuwen, F. E., *448*

van Leynseele, J., 92, *102*

Vannatta, K., 452, 460, 462, *465*

van Roosmalen, M. S., 307, 308, *320*

van Stolk, R. U., *35*

van Tienhoven, G., *359*

van't Veer, L., *319*

Van Vunakis, H., *182*

Van Willigan, J., 46, *55*

van Zuuren, F. J., *345*

Varian, H. R., 549, *557*

Varnell, S. P., 85, 89, 90, 91, 91n, 94n, 95n, 96, *101*, *102*

Varnes, J. D., *97*

Varni, J., *464*

Varni, J. W., 121, *128*

Vasey, J. J., 422, *430*

Vasterling, J., 350, *360*

Vatn, M. H., *298*

Velicer, W., *181*, *527*

Velicer, W. F., 70, 80, *83*, *274*, *558*

Venter, J. C., 535, *546*

Venturelli, E., *387*

Verbeek, J. H., 422, *430*

Verbeke, G., 79, *83*

Verhoef, L. C. G., 308, *320*

Verhoog, L. C., *318*

Verhulst, F. C., 454, *465*

Verkasalo, P. K., 503, 504, *514*

Verlicer, W. F., 550, *558*

Vermey, A., *345*

Verne, J., *298*

Vernon, S. W., 6, *22*, *102*, 256, 258, 269, 270, 272, 273, *275*, *276*, *277*

Verstappen, C. C., 440, *448*
Vess, J. D., 470, 471, 473, 474, *485*
Vesselago, M., *126*
Vessey, M., 295, *300*
Vickberg, S. M., 349, *355*
Vickers, K. S., *183*
Victora, C. G., 272, *277*
Videtic, G. M., 179, *188*
Vieira, M., 440, *447*
Viezemans, H., *408*
Viles, C., *207*
Vincent, L., 351, *356, 512*
Vinciguerra, V., *463*
Visser, M. R., 328, *359*
Visser, M. R. M., *345*
Vitaliano, P., 393, *408*
Voeks, J. H., *217*
Vogl, D., 416, *430*
Vogt, T. M., 64, *81*, 271, *277, 525, 528*
Vollono, J., *249*
von Eschenbach, A. C., *234*, 380, 388, 532, *546*
von Eye, A., 392, *408*
Von Hoff, A. L., *448*
Von Hoff, D. D., 433, *448*
Voorhees, C. C., *186*
Vu, H. T., 177, *183*
Vu, T., *202*
Vuckovic, N., 68, *83*, 171, *186*

Waber, D. P., 450, *461, 465*
Wagenaar, A. C., *163*
Wagner, A., *318*
Wagner, E. H., 100, *555*
Wagner, G., *388*
Wagner, P. J., 339, *346*
Wagner, T. H., 258, 261, 267, *278*
Wahl, E., *320*
Wakefield, M., 159, *165*
Walker, J., 407, *484*
Walker, L. B., 467, 469, *485*
Walker, P., *297*
Walker-Thurmond, K., 28, *36*
Walkosz, B. J., 213, 215, 217, *222*
Wall, J., 199, *205*
Wall, P. D., 351, *360*

Wallace, J. A., 329, *346*
Wallace, J. L., *247*
Wallace, R. B., *515*
Wallace, W. H., *446*
Wallack, L., 47, *55*
Wallander, J. L., *235*
Wallbanks, C., 211, *220*
Waller, J., 289, 299, *301*
Wallerstein, N., 46, *54*
Wallerstein, N. B., 105, *112*
Wallfisch, A., *182*
Wallston, K. A., 146, *148*
Walsh, B. T., *184*
Walsh, D. C., 46, *55*
Walsh, M. M., 92, *102*
Walsh, P. C., 381, *389*
Walter, A., *447*
Walter, F., 307, *314*
Walter, S. D., 124, *127*
Walters, E. E., *513*
Wang, C., 305, 312, *314, 321*
Wang, D. T., *201*
Wang, E. Y. I., *164*
Wang, H. J., 469, *481*
Wang, M. Q., 199, *203*
Wang, Q., *314*
Wang, T., *101, 206*
Wang, W. W., *101*
Wang, Y., 29, *41*
Warburton, R., *387*
Ward, D. S., *249*
Ward, E., 20, 233, *444*
Ward, H. E., *512*
Ward, P., 335, *343*
Ward, P. A., *319*
Wardle, J., 272, 278, 283, 285, 286, 286–287, 289, 290, 292, 294, 296, *299*
Ware, J. E., Jr., 118, 123, 128, 290, 300, *301*
Ware, J. H., 76, *83*
Warnecke, C., *98*
Warnecke, R., 17, *21*, 92, 100, 175, *185*
Warnecke, R. B., 269, 270, 271, *274, 275, 277, 278*
Warneke, C. L., 388, *447, 485*
Warner, J. T., 434, *448*

Warner, K., 160, *163*
Warr, D., *358, 511*
Waseda, M., 549, *555*
Washington, C., 98
Waskerwitz, M. J., *463*
Waters, A. J., 178, *187*
Watkins, L. R., 500, 501, *514*
Watson, A., 214, *219*
Watson, E., 281, *296*
Watson, M., 308, *316*, 505, *516*
Watson, P., *317, 320*
Watts, B. G., 275, *319*
Wayne, S. J., 488, 489, *494*
Webb, D. K., 434, *448*
Webber, B., *444*
Webber, C., *444*
Webber, G. C., 335, 340, *346*
Webber, L. S., *206*
Weber, B., *313*
Weber, B. E., 257, *278*
Weber, E. U., 135, *146*
Weber, M. D., *164*
Webster, P., *296*
Wechsler, H., 25, *39, 40*
Wee, C. C., *38*
Weeks, J., 488, *493*
Weeks, J. C., 17, *21, 514*
Wei, Q., 503, *511*
Weil, M., *54*
Weinberg, P. D., *220*
Weinberg, R. A., 509, *513*
Weinblatt, M., *463*
Weiner, B., *55*
Weiner, J., *99*
Weiner, S. L., 423, *427*
Weinstein, N., 134, *148*
Weinstein, N. D., 44, 55, 134, 135, 137,
        138, 139, 141, 142, *148*, 270, *278*
Weinstock, J. E., 215, *222*
Weinstock, M. A., 209, *222*
Weir, H. K., 532, *546*
Weisman, A. D., 415, *430*
Weiss, J., 215, *223*
Weiss, R., *465*
Weiss, R. B., *427*
Weiss, T., 479, *485*

Weissman, M. M., 468, *482*
Weitzner, M., 395, 408, *483*
Weizman, A., 194, *204*
Welch, E., 135, *146*
Welch, H. G., 134, 140, *149*, 281, *300*
Welch, L. C., *408*
Wellisch, D. K., 469, *481*
Wells, H. B., *232*
Wells, N., 398, *408*
Welsch, S. K., 175, *186*
Weltz, C., 352, *357*
Wender, D. B., *386*
Wender, R., *234*
Wengstrom, Y., 352, *360*
Wenrich, M. D., 331, *346*
Wensing, W., 242, *250*
Wenzel, L., 230, 231, *232*, 235, *316, 320*
Wenzel, L. B., *232*
Werkman, A., 192, *205*
West, J. A., 304, *320*
West, P., *112*
West, S. G., 138, *143*, 257, *273*
Westcombe, A. M., *300*
Westie, K. S., 383, *386*
Weston, R., 228, *234*
Wetle, T., *408*
Wetter, D. W., 174, 179, *182, 188*
Wever, L. D., 116, *125*
Whalen, C. K., *164*
Whaley, F. S., 433, *447*
Wheeler, C. M., 38, *299*
Whelan, T., *405*
While, D., 454, *464*
White, H., 92, *100*
White, K., *148*
White, M. M., 536, *544*
Whiteside, T., *513*
Whitman, S., 257, *278*
Whitt, J. K., 452, 462, *463*
Whittington, R., 557, *558*
Whitton, J., *447, 465*
Wickerham, D. L., *112, 125, 126*
Widner, B., *515*
Wiedrich-Smith, M. D., 70, *80*
Wilcox, S., *248*
Wildemuth, B., *207*

Wileyto, E. P., 544
Wilhelmsen, I., 290, 301
Wilkins, E. G., 429
Wilkinson, C., 286, 287, 289, 300, 301
Wilkinson, E. G., 417
Wilkinson, E. J., 285, 301
Wilkinson, G., 37
Will, S., 215, 219
Willems-Groot, A. F., 359
Willett, W. C., 20, 23, 26, 30, 31, 36,
    37, 38, 39, 40, 41, 222, 515
Williams, D., 399, 404
Williams, D. A., 368, 373
Williams, G. C., 358
Williams, J. E., 248
Williams, J. I., 513
Williams, P., 328, 343
Williams, T., 135, 149
Williamson, D. L., 47, 54
Williamson, S., 278, 290, 299, 301
Williams-Piehota, P., 295, 301, 552,
    558
Willis, G. B., 270, 273
Wilson, J. M. G., 255, 256, 278
Wilson, K. M., 269, 274, 275, 276
Wilson, M. H., 181
Wilson, P., 138, 146
Winawer, S., 275
Windschitl, P. D., 141, 149
Winefield, H. R., 428
Winer, E., 307, 320, 488, 493
Winett, R. A., 62, 83, 192, 207, 214,
    223
Wing, A. L., 39
Wing, R. R., 45, 54, 192, 207, 239, 250,
    551, 558
Wingo, P. A., 20, 23, 40, 546
Winkel, G., 349, 352, 357
Winkelstein, W., Jr., 226, 235
Winkleby, M. A., 171, 183
Winn, R. J., 414, 415, 427
Winter, L., 396, 404
Winzlenberg, A., 428
Wirth, A., 375
Wise, M., 557
Wiseman, S. M., 187

Wissler, K., 460
Witte, K., 213, 222, 223
Wobbes, T., 468, 481
Wojcik, C., 355
Wolchok, S., 427
Wolf, F. M., 183
Wolfe, C., 301
Wolfe, C. D. A., 288, 300
Wolfe, P., 204
Wolfinger, R. D., 92, 100
Wolfson, M., 92, 99, 163
Wolk, A., 36
Woloshin, S., 134, 140, 149, 281, 300
Women's Health Initiative Study
    Group, 191, 208
Wong, G., 181
Wood, J. V., 469, 483
Wood, M. C., 211, 221
Woodbury, W., 393, 407
Woodcock, A. A., 443
Wood-Dauphinee, S., 513
Woodman, C. B. J., 215, 219
Woods, N. F., 470, 473, 482, 483
Woodward, C. K., 138, 143, 257, 273
Wooldridge, J. A., 144
Wooley, T., 215, 223
Woolf, S. H., 269, 276, 528
Woolhandler, S., 185
Worden, J. K., 17, 22, 157, 163, 165,
    314
Worden, J. W., 415, 430
World Cancer Research Fund (WCRF),
    189, 208
World Cancer Research Fund &
    American Institute for Cancer
    Research, 29, 31, 40
Wortman, C. B., 420, 430
Wray, R. J., 271, 275
Wren, P. A., 426
Wright, E. B., 334, 346
Wright, K., 425
Wright, M. J., 434, 435, 448
Wright, T. C., Jr., 285, 301
Wrosch, C., 348, 360
Wu, A. W., 181, 516
Wu, K., 30, 41

Wujcik, D., 398, *408*
Wulf, H. C., 214, *222*
Wunder, J. S., *125*
Wyatt, G., *405*
Wyatt, G. E., 366, *374, 429, 469, 481*
Wylie, J. E., *314*
Wynings, C., *376, 430*

Xiong, X., *465*
Xistris, D., 417, *427*
Xu, J., *233*

Yabroff, K. R., 228, *235, 258, 261, 263,*
        265n(i), 266, 267, 269, 273, 275,
        278, 287, 296, 422, 430
Yager, G. G., *318*
Yalom, I., 350, *359*
Yam, B. M. C., 348, *357*
Yamagishi, K., 134, *149*
Yancik, R., *37*
Yanes, B., 349, *359*
Yang, J., 349, *355*
Yao, J. F., 228, *232*
Yarkin-Levin, K., 364, *375*
Yarnall, K. S., *234*
Yarnold, J. R., *430*
Yaroch, A. L., 197, *203, 207, 212, 216,*
        218, 220, 221, 223
Yarsevich, J., 159, *163*
Yasko, J., 370, *374*
Yasko, J. M., *112*
Yasui, Y., 387, *445, 446, 460, 461*
Yates, P., 396, *408*
Yaun, S. S., *39*
Ybema, J. F., 477, *482*
Ye, J., *387*
Yedidia, M. J., 172, *188*
Yee, D., 490, *493*
Yetman, R. J., *388*
Yin, D., *516*
Yost, L., *483*
Young, C., *315*
Young, J., 488, *494*
Young, M. A., *344*

Young, R. C., *235*
Young, Z. M., 179, *187*
Yung, H. P., 348, *357*
Yung, L., 433, *448*

Zahlis, E. H., 469, *471, 473, 485*
Zaidel, N., 456, *459*
Zaizov, R., 456, *459*
Zakeri, I., *201*
Zanetti, R., 215, *222*
Zanna, M. P., *148*
Zapart, S., *22*
Zapka, J., 173, *188*
Zapka, J. G., 172, *186*
Zauber, A., 226, *233*
Zawacki, K., 398, *405*
Zaza, S., 527, *527*
Zebrack, B., 451, *465*
Zeger, S. L., 76, *81*
Zehner, M. E., *183*
Zeller, P. K., 269, *276*
Zeltzer, L. K., 452, *460, 465*
Zetocha, K., *146*
Zhang, C., *427*
Zhang, J., 174, *185, 393, 408*
Zhang, Q., 29, 30, *41*
Zhang, S., *407*
Zhang, S. M., 31, *41*
Zhang, T. Y., *233*
Zhao, H., *356*
Zhou, J. N., *516*
Zhu, K., 92, *102*
Zibecchi, L., 385, *387*
Zick, C. D., 306, *320*
Ziegler, R. G., *37*
Ziegler, R. S., *442*
Zimmerman, R. S., 257–258, *276*
Ziogas, A., *112*
Zippe, C., 388, *447, 471, 484, 485*
Zolnoun, D., 255, *274*
Zucker, D. M., 89, *102*
Zuckerman, E., *427, 481*
Zuckerman, E. L., *427*
Zweifler, A. J., *183*

SUBJECT INDEX

Access-enhancing interventions, for
screening, 266
Accrual to clinical trials (ACT) framework, 104–105, 109–110
case study of, 105–111
future research needed on, 111
Acute lymphoblastic leukemia (ALL),
432
in adolescents, 452
in children, 450
and obesity, 433
Addiction
to alcohol and smoking, 176
transdisciplinary research on,
532–533
Adolescents, physical activity interventions for (female), 241
Adolescents' tobacco use, 151, 152–153
and antismoking campaign, 157–158
and self-regulation skills, 18
Advertising
of food and beverages (regulating of),
199–200
for tobacco use prevention, 157–158
See also Media
Advisory Committee on Cancer
Control of the National Cancer
Institute of Canada, 6
Advocates, and quality of life, 116
African American Cancer Survivor
Study, 105–111
African Americans
as breast cancer survivors (risk of
nonemployment), 423
and genetic-testing decision,
306–307
and inactivity, 27

and neighborhood physical activities, 537
and physical activity interventions
for female adolescents, 241
as smoking-cessation intervention
target, 175
Age
and cancer risk, 24
and family caregiver distress, 395
as predictor of reaction to cancer
diagnosis and treatment, 365
Agency for Healthcare Research and
Quality (AHRQ), 521–522, 523,
524, 526
Alcohol use
and cancer prevention, 31–32
and cancer survivors, 488–489
and smoking cessation, 176–177
ALL. See Acute lymphoblastic leukemia
Alzheimer's disease caregivers, depression of, 402
American Cancer Society
on age and cancer incidence, 24
and Cancer Control PLANET, 524
cancer reduction goals of, 61
and dietary interventions, 196
Look Good . . . Feel Better program
of, 421
*Nutrition and Physical Activity During
and After Cancer Treatment*,
487
on skin cancers, 33, 209
American College of Sport Medicine,
on physical inactivity, 237
American Dietetic Association, 198
American Heart Association, on physical inactivity, 237

American Indians, as smoking-cessation intervention target, 175

American Journal of Preventive Medicine, 543

American Journal of Public Health, 85, 90, 93, 97

American Society of Clinical Oncology, 339, 441

Amputation, cancer survivors with, 434

Analysis of covariance (ANCOVA), 91–92

Analysis of variance (ANOVA), 91–92

Androgen therapy, 384

Anemia, and CRF, 350

Angiogenesis, 503

Anthracycline class of chemotherapy, 433

Anticipatory nausea and vomiting (ANV), 349

Antiemetic medications, 348

Anxiety
   of cancer survivors, 414–415
      interventions for, 419
   and childhood cancer survivors, 451
   from expected nausea, 353
   over genetic testing, 307
   and HPV screening, 288–289
   in parents of childhood cancer survivors, 453
   of physicians in face of bad news, 329
   in reaction to diagnosis and treatment, 363
   and screening, 293, 295
      for cervical cancer, 288
      with fecal occult blood tests, 291
      positive breast cancer screening, 281–282, 284
   from screening invitation, 285, 286–287
   and treatment for reactions to cancer, 370

Asian Americans, as smoking-cessation intervention target, 175

Asplenic survivors, 436

Assessment intervals, 71

Attitude, definition of, 49

Audiotapes, as anti-MV intervention, 350

Australia, sun protection intervention in, 214

Australia (New South Wales), sun protection programs in, 211, 213–214

Australia (Queensland), sun protection policy in, 215

Bad news, oncologist's presentation of, 329, 330–331, 332–333

Beaches, sun protection intervention at, 215

Behavior (and behavior change)
   in cancer control, 9–10
   and cancer prevention, 24
   and cancer risk, 62, 79
      beliefs about, 136–138, 141–142
   and knowledge, 553
   knowledge about as critical, xix
   mechanisms linking with cancer, 502
   and risk assessment, 554
   and risk communication, 141–143
   and risk perception, 142
   See also Lifestyle

Behavioral assessment, for quality of life, 121–122

Behavioral causes of cancer, 3

Behavioral choice theory (BCT), 537–538

Behavioral epidemiology, 9

Behavioral intervention(s), 11, 12, 13, 347–348
   for cancer prevention and control, 62
      common approaches for, 63–64
      conceptual frameworks for, 63
      data analysis in, 74–79
      intervention design in, 64
   for cancer survivors, 487, 490–491
   efficacy and effectiveness of, 15–16
   for sexual rehabilitation after cancer, 383–385, 385–386

and treatment–outcome study
design, 68–74
for side effects, 353–354
fatigue, 350–351
nausea and vomiting, 348–350
pain, 351–352
Behavioral maintenance, 143
Behavioral and psychosocial factors in
cancer risk, xxi
Behavioral research, 17
Behavioral risk factors, difficulty of
influencing, 534
for tobacco use, 536
Behavioral Risk Factor Surveillance
Survey, 116
Behavioral Risk Factor Surveillance
System (1996), 27
Behavioral science, xxi, 6, 61
and cancer control (in integrative
framework), 11–15
in cancer control research, 5–6
and gynecologic cancers, 227–228
Behavioral theory, and behavioral intervention among cancer survivors,
490
Belgium, oophorectomy rate in, 308
Bereavement, and family caregivers,
401–402
Bias
in samples of breast cancer survivors,
413–14
in sandwich estimator, 92
selection bias, 86–87
Biobehavioral models, of psychosocial
variables and disease course in
cancer, 509
Biofeedback, as anti-NV intervention,
349
Bioinformatics and consumer, integrating of, 554
Biological mechanisms, as mediating
relation of psychological variables
to cancer etiology, 499–503
and biobehavioral models, 509
future directions for research on,
507–509

Biomarker feedback, 310
Blunters or blunting, of information
about cancer risks or diagnosis,
229–230
Body image
of cancer survivors, 416–417
interventions for, 420–421
patients' concern with, 363–364
Body and Soul program, 196–197
Bone marrow transplantation (BMT),
for children with leukemia and
solid tumors, 450
and siblings, 454
Borland, Ron, 210, 211
Boundary crossing, in transdisciplinary
research, 539
Brachytherapy, 381
Brain tumors, in children, 450, 451, 452
Breast cancer
and alcohol use, 489
behavioral factors in, 23
and cancer-survivor study, 106
and diet, 30, 31
genetic susceptibility to, 535
group psychological intervention
among women with, 504
husbands' failure to talk about, 470
and inactivity, 26
musculoskeletal late effects of, 434
and obesity, 28
and overestimation of risk, 136
preventive measures for, 137
and psychosocial telephone counseling, 230–231
and research on effects of cancer on
survivors, 413
screening for, 10, 34, 141
with mammography, 258,
260–264, 266, 309
population-based, 268
psychological consequences of,
280–284
and testosterone levels, 385
treatment of (and sexual dysfunction), 380–381

Breast cancer caregivers, psychoeducational support group for, 400
Breast Cancer Questionnaire, 121
Breast cancer survivors
    and body image, 416–417, 420–421
    depression in, 414
    diets of, 489
    fear of recurrence among, 415
    late effects with, 438
        from hormone therapy, 439
        and obesity, 433
    lymphedema in, 440
    reactions of, 363
Breast and Cervical Cancer Prevention and Treatment Act (2000), 34
Bupropion, 177, 178
Burden
    in family caregiving, 392, 397, 398
    response, 74

Calcium, and cancer risk, 30
Cancer
    causes of, xviii
        behavioral, 3 (see also Behavior; Lifestyle)
    deaths from, 23
        projected increase in, 24
    and depression, 504
        mechanisms linking with, 500–503
    as genetic disease, 534–535
    as heterogeneous group of diseases, 500
    interval cancers, 293
    prevalence of (various types), 414
    and psychological interventions in cancer survival, 505–507
    and psychological variables mediated by biological mechanisms, 499–503
    and biobehavioral models, 509
    future directions for research on, 507–509
    and psychosocial variables in cancer development, 503–504

and psychosocial variables in cancer progression, 504–505
    recovery from (domains of), 413
    survival rate for, 328
Cancer (publication), 90, 93
Cancer Care teleconference series, 423
Cancer clinical trials, participation in. See Participation in cancer clinical trials
Cancer control, 6, 11
    behavior in, 9–10
    behavioral interventions for, 62
        common approaches for, 63–64
        conceptual frameworks for, 63
        data analysis in, 74–79
        intervention design in, 64
        and treatment–outcome study design, 68–74
    and behavioral science (in integrative framework), 11–15
    disparities in, 19–20 (see also Gender differences; Racial or ethnic differences)
    emerging themes and directions in, 15–19
    goals of, 12, 13, 15
    and group-randomized trials, 85
    and patients, 10
Cancer control continuum, 7–9, 11
Cancer control interventions
    design of, 17–19
    dissemination of, 17
    evaluation of, 525
    See also Intervention(s); specific types of intervention
Cancer Control PLANET (Plan, Link, Act, Network with Evidence-Based Tools) web portal, 524
Cancer control research. See Research on cancer control
Cancer Epidemiology, Biomarkers & Prevention, 90, 93, 927
Cancer health disparities among population groups (NCI), 517–518
    elimination of as goal, 526
    See also Gender differences; Racial or ethnic differences

Cancer Health Disparities Progress
Review Group (CHD PRG), 519
Cancer immunoediting, 500
Cancer and Leukemia Group B
(CALGB), 105–106
Cancer prevention. *See* Prevention of
cancer
Cancer Prevention and Control
Research Network (CPCRN),
525–526, 527
Cancer registries, 116
Cancer Rehabilitation Evaluation
System (CARES), 119, 120
Cancer-related fatigue (CRF), behav-
ioral intervention for, 350–351
Cancer risk. *See* Risk of cancer
*Cancer Risk Communication: What We
Know and What We Need to Learn*
(journal volume), 133
Cancer screening. *See* Screening
Cancer survivors. *See* Survivors of
cancer
Cancer syndromes, hereditary, 303. *See
also* Genetic testing
Cancer treatment. *See* Treatment
Cardiac rehabilitation, physical-activity
interventions for, 240
Cardiovascular disease risk factors,
interventions for, 241
Cardiovascular late effects, 432–433
Caregivers, and sun protection inter-
ventions, 213–214
Caregiving, family. *See* Family caregiving
Carotenoids, and cancer risk, 31
Cataracts, from corticosteroid
chemotherapeutic agents, 439
Causes of chronic diseases, sociological
and environmental models of, xviii
CDC. *See* Centers for Disease Control
and Prevention
CD-ROM, tailored messages on, 192
Center on Budget and Policy Priorities,
on food taxes, 198
Center for Patient Partnerships,
University of Wisconsin Law

School, Cancer Legal Resource
Center, 423
Centers for Disease Control and
Prevention (CDC)
and Cancer Control PLANET, 524
and cervical cancer screening, 34
on physical inactivity, 237
on vaccination for HPV, 226
Cervical cancer
epidemiology and risk factors for,
226
population-based screening for, 268
prevention, detection and screening
of, 33, 228, 231
screening for
and colposcopy offer, 294
with Pap test
psychological consequences of,
284–289
rates of, 10, 256
and smoking, 179
Chemoprevention (tamoxifen), 310
Chemotherapy
anthracycline class of, 433
interventions for side effects of, 349
late effects of
endocrine, 435–436
gastrointestinal, 438
genitourinary, 437
neurologic, 438
neuropathy, 440
obesity, 433
pulmonary, 437
Child and Adolescent Trial for
Cardiovascular Health, 238
Child Behavior Checklist, 454
Childhood cancer, 449
Childhood cancer survivors, 431–432,
449–450
directions for future research on,
456–458
effects on families of, 452–455
interventions for, 455–456, 457
neurocognitive effects on, 450–451
psychological functioning of,
451–452

Childhood cancer survivors (*continued*)
  social functioning of, 452
  See also Pediatric cancer survivors
Children, sun protection interventions
      for, 210–212
Children's Oncology Group, 441
Chronic effect, 432
Chronic effects of cancer treatment, 440
Clinical Disease pathway, 11, 12, 14
Clinical trials, increasing participation
      in, 59. *See also* Participation in
      cancer clinical trials
Coalition building, 46
Cochrane Collaboration, 524
Cochrane Review(s), 524
  on academic detailing, 173
Cognitions, definition of, 49
Cognitive behavior and skill training
      therapy, for smoking cessation,
      170
Cognitive behavior therapy
  for cancer survivors, 419
  and motivational interviewing, 193
  in treatment of reactions to cancer,
      369
Cognitive-Social Health Information
      Processing (C-SHIP) framework
      or model, 18, 45, 141–142
  for prevention of gynecologic cancer,
      229–230
Collaborative filtering, 549–550
College-age adults, sun protection inter-
      vention for, 213
College student samples, 138n
Collins, Francis S., 303
Colon and colorectal cancer
  behavioral factors in, 23
  and cancer-survivor study, 106
  depression in survivors of, 414
  and diet, 29, 29–30, 30, 31
  with FOBT or sigmoidoscopy, 258
  genetic susceptibility to, 535
  and inactivity, 26
  and obesity, 28
  screening for, 10, 34, 137, 256, 534
    with fecal occult blood test,
      266–267

and genetic testing, 309–310
  population-based, 268
  psychological consequences of,
      289–292
  and smoking, 24
Colonoscopy, 279, 289, 290, 292, 309
Colposcopy, 285–286, 287–288, 294
Communication, across disciplines, 538
Communication (in patient's relation-
      ships), and reaction to cancer
      diagnosis and treatment, 364
Communication (practitioner–patient),
      327, 328–333, 341
  culture, ethnicity and language in,
      335–336
  and families of cancer survivors, 473,
      474–475
  with family of patient, 336, 338
  future research on, 340–341
  and informed consent, 336–337
  in marriages of cancer survivors, 470
  online, 553
  scientific study of, 328
  tailored, 550
  training of patients in, 339–340
  training of practitioners in, 337–339
  and treatment decision making,
      333–337
Communication–persuasion matrix, 46,
      48
Communications, 49
Community approaches to health
      behavior change, 45–47, 48
  in dietary change, 193–194, 200–201
  for physical activity, 240–242
  for sun protection, 211–212
  in tobacco use prevention, 156
    combined with media campaigns,
      159
Community-based care for childhood
      cancer survivors and families, 458
Community-based education, for smok-
      ing cessation intervention,
      172–173
Community development, 48
Community organizing, 48

Competency-based approaches, in research on childhood cancer survivors, 457
Complementary medicine, for cancer prevention, 310
Computer-driven interventions, 554
Computer-mediated support services, 550–551
Computers
    in smoking cessation programs, 173–174, 174
    sun safety instruction on, 211
Concept mapping, in transdisciplinary collaboration, 540
Conceptual models
    and gynecologic cancer prevention, 229–231
    and intervention components, 79
    translating of, 67–68
Concurrent stressors, on families of cancer survivors, 473–474
Conditioning theory, 48
Consolidated Standards for Reporting of Trials statement, 268
CONSORT (Consolidated Standards of Reporting Trials) statement, 77–78, 509
Consumer health informatics, 547
    integrating of with bioinformatics, 554
    integrating of with medical informatics, 553
    See also Interactive health communications
Consumers, and quality of life, 116
Contamination, of group randomized trials, 87
Continuum
    of cancer control, 7–9, 11
    of cancer prevention and control interventions, 64–66
    of care, 273
    of responses to genetic testing, 304
Control groups, 69
Control theory, 48

Coping
    and cancer etiology, 503
    and cancer progression, 505
    and family caregivers, 392, 396
    in processing bad news, 329
    and responses to genetic information, 308
    and stressful event or situation, 230
Coping With Cancer, 476
Coping skills interventions, in treatment of reactions to cancer, 368
Cortisol, 501
Cost, and genetic-testing decision, 305
Counseling
    for dietary change, 191
    for spouses of cancer victims, 476–477
Cranial radiation therapy (CRT), in children, 450
Cultural context
    in communication, 335–336
        future research on, 341
    and school-based prevention programs, 154
    and self-reports of screening, 269
    and tobacco use prevention, 161
Curative care, 10

Data analysis, 74–79
Data collection methods, in behavioral intervention studies, 70–71
Decision aids, 140
Decision making on treatment
    and communication, 333–337
    cultural variation in approach to, 335–336
    family-centered model of, 336
    participation styles in, 335
    in patient-centered model, 327
    as research theme, 15–16, 272
Definitions, clarity and consistency needed in, 269
Delivery, in implementation of intervention, 51
Demographic influences, on genetic-testing decisions, 305–307
Denial, 329

Department of Health and Human
Services, U.S. (USDHHS), 519
Department of Veterans Affairs, U.S.,
and electronic medical records
systems, 553
Depression, 501
and cancer, 500–503, 503–504, 504,
507, 508
of cancer survivors, 414–415
interventions for, 419
and childhood cancer survivors, 451
and CRF, 350
of family caregivers, 393, 395, 398
during bereavement period, 402
and hospice, 401
in parents of childhood cancer survivors, 453
in reaction to diagnosis and treatment, 363
and smoking cessation, 177–178
among women, 179
and treatment for reactions to cancer, 370
"Designing for Dissemination" (NCI
conference, 2002), 518
Detection, for gynecologic cancers,
227–228
Developmental phases of family, and
families of cancer survivors,
475–476
Diabetes, physical-activity interventions
for, 240
Diagnosis, and informed consent,
336–337
Diagnostic disclosure, 329–331
*Diagnostic and Statistical Manual of
Mental Disorders* (4th ed.), on
PTSD, 416, 451
and mothers of childhood cancer
survivors, 453
Diaries, on sexual practices or frequency, 383
Dietary improvement
and cancer prevention, 29–31
of cancer survivors, 489
difficulty of, 189–190

through physical-activity interventions at worksite, 239
See also Nutrition
Dietary interventions, 190–191,
200–201
environmental and policy-level,
197–200
individual-level approaches to,
191–193
interpersonal and social networks in,
193–94, 200–201
organizational settings for, 194–197
Differential history, for group randomized trials, 87
Differential maturation, for group randomized trials, 87
Diffusion, 17, 45–46
Diffusion of innovation, 45–46, 47, 48,
522–523
Diffusion of innovation model, 522–523
and sun protection interventions,
215
Discoveries, levels of, xix
Disease-related predictors of reaction to
cancer diagnosis and treatment
characteristics, 365–66
resources, 366–368
Dissemination, of cancer control interventions, 17, 523
Distress, of cancer survivors, 414–415
interventions for, 419
Diversity
need for in caregiver research samples, 479
and screening interventions, 271
and self-reports of screening, 269
Diversity Enhancement Program (DEP),
108
"Dot-bomb" bubble, 548
Drug Abuse Resistance Education–type
programs, 154
Drug prevention programs, school-
based, 154
Drug use, and needle exchange programs, 33

Early disease pathway, 11, 12, 13–14
Eating for a Healthy Life program, 197
Ecological momentary assessments, 70–71
Ecological perspectives, on behavior change, 45
Education
    for dietary change, 191
    and inactivity, 27
    as predictor of reaction to cancer diagnosis and treatment, 365
    See also Socioeconomic status
Educational interventions
    and cancer survival, 506–507
    for childhood cancer survivors and families, 457
    for family caregivers, 398–399
    on genetic testing, 311–312
Education of health care providers. *See* Training of health care providers
Effectiveness studies
    vs. efficacy studies, 17, 68–69, 519
    and response burden, 74
Effect moderator, 77
Efficacy studies
    vs. effectiveness studies, 17, 68–69, 519
    and response burden, 74
Efficacy of test, 256
eHealth, 547. *See also* Interactive health communications
Electrical stimulation, as anti-NV intervention, 349
Electronic medical records systems, in Department of Veterans Affairs, 553
Emotional distress, for families of cancer survivors, 473
Emotional repression, and cancer progression, 505
Emotional well-being
    and families of cancer survivors, 468–469
    of family caregivers, 392–393
Emotions, in reaction to cancer diagnosis and treatment, 362–363

Employment, after cancer, 422–423
End-of-life care
    transition to, 331–332
    See also Palliative care
Endocrine late effects, 435–436
Endometrial cancer
    epidemiology and risk factors for, 227
    future research on, 231
    and obesity, 28
    prevention, detection and screening of, 227
Environment, medical, 368
Environment, and physical activity, 244–245
Environmental dietary interventions, 197–200
Environmental exposures, 535. *See also* Behavior; Lifestyle
Environmental hazards, 35
Environmental theory, for physical activity interventions in work sites, 239
EORTC Quality of Life Questionnaire—Cancer 30 Items (QLC–C30), 119, 120
Epidemiology, of gynecologic cancers, 225–227
Epigenetics, xxi
Erectile dysfunction (ED), from cancer treatment, 380
    for prostate cancer, 381
Error, Type I, 88, 89, 92, 96
Error, Type II, 73, 369
Ethnicity, in communication, 335–336
    future research on, 341
Ethnic minorities, 19. *See also* Minorities; Racial or ethnic differences
European Organisation for Research and Treatment of Cancer Quality of Life Questionnaire—Cancer 30 Items (EORTC QLQ–C30), 119, 120
Evidence-based cancer control interventions
    adoption of, 524
    dissemination of, 523

Evidence-based public health practice, 520–522
  growth of, 526
Exercise, 240, 240n
  for fatigue, 350
  See also Physical activity
Expectations of patients
  and reaction to cancer diagnosis and treatment, 366, 367
  and side effects, 352–354
    nausea or vomiting, 348
Expert system interventions, 243–244
Expert systems, 550, 551
Exposure, in implementation of intervention, 51

Facing Forward (educational material), 423
False assurance, from negative screening, 293
False negative results of screening, 294, 295
  of breast cancer screening, 281
False positive results of screening, 293
  of breast cancer screening, 281–284
  of fecal occult blood tests, 291
Family
  communicating with, 336, 338
  in dietary change interventions, 193–194
  genetic-testing communication among, 312–313
  and genetic-testing decision, 306
  in patient-centered model, 327
Family(ies) of cancer survivors, 467
  directions for future research on, 478–480
  interventions to improve coping of, 476–478
  quality-of-life issues of, 468–476
Family caregiving, 391, 402–403
  and bereavement, 401–402
  caregiver responses, 392–394
  conceptual frameworks for, 392
  interventions for improvement of, 398–401

research on, 394, 398, 401, 402–403
  and risk factors for caregivers, 394–396
  skills and needs of, 397–398
Family(ies) of childhood cancer survivors
  interventions on behalf of, 455–457
  psychological effects on, 452–455
Family prevention programs (tobacco), 155–156
  and Family Matters program, 156
Family stress theory, 468
Fat, dietary, and cancer rates, 30
Fatigue
  behavioral interventions for, 350–351
  among family caregivers of cancer patients, 471
Fears
  in reaction to cancer diagnosis and treatment, 363–364
    of recurrence, 363, 415–416, 420
  See also Anxiety
Fecal occult blood test (FOBT), 266–267, 279
  false positive results of, 291
  negative results from, 290
  review of determinants of, 257
Fertility
  and marriages of cancer survivors, 470
  and quality of life, 117
  See also Infertility
Fiber, and cancer prevention, 30
Filtering, collaborative, 549–550
Finland, and selenium fortification, 31
Flexible sigmoidoscopy (FS), 289
  negative results from, 290
  positive results from, 292
  See also Sigmoidoscopy
Florida, antismoking campaign in, 158
FOBT. *See* Fecal occult blood test
Folate, and cancer risk, 29–30
Follow-up examinations, 433
Food pricing, 198–199
Food taxation, restrictive, 197–198

Fruits, and cancer risk, 29
FS. *See* Flexible sigmoidoscopy
Functional Assessment of Cancer
    Therapy—General (FACT–G),
    119, 120
Funding initiatives, for transdisciplinary
    collaborations, 543

Gamble technique, for quality-of-life
    assessment, 122
Gastrointestinal late effects, 438–439
Gender differences
    in alcohol use, 32
    in caregiver distress, 395
    in effect of antismoking campaign,
        157
    in focus of research on reactions to
        cancer, 362
    in inactivity, 27
    in overweight/obesity, 28
    and psychosocial adaptation to can-
        cer, 415
    and screening, 272
    in sexual dysfunction from cancer
        treatment, 381
    and smoking cessation, 178–179
    in smoking rates, 25, 26
General Health Questionnaire (GHQ),
    and management choices after
    Pap results, 286
Generalized estimating equations
    (GEE), 91
Generic instruments, for quality-of-life
    assessment, 118–120
Genetic factors
    in cancer process, 534–535
    and impact of genetic risk informa-
        tion, 307–310
    and nicotine dependence, 536
    and physical activity, 246
Genetic testing, 303–304, 311–314
    barriers to access to, 312
    educational interventions on,
        311–312
    and lifestyle changes, 310, 313
    predictors of uptake in, 304–307

and screening behaviors, 309–310
Genomics research, 303
Geographical differences, in reatten-
    dance after breast cancer screen-
    ings, 283
Goals of cancer control, 12, 13, 15
Go Sun Smart program, 214
Graduate education, for smoking cessa-
    tion intervention, 172
Great Britain (United Kingdom)
    1980s apprehension over abnormal
        Pap smears in, 295
    oophorectomy rate in, 308
Group interventions, 369–370
    for sexual rehabilitation after cancer,
        383
Group-level factors, in screening behav-
    ior, 270
Group-randomized trials (GRT), 85
    analytic issues for, 87–90
        and inappropriate analytic meth-
            ods, 95–96
        and misguided strategies, 88–89
    design issues for, 86–87
    recent developments in, 90
    recommendations on, 96–97
    review of literature on, 90–96
Group therapy, for cancer survivors, 419
Growth hormone (GH), secondary, 433
Guide to Clinical Preventive Services, 524
Guide to Community Preventive Services,
    524, 527
Guided imagery, as anti-NV interven-
    tion, 349
Gynecologic cancer
    conceptual models applied to pre-
        vention of, 229–231
    depression in survivors of, 414
    epidemiology and specific risk factors
        of, 225–227
        fear of recurrence among sur-
            vivors of, 415
    future research on, 231
    prevalence of, 225
        for cervical cancer, 226

Gynecologic cancer (*continued*)
    prevention, detection and screening
        of, 227–228
    See also Breast cancer; Cervical can-
        cer; Human papillomavirus;
        Ovarian cancer

Health belief model, 44, 47, 48, 134,
    522
    for sun protection intervention, 212
Health care providers, and smoking ces-
    sation, 170–174, 180
Health care system, challenge to, xviii
Health Education & Behavior, 90, 93
Health Interview Survey, 116
    on cervical cancer screening, 34
Health-related problems, and interven-
    tions for childhood cancer sur-
    vivors, 456
Health-related quality of life (HRQOL),
    117
Health Works for Women, 196
Healthy People 2010, 238
Healthy People 2010 goals, 189, 526
Hepatitis, 437
Hereditary cancer syndromes, 303. *See
    also* Genetic testing
Hispanics
    and inactivity, 27
    and smoking cessation, 175
Hispanic women, and cervical cancer
    screening, 34
Hodgkin's disease (HD)
    and asplenia, 436
    and cardiovascular disease 432
    mood disorders in survivors of, 414
    and secondary cancer, 439
    and thyroid disease, 436
Hodgkin's lymphoma, and cancer-
    survivor study, 106
Home health care interventions, and
    family caregiving, 400
Hopelessness
    and cancer, 503, 505, 507
    among families of cancer survivors,
        474

Horse-race studies, 65
Hospice, and family caregiving, 401
Hospitals, sun protection for small chil-
    dren through, 210
Human genome discoveries, 531,
    534–535
    and health risks, 554
Human Genome Project, 303
Human papillomavirus (HPV), 32, 61,
    226, 231, 284–285
    testing for, 231, 288–289, 294
    vaccination against, 33, 285, 289
Hyperthyroidism, 436
Hypnosis, as anti-NV intervention, 349

ICC (intraclass correlation coefficient),
    88–89, 93
Identifiable group, 85
Illness demands, on families of cancer
    survivors, 473, 473–474
Illness representation model, 141
Image, body. *See* Body image
Imagery, as anti-NV intervention, 349
Immigrants, and cancer risk, 34
Immunity, and psychosocial factors,
    500–501
Immunoediting, cancer, 500
Implementation, 17, 51, 64
    of antismoking policy, 160
    of cardiovascular disease interven-
        tions, 241
    of innovation, 523
    of physical-activity intervention in
        schools, 238
    and school-based prevention, 153,
        155
Incentives, in cancer prevention and
    control trials, 74
Income
    as predictor of reaction to cancer
        diagnosis and treatment, 365
    See also Socioeconomic status
Individual differences, 11
    in integrative framework, 15
    and personalized medicine based on
        DNA, 535

and research on psychology–cancer link, 509–510

Infants, sun protection interventions for, 210

Infectious late effects, 436–437

Infertility
and cancer during young adulthood, 475
as late effect
from chemotherapy, 435
from gonadal tissue damage, 436
See also Fertility

Informational support, and reaction to cancer diagnosis and treatment, 368

Information needs, 333–335

Informed consent
and communication, 336–337
and conveying of information, 330

Innovation, 46
and diffusion of innovations model, 45–46, 47, 522–523
and knowledge sharing, 540

Innovative advances in cancer prevention and control, xxii

Institute of Medicine
on behavioral risk factors, 61
cancer survivorship reports of, 423
on dietary improvement intervention, 190
Unequal Treatment . . . report of, 517

Insurance discrimination, and genetic-testing decision, 305

Integrative framework, for cancer control and behavioral science, 11–15

Intention-to-treat principle, 77–78

Interactive health communications (IHC), 547, 554–555
effectiveness of, 549–551
future directions for, 549–554
reach of, 548

Interactive interventions, 243, 244

Interdisciplinary focus, for physical activity interventions, 245–246

Interdisciplinary and transdisciplinary approach, xvii

International Index of Erectile Dysfunction, 383

Internet
cancer support groups on, 418–419
and family caregiving information, 397
and interactive health communications, 547, 548, 549
for screening interventions, 271
and smoking cessation, 174
tailored messages on, 192
tobacco use promotion in, 161

Interpersonal dimensions of patient care, and oncologist training, 328

Interpersonal influences, on genetic-testing decisions, 305–307

Interval cancers, 293

Intervention(s)
addressing quality of life, 124
dissemination of, 523
and efficacy studies vs. effectiveness studies, 17, 68–69, 519
evaluation of variables in, 51–52
family-based (of cancer survivors), 476–478
impact of, 525
implementation of, 51, 64
and school-based tobacco prevention, 153, 155
research categories providing evidence base for, 268
and smoking cessation, 174
tailoring and targeting of, 15, 16–17
See also Cancer control interventions

Intervention design, 64–8

Intervention outcomes, 12, 13

Intervention research, 6, 62
study design in, 59

Interviewing, motivational, 64, 170, 193

Intraclass correlation coefficient (ICC), 88–89, 93

Israel, sun protection intervention in, 214

Item response theory (IRT), and quality-of-life assessment, 123

Job lock, 422
Journal of the National Cancer Institute, 90, 93, 133

Kaiser Permanente and Group Health Cooperative, and information integration, 553
Karnofsky score, 121
Knowledge, and behavior, 553
Knowledge transfer, 17
Korean Americans, communication values of, 336

Language, in communication, 335–336
   future research on, 341
Late effect, 432
Late effects of cancer treatment, 432–439
   follow-up activities and surveillance for, 440–441
   medical, 432–439
Late effects of cancer and treatment for cancer in children, 449–450
   among family, 452–455
   neurocognitive, 450–451
   psychological, 449, 451–452
   in social functioning, 452
Latina women
   and cervical cancers, 226
   HPV status among, 231
   and physical activity interventions for female adolescents, 241
Laws, in tobacco use prevention, 159–160
Leadership, shared, in transdisciplinary collaboration, 540
Learning model, for pretreatment side effects, 349
Legacy Media Tracking Survey, 158
Leisure, for cancer survivors, 422
Leukemia
   and cancer-survivor study, 106
   secondary, 43

Leukemia (acute), mood disorders in survivors of, 414
Leukoencephalopathy, 438
Levels of discovery and treatment, xix
Library, Internet as, 549
Life events
   and cancer etiology, 503
   measure of, 507
Life Events and Difficulties Scale, 507
Life Skills Training Program (LST), 153, 154
Lifestyle, 23
   and cancer etiology, 504
   for cancer prevention, 35
   in cancer-related deaths, 61
   and cancer survivors, 487, 488–490
   and community's rules of conduct, 45
   and genetic testing, 310, 313
   mechanisms linking with cancer, 502
   and research on late effects, 441
   See also Behavior
Likelihood risk judgments, 134, 142
Liquid-based cytology, 284
Literature on group randomized trials, review of, 90–96
Literature on reactions to cancer diagnosis and treatment, 362
Locus of control theory, and expectations, 353
Logic map, in transdisciplinary collaboration, 540–541
Longitudinal learning programs, in training for communication, 338
Longitudinal randomized trials, on family caregiving, 394
Low-income population
   and occupational or environmental hazards, 35
   and physical activity, 27
   and workplace dietary intervention, 196
   See also Socioeconomic status
Lumpectomy, 380, 417

Lung cancer
    behavioral factors in, 23
    biomarket feedback on, 310
    and cigarette smoking, 23, 24
    and diet, 29, 31
    and physical activity, 26–27
    screening for, 137, 268
Lung cancer survivors, depression in,
    414
Lymphedema, 440
Lymphoma, depression in survivors of,
    414

Maintenance of behavior, 143
Making Cancer Health Disparities History
    (USDHHS), 519
Mammography, 256, 258, 260–264, 266,
    279, 280–281, 309
    adherence rates for, 534
    review of determinants of, 257
Marriages
    of cancer survivors, 469–471
    as stressed by cancer, 364
    See also Family
Massachusetts, antismoking campaign
    in, 157–158
Mastectomy, 308, 380, 417
Master Settlement Agreement, 25
Measures
    development of as research category,
        268–269
    process and outcome, 71–72
    self-report, 70–71
Meat, red, and cancer risk, 30
Media, dietary education over, 200
Media approaches to tobacco use pre-
    vention, 157–159
Media-based interventions, for physical
    activity improvement, 239
Mediation hypotheses, 18
    in intervention design, 17–19
Mediator variable, 77
    of physical activity interventions,
        244
    and screening behaviors, 257

and tobacco use prevention pro-
    grams, 153, 155
in treatment for reactions to cancer,
    370–371
Medical and consumer informatics,
    integrating of, 553
Medical environment, and reaction to
    cancer diagnosis and treatment,
    368
Medical late effects of cancer treatment,
    432–439
Medically ill populations, and smoking
    cessation, 179–180
Medical Outcomes Study Short Form—
    36 (SF-36), 118, 119
    and colonoscopy impact, 290
Medical schools, and tobacco cessation
    techniques, 172
Medicine, evidence-based, 520, 521
Melanoma, 33–34, 209, 214. *See also*
    Sun protection interventions
Memorial Sloan Kettering Cancer
    Center, Post-Treatment Resource
    Program of, 423
Mental representations, 48
Mexican Americans, communication
    values of, 336
Minnesota Heart Health program, 241
Minorities
    as cancer survivors (unemployed risk
        of), 422–423
    as excluded from research on child-
        hood cancer survivors, 458
    recruitment of into cancer clinical
        trials, 105, 110
    and screening, 257
    smoking cessation interventions for
        (racial/ethnic), 175–176
    as underrepresented in research on
        psychosocial response (eth-
        nic), 19
    as underserved by physical activity
        interventions, 243
    unequal burden of cancer among,
        517

Minorities (*continued*)
  and workplace dietary intervention,
    196
Missing outcome data, 78, 124
Moderator, effect, 77
Moderating factors
  and screening behaviors, 257
  and tobacco use prevention pro-
    grams, 153
  in treatment for reactions to cancer,
    370–371
Molecular and behavioral signature, 11,
  12
Monetary incentives, for physical activity, 244
Monitoring attentional style, 280
Monitoring the Future study, and ciga-
  rette smoking, 152
Monitors, of information about cancer
  risks, 229–230
Mood, in reaction to cancer diagnosis
  and treatment, 362–363
Motivational interviewing, 64, 193
  for dietary change, 193
  for smoking cessation, 170
Multicomponent treatment, 69
Multilevel intervention
  for physical activity (research on), 537
  for recruitment into cancer clinical
    trial, 104–110, 111
Multilevel and population-level (public
  health-level) interventions, 19
Multiphase optimization strategy
  (MOST) designs, 552
Multiple comparison problem, 75
Multiple screening tests, 264–265, 267
Multiunit interventions, for sun protec-
  tion, 211
Musculoskeletal late effects, 434–435

National Cancer Act (1971), 531
National Cancer Institute (NCI)
  on age and cancer incidence, 24
  and Cancer Control PLANET, 524
  and cancer health disparities, 517,
    518

Cancer Information Service of, 311
on definition of "cancer control," 6
"Designing for Dissemination" conference of, 518
and dietary interventions, 196
on dissemination , 17
Facing Forward program of, 423
family-caregiving focus groups of,
  397
and "team science" approach, xvii
as TTURC sponsor, 536
National Cancer Institute of Canada,
  Advisory Committee on Cancer
  Control of, 6
National Coalition for Cancer
  Survivorship, Toolbox and
  Almanac program of, 423
National Health Interview Survey
  on drinkers, 32
  and factors behind screening behav-
    ior, 257
  an race and smoking incidence, 25
National Health and Nutrition
  Examination Surveys, on SES
  and obesity, 29
National Institute for Drug Abuse, as
  TTURC sponsor, 536
National Institutes of Health (NIH)
  and QOL research, 123
  and transdisciplinary collaboration
    542
Nausea, behavioral interventions for,
  348–350
Needle exchange programs, 33
Neoplasms, second malignant, 439
  screening for, 441
Netherlands, oophorectomy rate in, 308
Neurocognitive effects, on childhood
  cancer survivors, 450–451
Neurocognitive interventions, for child-
  hood cancer survivors and fami-
  lies, 455
Neurologic late effects, 437–438
Neuropathy, 440
  peripheral, 438

Nicotine replacement therapy (NRT), 174, 176–177, 178

Nonrandom missing data, as methodological issue, 78, 124

Norms, and antismoking campaigns, 160

Norway, media antismoking campaign in, 157

Nottingham Health Profile, 118, 119

Nutrition
deficiency in, 534
See also Dietary improvement

Nutrition education
computer-based interactive, 192
See also Dietary interventions

Nutrition and Physical Activity During and After Cancer Treatment (American Cancer Society), 487

NV. *See* Nausea; Vomiting

Obesity
and cancer incidence, 26
in cancer survivors, 489
and cardiovascular late effects, 432–433
as late effect of cancer, 433–434

Obesity prevention, and cancer prevention, 28–29

Occupational hazards, 35

Ohio State University (OSU), in recruitment case study, 109

Older people
depression–cancer association among, 501
as excluded from survivorship studies, 414
physical inactivity among, 242
and research on late effects, 441
as underserved by physical activity interventions, 243

Oncology Interactive Education Series, 340

Oncotalk program, 338–339

Online communication, between clinicians and patients, 553

Online support groups, 550–551

Online therapists, 551

Oophorectomy, 308–309
and worry, 136

Optimism
of family caregivers, 396
in reaction to cancer diagnosis and treatment, 367

Organizational settings, for dietary interventions, 194–197

Oropharyngeal cancer, depression in survivors of, 414

Osteopenia, 434

Osteoporosis, 434

Outcome efficacy, 45

Outcome measures, 71–72

Outcome studies, treatment, 65, 68–74

Outcome targets, 67

Ovarian cancer
epidemiology and risk factors for, 226–227
fear of recurrence among survivors of, 415
future research on, 231
genetic susceptibility to, 535
and oophorectomy, 308–309
prevention, detection and screening of, 227
and psychosocial telephone counseling, 230–231
screening for, 309
and VEGF, 503
and worry in decision to remove ovaries, 136

Pain
behavioral interventions for, 351–352
chronic, 440

Palliative care, 10
transition to, 331–332

Palliative care specialists, and terminal prognoses, 330

Pancreatic cancer, depression in survivors of, 414

Papaniculou (Pap) smear test, 23, 228, 255, 256, 259–260, 266, 279, 284, 285

Papaniculou (Pap) smear test (*continued*)
    and follow-up attending, 286
    and HPV, 289
    review of determinants of, 257
    studies on use of, 258
Parental effects on adolescent smoking,
    155–156
Parents, sun protection interventions
    for, 213–214
Parents of childhood cancer survivors
    interventions on behalf of, 456
    psychological effects on, 452–453
Participation in cancer clinical trials,
    103–104, 110–111
    recruitment for, 104, 110
    recruitment framework (ACT) for,
        104–105, 111
        case study of, 105–111
        future research needed on, 111
Participation styles, in decision making,
    335
Participatory learning principles, 212
Patient-centered model, 327
Patient populations, physical-activity
    interventions for, 240
Patient-reported outcome (PRO), 117
Pawtucket Heart Health Program, 241
Pediatric cancer survivors, 431–432
    clinical practice guidelines for, 441
Pediatric Quality of Life Inventory, 121
Peer discussion, and treatment for reac-
    tions to cancer, 370
Performance status scale for head and
    neck cancer patients, 122
Peripheral neuropathy, 438
Personal characteristics, as predictor of
    reaction to cancer diagnosis and
    treatment, 365–366
Personality style, and cancer etiology,
    503
Personal resources, as predictor of reac-
    tion to cancer diagnosis and
    treatment, 366–368
Persuasive communication, 46, 48
Pew Internet and American Life
    Project, 548

Phantom limb pain, 434
Philip Morris tobacco company, Think,
    Don't Smoke campaign of, 159
Physical activity, 237n
    benefits of, 237, 246
    and cancer prevention, 26–27
    among cancer survivors, 489
    lack of, 237, 238, 246
    recommendation for increase of,
        237–238
*Physical Activity and Cardiovascular
    Health*, 237–238
*Physical Activity and Health: A Report of
    the Surgeon General*, 237
Physical activity interventions, 246, 537
    community-based, 240–242
    large-group vs. small-group focus for,
        242–243, 246
    new directions for, 242–246
    population based, 238–240
    successes among, 242
Physical inactivity, microlevel and
    macrolevel interventions for,
        537–538
Physical well-being
    of families of cancer survivors,
        471–472
    of family caregivers, 393
Placebo effect, as expectancy, 352
Planned behavior, theory of, 44, 48, 49,
    490
Planning
    in recruitment for clinical trials, 111
    of studies, 97
Point-of-decision prompts, for encour-
    aging physical activity, 240, 242,
    245
Policies, 49
Policy advocacy, 48
Policy approaches
    to dietary change, 197–201
    and indoor tanning facilities, 216
    and physical activity, 245–246
    to tobacco use prevention, 159–160
Polygenic disorders, 230
Polyp Prevention Trial, 191
Population sciences, 6

Population-wide prevention, 23
    in dietary improvement, 190
    for sun protection, 34
Positive screening results, from flexible
    sigmoidoscopy, 292
Postgraduate education, for smoking
    cessation intervention, 172–173
"Posttraumatic growth," 479
Posttraumatic stress disorder (PTSD)
    and cancer survivors, 416
        interventions for, 420
    in childhood cancer survivors, 451,
        452
    and mothers of childhood cancer
        survivors, 453
Posttraumatic stress symptoms (PTSS)
    in childhood cancer survivors, 451
    interventions against, 456
    and parental distress, 457
    among siblings of children with can-
        cer, 454
Practice. See Public health practice
Practice-based research networks
    (PBRNs), 526
Precaution adoption model, 44, 48
Predisease pathway, 11, 12, 13
Pre–post observational studies, 70
Preschool children, sun protection
        interventions for, 210
President's Cancer Panel, cancer sur-
        vivorship reports of, 423
Prevention of cancer, 23–24, 35
    and alcohol use limitation, 31
    behavioral interventions for, 62
        common approaches for, 63–64
        conceptual frameworks for, 63
        data analysis in, 74–79
        intervention design in, 64
        and treatment–outcome study
            design, 68–74
    and diet, 29–31
    follow-up activities for, 440–441
    and group-randomized trials, 85
    and gynecologic cancers, 227–228
        conceptual models of, 229–231

through oophorectomy and mastec-
        tomy, 308–309
    phases of
        primary, 7, 8, 9, 18, 34, 131, 256
        secondary, 7, 8, 9–10, 18, 34, 253
        tertiary, 7, 8, 10, 18, 325
        quaternary, 7, 8, 10, 18, 411
    and physical activity, 26–27
    through screening, 34
    and sex and viral transmission,
        32–33
    of skin cancer, 209, 216
        through sun protection, 33–34
            (see also Sun protection
            intervention)
    and tobacco use cessation, 24–26
    and weight control/obesity preven-
        tion, 28–29
    See also Intervention(s); specific types
        of intervention
Prevention of cancer, phases of. See
        Primary prevention; Quaternary
        prevention; Secondary preven-
        tion; Tertiary prevention
Preventive Medicine, 85, 90, 93
Price increases, for tobacco use, 160
Primary appraisal, of stressful event or
        situation, 230
Primary prevention, 7, 8, 9, 131
    for colorectal and cervical cancers,
        34
    and screening, 256
    as theory driven, 18
Princess Margaret Hospital (PMH),
        computer-based patient educa-
        tion program of, 340
Print communications, tailored, 16–17
Problem-solving skills, for family care-
        givers, 399
Process measures, 71–72
Process targets, 67
Professional specialization, 538
Prognosis, discussions about, 329–331
Progressive muscle relaxation (PMR), as
        anti-NV intervention, 349
Project ALERT, 153, 154, 161

Prompts, for encouraging physical activity, 240, 242, 245
Prostate cancer
behavioral factors in, 23
and cancer-survivor study, 106
and diet, 29, 30, 31
and obesity, 28
and physical activity, 26–27
screening for, 34, 268
and smoking, 24
Prostatectomy, 381
Protection motivation theory, 44, 48
for sun protection intervention, 212
Proxy ratings, for quality-of-life assessment, 121
Psychiatric comorbidity, and smoking cessation, 177–178
Psychoeducational group meetings, for partners of breast cancer patients, 477
Psychoeducational interventions, for family caregivers, 399–400
Psychological consequences of cancer screening, 279–280, 292–295
for breast cancer, 280–284
for cervical cancer, 284–289
for colorectal cancer, 289–292
Psychological Consequences Questionnaire (PCQ), 281, 282
Psychological distress, decreasing of as goal, 510
Psychological functioning, of childhood cancer survivors, 451–452
Psychological interventions, and cancer survival 505–507
Psychological issues, for families of cancer survivors, 475
Psychological–physiological connection, 352–353
Psychological variables, as linked to cancer etiology
through biological mechanisms, 499–503
and biobehavioral models, 509
future directions for research on, 507–509

and cancer survival, 505–507
psychosocial variables and cancer development, 503–504
psychosocial variables and cancer progression, 504–505
Psychometric standards, for validity and reliability, 72
Psychoneuroimmunology, 499
Psychosocial influences, on genetic-testing decision, 304–305
Psychosocial interventions, on behalf of cancer survivors, 418–421, 423,424–425
Psychosocial issues in cancer control continuum, 7–9
Psychosocial reactions to cancer diagnosis and treatment, 361–362
benefits from understanding of, 371
emotions and mood, 362–363
predictors of (personal, social, disease-related), 365
characteristics, 365–366
resources, 366–368
research recommendations on, 371–372
and social well-being, 364
thoughts and fears, 363–364
treatment of, 368–371
Psychosocial and spiritual effects of cancer, 414–418
Psychosocial telephone counseling (PTC), and transactional model of stress and coping, 230–231
Psychosocial variables
and biobehavioral models, 509
and cancer development, 503–504
and cancer progression, 504–505
and immunity, 500–501
Public health-level interventions, 19, 64–65
group-randomized trials for, 85–97
Public health policy, 47
Public health practice, translation of research into, 517–519

and evidence-based approach, 518–519, 520–522

and evidence-based cancer control interventions, 523–25

new initiatives for, 525–526

theoretical frameworks for, 522–523

Public Health Service, clinical practice guidelines for smoking cessation, 170

Pulmonary late effects, 437

Put Prevention Into Practice program, 524

Quality-adjusted life year (QALY), 122

Quality of life (QOL), 117, 468

of cancer survivors, 414–415

as goal, 510

interventions for, 419

and cervical cancer, 231

and families of cancer survivors, 468–476

Quality of Life of African American Cancer Survivors study, 105–110

Quality-of-life assessment, 59, 115–116, 117, 124–125

absence of theory in, 117

through behavioral assessment, 121–122

challenges for research on, 123–124

core questionnaire plus module for, 121

through generic cancer questionnaires, 120

through generic instruments, 118–120

in measures of psychological consequences of screening, 290

through proxy ratings, 121

through self-report questionnaires, 117–118

through specific cancer questionnaires, 119, 120–121

through utility assessment, 122–123

Quasi-experimental designs, 69

Quaternary prevention, 7, 8, 10, 411

as theory-based, 18

Question asking, by patients (intervention to increase), 339

Questionnaires

cancer site–specific or treatment-specific, 119, 120–21

generic cancer, 120

self-report, 117–118

Questions, retrospective, 381

Quit lines, 548

for smoking cessation, 173

Racial and Ethnic Approaches to Community Health 2010 (REACH), 526

Racial or ethnic differences

in alcohol use, 32

in caregiver's role, 479

in effect of family smoking prevention program, 156

in genetic-testing decision, 306

in inactivity, 27

in overweight/obesity, 28

and side-effect control, 352

and skin cancer, 33–34

in smoking rates, 25, 26

Racial/ethnic minorities, smoking cessation interventions for, 175–176

Radiation, late effects of

cardiovascular, 433

cataracts, 439

in central nervous system, 435

on child or adolescent survivors, 450, 452

dental, 439

genitourinary, 437

gonadal tissue damage, 436

musculoskeletal abnormalities, 434

neurologic, 437, 438

neuropathy, 440

second malignant neoplasms, 43

thyroid disease, 436

Randomized clinical trials (RCTs), 272

vs. group randomized trials, 85, 86, 88

Randomized (experimental) trials, 68–69, 73

RE-AIM (reach, effectiveness, adoption, implementation and maintenance) framework, 64, 65, 525
Reasoned action, theory of, 44, 48, 49
Reattendance, 293
    and false positive screening outcomes, 282–284
    and positive screening outcomes, 287
Recreation centers, sun protection intervention at, 213, 214
Recruitment for cancer clinical trials, ACT framework for, 104–105, 111
    case study in, 105–111
    future research needed on, 111
Recurrence of cancer, 10
    fear of, 363, 415–416
        intervention for, 420
    lack of studies on, 479
Relapse, posttreatment, 534
Relaxation, as anti-NV intervention, 349
Reliability, 72
    psychometric standards for, 72
Religious identity, and genetic-testing decision, 305
Religious organizations, dietary interventions in, 196–197
Reprioritizing, by cancer survivors, 422
Research
    basic vs. applied, 6
    behavioral, 17
    on coping, 476
Research on cancer and cancer control
    on barriers to provider readiness for smoking cessation, 173
    behavioral science in, 5–6
    on childhood cancer survivors, 456–458
    on communication of prognosis, 330
    on content of information on colonoscopy, 292
    on dietary improvement, 200, 201
    on faith-based dietary interventions, 197

    on families of cancer patients, 478–480
    on family caregiving, 394, 398, 401, 402–403
    fundamental research, 6
    on genetic testing, 311, 313
    for gynecologic cancer, 231
    on impact of false positive results on reattendance, 293
    intervention research, 6, 59, 62
        behavioral, 79 (see also Behavioral interventions)
        on interventions to improve physical activity, 433–434
    on late effects, 441–442
    minorities underrepresented in, 19–20
    phases of, 62
    on physical activity, 242–243
    and practice, 272
    on practitioner–patient communication, 340–341
    and prevention, 61
    psychosocial (uneven representation in), 362
    on PTSD in cancer survivors, 420
    and quality-of-life assessment, 115–116
    on relationship of psychological variables to cancer, 507–510
    on screening interventions, 268–272, 273
        methodological issues in, 267–268
    and sexual dysfunction
        on sexual outcomes, 380–382
        and treatment after cancer, 384
    on smoking cessation, 176–177
    on strategies for breaking bad news, 332
    on sun protection programs
        for adults, 216
        for children, 212
        for college students, 213
    surveillance research, 6
    on survivors of cancer, 424

themes of, 15–16
on tobacco use (smoking) cessation, 168, 180
on tobacco use (smoking) prevention, 161–162
translation of into practice, 517–519
and evidence-based approach, 518–519, 520–522
and evidence-based cancer control interventions, 523–25
new initiatives for, 525–526
theoretical frameworks for, 522–523
Resources, 49
Response burden, 74
Restrictive food taxation, 197–198
Retrospective questions, in research, 381
Reviewers, and study methodology, 97
Risk assessments, and behavior, 554
Risk of cancer
and age, 24
and behaviors, 79
as related to beliefs about, 136–138, 141–142
comparative judgments of, 142
and diet, 189 (see also Dietary interventions)
genetic information about, 307–310 (see also Genetic)
for gynecologic cancers, 225–227
and testosterone levels, 385
for immigrants, 34
multiple features of, 142
presenting information about, 140–141
understanding of, 134–136
Risk communication, 136, 137–138
and behavior, 141–143
cancer diagnosis as, 137
defensive response to, 143
differing from original beliefs, 139
as individualized, 140
for informed decision making, 552–53

persuasion vs. information-providing focus in, 136
stages of, 138
Risk perceptions
changing of, 138–139
and larger environment of perceptions, 141
Robert Wood Johnson Foundation, as TTURC sponsor, 536
Role problems, for families of cancer survivors, 474
Rotterdam Symptom Checklist (RSCL), 119, 120

Samples, self-selected vs. nonvolunteer, 73–74
Sandwich estimator, bias in, 92
SCCIP (Surviving Cancer Competently Intervention Program), 456
Scheduled reduced smoking (SRS), 174
Schemas, 353
Schizophrenia, and smoking, 177
School-based care for childhood cancer survivors and families, 458
School-based dietary interventions, 195–196
School-based drug prevention programs, 154
School-based tobacco prevention programs, 153–155, 160
combined with mass media campaigns, 157, 159
Schools
physical activity interventions in, 238
sun safety interventions in, 210
Science
"team science" approach in, xvii
transdisciplinary, 533 (see also Transdisciplinary collaborative research)
Scientific evidence, 520–522. *See also* Public health practice
Scientific meetings, for transdisciplinary collaboration, 542–543

Scotland, sun protection program in, 212

Screening, 34, 255–257, 272, 273
  aim of, 279
  behavioral research in, 255
  of blood donors, 33
  for colorectal cancer, 534
  conditions around, 294
  criteria for, 256
  future research directions on, 268–272
  for gynecologic cancers, 227–228
  high uptake vs. informed participation in, 295
  organized vs. opportunistic systems of, 295
  for precancerous conditions, 279
  psychological consequences of 279–280, 292–295
    for breast cancer, 280–284
    for cervical cancer, 284–289
    for colorectal cancer, 289–292
  public understanding of, 295
  rates of, 10
  for survivors in need of intervention, 424
  as teachable moment, 294
Screening adherence, 9
Screening behaviors, 309–310
  correlates, predictors, and determinants of, 257–258
  developing measures of, 268–270
  evaluating interventions to change, 271–272
  identifying influences on, 270
  linking of with health, 268
Screening interventions, 258–268, 272–273
  cost-effectiveness of, 272
  evaluation of, 271–272
  recall distress reduced by, 284
Secondary appraisal, of stressful event or situation, 230
Secondary cancers, 10
Secondary growth hormone (GH), 433
Secondary prevention, 7, 8, 9–10, 253

colorectal and cervical screening as, 34
  theoretical models in, 18
Second malignant neoplasms, 439
  screening for, 441
SEER (Surveillance Epidemiology and End Results), 103
Selection bias, for group-randomized trials, 86–87
Selenium, and cancer risk, 31
Selenium and Vitamin E Cancer Prevention Trial study, 110
Self-determination theory
  and dietary intervention, 194
  and motivational interviewing, 193
Self-efficacy, 45
Self-examination, breast, 280
Self-regulation model or theory, 44, 47, 48
Self-report measures, 70–71
  of cancer screening behaviors, 269
  on quality of life, 117–118
  on sexual function, 382, 383
  and sun protection, 216
  validation of outcomes for, 72–73
Self-selected sample, 73–74
Sequentially rejective Bonferroni method, 75
Sex, and cancer incidence, 32–33
Sexual dysfunction and dissatisfaction
  and cancer survivor families' quality of life, 470–471
  from cancer treatment, 379–382
    and assessment of sexual function, 382–383
    behavior therapy for, 383–385, 385–386
  collaborative treatment programs needed for, 385
  in reaction to cancer diagnosis and treatment, 364
Sexuality, during posttreatment phase
  and quality of life for dyads, 470–471
  research needed on, 479
Sexuality, and quality of life (prostate cancer), 117

Sexually transmitted infection (STI), 288
Sibling Adaptation to Childhood Cancer Collaborative Study (SACCCS), 454
Siblings of childhood cancer survivors interventions on behalf of, 456 psychological effects on, 454
Sickness Impact Profile, 118, 119
Side effects, 347
    behavioral interventions for, 353–354
        fatigue, 350–351
        nausea and vomiting, 348–350
        pain, 351–352
    and patient expectations, 352–354
Sigmoidoscopy, 266, 279, 289
    flexible (FS), 289, 290, 292
Ski areas, sun protection interventions at, 213, 214, 215
Skills, for behavior change, 49
Skills training, 64
Skin cancer, 33–34, 209
Skin cancer prevention interventions, 209, 216. See also Sun protection
Smokeless tobacco, 152
Smoking
    and cervical cancer, 287
    and genetic testing, 310
    See also Tobacco use
Smoking cessation, 167
    application guidelines on, 17
    Internet for information about, 548
    relapses from, 168
    and risk beliefs, 137
    unassisted, 168
    See also Tobacco use cessation
Smoking cessation interventions, 180
    background of, 167–169
    challenges to, 167, 180
    and population subgroups, 174–80
    provider readiness for, 170–171, 180
        barriers to, 173–174
        enhancing of, 174
        training for, 171–173

timing of, 67
    See also Tobacco use prevention programs
Smoking and Health (Surgeon General's report), 167
Snack foods, taxes on, 198
Social change, research needed on, 273
Social characteristics, as predictor of reaction to cancer diagnosis and treatment, 365–366
Social-cognitive theory
    and behavioral intervention among cancer survivors, 490
    for cancer survivors, 419
    for physical activity interventions in work sites, 239
    for sun protection intervention, 212, 215
    and treatment for reactions to cancer, 370
Social comparison, 142
Social functioning, of childhood cancer survivors, 452
    interventions for, 455–456
Social influence programs, for tobacco use prevention, 153, 154
Social learning theory, 45, 48
    and expectations, 353
Social marketing, 46, 48
Social norms, and antismoking campaigns, 160
Social resources, as predictor of reaction to cancer diagnosis and treatment, 366–368
Social support, 48
    and cancer progression, 505, 508
    and dietary interventions, 193–194, 196, 200–201
    and families of cancer survivors, 473, 475
    and family caregiving, 396
        interventions for, 399
    human-to-human interaction for, 550–551
    and reactions to cancer diagnosis and treatment, 367–368

Social support (*continued*)
   in successful adaptation to cancer, 415
   support groups
      for cancer survivors, 418
      online, 550–551
Social well-being
   and families of cancer survivors, 469–471
   and reactions to cancer diagnosis and treatment, 364
Socioecological model, of dietary interventions, 190–191
Socioeconomic effects of cancer, 421–423
Socioeconomic status (SES)
   and overweight/obesity, 29
   and research on psychology–cancer link, 510
   and screening, 257
   and side-effect control, 352
   and smoking rates, 25–26
Specialization, professional, 538
Spiral computed tomography, and psychosocial factors, 268
Spiritual effects of cancer, 414–418
   and quality of life, 117
Spiritual faith, and genetic-testing decision, 305
Spiritual well-being, and families of cancer survivors, 472
Spouse caregivers, 396, 399. *See also* Family caregiving
SRS (scheduled reduced smoking), 174
Standardized Nursing Intervention Protocol, 478
State Tax Handbook, on food taxes, 198
Stem cell transplantation (SCT), for children with leukemia and solid tumors, 450
Stepped-care approaches, for smoking cessation, 169, 170
Stomach cancer
   and diet, 29, 31
   and obesity, 28
Stress
   and cancer, 502, 503, 505, 507
   and immunity, 500–501
   measures of, 507
   physical changes from, 372
Stress-coping theory, 468
Stress reduction techniques, for mothers of patients undergoing BMT, 456
Stress syndromes, and cancer survivors, 416
   interventions for, 420
Structures, 49
Study design, treatment–outcome, 68
Study population and participants, 73–74
Subgroup analysis, 76–77
Substance abuse, and tobacco cessation, 177
Substance Abuse and Mental Health Services Administration, and Cancer Control PLANET, 524
Suggestive therapy, as anti-NV intervention, 349
Sun exposure, measuring of, 216
Sun protection, and cancer prevention, 33
Sun protection interventions, 209–210, 217
   for adults, 212–216
   for children, 210–212
Support groups
   for cancer survivors, 418
   online, 550–551
   See also Social support
Supportive–expressive interventions, in treatment of reaction to cancer, 368
Supportive therapy, for smoking cessation, 170
Support theory, 140–141
Surveillance, 9
Surveillance research, 6
Survival, quality along with duration of, 361
Surviving Cancer Competently Intervention Program (SCCIP), 456

Survivors of cancer, 431
 behavioral interventions for, 487,
  490–491
 child vs. adult, 431–432
 educational materials on, 423
 future directions for study of,
  423–425
 interventions on behalf of, 418–421,
  423, 424–425
 lifestyle practices among, 488–490
 and posttreatment phase, 467
 psychological and spiritual effects
  on, 414–418
 research on (biased samples of),
  413–414
 risk of disease among, 487
 socioeconomic effects on, 421–423
Survivorship/End of Life pathway, 11,
 12, 14–15
Sweden, sun protection interventions
 in, 214
Synergy, in interventions, 51

Tailoring, 15, 16–17, 191–193
 of anti-NV interventions, 350
 of communications for cancer prevention and control, 550
 computer-based, 192
 of diet-change intervention, 192
 of information to educational level
  and attentional style, 294
 of information on genetic testing,
  311
 of information to information-
  processing style, 292
 of physical-activity intervention for
  underserved populations, 241
 of risk message, 140
 of screening interventions, 267, 271
 for smoking cessation interventions,
  170, 173–174
 of tobacco use prevention, 154, 161
Taloxifene, 310
Tamoxifen, 310
Tanning facilities, indoor, 216

Targeting of intervention, 16–17
Targets, outcome vs. process, 67
Task Force on Community Preventive
 Services, 217, 242, 258
Taxation
 on food, 197–198
 and youth smoking, 160
Teachable moment, screening participa-
 tion as, 294
"Team science" approach, xvii
Telecounseling services, 551
Telemark Study, on negative FS screen-
 ing results, 290
Telephone counseling
 for cervical cancer screening follow-
  up, 287
 as screening intervention, 271
Telephone counseling, psychosocial
 (PTC), and transactional model
 of stress and coping, 230–231
Telephone quit lines, for smoking cessation, 173, 548
Telephone systems, automated, tailored
 messages on, 192, 193
Television, and children's behavior, 199
Terminal care, 10
Tertiary prevention, 7, 8, 10, 325
 and expectancy, 18
Test efficacy, 256
Testicular cancer, mood disorders in survivors of, 414
Testosterone, for sexual dysfunction
 after cancer, 384–385
Theoretical framework or models for
 public health intervention
 design, 17–19, 43
 and existing theories, 44–47
 models combined for, 47–51
 testing of variables in, 51–52
Theory(ies), 63
 in intervention design, 17–19
Theory of planned behavior, 44, 48, 49,
 490
Theory of reasoned action, 44, 48, 49
Therapists, online, 551

Thoughts, in reaction to cancer diagnosis and treatment, 363–364
Time trade-off, for quality-of-life assessment, 122
Timing, of delivery of intervention components, 67
Tobacco use
    during adolescence, 151, 152–153
        and antismoking campaign, 157–158
    as biopsychosocial phenomenon, 535–537
    among cancer survivors, 488–489
    morbidity and mortality from, 131, 151
    multiple factors in, 161
    prevalence of, 534
    of smokeless tobacco, 152
    stages of, 152
    See also Smoking
Tobacco use cessation
    and cancer prevention, 24–26
    components of interventions for, 63
    See also Smoking cessation
Tobacco use prevention programs, 153
    community approaches in, 156
        combined with media programs, 159
    family-based, 155–156
    media approaches in, 157–159
    policy approaches in, 159–160
    research on, 161–162
    school-based, 153–155, 160
        combined with mass media campaigns, 157, 159
    transdisciplinary perspective on, 162
    and transitions through stages, 161
    See also Smoking cessation interventions
Toolbox and Almanac program, 423
Towards No Tobacco Use (TNT) program, 153, 154
Training of health care providers
    in communication and interpersonal dimensions, 328, 337–39

for smoking cessation interventions, 171–173
Transactional model of stress and coping, 18, 44, 48, 49
    for prevention of gynecologic cancer, 230–231
Transdisciplinary collaborative research, 531–533
    attainment of, 538–540, 541
    and behavioral risk factors, 534
    cancer control research questions for, 535–538
    evaluation of, 540–542
    future directions for, 542–543
    and genetics, 534–535
    levels of, 533
    need for, 543
Transdisciplinary Tobacco Use Research Centers (TTURCs), 536
    emotional responses for participants in, 541–42
    model for evaluating, 540–541
Transtheoretical model of behavior change, 44, 47, 48, 49
    and behavioral intervention among cancer survivors, 490
    and motivational interviewing, 193
    for physical activity interventions in work sites, 239
    for sun protection intervention, 212, 215
Traumatic stress model, and parents of children with cancer, 18, 453
Treatment
    of cancer
        chronic effects of, 440
        sexual dysfunction from, 379–386
    of psychosocial reactions to diagnosis and treatment of cancer, 368–371
    See also Intervention(s); *specific types of intervention*
Treatment adherence, 9
Treatment matching approaches, for smoking cessation, 169–170

Treatment–outcome research design, and study population, 73–74
Treatment outcome studies, 65, 68–74
"Triage," and QOL score, 124
TTURCs. *See* Transdisciplinary Tobacco Use Research Centers
Type I error, 88, 89, 92, 96
Type II error, 73, 369

UCLA Prostate Cancer Index Prostate Cancer Treatment Outcome Questionnaire, 121
Uncertainty
    and families of cancer survivors, 469, 473, 474
    intervention for management of, 420
Underserved populations, and physical activity interventions, 241–242, 243–244
Unequal Treatment: Confronting Racial and Ethnic Disparities in Health Care (Institute of Medicine), 517
United Kingdom (Great Britain)
    1980s apprehension over abnormal Pap smears in, 295
    oophorectomy rate in, 308
University of Illinois at Chicago, in participant study, 106
User navigation, as IHC strategy, 549
Utility assessment, for quality of life, 122–123

Vaccinations, for HPV, 33, 285, 289
Validation, of self-reported outcomes, 72–73
Validity, 72
    internal vs. external, 17, 272
    psychometric standards for, 72
    and RCTs, 272
Values, and genetic-testing decision, 305
Variance Inflation Factor (VIF), 88
Vascular endothelial growth factor (VEGF), 503
Vegetables, and cancer risk, 29
Video, for colposcopy education, 287

Viral transmission, and cancer incidence, 32–33
Vitamin A, and cancer risk, 31
Volunteerism, 48
Vomiting, behavioral interventions for, 348–350
Vouchers, for screening, 266
Vulnerability
    of cancer survivors to emotional distress, 415
    sense of (in reaction to cancer diagnosis and treatment), 364

War on Cancer, 531
Weather reports, UV indexes in, 215
Weight control
    and cancer prevention, 28–29
    physical-activity interventions for, 240
Weight loss materials, group-targeted vs. individually tailored, 192
Weight-related interventions, family members in, 194
Whole grains, and cancer risk, 31
Women
    with dependent children (physical activity interventions for), 241–242
    as disproportionately represented in research on reactions to cancer, 362
    Hispanic women (and cervical cancer screening), 34
    and information needs, 334
    and population-based screening, 272
    and smoking cessation, 178–179
    working with breast cancer, 422
    See also Breast cancer; Cervical cancer; Gender differences; Ovarian cancer
Women's Health Initiative (WHI), 110
Women's Healthy Eating and Living Study, 491
Women's Intervention Nutrition Study, 491

Working Healthy Project, 239
Work roles, of family caregiver, 393
Worksites
   dietary interventions in, 196
   physical activity interventions in,
      238–239, 244

sun protection interventions at,
   214–215
World Health Organization, and cancer
   screening guidelines, 256, 279
Wristbands, as anti-NV intervention,
   349

ABOUT THE EDITORS

Suzanne M. Miller, PhD, is senior member of the Division of Population Science at Fox Chase Cancer Center and the director of the Psychosocial and Biobehavioral Medicine Program, the Behavioral Core Facility, and the Behavioral Center of Excellence in Breast Cancer. She is also the director of the Intervention Development and Measurement Core of the Cancer Information Service Research Consortium. Her funded research focuses on applying biobehavioral principles to promote the uptake of cancer prevention and control technologies. She is a fellow of the American Psychological Association and the Society of Behavioral Medicine and serves in leadership positions in the Society of Behavioral Medicine, the American Society of Preventive Oncology, and the American Psychosocial Oncology Society. She received the Partners in Research Award from the National Cancer Institute's Cancer Information Service and the Cancer Control Award from the American Cancer Society. Her most recent published volume, *Individuals, Families, and the New Era of Genomics: Biopsychosocial Perspectives* (2006), received a number of book awards.

Deborah J. Bowen, PhD, is a full professor and chair in the Department of Health Services, School of Public Health, at Boston University. Dr. Bowen is currently an investigator in the regional Cancer Prevention Network, focused on community-based research on cancer prevention targets. She is a coinvestigator on the regional Native American Community Health Network, a group of investigators and community health experts working to conduct research and training in Native American communities in the western United States. Dr. Bowen has been an investigator in the coordinating centers of three large multicenter prevention trials of health behavior change.

Robert T. Croyle, PhD, is the director of the Division of Cancer Control and Population Sciences at the National Cancer Institute. Previously, he was the division's associate director for behavioral research. Before moving to the National Cancer Institute in 1998, Dr. Croyle was a professor of psychology and member of the Huntsman Cancer Institute at the University of Utah. Dr. Croyle received his PhD in social psychology from Princeton University and his BA in psychology from the University of Washington. His research has focused on psychological responses to risk-factor testing and screening. In

2002, Dr. Croyle received a Meritorious Research Service Commendation from the American Psychological Association Board of Scientific Affairs.

Julia H. Rowland, PhD, is the director of the Office of Cancer Survivorship at the National Cancer Institute (NCI) as well as a long-time clinician, researcher, and teacher in the area of psychosocial aspects of cancer. She has worked and conducted research among both pediatric and adult cancer survivors and their families, published broadly in psychooncology, and coedited the groundbreaking text *Handbook of Psychooncology: Psychological Care of the Patient With Cancer* (1989). Dr. Rowland received her PhD in developmental psychology from Columbia University and trained and worked at Memorial Sloan-Kettering Cancer Center in New York City for many years. She served as founding director of the Psycho-Oncology Program at Georgetown University and the Lombardi Cancer Center prior to joining the NCI.